OXFORD MEDICAL PUBLICATIONS
Infectious complications of renal disease

Other related titles

The spectrum of renal osteodystrophy
Edited by Tilman B. Drüeke and Isidro B. Salusky

Rheumatology and the kidney
Edited by Dwomoa Adu, Paul Emery, and Michael P. Madaio

Analgesic and NSAID-induced kidney disease
Edited by J. H. Stewart

Dialysis amyloid
Edited by Charles van Ypersele and Tilman B. Drüeke

Infections of the kidney and urinary tract
Edited by W. R. Cattell

Polycystic kidney disease
Edited by Michael L. Watson and Vicente E. Torres

Treatment of primary glomerulonephritis
Edited by Claudio Ponticelli and Richard J. Glassock

Inherited disorders of the kidney
Edited by Stephen H. Morgan and Jean-Pierre Grünfeld

Complications of long-term dialysis
Edited by Edwina A. Brown and Patrick S. Parfrey

Lupus nephritis
Edited by E. Lewis, M. Schwartz, and S. Korbet

Nephropathy in type 2 diabetes
Edited by Eberhard Ritz and Ivan Rychlik

Hemodialysis in vascular access
Edited by Peter J. Conlon, Michael Nicholson, and Steve Schwab

Mechanisms and clinical management of chronic renal failure (Second edition; formerly Prevention of progressive chronic renal failure)
Edited by A. Meguid El Nahas with Kevin Harris and Sharon Anderson

Cardiovascular disease in end-stage renal failure
Edited by Joseph Loscalzo and Gérard M. London

Infectious complications of renal disease

Edited by

PAUL SWENY
Consultant Nephrologist
Royal Free NHS Trust
UK

ROBERT RUBIN
Chief of Infectious Disease for Transplantation
Massachusetts General Hospital
Boston, USA

and

NINA TOLKOFF-RUBIN
Department of Nephrology
Massachusetts General Hospital
Boston, USA

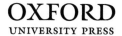

OXFORD
UNIVERSITY PRESS

OXFORD

UNIVERSITY PRESS

Great Clarendon Street, Oxford OX2 6DP

Oxford University Press is a department of the University of Oxford.
It furthers the University's objective of excellence in research, scholarship,
and education by publishing worldwide in

Oxford New York

Auckland Cape Town Dar es Salaam Hong Kong Karachi
Kuala Lumpur Madrid Melbourne Mexico City Nairobi
New Delhi Shanghai Taipei Toronto

With offices in

Argentina Austria Brazil Chile Czech Republic France Greece
Guatemala Hungary Italy Japan South Korea Poland Portugal
Singapore Switzerland Thailand Turkey Ukraine Vietnam

Oxford is a registered trade mark of Oxford University Press
in the UK and in certain other countries

Published in the United States
by Oxford University Press Inc., New York

© Oxford University Press 2003

The moral rights of the author have been asserted

Database right Oxford University Press (maker)

First published 2003

Reprinted 2005

Library of Congress Cataloging in Publication Data

The infectious complications of renal disease/edited by Paul Sweny,
Robert Rubin, Nina Tolkoff-Rubin.

(Oxford medical publications)

Includes bibliographical references and index.

ISBN 0 19 263294 9 (Hbk)

1. Kidneys–Infections. 2. Kidneys–Diseases–Complications. I. Sweny, Paul.
II. Rubin, Robert (Robert H) III. Tolkoff-Rubin, Nina. IV. Series.

RC918.I53 I53 2002 616.6'1–dc21 2002075406

10 9 8 7 6 5 4 3 2

Typeset by Cepha Imaging Pvt Ltd
Printed in Great Britain on acid-free paper
by Antony Rowe Ltd, Chippenham, Wiltshire

PREFACE

The book is divided into three parts: I, *Basic mechanisms*; II, *Infectious complications of common renal conditions, renal failure*, and *transplantation*; III, *Prevention and management*.

The uraemic condition as a state of immunosuppression is discussed to set the scene for why renal patients are prone to so many diverse infections. Increasingly potent immunosuppressive drugs are being deployed in a variety of primary conditions and also to prevent renal allograft rejection. The mechanisms by which these drugs predispose to infection are discussed. A chapter deals specifically with peritoneal defence mechanisms of critical importance in the management of infection complicating continuous ambulatory peritoneal dialysis.

The second section of the book deals specifically with infectious complications in defined situations. For example, diabetes mellitus is discussed in detail, as this is now the major cause of end-stage chronic renal failure. Infectious complications of glomerulonephritis and vasculitis are discussed, and this relates to the effects of the potent immunosuppressive agents now used. Specific chapters are devoted to infectious complications of peritoneal dialysis and there is a section on mucormycosis. Hepatitis B and hepatitis C have each been given a chapter and the impact of these hepatitis viruses on the renal patient from chronic renal failure through dialysis to transplantation is discussed. A discussion of infectious complications of transplantation follows and there is a review of the common infections, as well as a presentation of current views on virus-induced tumours.

In the final section of the book, prevention of infection is discussed with particular emphasis on vascular access and the care of the uraemic ischaemic/diabetic foot. The general principles relating to limiting the spread infection within the renal unit are discussed in detail. Increasing patient mobility and travel requires that travel and vaccination in renal patients are explored. The book ends with a practical chapter on prescribing advice for the use of common antimicrobial agents.

CONTENTS

LIST OF CONTRIBUTORS

P.L. Amlot MD
Department of Immunology and
Molecular Pathology
Royal Free and University College
Medical School
Rowland Hill Street
London NW3 2PF
UK

D. Craig Brater MD
Department of Medicine
Indiana University School of Medicine
545 Barnhill Drive
Emerson Hall 317
Indianapolis, IN 46202–5124
USA

Aine Burns MD
Renal Unit
The Royal Free Hospital
Pond Street
London NW3 2QG
UK

Jack W. Coburn MD
Department of Medicine
UCLA School of Medicine
Los Angeles, CA
(Nephrology Section (111L)
V.A. West Los Angeles Healthcare Center
11301 Wilshire Blvd.
Los Angeles
CA 90073
USA

Allan Cumming MD
Department of Renal Medicine
Royal Infirmary of Edinburgh
Edinburgh, EH3 9YW, UK

Mrinal K. Dasgupta MD
2E3.22 Walter C. Mackenzie Health
Sciences Centre
University of Alberta School of Medicine
Edmonton, Alberta
CANADA T6G 2B7

Andrew Davenport MD
Renal Unit
The Royal Free Hospital
Pond Street
London NW3 2QG
UK

A. Dhondt MD
Nephrology Department
University Hospital
De Pintelaan 185
B9000 Gent
BELGIUM

M.E. Edmonds MD
Diabetic Foot Clinic
King's College Hospital
Denmark Hill
London SE5 9RS
UK

Vincent C. Emery PhD
Royal Free and University College
Medical School
London NW3 2QG
UK

Ken Farrington MD
Lister Hospital
Stevenage
Herts SG1 4AB
UK

Jay A. Fishman MD
Infectious Disease Division
Massachusetts General Hospital
55 Fruit Street
Boston, MA, 02114
USA

A.V.M. Foster
Diabetic Foot Clinic
King's College Hospital
Denmark Hill
London SE5 9RS
UK

Gill Gaskin MD
Imperial College School of Medicine
Hammersmith Hospital
London W12 0NN
UK

Jane Goddard MD
Department of Renal Medicine
Royal Infirmary of Edinburgh EH3 9YW
UK

Paul D. Griffiths MD
Royal Free and University College
Medical School
London NW3 2QG
UK

Alan Macdonald MD
Lister Hospital
Stevenage
Herts SG1 2AB
UK

Glenn E. Mathisen MD
Clinical Professor of Medicine
University of California at Los Angeles
Department of Medicine, Division of
Infectious Diseases
14445 Olive View Drive, 2B182
Sylmar, CA 91342,
USA

Hla M Maung MD
Department of Medicine,
UCLA School of Medicine
Los Angeles, CA 90073
USA

Svetlozar N. Natov, MD
Tufts University School of Medicine
St Elizabeth's Medical Center of Boston
2310, Commonwealth Ave,
Newton, MA 02466
USA

Brian J.G. Pereira MD
Division of Nephrology
Box 391
New England Medical Center
750 Washington Street
Boston, MA 02111
USA

Phoung-Chi T. Pham MD
Assistant Clinical Professor of Medicine
University of California at Los Angeles
Olive View-UCLA Medical Center
Department of Medicine,
Nephrology Division,
14445 Olive View Drive, 2B182
Sylmar, CA 91342
USA

Phuong-Thu T. Pham MD
Assistant Clinical Professor of Medicine
University of California at Los Angeles
Department of Medicine
Kidney and Pancreas Transplantation
7-155 Factor 168917
Los Angeles, CA 90095
USA

T.K. Sreepada Rao MD
SUNY Downstate Medical Center
450 Clarkson Avenue
Box 52, Brooklyn, NY 11203
USA

Robert H. Rubin MD
Massachusetts General Hospital
55 Fruit Street
GRB-858
Boston, MA 02114-2696
USA

Jon Stratton MD
Lister Hospital
Stevenage
Herts, SG1 4AB
UK

P Sweny MD
Renal Unit
The Royal Free Hospital
Pond Street
London NW3 2QG
UK

Ban-Hock Tan MD
Senior Registrar
Department of Internal Medicine
Singapore General Hospital
SINGAPORE

Nina E. Tolkoff-Rubin MD
Massachusetts General Hospital
55 Fruit Street
GRB-858
Boston, MA 02114-2696
USA

R. Vanholder MD
Nephrology Department
University Hospital
De Pintelaan 185
B9000 Gent
BELGIUM

Prem P. Varma MD
Classified Spl Medicine and Nephrology
Command Hospital (EC)
Alipore
Calcutta 700027
INDIA

ABBREVIATIONS

$1,25(OH)_2D_3$	1,25 Dihydroxycholecalciferol
2DEHP	2-diethylhexylphthalate
A	Adenosine
AA	Arachidonic acid
AAMI	Association for the Advancement of Medical Instrumentation
Ab	Antibody
ACE-I	Angiotensin converting enzyme–inhibitor
ACV	Acyclovir
ADA	Adenosine deaminase
ADH	Antidiuretic hormone
Ag	Antigen
AIDS	Acquired immunodeficiency syndrome
ALG	Antilymphocyte globulin (antibodies)
ALP	Alkaline liver phosphatase
ALT	Alanine aminotransferase
ANCA	Antineutrophil cytoplasmic antibodies
Ang II	Angiotensin II
AP	Activator protein
ARDS	Adult respiratory distress syndrome
ARF	Acute renal failure
ATG	Antithymocyte globulin (antibodies)
AV	Arteriovenous
AVP	Arginine vasopressin
AZT	Zidovudine
βFGF	Beta fibroblast growth factor
BAL	Bronchoalveolar lavage
BCG	Bacillus Calmette-Guérin
BCRF1	EBV interleukin-10 homologue
bDNA	Branched-chain DNA
bFGF	Basic fibroblast growth factor
BFGF	Basic fibroblast growth factor
BHRF 1	EBV bcl-2 anti-apoptotic homologue
BRMS	Biological response modifier substance
C	Complement protein (1-9)
C AMP	Cyclic adenosinemonophosphate
CaM	Calmodulin
CAPD	Continuous ambulatory peritoneal dialysis
CARM	Coactivator-associated arginine methyltransferase

CBP	Creb binding protein
CD	Cluster determinant
CDC	Centres for Disease Control and Prevention
cfu	Colony-forming units
CHOP	Cyclophosphamide, adriamycin, oncovin, prednisolone
CIFN	Consensus interferon
CIN	Cervical intraepithelial neoplasia
CK	Cytokine
CKR	Cytokine receptor
CM	Cell membrane
CMV	Cytomegalovirus
CN	Calcineurin
CNS	Central nervous system
CO	Cardiac output
COSHH	Control of substances hazardous to health
COX	Cyclo-oxygenase
CR	Complement receptor
CREB	CAMP response element B
CRP	C-reactive protein
CSA	Cyclosporine A
CSF	Cerebrospinal fluid
CSS	Churg-Strauss syndrome
CT	Computerised tomography
CTL	Cytotoxic lymphocytes
CyP	Cyclophilin
CYP	Cytochrome P450 oxidases
D	Donor
DAG	Diacylglycerol
DDI	Didanosine
DEAFF	Detection of early antigen by fluorescent foci
DFMO	Difluoromethyl ornithine
DFO	Desferrioxamine
DIP	Degranulation inhibitory protein
DKA	Diabetic ketoacidosis
DNA	Deoxyribonucleic acid
DTP	Diptheria, tetanus, pertussis
EBER	Epstein Barr virus encoded RNA
EBNA	Epstein–Barr nuclear antigen
EBV	Epstein–Barr virus
ECM	Extracellular matrix
EDGF	Endothelial growth factor
EDTA	European Dialysis and Transplantation Association
EIA	Enzyme immunoassay
ELISA	Enzyme-linked immunosorbent assay
EMRSA	Epidemic methicillin resistant staphylococcus aureus

ENT	Ear, nose and throat
ESRD	End-stage renal disease
ESRF	End-stage renal failure
ET-1	Endothelin 1
ETR	End of treatment response
Fc	Fraction crystallizable
FcR	Fc receptor
FKBP	FK506 binding protein
Flip	FLICE-inhibitor protein
FMLP	F met-leu-Phe protein
FSGS	Focal and segmental glomerulosclerosis
G	Guanine
GBM	Glomerular basement membrane
Gc	Glucocorticoid
GCR	G-protein coupled receptor
GCV	Ganciclovir
GFR	Glomerular filtration rate
GI	Gastrointestinal
GIP	Granulocyte inhibitory protein
GM-CSF	Granulocyte–macrophage colony-stimulating factor
GMP	Guanosine monophosphate
GP120	Glycoprotein 120
GPI	Glycosyl-phosphatidylinositol
GPMS	GMP synthase
GR	Glucocorticoid receptor
GRE	Glucocorticoid response elements
GRE	Glycopeptide-resistant enterococci
GRIP-1	Glucocorticoid receptor interacting protein-1
GVHD	Graft venous host disease
H	Hypoxanthine
HAART	Highly active antiretroviral therapy
HAMA	Human antimonoclonal antibody
HAT	Histone acetyl transferase
HB	Hepatitis B
HBcAb	Hepatitis B core antibody
HBcAg	Hepatitis B core antigen
HBeAg	Hepatitis E antigen
HBIG	Hepatitis B immune globulin
HBsAg	Hepatitis B surface antigen
HBV	Hepatitis B virus
HCC	Hepatocellular carcinoma
HCG	Human chorionic gonadotrophin
HCO_3	Bicarbonate
HCV	Hepatitis C virus
HD	Haemodialysis

HDAC	Histone deacylase
HGPRT	Hypoxanthine-guanine phosphoribosyltransferase
HHV	Human herpesvirus
HIB	Heamophilus influenzae B
HIC PAC	Hospital Infection Control Practices Advisory Committee
HIV	Human immunodeficiency virus
HIVAN	HIV-associated nephropathy
HLA	Human leucocyte antigen
HNIG	Human normal immunoglobulin
HPV	Human papillomavirus
HSP 90	Heat shock protein 90
HSV	Herpes simplex virus
HTLV	Human T cell leukaemia virus
HUS	Haemolytic uraemic syndrome
HVS	Herpes virus simian
ICAM-1	Intercellular adhesion molecule-1
IFN	Interferon
Ig	Immunoglobulin (A, G, M, D, E)
IL	Interleukin
IL-2R	IL-2 receptor complex
IMP	Inosine monophosphate
IMPD	Inosine monophosphate dehydrogenase
INH	Isoniazid
iNOS	Inducible nitric oxide synthase
IP	Immunophilin
IP	Intraperitoneally
IP_3	Inositol triphosphate
IRF	Interferon regulatory protein
ITU	Intensive therapy unit
IV	Intravenously
KCO	Diffusing capacity for carbon monoxide
KS	Kaposi's sarcoma
KSHV	Kaposi's sarcoma herpes virus
KSV	Kaposi's sarcoma virus
KUF	Ultrafiltration coefficient
L-NAME	L-arginine analogue N-nitro-L-arginine methyl ester
LAK	Lymphokine-activated killer cells
LAL	Limulus amoebocyte lysate test
LANA	Latency-associated nuclear antigen
LFA - 1	Leucocyte function antigen-1
LFT	Liver function test
LMPs	Latent membrane proteins
LPS	Lipopolysaccharide
LT	Leucotriene
Mab	Monoclonal antibodies

MCP	Monocyte chemotactic protein
MH	Maintenance haemodialysis
MHC	Major histocompatibility complex
MIC	Minimal inhibitory concentration
MIP	Monocyte inhibitory protein
MMF	Mycophenolate mofetil
MMR	Measles, mumps, rubella
MØ	Macrophage
MP	Microscopic polyangiitis
MPA	Mycophenolic acid
MRI	Magnetic resonance imaging
MRSA	Methicillin-resistant *Staphylococcus aureus*
MU	Million units
MZ	Mizoribine
MZ-5-P	Mizoribine-5-monophosphate
NA	Not applicable or not available
Na RTI	Nucleotide reverse transcriptase inhibitor
NAD P(H)	Nicotinamide adenine dinucleotide phosphate (reduced formula)
NANBH	Non-A, non-B hepatitis
NC	No change
nCoA	Nuclear receptor coactivators
nCoR	Nuclear receptor corepressors
NCR	Non-coding regions
NFAT	Nuclear factors of activated T cells
NFκB	Nuclear factor κ Beta
NK	Natural killer
NOS	Nitric oxide synthase
NM	Nuclear membrane
NNRTI	Non-nucleoside analogue reverse transcriptase inhibitor
NO	Nitric oxide
NRTI	Nucleoside reverse transcriptase inhibitor
OG	Oncogene
ORF	Open reading frame
p/CIP	p300/CBP/cointegrator-associated protein
PAF	Platelet activating factor
PAN	Polyarteritis nodosa
PAN	Polyacrylonitrile
PBL	Peripheral blood lymphocytes
PCAF	p300/CBP associated factor
PCP	Pneumocystis carinii pneumonia
PCR	Polymerase chain reaction
PD	Peritoneal dialysis
PE	Pulmonary embolus
PEL	Primary effusion lymphoma

PFB	Peritoneal fibroblast
PG	Prostaglandin
PGE_2	Prostaglandin E_2
PGI_2	Prostacyclin
PHA	Phytohaemagglutinin
PI-3K	Phosphtidylinositol-3 kinase
PIP_2	Phosphatidylinositol-4,5-biphosphate
PKC	Protein kinase C
PLA_2	Phospholipase A_2
PLC	Phospholipase C
PMC	Peritoneal mesothelial cell
PMN	Polymorphonuclear neutrophils
PMØ	Peritoneal macrophage
PNP	Purine nucleoside phosphorylase
PO	Per os
POEMS	Peripheral neuropathy, organomegaly, endocrinopathy, monoclonal plasma proliferative disorder, skin changes
PPD	Purified protein derivative
PRPP	Phosphoribosyl pyrophosphate
PRPP-S	PRPP-synthase
PTFE	Polytetrafluoroethylene
PTH	Parathyroid hormone
PTLD	Post-transplant lymphoproliferative disease/disorder
PUO	Pyrexia of unknown origin
QC PCR	Quantitative-competitive polymense chain reaction
R	Ribosyl
RAFT	Rapamycin associated functional target
RANTES	Regulated-upon-activation normal T-cell expressed and presumably secreted protein
RAPA	Rapamycin
RBF	Renal blood flow
RFLP	Restriction fragment length polymorphism
rHuEPO	Recombinant human erythropoietin
RIA	Radio immunoassay
RIBA	Recombinant immunoblot assay
RMP	Rifampicin
RNA	Ribonucleic acid
RO	Reverse osmosis
RRI	Ribonucleotide reductase inhibitor
RSV	Respiratory syncytial virus
RTI	Reverse transcriptase inhibitor
SC	Spindle cell
SCC	Squamous cell carcinoma
sCD25	Soluble IL-2 receptor
SIR	Sirolimus

SIRS	Systemic inflammatory response syndrome
SLE	Systemic lupus erythematosus
Spp	Species
SR	Sustained response
SRA	Steroid receptor RNA coactivator
SRC	Steroid receptor coactivator superfamily
SRU	SRU responsive unit
SVR	Systemic vascular resistance
T-IMP	Thio-IMP
TAC	Tacrolimus
TATA	'Thymidine adenine'-refers to repeated sequence of TATA in DNA that positions start of transcription
TB	Tuberculosis
TCR	T-cell receptor
TGF	Transforming growth factor
TH	T-helper
TMP-SMX	Trimethoprim-sulphamethoxazone
TNF-α	Tumour necrosis factor-α
TOR	Target of rapamycin
TRAFs	TNF receptor associated factors
TRI	Tubuloreticular inclusions
TRIP	TGFβ-receptor-interacting protein
TSG	Tumour suppressor gene
TTP	Thrombotic thromocytopaenic purpura
TVC	Total viable count
Tx	Transplant
TxA$_2$	Thromboxane A$_2$
UL	Unique long
UNOS	United network for organ sharing
US	Unique start
UTI	Urinary tract infection
UV	Ultraviolet
UVS	Unique startq
V	Valve
VACV	Valaciclovir
Vd	Volume of distribution
VEGF	Vascular endothelial growth factor
VGC	Valganciclovir
VRE	Vancomycin-resistant enterococci
VZV	Varicella zoster virus
WG	Wegener's granulomatosis
X	Xanthine

PART I
BASIC MECHANISMS

1

Renal failure as an immunodeficiency state

R. Vanholder and A. Dhondt

Introduction

Infectious diseases remain one of the major causes of morbidity and mortality in patients with end-stage renal disease (ESRD), especially in those on dialysis treatment. This susceptibility to infection is attributed to immune dysfunction (Cohen *et al.* 1997). Other clinical observations also support the thesis that ESRD induces immune deficiency:

(1) an enhanced risk for cancer,
(2) attenuation of autoimmune disorders,
(3) skin anergy, and
(4) a depressed response to vaccination.

Infection, however, remains the factor which affects the largest number of patients. Dysfunction of the host defence mechanisms has major clinical and socioeconomic implications. Life expectancy, hospitalization rate and duration, and treatment costs may all be adversely affected since the application of expensive and prolonged courses of antibiotics, vasopressors, haemodynamic monitoring, and ventilation may be necessary.

The pathophysiology of immune dysfunction in dialysed patients can be attributed to two different factors: the influence of renal failure *per se* and the influence of dialysis. Patients with renal failure who are not yet dialysed and kidney transplant recipients also have a higher risk for infection. Endogenous and/or iatrogenic immune suppression play a role. In addition it should be stressed that patients with ESRD often have associated diseases which have a negative impact on the immune system (Table 1.1).

Knowledge about the pathophysiological interference between immune function, the uraemic syndrome, and renal replacement therapy should allow more focused treatment and improved preventive measures.

In this chapter we review the conditions which cause the immune deficiency. As these infectious complications become more preponderant once dialysis treatment is started, most attention will be paid to dialytic therapy.

Importance of infectious disease

Several studies address the morbidity and mortality from infection in renal failure. Reported mortality figures are probably underestimated, since patients may be hospitalized because of infection but may die from a different aetiology (e.g. cardiac arrest, multiorgan failure).

Table 1.1 Comorbid factors increasing the risk of infection in renal disease

Primary causes increasing the risk of infection	Diabetes mellitus
	Hepatic failure
	Cancer, leukaemia, lymphoma, multiple myeloma
	Reflux nephropathy
	Polycystic kidney disease
	Obstructive nephropathy
	Nephrolithiasis
Coexisting conditions causing immune dysfunction	Autoimmune disorders
	Immunosuppressive treatment
	Kidney transplantation
	Graft rejection
Complications affecting host defence	Heart failure
	Hepatic failure
	Cancer
	Hyperparathyroidism
	Hypovitaminosis D, other vitamin deficiencies
	Iron overload
	Granulocytopenia

Data collected in the early 1970s pointed to an infectious mortality in the haemo-dialysed population in the range of 40% (Blagg *et al.* 1970). Patient case mix and treatment modalities in that study, however, were too different from those found today to allow extrapolation to current conditions. Lower figures are reported in the more recent literature, although in the careful analysis by Mailloux *et al.* (1991) an overall mortality due to infection of 36% was found. Therefore, even today, despite all the achievements of optimized intensive care, diagnostic procedures, dialysis, and antibiotic treatment, bacterial infection remains a major cause of death in the dialysed population. Data on the incidence of infection in the predialytic stage are scant, but the endogenous immune suppression observed causes an enhanced risk for infection.

Alterations of host defence

Immune defence against infection involves a complex network of mechanisms effected by numerous participants:

(1) circulating (lymphocytes, monocytes, polymorphonuclear cells) and tissue immuno-competent cells (lymphocytes, macrophages),

(2) humoral substances (cytokines, chemokines, leucotrienes, prostaglandins, growth factors, complement factors, platelet activating factor, soluble receptors, and receptor antagonists).

All these elements combine to reach a single end-point: the destruction of infectious agents with minimal damage to the host.

In renal failure and dialysis both innate (natural) and adaptive (acquired) immunity are impaired. Remarkably, this deficient state is almost invariably accompanied by signs of activation as well.

Lymphocytes

The total number of circulating lymphocytes in uraemic dialysis patients is reduced.

T cells

Uraemic T cells exhibit an impaired response to most stimuli. The defective proliferation of T cells is associated with a decreased production of interleukin 2 (IL-2) and interferon-γ (IFN-γ). Uraemic plasma has also been demonstrated to reduce the proliferative response of normal T cells. Furthermore, it has been hypothesized that a blunted T-cell response to antigens is due to down-regulation of the T-cell receptor/CD3 antigen receptor complex in the uraemic milieu.

Despite this impaired response, T cells also show signs of activation: elevated levels of soluble IL-2 receptor (sCD25) are present in both dialysed and non-dialysed chronic uraemic patients (Descamps-Latscha *et al.* 1995). Dialysis with complement-activating membranes induces an increase in sCD25. Dialysis with complement-activating membranes also induces an up-regulation of the expression of IL-2 receptor (CD25) on lymphocytes, which can be reversed by dialysis with more biocompatible membranes.

B cells

Uraemic patients develop inadequate and retarded antibody formation after hepatitis B vaccination and show rapid disappearance of these antibodies (see Chapter 20). Some authors advise giving vaccination as soon as possible in the course of kidney disease. A blunted response may equally be observed after vaccination against pneumococcus, tetanus, diphtheria, and influenza. Vaccines can usually be administered safely to patients with renal failure (although live vaccines are best avoided in the presence of impaired cell-mediated immunity). Inoculation with attenuated micro-organisms can result in persistent or even fatal infection in patients taking immunosuppressive drugs. All vaccination should be avoided in the early post-transplantation period.

The impaired antibody response in the uraemic patient could be the consequence of an intrinsic B-cell defect. However, T helper cells and monocyte antigen-presenting cells are important for antibody formation and hence could also be responsible.

As a sign of B-cell activation, the level of soluble CD23 (sCD23) is increased both in uraemic and haemodialysis patients (Descamps-Latscha *et al.* 1995). CD23 is the low-affinity crystallizable fragment (Fc) receptor of immunoglobulin E (IgE) predominantly expressed on activated B cells. In undialysed patients, the level of sCD23 increases with the progression of renal failure (Descamps-Latscha *et al.* 1995). Dialysis with complement-activating membranes induces an increase of sCD23 (Descamps-Latscha *et al.* 1995).

Natural killer (NK) cell activity

Cytolytic activity of NK cells is depressed after chronic *in vivo* exposure to unmodified cellulosic dialyser membranes, which may be related to the immune defects and the increased incidence of malignancy in uraemia. This alteration was less pronounced with other dialyser membranes.

Monocytes

During haemodialysis with complement-activating membranes the total number of circulating monocytes decreases dramatically.

A defective Fc receptor-mediated internalization of opsonized particles has been demonstrated in the monocytes of chronic dialysis patients, which could lead to an impaired antigen-presenting function.

Monocyte activation in undialysed patients with renal failure has been demonstrated by increased plasma levels of neopterin (Descamps-Latscha *et al*. 1995). In patients on dialysis, monocyte activation has been illustrated by the enhanced capacity to synthesize proinflammatory cytokines. Increased levels of cytokines in the serum of haemodialysis patients are attributed to two triggers: complement activation by the dialyser membrane and backfiltration of lipopolysaccharide (LPS) fragments from the dialysate. A rise in postdialysis plasma IL-1β is mainly observed in patients on chronic maintenance dialysis and not during the first dialysis, suggesting a progressive triggering of the inflammatory response. A similar rise was reported for IL-6 and tumour necrosis factor-α (TNF-α). Simultaneously with the cytokine increase, the concentration of specific inhibitors such as the TNF-α soluble receptor and the IL-1 receptor antagonist is enhanced, and these might counteract the proinflammatory cytokines.

However, not all studies demonstrate differences in *in vivo* cytokine release between membranes with different complement-activating capacities.

Neutrophil granulocytes

During haemodialysis sessions with complement-activating membranes, the total number of circulating neutrophils decreases dramatically.

Phagocytosis and metabolic pathways

The penultimate step in the destruction of bacteria is their ingestion and killing by phagocytes. Disturbances of phagocytosis will in part result from defects at other levels of the immunological cascade, such as lymphocyte dysfunction and/or the deficient production of humoral factors, phagocytosis being the end-point of host defence.

The response of phagocytic leucocytes is dependent on different steps and aspects of functional capacity:

(1) the attraction of phagocytic cells and their movement towards the focus of infection (chemotaxis);
(2) the ingestion of bacteria (phagocytosis);
(3) the digestive destruction of ingested bacteria by enzymatic processes (lysozyme and elastase release) and by the production of oxygen free radical species (hydrogen peroxide, superoxide, hypochlorite).

Functional disturbances may occur at each of these levels.

Phagocytic function in the uraemic state has been submitted to repeated study. A decrease in the functional capacity of phagocytic cells is described in the vast majority of studies (Vanholder and Ringoir 1993). In a large study population, phagocytic response was markedly depressed from the moment that residual renal function, as estimated by creatinine clearance, decreased below 15 ml/min (Vanholder *et al.* 1991). Furthermore, phagocyte function upon stimulation was depressed during dialysis sessions with complement-activating membranes (Vanholder and Ringoir 1993). This functional disturbance, per phagocytic cell, is further intensified by the presence of marked leucopenia during haemodialysis with unmodified cellulose membranes. Apart from an acute decrease of granulocyte functional capacity during each dialysis with unmodified cellulose the authors could also demonstrate a progressive decline in basic function in predialysis blood samples in patients starting with haemodialysis on unmodified cellulose membranes (Vanholder *et al.* 1991). This combination of factors suggests a profound decline in phagocytic functional capacity, especially during the first weeks after the start of dialysis.

Key metabolic pathways of the immune system, such as the hexose monophosphate shunt, the production of free radicals by NADPH oxidase, and their further transformation by myeloperoxidase, are disturbed in the uraemic condition.

Receptor expression

The expression of adhesion molecules, such as CD11b/CD18, has been reported to be enhanced during dialysis with complement-activating membranes. This may be related to the increased tendency of leucocytes to adhere and to aggregate, eventually resulting in their entrapment in capillary beds, especially of the lungs, and in early dialysis neutropenia. Although up-regulation of surface molecules is present on phagocytic cells in their basic ('resting') state after contact with leucocyte-activating membranes, their *ex vivo* response to additional stimuli is blunted (Dhondt *et al.* 1996, 1998). Whether this decreased receptor expression is also related to the propensity to infection needs to be confirmed.

Only limited data are available about the effect of accumulation of uraemic toxins on the expression of adhesion molecules. It has been demonstrated that granulocytes from patients with chronic renal failure display a lower expression of L-selectin and a higher expression of CD11b, suggesting an activation state (Dou *et al.* 1998).

Aetiological factors in the alteration of host defence

The contributing factors are multiple, and may be influenced by the uraemic status *per se*, by the dialysis treatment, by a combination of both, or by active immune suppression (Fig. 1.1).

Uraemic toxicity

Uraemic serum and/or ultrafiltrate have repeatedly been demonstrated to alter aspects of the immune function. Knowledge concerning the factors that are responsible for this failure remains in part speculative but several compounds have been incriminated, as listed in Table 1.2.

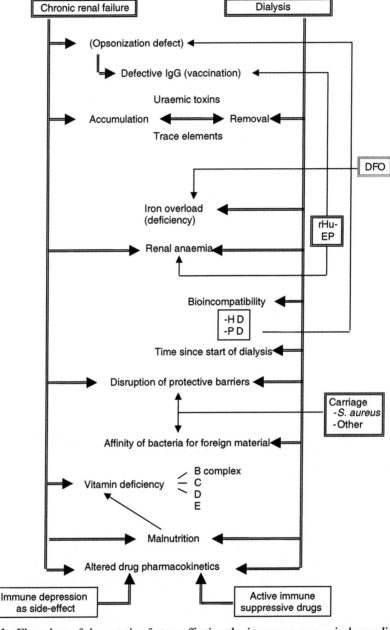

Fig. 1.1 Flow chart of the putative factors affecting the immune response in haemodialysed patients. Double lines: primary events playing a role in virtually all patients, either related to uraemic status (left) or dialysis (right). Single lines: secondary events, not necessarily applying in all patients. Several factors interact. Abbreviations: DFO, desferrioxamine; rHuEPO, recombinant human erythropoietin; HD, haemodialysis; PD, peritoneal dialysis; IgG, immunoglobulin G; *S. aureus, Staphylococcus aureus.*

Table 1.2 Uraemic retention products with potential impact on immune function

Degranulation inhibitory protein (DIP)
Endorphins
Granulocyte inhibitory proteins I and II (GIP I and II)
Guanidino succinic acid
Indoles
Parathyroid hormone
p-cresol
Phenols/phenolic acids
Phosphate
Spermidine
Spermine
Ubiquitin (modified variant)
Urea
Uric acid*

*The only compound that has a kinetic behaviour comparable to that of urea.

A negative impact of the phenolic compound *p*-cresol on the capacity of granulocytes to destroy bacteria has been described. Most interestingly, several middle molecular peptidic structures have been described which have inhibitory characteristics on granulocytes. Recently one of these compounds was characterized by structural homology with β_2-microglobulin. Phagocytosis was also more affected in renal patients with hyperparathyroidism. In parallel, enhanced release of elastase by granulocytes was found after *in vitro* contact with parathyroid hormone (PTH) at concentrations exceeding those currently encountered in the clinical condition. T-cell proliferation in response to phytohaemagglutinin (PHA) was enhanced in hyperparathyroid but not in parathyroidectomized uraemic rats.

Infection-related mortality in haemodialysis patients is inversely correlated with the dose of dialysis as measured by K_t/V. It is thus conceivable that uraemic toxicity plays a role in the functional disturbances of the leucocytes in uraemia. The compounds responsible are, however, not clearly delineated. We are probably confronted with several factors in combination. It is interesting to note that most of the compounds claimed to interfere with host defence are larger than urea and creatinine, and/or partly hydrophobic, and/or protein bound. Their retention pattern and kinetic behaviour during dialysis should therefore differ from that of urea and creatinine, the classical uraemic marker molecules.

Iron overload and anaemia

Although it is currently accepted that iron deficiency is associated with immunodeficiency and a higher risk of infection, iron overload has been the most frequent problem in patients undergoing dialysis. This may be due to excessive iron administration, haemolysis, and overtransfusion.

Patients with a high serum ferritin show a markedly suppressed granulocyte response upon activation, compared with patients with lower serum ferritins (Flament *et al.* 1986). Using *Yersinia enterocolitica* as a particle for stimulation, it was demonstrated that the phagocytic index, the phagocytosis percentage, and the killing capacity were lower in a group of haemodialysed patients with a high serum ferritin. Bacteraemia per year is three times higher in patients with a serum ferritin above 1000 µg/litre.

A way to lower body iron stores is by the administration of recombinant human erythropoietin (rHuEPO). In a group of patients with excessive body iron (average serum ferritin 1860 µg/litre), an improvement of phagocytosis together with a decrease of serum ferritin was found after the start of rHuEPO. Note that a beneficial effect of rHuEPO has also been demonstrated for other aspects of the immune system, such as the composition of the subpopulation of lymphocytes, cytokine production, response upon vaccination, and immunoglobulin production. Improvement of cellular immunity was also observed when rHuEPO was used in indications other than nephrological ones.

Renal anaemia *per se* may result in inadequate tissue oxygenation, and subsequently in functional disturbances. A gradual increase in phagocytotic response under rHuEPO treatment has been observed, even if body iron stores are unaltered (Veys *et al.* 1992).

Another manoeuvre to reduce iron overload, the administration of desferrioxamine (DFO), in turn may lead to a defective immune response. DFO especially depresses the fungistatic effect of serum against the yeast *Rhizopus*, resulting in an increased incidence of fatal events due to mucormycosis (see Chapter 9). This problem is especially important in dialysed patients, which may be attributed to the altered pharmacokinetics of DFO in uraemia, resulting in its prolonged accumulation. The desferrioxamine–iron chelate, feroxamine, can function as a siderophore for *Rhizopus*. This siderophore-mediated iron uptake can stimulate *in vitro* growth, as well as *in vivo* pathogenicity of *Rhizopus*.

Trace elements

Significant alterations in the concentration of various trace elements have been demonstrated in renal failure. Among the factors that could interfere with immune function, are cadmium, mercury, and copper accumulation and zinc depletion. Zinc therapy may improve impaired cell-mediated immunity in chronic uraemic patients.

One of the problems with trace elements is that exposure-related variations may occur in the concentration of various inorganic and organic metabolites, all with a different degree of toxicity. Intra- and extracellular protein binding may further influence free concentration and hence toxicity.

Vitamin deficiency

Some authors have reported subnormal vitamin E levels in patients undergoing haemodialysis, which has been related to a blunted immune response. Supplementation of vitamin E in patients with a decreased blood level resulted in a reduction in the number of CD8 lymphocytes.

In non-supplemented haemodialysis patients, a depletion of folic acid, vitamin C, and pyridoxine has been recorded. Deficiencies in folic acid may impair humoral immune responses. Vitamin C deficiency affects cellular immunity. In animal studies, pyridoxine deficiency resulted in the depression of antibody response and impaired cellular immunity. Since supplementation of these vitamins is current practice in many dialysis units, deficiencies will rarely play a role in the immune dysfunction of uraemia. Too high doses of vitamin C may, however, lead to oxalate retention.

Receptors for 1,25-dihydroxycholecalciferol $(1,25(OH)_2D_3)$ have been identified on human monocytes and T and B lymphocytes. The vitamin D deficiency of chronic uraemia may affect immune response, especially since $1,25(OH)_2D_3$ acts as an immune-modulating agent. Intravenous calcitriol therapy in deficient patients restores the reduced antigen-induced T-lymphocyte response.

Chronic renal failure not only results in deficient $1,25(OH)_2D_3$ production, due to a decrease in renal mass with lack of 1α-hydroxylase, but also in changes in the cellular response to $1,25(OH)_2D_3$. The latter effects may at least in part be attributed to a deficient receptor binding affinity for DNA, subsequently impeding the biological actions of $1,25(OH)_2D_3$ in renal failure. Hence, vitamin D deficiency and resistance may have important consequences, not only on the bone and calcium/phosphorus status, but also on other vitamin D-dependent metabolic processes, of which immunocompetent mononuclear cell function is one of the targets.

Bioincompatibility

Recurrent complement activation

Complement-activating dialyser membranes may have a negative impact on the response of phagocytes in addition to their effect on the circulating leucocyte count. The repetitive exposure of blood to these membranes leads to degranulation of neutrophils, and release of oxygen free radical species (Hakim 1993). Although these reactive oxygen species are bactericidal, their unintended release results in decreased responsiveness to further stimuli. The reduced response upon stimulation is associated with an increased baseline activity of leucocytes, pointing to exhaustion of the immune system. In addition, a chronic progressive inhibition of immune response during repeated contact with complement-activating dialysis membranes has also been described. These findings parallel the poor response of granulocyte function to various stimuli in other chronic inflammatory states such as infection, burns, or trauma. Additional immunoalteration may be created by the production/release of cytokines, although not all studies demonstrate differences in *in vivo* cytokine release between membranes with different complement-activating capacities.

Although it is clear from the above mentioned data that the structure of dialyser membranes and its interference with various aspects of immune function may cause alterations that eventually result in defective immune response and hence infectious disease, the ultimate proof of the influence of bioincompatibility on infectious suscepti-bility should be the demonstration of differences in infectious incidence, morbidity, and mortality dependent on the membrane used.

No evidence based on prospective study is yet available. Retrospective analyses, however, show a higher mortality due to infection and a higher incidence of hospitalization for infection in patients treated by cellulosic dialysers (Levin *et al.* 1991; Hornberger *et al.* 1992; Hakim *et al.* 1994; Schiffl *et al.* 1994). The present authors found that metabolic response to phagocytic stimuli was depressed in patients treated by unmodified cellulose membranes, compared with polysulfone (Vanholder *et al.* 1991). Interestingly, during a follow-up of 6 months, there was also a higher incidence of clinical infections in the patients treated by unmodified cellulose. However, only marginal significance was reached, in view of the small number of patients.

Endotoxin transfer to the bloodstream

A host of mostly Gram-negative species have been identified in dialysate circuits (Klein *et al.* 1990). Although bacteria and endotoxins classically are supposed not to cross intact dialyser membranes, they may enter the circulation through microscopic defects. Moreover, endotoxin might be broken down into smaller fragments with monocyte- and complement-activating properties, that may cross smaller pores. The transfer of LPS or LPS fragments may be responsible for a chronic inflammatory response. Backfiltration/backdiffusion of endotoxin fragments is especially suspected with large-pore dialysers, in the presence of a low or negative transmembrane pressure. Passage of monocyte-activating material has been demonstrated even through low-flux cellulose membranes. The risk for these events has been reduced by the introduction of better purification systems for dialysate water and of sterile electrolyte concentrates for the production of dialysate.

Bacterial contamination is a potential risk in dialyser reprocessing if sterilization is incomplete. Bacteraemia may also result from the infusion of contaminated fluids, e.g. heparin solutions. Another source may be infected dialysate transferred through dialysers with a damaged surface.

The specific problem of peritoneal dialysis

Peritonitis is the most frequent cause of infectious disease in peritoneal dialysis patients, and the most common cause of morbidity and mortality in this group of patients. According to some studies, hospitalization might be more frequent in peritoneal dialysis patients than in haemodialysis patients, and this difference is at least in part related to a high incidence of peritonitis (Maiorca *et al.* 1993).

The risk for peritonitis in peritoneal dialysis is enhanced in immunosuppressed patients. The contents of peritoneal fluid also play a role in altered host defence in the peritoneal cavity. As these events may be related to the instillation and/or the unphysiological composition of the peritoneal dialysate, as well as to the presence of a catheter composed of foreign material entering the peritoneal cavity through the skin barrier, this can also be considered as a biocompatibility problem. Fresh dialysate as it is instilled into the peritoneal cavity has a depressive effect on immunoreactive cells: low dialysate pH, the combination of lactate and low dialysate pH, dextrose content, and increased osmolality all have been suggested as potential culprits, and result in a negative impact on multiple functions of the phagocytic cells. A major defect is opsonic deficiency, especially recognized in the peritoneal dialysis effluent of patients with a high incidence of infection. The concentration of fibronectin in peritoneal dialysis fluid has been found to be significantly lower in peritoneal dialysis patients with a high infection rate. Additional factors may be the presence of uraemic toxins, especially as dwell-time progresses. Peritoneal leucocytes might contain increased intracellular calcium and show shifts in intracellular pH, resulting in an inadequate cellular response.

Although ingestion of bacteria by peritoneal macrophages harvested from peritoneal dialysis effluent may be normal, suppression of bactericidal activity by leucocytes is the main pathophysiological event.

A decreased capacity of phagocytes to kill bacteria may result in the intracellular sequestration of bacteria without destruction, resulting in a risk of relapse, especially if peritonitis is treated by antibiotics (e.g. vancomycin) that do not readily penetrate white blood cells. Peritoneal defence mechanisms are discussed in more detail in Chapter 3.

Prolongation of intraperitoneal dwell-times results in a larger number of more effective macrophages in the effluent fluid, as well as an increase in opsonic capacity. On the other hand, release of IL-6 and TNF-α by mononuclear leucocytes and granulocyte NADPH oxidase response are inhibited in the presence of spent peritoneal dialysate, and this inhibition increases with dwell-time.

An additional role may be played by $1,25(OH)_2D_3$ since peritoneal macrophages of patients with a high incidence of peritonitis are insensitive to the cytokine effect of $1,25(OH)_2D_3$, especially after short incubation times (24 h), whereas they also produce a high amount of prostaglandin E_2 (PGE_2) (Levy *et al.* 1990). Addition of indometacin, however, improved the killing capacity of peritoneal macrophages, even after 24 h, whereas PGE_2 had a depressive effect, pointing to the modulatory capacity of PGE_2 on the effect of $1,25(OH)_2D_3$ on macrophage function.

Various structural modifications have been introduced in the access systems for peritoneal dialysis in the hope of reducing the number of infections. Also the manipulations at the moment of the connection of the dialysate have been simplified and optimized, decreasing the risk of infection (see Chapter 8).

Disruption of protective barriers

For all dialysis procedures the access must be manipulated repeatedly, which increases the risk for infection. In haemodialysis an acute inhibition may occur immediately after the vascular access has been connected to the extracorporeal circuit. If bacteria are introduced, the performance of the immune system is at its weakest at that moment.

For central vein catheter dialysis either permanent or temporary catheters are used. For permanent catheters either stiff small-bore catheters (polyurethane or Teflon) can be used for a relatively short period of time (maximum 6–8 weeks), or soft large-bore catheters (silicone) for longer periods (up to several years). As the soft large-bore catheters are tunnelled during the introduction procedure, and as they contain a protective cuff, the incidence of infection per application period will be significantly lower than for the stiffer variants (see Chapter 18).

Affinity of bacteria for foreign material

Bacteria have a special affinity for artificial devices and synthetic material. Once bacterial contamination occurs, bacteria may easily stick to the polymer materials and to the fibrin sheath that covers them.

Modification of the surface of catheters may be of help in coping with this problem. Coating of catheters with silver has been used, and was claimed to decrease infection risks. Well-controlled studies are, however, lacking. Bonding of the surface with antibiotics may be another way of preventing infectious overgrowth. The few studies with catheters bonded with antibiotics have been undertaken in indications other than dialysis. Catheters may be maintained for a much longer period in the dialysis setting than in other conditions. Shear conditions are much more marked and the loss of antibiotic from the catheter surface during long-term application might be a drawback if bonded catheters were to be applied in dialysis.

Carriage

A substantial number of dialysis patients are carriers of *Staphylococcus aureus*, mostly in the anterior nares. The link between *S. aureus* nasal carriage and development of subsequent *S. aureus* infection has been established in patients on both on haemodialysis and peritoneal dialysis. Check-up for carrier state in dialysis patients and for methicillin-resistant *S. aureus* (MRSA) should be performed in all patients at least once every 3 months, and samples should be collected from the nose, throat, and perineum. Caregivers should be screened as well, although benefit of treatment is only expected in units where the number of MRSA carriers is limited among the patients. This type of carriership can be eliminated by local intranasal antibiotic treatment (e.g. mupirocin). This drug should be applied at given intervals, e.g. for 5 days every month or one day a week. Such strategies help to reduce the number of infectious and peritonitis episodes, and on the other hand prevent the development of bacterial resistance to mupirocin.

The problem of carriership of glycopeptide-resistant enterococci (GRE) emerged only recently, and is potentially dangerous for patients who are at the same time contaminated with MRSA, since the transfer of genetic material may result in a strain resistant to both methicillin and vancomycin.

The incidence of MRSA in the dialysis population now stands at 15% or more in many countries, in a population that is already highly susceptible to *Staphylococcus aureus* carriage. No convincing data exist for GRE, but it should be taken into account that GRE carriership is consistently present even in the normal healthy population.

The question should be raised of whether carriers of MRSA and GRE need to be isolated in the dialysis unit. Whereas there is not much debate that this should be the case for MRSA, the options are less clear with regard to GRE. Nevertheless, it seems wise to separate GRE carriers from other patients as well. In any case, MRSA and GRE carriers should be separated from each other (see Chapter 17).

Hepatitis B and C carriership implies the potential risk of patient to patient transmission. Here isolation is also indicated. The consequence of this trend for isolation is that at least five subgroups have to be created in the haemodialysis population: patients with GRE, MRSA, hepatitis B and C, and non-carriers. Such strategies pose a major practical problem for dialysis units. Additional isolation is necessary in patients with combinations of carriership.

Time since start of dialysis

It is possible that shifts in host defence function occur during the long-term follow-up of dialysed patients. A severe suppression of phagocyte response follows in the first weeks after the start of dialysis. Both in cross-sectional and in prospective studies, this functional capacity improved when dialysis treatment was prolonged (Vanholder *et al.* 1993).

The functional improvement over time may be attributed to the development of compensatory mechanisms. Patients after long-term dialysis show higher values of IL-1 secretion than do not-yet-dialysed uraemics. Also the levels of circulating soluble IL-2 receptors are positively correlated to the duration of haemodialysis.

Malnutrition

A substantial number of patients with ESRD are malnourished, which can lead to delayed wound healing, depression of secretory immunity, impaired macrophage function, reduced NK cell activity and IL-2 production, and impaired respiratory burst activity and free radical production in response to phagocytosis. Low serum albumin, as a result of undernourishment, is associated with an extra risk for infection.

Attempts to retard the progress of ESRD by imposing protein restriction may at the same time induce undernourishment, especially if dietary restriction is prolonged after the start of dialysis. The use of all-protein restricting diets has been associated with non-specific decreases in numbers of circulating leucocyte and with an effete *in vitro* response of mononuclear cells to various mitogens (Field *et al.* 1991).

Correction of anaemia by rHuEPO also has a positive effect on malnutrition, and this may be one of the reasons why erythropoietin improves several aspects of immune function.

Associated diseases

Several diseases causing immune deficiency can be accompanied by renal failure. This is the case for alcoholism (IgA nephropathy), cirrhosis (IgA nephropathy, hepatorenal syndrome), hepatitis B (membranous nephropathy, polyarteritis nodosa), malignancy (obstructive nephropathy, membranous nephropathy), diabetes mellitus, myeloma, or lymphoma.

In addition, chronic renal failure may also be complicated by diseases such as cancer and hepatitis, providing an additional weakening of the immune system.

Finally, some renal diseases may necessitate the administration of drugs with an inhibitory effect on the immune function (see Chapter 2).

Diabetic patients are at risk for infectious disease (see Chapter 6). Diabetes mellitus has become one of the major causes of ESRD leading to dialysis, and the prevalence of diabetes as a primary cause of renal failure is still increasing. Diabetes is an extra source of immune deficiency superimposed on the uraemic mechanisms. This condition increases the risk for serious opportunistic infections such as fungal disease, in addition to the fact that several barrier functions work insufficiently. Finally, these patients are also prone to vascular occlusion. Infection of ischaemic diabetic lesions is one of the leading causes of morbidity and even mortality in this population, see Chapter 19. Focal infections, e.g. of access systems, also tend to metastasize more easily throughout the body.

Many diseases associated with renal failure are by themselves a cause of local infection of the kidney and/or the urinary tract: polycystic kidney disease, nephrolithiasis, anatomical anomalies, urinary tract obstruction, reflux, and papillary necrosis. These local infections may become systemic and disseminate throughout the body. Other associated disorders which occur frequently in renal failure, such as vascular ulcers of the limbs (Johnson *et al.* 1995) or pulmonary oedema, are a prominent cause of infection.

Drug treatment

A number of alternative causes of defective immune function that are not directly related to uraemia should not be neglected. These include the use of immunosuppressive agents in renal transplant recipients and in autoimmune disorders, and the use of antibiotics with immunosuppressive characteristics. These negative influences may be enhanced by altered pharmacokinetics, protein binding, and increased retention of drug and drug metabolites due to renal failure. Even low-dose immunosuppression in combination with renal failure (e.g. during chronic renal allograft rejection), is associated with an increased incidence of infection.

Corrective measures

The defect in immune function in uraemia is multifactorial. It is related to uraemic toxicity, bioincompatibility of dialyser membranes, deficiencies of vitamins and trace elements, anaemia, iron overload, and malnutrition. The changes in immune function are an illustration of the interference between a biological system, uraemic toxicity, and the strategies employed to reduce this toxicity. Dialysis removes potential toxins, but may exhibit its own toxicity due to bioincompatibility. The main causative factors of dysfunction of the immune system, together with the possible preventive and therapeutic measures, are summarized in Table 1.3.

Several pharmacological strategies are available to improve immune function. Erythropoietin may be one of those. The response to vaccination may be improved in long-term haemodialysis patients by the administration of recombinant human IFN-γ. Administration of interferon in patients with chronic hepatitis C is effective in controlling disease activity. The question is whether these measures when used in patients with chronic renal failure enhance bioincompatibility reactions and/or the risk of rejection in the case of transplantation. The point is that circulating and intracellular levels of cytokines are increased in exactly those conditions in which a decreased immune response has been suspected, but their accumulation is associated with increased concentrations of anti-inflammatory agents as well, such as soluble receptors and cytokine antagonists.

Iron and blood products should be administered with care. This can be realized more easily since the advent of proper methods for estimating body iron stores and the availability of rHuEPO. On the other hand, extra iron supplementation to levels above normal is often needed to induce an appropriate response to rHuEPO. Treatment of iron

Table 1.3 Causes of immune dysfunction in uraemia: preventive and therapeutic measures

Cause	Preventive and therapeutic measures
Dialysis bioincompatibility	Non-complement-activating dialyser membranes Sterile dialysate PD* fluid solutions with minimal negative effect on the immune system
Uraemic toxicity	Optimum solute removal. Adequate K_t/V Elimination of both hydrophilic and hydrophobic compounds Better definition of responsible toxins
Uraemic anaemia	Erythropoietin
Interference by medication	Erythropoietin Vitamin D analogues Avoid (if possible) immunosuppressive medication Use immune stimulation?
Iron overload	Erythropoietin Avoid unnecessary iron and blood transfusions Desferrioxamine (use carefully because of immunosuppressive risks)
Infection of dialysis access	Rigid asepsis Materials with low affinity for bacteria Protective coating of materials
Chronic infection carrier state	Preventive chronic antibiotics (local or systemic)
Malnutrition	Hyperalimentation Growth hormone Erythropoietin
Vitamin deficiency	Usual substitution
Resistance to 1,25(OH)$_2$D$_3$	Removal of responsible toxins?

*PD = peritoneal dialysis.

overload with desferrioxamine may induce immune dysfunction by itself. This has especially enhanced the risk for infection with a specific morbid yeast, *Rhizopus*.

Care should be taken to avoid introduction of bacteria at insertion sites of dialysis catheters. In-dwelling catheters for long-term use (in either peritoneal or haemodialysis) should be developed in materials with a low affinity for bacteria, or materials might be coated with compounds that are destructive (antibiotics) or reflective (silver) for bacteria.

Patients at a sustained chronic risk of infection might be treated with prophylactic long-term low-dose antibiotics, as has been proposed for chronic granulomatous disease. Antibiotic unguents have successfully been administered to nasal carriers of *Staphylococcus aureus*, resulting in a decrease of infection of access sites, skin, and soft tissue. This effect is optimal if prevention is applied on an intermittent basis, e.g. by application of intranasal unguents one week per month, to avoid development of resistance.

Malnutrition may be underestimated as a cause of immune deficiency, and should be corrected by peroral or parenteral hyperalimentation and/or the use of hormones stimulating tissue anabolism, e.g. growth hormone or erythropoietin. Although vitamin deficiency may cause immune dysfunction, incidence is low since most vitamins are adequately substituted or even oversubstituted in uraemic dialysis patients. A specific problem may, however, arise with $1,25(OH)_2D_3$, whereby even adequate substitution may be inefficient since relative resistance occurs.

The factors summarized in Table 1.3 contribute to the propensity of infection in the continuously growing population with renal failure and/or on renal replacement therapy. Taking these factors into account and counteracting them should necessarily decrease the number and severity of these infections and consequent mortality, improving the quality of life and survival of ESRD patients.

References

Alter MJ, Favero MS, Moyer LA, and Bland LA (1991). National surveillance of hemo-dialysis associated diseases in the United States. *American Society of Artificial Internal Organs Journal*, **37**: 97–109.

Blagg CR, Hickman RO, Eschbach JW, and Scribner BH (1970). Home hemodialysis: Six years' experience. *New England Journal of Medicine*, **283**: 1126–31.

Cohen G, Haag-Weber M, and Horl WH (1997). Immune dysfunction in uremia. *Kidney International*, **25**: S79–S82.

Descamps-Latscha B, Herbelin A, Nguyen AT, *et al.* (1995). Balance between iL-1β, TNF-α, and their specific inhibitors in chronic renal failure and maintenance dialysis. *Journal of Immunology*, **154**: 882–92.

Dhondt A, Vanholder R, Waterloos MA, Glorieux G, and Ringoir S (1996). Leukocyte CD14- and CD45-expression during hemodialysis: polysulfone versus cuprophane. *Nephron*, **74**: 342–8.

Dhondt A, Vanholder R, Waterloos MA, Glorieux G, De Smet R, and Lameire N (1998). Citrate anticoagulation does not correct cuprophane bioincompatibility evaluated by expression of granulocyte surface molecules. *Nephrology Dialysis and Transplantation*, **13**: 1752–8.

Dou L, Brunet P, Dignat-George F, Sampol J, and Berland Y (1998). Effect of uremia and hemodialysis on soluble L-selectin and leukocyte surface CD11b and L-selectin. *American Journal of Kidney Diseases*, **31**: 67–73.

Field CJ, Gougeon R, and Marliss EB (1991). Changes in circulating leukocytes and mitogen responses during very-low-energy all-protein reducing diets. *American Journal of Clinical Nutrition*, **54**: 123–9.

Flament J, Goldman M, Waterlot Y, Dupont E, Wybran J, and Vanherweghem JL (1986). Impairment of phagocyte oxidative metabolism in hemodialyzed patients with iron overload. *Clinical Nephrology*, **25**: 277–30.

Hakim RM (1993). Clinical implications of hemodialysis membrane bioincompatibility. *Kidney International*, **44**: 484–94.

Hakim RM, Wingard RL, Parker RA, Vanholder R, Husni L, and Parker TF (1994). Effects of biocompatibility on hospitalization and infectious morbidity in chronic hemodialysis patients (CHD)(abstract). *Journal of the American Society of Nephrology*, **5**: 443.

Hornberger JC, Chernew M, Petersen J, and Garber AM (1992). A multivariate analysis of mortality and hospital admissions with high-flux dialysis. *Journal of the American Society of Nephrology*, **3**: 1227–37.

Johnson BL, Glickman MH, Bandyk DF, and Esses GE (1995). Failure of foot salvage in patients with end-stage renal disease after surgical revascularization. *Journal of Vascular Surgery*, **22**: 280–6.

Klein E, Pass T, Harding GB, Wright R, and Million C (1990). Microbial and endotoxin contamination in water and dialysate in the central United States. *Artificial Organs*, 14: 85–94.

Levin NW, Zasuwa G, and Dumler F (1991). Effect of membrane type on causes of death in hemodialysis patients (abstract). *Journal of the American Society of Nephrology*, 2: 335.

Levy R, Klein J, Rubinek T, Alkan M, Shany S, and Chaimovitz C (1990). Diversity in peritoneal macrophage response of CAPD patients to 1,25-dihydroxyvitamin D₃. *Kidney International*, 37: 1310–15.

Mailloux LU, Bellucci AG, Wilkes BM, *et al.* (1991). Mortality in dialysis patients: analysis of the causes of death. *American Journal of Kidney Diseases*, 18: 326–35.

Maiorca R, Cancarini GC, Brunori G, Camerini C, and Manili L (1993). Morbidity and mortality of CAPD and hemodialysis. *Kidney International*, 43 (Suppl. 40): S4–S15.

Schiffl H, Lang M, König A, Strasser T, Haider MC, and Held E (1994). Biocompatible membranes in acute renal failure: prospective case-controlled study. *The Lancet*, 344: 570–2.

Vanholder R and Ringoir S (1993). Infectious morbidity and defects of phagocytic function in end-stage renal disease. A review. *Journal of the American Society of Nephrology*, 3: 1541–54.

Vanholder R, Ringoir S, Dhondt A, and Hakim R (1991). Phagocytosis in uremic and hemodialysis patients: a prospective and cross sectional study. *Kidney International*, 39: 320–7.

Vanholder R, Van Biesen W, and Ringoir S (1993). Contributing factors to the inhibition of phagocytosis in hemodialyzed patients. *Kidney International*, 44: 208–14.

Veys N, Vanholder R, and Ringoir S (1992). Correction of deficient phagocytosis during erythropoietin (EPO) treatment in maintenance haemodialysis patients. *American Journal of Kidney Diseases*, 19: 358–63.

2

The effect of immunosuppressive agents on the defence against infection

P.L. Amlot

Susceptibility to infection is characteristic of patients with immune deficiency. Deficiencies of B cells and polymorphonuclear phagocytes affect antibody responses thereby preferentially increasing bacterial infection. Deficiencies affecting T cells and mononuclear phagocytes increase viral and intracellular pathogenic infections preferentially. There is a great deal of overlap between these two arms of the immune system, and effective control of particular infectious diseases requires the coordination of both arms of the immune system. For example, deficiency of T helper cells can increase the risk of bacterial infection because of a requirement for T helper cells in providing growth factors for B cells involved in antibody production.

This chapter will attempt to analyse the known effects of immunosuppressive drugs in clinical practice upon immune mechanisms and the potential that such drugs have in predisposing to infection. It has to be remembered throughout that the immunosuppressive drug or drugs employed contribute to the total effect upon immunity in any individual. In patients with allogeneic renal transplants it is rare that a single immunosuppressive drug is administered alone and many immunosuppressive drugs or drugs that influence immunosuppressive drug therapy are now used together to control allograft rejection. During hospital procedures the patient on immunosuppressive therapy is exposed to nosocomial infection as a result of the invasive diagnostic and therapeutic mechanisms (catheterization, intravenous cannulation, urinary, biliary, or wound drains, etc.). Immunosuppressive drugs may predispose to viral or other infection, which in turn contribute to a heightened immune deficiency. One immunosuppressive drug may act synergistically, additively, or antagonistically with other drugs used in the patient's therapy. These effects contribute to what has been termed the 'net immunosuppressive' effect making it difficult to attribute to immunosuppressive drugs the selective susceptibility to defined infectious agents. In over 90% of renal transplant patients who developed opportunistic infections (*Aspergillus, Nocardia, Cryptococcus*, and *Pneumocystis*) at one centre there was a concurrent viral infection (Rubin 1993). The combination of immunosuppressive drugs has certainly been of benefit in renal transplantation and the use of steroid-sparing immunosuppressive drugs in autoimmune diseases of the kidney has likewise tried to avoid the damaging effects of overuse of single agents. All of these effects blur the direct influence of individual immunosuppressive drugs on infection. Nonetheless, by understanding how immunosuppressive drugs act upon the immune system the clinician is in a better position to assess the risk of certain types of infection. Radiation therapy will not be evaluated, as it is a poor immuno-suppressive modality and the morbidity from total body irradiation or total lymphoid irradiation is unacceptably high, and, although used experimentally, these methods have not found a place in standard practice except for allogeneic bone marrow transplantation.

Five principal points concerning immunosuppression need to be borne in mind. The severity of immunosuppression is a function of:

(1) the dose of immunosuppressive agent used;
(2) the duration of treatment with an immunosuppressive agent;
(3) the number of immunosuppressive agents used in combination;
(4) the immunosuppressive impact of concurrent infection (e.g. cytomegalovirus (CMV));
(5) the susceptibility of the recipient's immune system to the immunosuppression used.

The clinician has control of the first three points above and will need to reassess their use if concurrent infection arises. Unfortunately in most cases there is no easy way other than trial and error to assess the patient's susceptibility.

Corticosteroids

Corticosteroids have a widespread effect on the body, affecting both metabolic (miner-alocorticoid) and the immune system (glucocorticoid). Glucocorticoids (Gc) are the forms that will be considered here. The therapeutic Gc most commonly used are prednisolone, prednisone, and methyl prednisolone because they have the fewest mineralocorticoid effects of all Gc. The latter two forms need to be metabolized in the liver and Gc are dependent upon cytochrome P-450. Drugs that upregulate P-450, such as phenytoin, phenobarbital, and rifampicin, will increase the speed with which Gc are metabolized and will affect their immunosuppressive effect. Renal transplant patients taking anticonvulsants have a poorer allograft survival (Wassner *et al.* 1977).

Glucocorticoid regulation of immune responses

Glucocorticoids initiate their action by binding to glucocorticoid receptor (GR) in the cytoplasm. Glucocorticoid receptor is a single molecule with no alleles or polymorphism but there is a splice variation, GRβ, this is unable to bind to Gc and which therefore may interfere with the action of GR. There are extremely rare familial mutations of GR causing glucocorticoid resistance and characterized by high blood cortisol levels without Cushing's syndrome. The GR has a Gc binding domain at the C-terminal, two zinc finger motifs that interact with DNA, two *trans*-activating regions, τ1 and τ2, that transcribe genes bound to DNA, and a heat shock protein, hsp90, binding region. Between 10 and 100 genes are directly or indirectly regulated by Gc. Direct regulation occurs when GR–Gc homodimers bind to glucocorticoid response elements (GRE) on DNA and initiate gene transcription or to negative GRE (nGRE) and repress gene transcription (Fig. 2.1). Repression via nGRE is due to the binding site lying over the TATA box of the involved gene and preventing initiation of transcription.

Most genes are directly or indirectly repressed by Gc and involve mechanisms other than the interaction between GR and GRE. GR–Gc complexes interact with

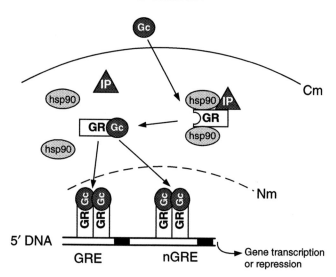

Fig. 2.1 Glucocorticoid regulation of gene *trans*-activation via glucocorticoid response elements (GRE). Solid bars in DNA represent steroid responsive genes. The Gc–GR complex cannot cross the nuclear membrane until Gc binds to it, whereupon hsp90 and IP dissociate allowing the Gc–GR complex to cross into the nucleus. Abbreviations: Cm = cell membrane; Gc = glucocorticoid; GR = glucocorticoid receptor, 300 kDa; GRE = glucocorticoid response element; hsp90 = heat shock protein 90 kDa; IP = immunophilin; nGRE = negative GRE; Nm = nuclear membrane.

transcription factors via leucine zipper molecules, enhancement of ribonucleases, AP-1 (a heterodimer of Fos and Jun oncoproteins), or nuclear factor κB (NFκB) (Fig. 2.2). For example, Gc are potent inhibitors of collagenase gene transcription induced by TNF-α and PE via AP-1. Most Gc-induced inhibition of cytokine or chemokine transcription is indirectly due to blocking AP-1 or NFκB (Fig. 2.2).

Lastly, Gc are known to influence chromatin structure via effects on nucleosomes and the degree to which chromatin is open or closed. These effects are mediated through histone acetylation or deacetylation respectively by the large protein complexes shown in Fig. 2.3. The cAMP response element (CREB) binding protein CBP complexed with a p300 protein is able to acetylate chromatin and this causes it to unwind from the histones facilitating gene transcription. Many proteins compete for binding to the CBP/p300 complex and thereby influence whether acetylation or deacetylation occurs leading to transcription or repression of genes. Gc can enhance acetylation via the steroid receptor coactivator superfamily (SRC). Other proteins, such as PCAF (p300/CBP associated factor) and SRA (steroid receptor RNA activator), interact to enhance acetylation in association with SRC and CBP/p300 and drive unravelling of the chromatin via nuclear receptor coactivators (nCoA). There are many other proteins (glucocorticoid receptor interacting protein-1 or GRIP-1, transcription factor intermediary factor 2 or TRIP-2, cointegrator associated protein or p/CIP) that influence SRC by determining the tissues or target cells or the type of activation. On the other hand, a molecule such as CARM (coactivator-associated arginine methyltransferase) will suppress transcription by enhancing deacetylation or methylation of DNA via nuclear receptor corepressors (nCoR).

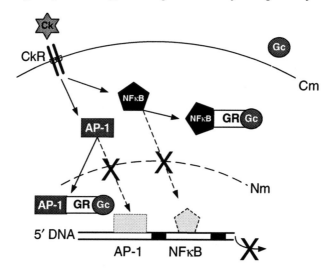

Fig. 2.2 Glucocorticoid regulation of gene *cis*-activation via AP-1 and NFκB. The crosses indicate that direct binding between the Gc–GR complex and AP-1 or NFκB components preventing them binding to the DNA thus blocking transcription. Abbreviations: Cm = cell membrane; Gc = glucocorticoid; GR = glucocorticoid receptor, 300 kDa; Nm = nuclear membrane; AP-1 = activator protein-1; Ck = cytokine; CkR = cytokine receptor; NFκB = nuclear factor κB.

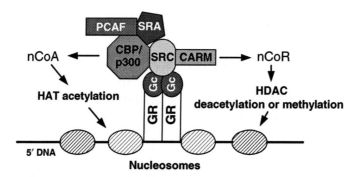

Fig. 2.3 Glucocorticoid effects upon histone acetylation and deacetylation. DNA is tightly wound around histones in the outer nucleosomes and forms dense chromatin, while it is unravelled in the inner nucleosomes. Abbreviations: CARM = coactivator-associated arginine methyltransferase; CBP/p300 = CREB binding protein (CREB = cAMP response element); HAT = histone acetyl transferase; HDAC = histone deacetylase; nCoA = nuclear receptor coactivators; nCoR = nuclear receptor corepressors; PCAF = p300/CBP-associated factor; SRA = steroid receptor RNA activator; SRC = steroid receptor coactivator superfamily.

Gc therefore influence immune-mediated inflammation and damage by either enhancing transcription of anti-inflammatory proteins or decreasing transcription of inflammatory proteins. Its effects are modified by the responsiveness of different types of cells to the actions and targets of Gc.

Table 2.1   Glucocorticoid effects on transcription of immunoregulatory molecules

Increased transcription	Inhibition of transcription
Lipocortin-1	Cytokines: IL-1 to IL-6, IL-11 to IL-13, TNF-α and GM-CSF
β$_2$-adrenoceptor	Chemokines: IL-8, RANTES, MIP-1α, MCP-1, MCP-3, MCP-4, eotaxin
Secretory leucocyte inhibitory protein	iNOS
IL-1 receptor antagonist	COX-2
IL-1R2 (non-signalling receptor)	PLA$_2$
IκB-α	Endothelin-1
Endonucleases → apoptosis	NK$_1$ and NK$_2$ receptors on smooth muscle. Adhesion molecules: ICAM-1, E-selectin

Abbreviations: IL=interleukin; TNF=tumour necrosis factor; GM-CSF=granulocyte–macrophage colony-stimulating factor; MIP=macrophage inflammatory protein; MCP=monocyte chemoattractant protein; INOS=inducible nitrous oxide synthase; COX=cyclo-oxygenase; PLA=phospholipase A; NK=natural killer; ICAM=intercellular adhesion molecule. RANTES=regulated upon activation normal T-cell expressed and secreted.

The enormous range of molecules involved in immune responses and inflammation affected by Gc is shown in Table 2.1 and account for the broad immunosuppression achieved with Gc. The range of anti-inflammatory and immunosuppressive effects include interference of intracellular signalling in lymphocytes (e.g. lipocortin-1 inhibits phospholipase A$_2$ (PLA$_2$)), inhibition of cellular synthesis (e.g. Clara cell protein inhibits epithelial cell secretion), increase of anti-inflammatory cytokines (e.g. IL-10), decrease of inflammatory cytokines that enhance inflammation either by their intercellular effects or because they affect migration of inflammatory cells into the site or by enhancing enzyme secretion (neutral endopeptidases that degrade inflammatory peptides such as substance P or bradykinin) and induce apoptosis in lymphocytes and eosinophils (Table 2.1). The mode of action and molecular mechanisms have recently been reviewed (Barnes 1998; Giordano and Avantaggiata 1999; Leo and Chen 2000).

At the cellular level Gc suppress T and B cells, macrophages, and eosinophils and alter epithelial cells. T cells are affected because of the reduction of IL-2 to IL-5, IL-13 and GM-CSF as well as a direct apoptotic effect of Gc on sensitive cells. Via IL-3 there may also be an effect on mast cells. Macrophages are affected because of the blockade of IL-1 and IFNγ. In addition the upregulation of IL-10 synthesis by macrophages contributes to switching off of proinflammatory cytokines. The reduction of granulocyte–macrophage colony-stimulating factor (GM-CSF) and IL-4 impairs maturation of early monocytes in the bone marrow into antigen-presenting dendritic cells. Eosinophil mediator release is suppressed directly by Gc and the reduction of GM-CSF and IL-5 reduces eosinopoiesis. Gc enhances neutrophils. Finally, there is a wide range of effects upon epithelial and endothelial cells, including the production of protease inhibitors to depress inflammation and chemokines to decrease leucocyte migration.

This potent and wide-ranging activity means that almost every kind of infection has been seen in patients treated with glucocorticoids and the severity of immunosuppression is dose related. In the early days of transplantation, prior to the availability of calcineurin inhibitors and azathioprine, corticosteroids were often used at high doses for prolonged periods of time. As a result about 50% of deaths were due to infection, with clinical fungal infections peaking 2–3 months post-transplant when the average dose of prednisolone was 60 mg/day. The use of steroid-sparing drugs has reduced the risk of infection associated with Gc while they continue to be used because of their potent anti-inflammatory, immunosuppressive, and synergistic effects with other immuno-suppressive drugs. The chronic use of Gc leads to a fall in serum IgG levels and a decrease in circulating B cells both of which predispose to bacterial infection (Butler and Rossen 1973b). Susceptibility to bacterial infection is high in patients given pulsed high doses of methyl prednisolone for allograft rejection episodes (Butler and Rossen 1973a).

Inhibitors of DNA synthesis

Purine Inhibitors

Azathioprine

In the late 1950s and early 1960, 6-mercaptopurine was shown to have immunosuppressive properties in addition to its known antileukaemic effects. It reduced antibody responses in rabbits and prolonged skin grafts in mice and renal grafts in dogs. Cortisone had already been shown to prolong skin grafts, and it was not long before azathioprine, a formulation that is metabolized to 6-mercaptopurine (Fig. 2.4) was combined with Gc to form the standard immunosuppressive drug regime used for renal transplantation

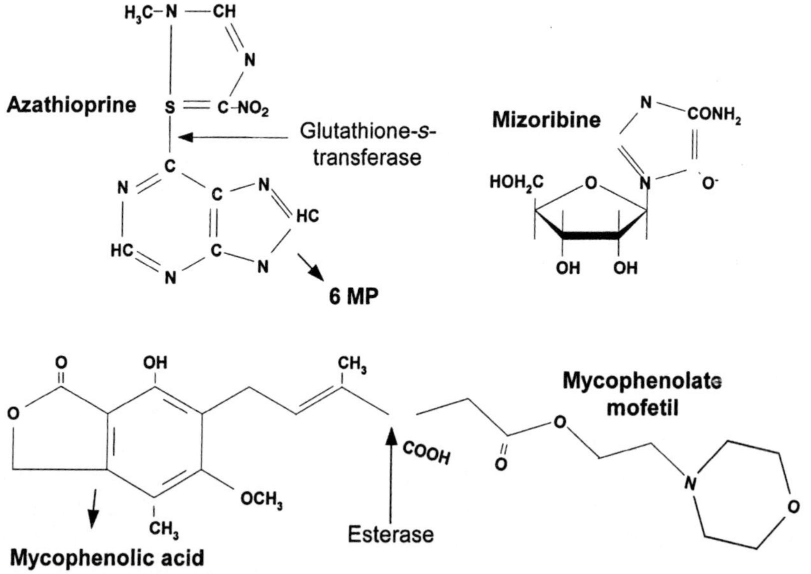

Fig. 2.4 Structure and active metabolites of purine inhibitors. Active metabolites of the drugs are produced by cleaving azathioprine to release 6-mercaptopurine (6 MP), phosphorylation of mizoribine and esterase action to release mycophenolic acid.

throughout the 1960s and 1970s. Outside of transplantation, the use of azathioprine as a glucocorticoid-sparing agent is well known. Azathioprine is converted to 6-mercaptopurine by glutathione present in erythrocytes. 6-mercaptopurine integrates into nucleotides including thioguanylic acid, which interfere with DNA synthesis and polyadenylate-containing RNA. Most of azathioprine's immunosuppressive effect is attributed to impaired proliferation of leucocytes and lymphocytes, but its mode of action is still poorly understood. It causes chromosomal breakages and interferes with lympho- cyte mitosis and the synthesis and action of coenzymes. Azathioprine is a relatively weak immunosuppressive drug but it increases the susceptibility to bacterial infection largely because of its myelosuppressive properties. Skin fragility and chromosomal breakage caused by long-term use of azathioprine predisposes to skin cancer (Gaya *et al.* 1995), which may have an underlying viral origin. Azathioprine suppresses primary more than secondary immune responses, even though proliferation of lymphoid cells is more depressed in the latter. It has relatively feeble effects upon antibody production with a most marked effect upon cellular immunity and inflammation. Humoral suppression is only seen in T-dependent antibody responses. Azathioprine is of no value in reversing ongoing immune responses such as acute rejection episodes or in acute vasculitic diseases.

The discrepancy between azathioprine's antiproliferative effect and immunosuppres- sion is seen clearly when dosage has to be reduced because of myelosuppression. Those myelosuppressed patients whose dosage is reduced have a higher incidence of rejection (Haesslein *et al.* 1972). This suggests that it is not only impaired proliferation that contributes to immunosuppression, because those patients who were more sensitive to myelosuppression ought to be better immunosuppressed. Contributing to this problem is the poor bioavailability and large interindividual variability in the absorption of azathioprine (Ohlman *et al.* 1994). Renal transplant patients maintained on higher doses of azathioprine ($> 1.5\,\text{mg/kg/day}$) had a significantly longer graft survival than those on lower maintenance doses (Opelz and Dohler 2000). Concerning azathioprine dosage, it should be remembered that the effect of concomitant allopurinol is important because of its inhibition of xanthine oxidase, which potentiates azathioprine's myelosuppression enormously. In the presence of allopurinol it is necessary to reduce azathioprine to a quarter of its usual dose. This is insufficient to control renal transplantation on its own but combined with corticosteroids it is effective.

Mycophenolate mofetil

Mycophenolic acid (MPA) was initially used to treat psoriasis but this was complicated by an unacceptably high level of serious infection and a questionable increase in cancer that led to its withdrawal (Lynch and Roenigk 1977). Subsequently, an esterified form of MPA, mycophenolate mofetil (MMF) was developed with better intestinal absorption than MPA, which converted into the active MPA upon absorption. MMF is a logical step in the further development of inhibition of purine synthesis following azathioprine, with the aim of making a more specific and potent immunosuppressive drug. The chemical structures of azathioprine, MMF, and mizoribine (MZ) are shown in Fig. 2.4, with the purine biosynthetic pathways and enzyme inhibition induced by these drugs in Fig. 2.5. Lymphocytes are dependent upon the *de novo* pathway of purine synthesis while there is variable use of the salvage pathway by other tissues. Deficiency of the enzyme adenosine deaminase (ADA), which impairs the *de novo* pathway of purine synthesis, has been

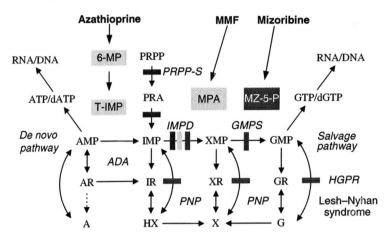

Fig. 2.5 Blockade of enzymes involved in purine biosynthesis by azathioprine, mizoribine, and mycophenolate mofetil. Drugs are in bold type, active metabolites in shaded boxes, and enzymes in italics. Abbreviations: A = adenosine; *ADA* = adenosine deaminase; G = guanine; *GMPS* = GMP synthase; H = hypoxanthine; *HGPRT* = hypoxanthine–guanine phosphoribosyltransferase; *IMPD* = inosine monophosphate dehydrogenase; MMF = mycophenolate mofetil; MP = monophosphate; MPA = mycophenolic acid; MZ-5-P = mizoribine-5′-monophosphate; *PNP* = purine nucleoside phosphorylase; PRPP = phosphoribosyl pyrophosphate; PRPP-S = PRPP synthase; R = ribosyl; T-IMP = thio-IMP; X = xanthine; 6-MP = 6 mercaptopurine.

linked to a severe combined immunodeficiency that does not impair myelopoiesis, erythropoiesis, platelet production, or neuronal development (Giblett *et al.* 1972). On the other hand, deficiency of hypoxanthine-guanine phosphoribosyltransferase (HGPRT) leads to the Lesch–Nyhan syndrome with normal lymphocyte function but progressive neurological degeneration; it is an essential enzyme for the salvage pathway. Impairment of ADA, inosine monophosphate dehydrogenase (IMPD), or GMP synthase affects the production of nucleotides essential for lymphocyte proliferation without affecting the salvage pathway. Guanosine nucleotides are important regulators of rate-limiting enzymes catalysing inosine synthesis (Franklin and Cook 1969) accounting for the importance of these enzymatic pathways. In addition to the dependence of lymphocytes upon the *de novo* pathway, there are two isoforms of the MPA-susceptible enzyme IMPD—type I is found predominantly in resting lymphocytes and type II in activated lymphocytes. The latter is five times more sensitive to MPA, making it an appropriate target for immunosuppression (Nagai *et al.* 1992).

MMF at clinically achievable levels suppresses both T- and B-cell proliferation *in vitro* by suppression of DNA synthesis and mitosis. The suppression is reversed by guanosine or guanosine derivatives but not adenosine. None of the purine synthesis inhibitors have any influence upon the early stages of lymphocyte activation or upon cytokine synthesis (IL-1 or IL-2). As a result of the restricted inhibition of purine synthetic pathways, both MMF and MZ are more selective inhibitors of lymphocyte function than azathioprine and they leave phagocytic leucocytes largely unaffected, unlike azathioprine. The numerous sites at which azathioprine inhibits purine synthesis lead to depletion of adenosine rather than guanosine. MMF is a more potent immunosuppressive drug than azathioprine and reduced acute renal allograft rejection significantly more than azathioprine in several phase III trials (Mathew *et al.* for the Tricontinental Mycophenolate Mofetil Renal Transplantation Study Group 1998). MMF is much more effective at reducing antibody responses than azathioprine (Kimball *et al.* 1995; Smith *et al.* 1998). Consequently there is an increased incidence of infection, particularly tissue-invasive CMV, when MMF is used. Since MMF suppresses growth of Epstein–Barr virus (EBV) transformed B-cell lines, it was hoped that the incidence of lymphoproliferative disease would decrease with the use of MMF in transplantation, but that has not been realized. Mizoribine is a very similar drug to MMF but they have never been compared directly with each other. It is interesting that mizoribine has a marked synergism with cyclosporine A whereas the effect of combining MMF or azathioprine and cyclosporine A is only additive.

Finally, the broad T- and B-cell immunosuppression produced by blockade of the IMPD and GMP synthase pathways (Fig. 2.5) could be made more selectively T-lymphocyte restricted if a purine nucleoside phosphorylase (PNP) inhibitor were developed, because patients with PNP deficiency have a severe T-cell deficiency with normal B-cell function.

Alkylating agents

Cyclophosphamide

Cyclophosphamide is an alkylating agent derived from mustine in which the methyl group has been replaced by phosphamide. This creates an inert, bioavailable form, which can be taken orally. Phosphorylation of the phosphor-nitrogen bond in the liver leads to release of active metabolites. It is activated by reactions catalysed by cytochrome P-450 in the liver. The alkylating agent blocks cells during DNA synthesis and this may lead to cell death. It is a much more powerful immunosuppressant than azathioprine and is particular effective in suppressing humoral immunity. B cells are particularly sensitive to cyclophosphamide and it is an effective drug in treating antibody-mediated autoimmune disorders and myeloma. Cyclophosphamide is particularly effective in treating Wegener's disease. Early use of cyclophosphamide in transplantation showed no superiority over azathioprine but there were no controlled studies and the more significant side-effects associated with cyclophosphamide did not encourage further investigation in transplantation. The combination of azathioprine and cyclophosphamide can have devastating myelosuppressive effects (Berlyne and Danovitch 1971). Although these agents and no longer used together for immunosuppression, the same effect may be seen when lymphoproliferative disease is treated by alkylating agents in patients who have received long-term azathioprine therapy. Because of its potent immunosuppressive activity, prolonged usage is associated with virtually every infectious complication that can be seen with immunosuppressive drugs.

Calcineurin inhibitors

Two immunosuppressive drugs affect the early stages of lymphocyte activation by interfering with a cell-signalling pathway that requires calcium (Ca^{2+}) and a calcium-binding molecule called calcineurin, also known as phosphatase 2B. The first of these drugs, cyclosporine A (CSA) revolutionized transplantation. Prior to its introduction, immuno-suppression with azathioprine and prednisolone was effective in about 50% of all renal allografts but for other organs transplantation could only be regarded as experimental. Following the introduction of CSA in the 1970s a wide range of organ transplantation became possible, including heart, liver, lung, and pancreas, with 1-year graft survival in kidney transplantation rising from 50% to 90%. Tacrolimus (TAC) was subsequently introduced and is more potent than CSA. Unfortunately, TAC shared with CSA the unwanted side-effect of nephrotoxicity and the therapeutic index is similarly narrow to that of CSA. The nephrotoxicity limits the use of CSA and TAC as general immunosuppressive agents outside of transplantation.

The mode of action of these calcineurin inhibitors is shown in Fig. 2.6. When the T-cell receptor (TCR) binds to antigen presented by the major histocompatibility complex (MHC) or to allogeneic MHC, it triggers transmembrane signals that lead to an increase in cytoplasmic Ca^{2+}. The initial pathway via phospholipase C (PLC), phosphatidylinositol-4,5-biphosphate (PIP_2), inositol triphosphate (IP_3), and diacyl-glycerol (DAG) is common to both T and B cells (Fig. 2.6). The free Ca^{2+} is rapidly

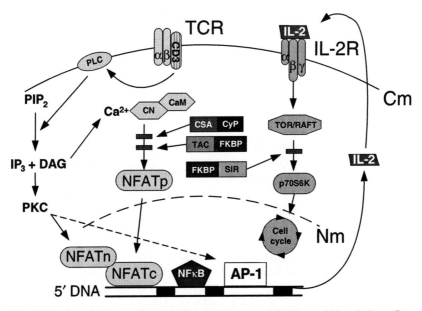

Fig. 2.6 Inhibition of cell signalling by CSA, tacrolimus, and sirolimus. Abbreviations: Cm=cell membrane; Nm=nuclear membrane; NFκB=nuclear factor κB; CaM=calmodulin; CN= calcineurin; CSA=cyclosporine A; CyP=cyclophilin; DAG=diacylglycerol; FKBP=FK506 binding protein; IL-2=interleukin 2; IL-2R=interleukin 2 receptor; IP_3=inositol triphosphate; NFAT=nuclear factor of activation of T cells; NFATc=cytoplasmic NFAT; NFATn= nuclear NFAT; NFATp=precursor of NFAT; p70S6K=p70S6 kinase; PIP_2=phosphatidylinositol-4,5-biphosphate; PKC = protein kinase C; PLC=phospholipase C; RAFT=rapamycin; SIR= sirolimus (rapamycin); TAC=tacrolimus (FK506); TCR=T cell receptor; TOR=target of rapamycin.

captured by a complex of calcineurin and calmodulin, which together with Ca^{2+} greatly enhances the serine/threonine phosphatase activity. The activated complex controls the phosphorylation of transcription factors important for the expression of immune response genes, the nuclear factors of activated T cells (NFAT). Dephosphorylation of the cytoplasmic precursor of NFAT allows it to cross the nuclear membrane and bind to and transactivate genes leading to the transcription and synthesis of interleukin 2 (IL-2) among other cellular activators. This early event in T-cell activation leads to secretion of IL-2 and concurrently the IL-2α chain of the IL-2 receptor complex (IL-2R) is upregulated on the membrane of T cells. These cytokine and cytokine receptors have, until recently, been regarded as the most important signals for T-cell growth. These events will normally take the T cell from G_0 to G_1 of the cell cycle and do not involve proliferation or DNA synthesis. Once IL-2 has been synthesized and the IL-2R expressed on the surface of the cell, binding of IL-2 to IL-2R initiates a transmembrane signal that leads to proliferation with DNA synthesis (S phase) and mitosis (Fig. 2.6).

Inhibition of this signalling occurs when a complex of CSA and cyclophilin (CyP) binds to calcineurin and prevents phosphorylation of the NFAT precursor in the cytoplasm and its subsequent translocation to the nucleus. A similar inhibition occurs when TAC complexes with FK506 binding protein (FKBP). Cyclophilin and FKBP belong to a large group of ubiquitous cytoplasmic proteins called immunophilins (because they bind the immunosuppressive drugs) and they function as peptidyl-prolyl *cis–trans* isomerases. This function involves the correct folding of nascent proteins. Although it is tempting to link the function of these cytoplasmic proteins to the immuno-suppressive effects of CSA and TAC, there is no support for this concept. It appears to be a purely fortuitous interaction but one that is essential for the creation of a drug–immunophilin complex such that it blocks the enzymatic activity of activated calcineurin. The outcome is that transcription of essential cytokines for T-cell expansion is inhibited and expansion of specific T cells is essential for an effective immune response. The development of these immunosuppressive drugs, like the development of MMF, made immunosuppression more specific and largely limited to cells of the immune system. There is no evidence that myelopoiesis or other rapidly dividing cells are affected. This means that unlike azathioprine, and to a lesser extent MMF, there is no risk of significant neutropenia and neutropenic sepsis or infection. However, the more potent lymphocyte-specific immunosuppression, which permits a wide range of organ transplantation, carries with it a greater susceptibility to viral, intracellular, and other opportunistic pathogens.

Cyclosporine

Cyclosporine's pharmacology has been well reviewed (Faulds *et al.* 1993) and only those aspects relevant to infection and immunosuppression will be addressed here. Cyclosporine is a cyclic undecapeptide; there are 25 natural species and over 2000 derivates have been made. The natural cyclosporines were originally obtained from *Tolypocladium inflatum Gans*. Only CSA and those analogues with substitution of α-amino butyric acid at the 2 position produce immunosuppression (CSA, CSC, CSD,

CSG, and CSM). None have been superior to CSA. Most cyclosporines bind to a wide range of cyclophilins (CyP), whether the cyclosporines have immunosuppressive activity or not. CSA is known to bind to many different types of cyclophilin but the effects of the interaction are largely unknown except that is obligatory for its immuno-suppressive effect. All cyclophilins tend to be small molecules, 18–23 kDa in size, and consist of types A, B, C, D, and 40. CyP A is the most abundant cytoplasmic protein; CyP B is found in the endoplasmic reticulum; CyP C is found abundantly in the kidney; and CyP D is in mitochondria. It is not known whether the abundance of CyP C is associated with the nephrotoxicity associated with CSA. CyP 40 is an interesting cyclophilin because it is a component of the inactive steroid receptor, which can bind to glucocorticoids, CSA, and the macrolides (TAC and sirolimus).

Inhibition of the enzymatic activity of calcineurin by CSA prevents dephosphorylation of NFATp as described above for CSA and TAC, but in addition it affects elk1 and CREB; these are DNA binding proteins, and their translocation to the nucleus is inhib-ited by CSA. In addition to the inhibition of IL-2 transcription there is suppression of proto–oncogenes, c-*myc*, c-*fos*, and n-*ras*. CSA has variable effects upon IL-6 synthesis with up-regulation in some cells (blood lymphocytes) but down-regulation of others (mast and epithelial cells). At high concentrations of CSA secretion of IL-6 by gingival fibroblasts may increase and this could be relevant to the gingival hypertrophy often seen with this drug. CSA is able to suppress T-dependent antibody production more effectively than azathioprine.

Immunosuppression with CSA affects cell-mediated immunity predominantly. In transplantation the beneficial effects are attributed to the inhibition of cytotoxic precursor cells becoming activated and the reduced proliferation of effector T cells.

Metabolism of CSA is under the control of the cytochrome P-450 and is affected by the concurrent use of drugs affecting cytochrome P-450. Induction of cytochrome P-450 by drugs such as phenytoin, rifampicin, or nafcillin will increase catabolism of CSA, decrease its levels in the blood, and decrease immunosuppression; inhibition of cytochrome P-450 by drugs such as erythromycin, ketoconazole, or diltiazem will decrease catabolism, increase CSA levels, and increase immunosuppression. CSA and steroids are metabolized by the same cytochrome P-450 and show bidirectional inhibition. CSA and steroids or CSA and MMF have additive effects of immuno-suppression while CSA and mizoribine have synergistic effects. The antibiotic ciprofloxacillin has the potential of antagonizing CSA because it leads to increased transcription of IL-2. Altogether, these observations on pharmacology and drug inter-actions mean that against a background of CSA use, many other drugs may influence the intensity of immunosuppression even though the drugs have no immuno-suppressive properties themselves. Even when additional immunosuppressive drugs are used there is a variable increase in the overall intensity of immunosuppression. Unfortunately, there is no overall measure or index of immunocompetence except for the pragmatic assessment of the response of autoimmune diseases to therapy or to allografting of organs or to the development of significant or severe infection. Almost every kind of opportunistic infection has been described with CSA but it has often been used in combination with other immunosuppressive drugs, particularly prednisolone or azathioprine.

Tacrolimus

The pharmacology of tacrolimus has recently been reviewed (Plosker and Foster 2000; Spencer *et al.* 1997). Tacrolimus is a macrolide compound isolated from a soil fungus *Streptomyces tsukubaensis* in northern Japan. It shares many of the immunosuppressive properties of CSA but is ten to a hundred times more potent. In addition to inhibition of IL-2 transcription it inhibits IL-3, IL-4, IL-5, TNF-α, and GM-CSF. It has been claimed that tacrolimus does not stimulate transforming growth factor-β (TGF-β) to the same extent as CSA and therefore might be less likely to predispose to chronic graft loss and arteriopathy. Absorption is not affected by bile salts and the drug appears to be hepatotrophic; these features contribute to its superiority over CSA in liver transplantation. Metabolism of tacrolimus, like CSA, is under the control of cytochrome P-450 and the same cautions relate to the effects of drugs using cytochrome P-450.

It is almost axiomatic that any increase in immunosuppressive potency will increase infection, but this has not been clearly demonstrated with tacrolimus. However, there are a number of publications suggesting that post-transplant lymphoproliferative disease (PTLD) is increased by tacrolimus. The same was claimed about CSA when it replaced azathioprine for transplant immunosuppression. Two issues influence PTLD in this setting. First, the need to increase immunosuppressive potency to prevent graft loss may lead to the point where a PTLD arises, and second, initial inexperience in the safe way to handle a new immunosuppressive drug leads to over immunosuppression. Nothing inherently should cause tacrolimus to increase PTLD and EBV infection, although it has been claimed that there may be inherent reasons why CSA can predispose to cancer related to TGF-β expression (Hojo *et al.* 1999).

Sirolimus (rapamycin)

Sirolimus, like TAC, is a macrolide and was originally obtained from a soil fungus *Streptomyces hygroscopicus*, on Easter Island (the indigenous name of which is Rapa Nui and hence the original name of the drug was rapamycin). Sirolimus (SIR) shares with TAC the ability to bind to FKBP but thereafter the similarity ends. Unlike TAC–FKBP, SIR–FKBP does not affect calcineurin activity but inhibits the signalling pathway from cytokine receptors leading to cellular proliferation. After a cytokine such as IL-2 binds to its receptor this leads to transmembrane signalling that activates TOR (target of rapamycin). TOR is known by many names (FRAP, RAFT1, SEP, or RAPT1). Mammalian TOR (mTOR) is a large protein, 289 kDa, and is homologous with the catalytic subunit of phosphtidylinositol-3 kinase (PI-3K) and mammalian PI-4K. TOR becomes activated by autophosphorylation and this is inhibited by the drug–immunophilin complex, SIR–FKBP. This inhibition interferes with the pathway that leads to p70 S6 kinase initiating the cell cycle (Fig. 2.6). The inhibition of the cytokine–cytokine receptor pathway explains why sirolimus affects lymphocytes in the S phase rather than early in the G_0 to G_1 stage like the calcineurin inhibitors (Sehgal 1998). The signalling pathways affected by sirolimus are shown in Fig. 2.7. It can be seen that the effects are very broad and are predominantly related to the cell cycle and protein synthesis.

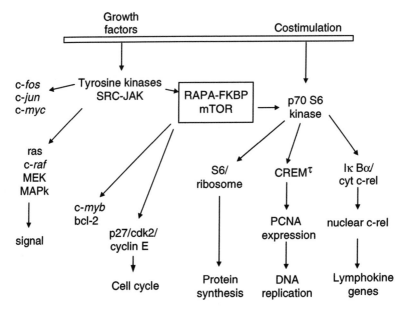

Fig. 2.7 Signalling pathways inhibited by sirolimus (SIR) (rapamycin (RAPA)). Abbreviations: TOR=target of rapamycin; mTOR=mammalian TOR; FKBP=FK506 binding protein.

Sirolimus has proven to be effective for transplant-related immunosuppression, both alone and in combination with CSA. It has shown no evidence of nephrotoxicity and since it binds to FKBP this suggests that it is the interaction with calcineurin that makes tacrolimus a nephrotoxic drug like CSA. The effect of sirolimus on risk of infection was assessed in a controlled clinical trial that compared sirolimus with CSA in first cadaveric renal transplants (Groth *et al.* 1999). Both sirolimus and CSA were used in combination with azathioprine and glucocorticoids and achieved similar graft survival, patient survival, and incidence of acute rejection in the first year. However, sirolimus was associated with a significantly greater incidence of thrombocytopenia (37% compared with 0%), leucopenia (39% compared with 14%), and both herpes simplex infections (24% compared with 10%) and pneumonia (17% compared with 2%). Sirolimus, at least under these conditions, carries a greater risk of infection than CSA for the same degree of immunosuppression. This does not mean that CSA is a superior immunosuppressive drug but that the 'learning curve' for handling sirolimus is in an early stage compared with CSA. However, the sirolimus-induced leucopenia probably contributes to the increase in pneumonic infection and relates to the drug's effect upon proliferating cells.

Serotherapy

The use of antibodies for immunosuppression outside transplantation has been rare until recently. There is still very little indication for the use of serotherapy for renal disease apart from transplantation. Antibodies have a long history of use in transplantation but the benefits have been difficult to establish until the advent of monoclonal antibodies (Mab). The problem before Mab was one of specificity and quality control. Polyclonal

antibodies raised conventionally in horses, sheep, or rabbits have to be extensively purified by absorbing out all the reactivity that is not desired and testing that the desired
specificity is adequate and not lost in the purification process. This makes it a process-
driven product with immunization, absorption, and accurate measurement of the
components in the polyclonal antibody mix crucial to the quality of the final product.
The results with polyclonal antithymocyte (ATG) or antilymphocyte (ALG) antibodies
are difficult to assess historically because 'good' batches of antibody may have produced
effective results while 'poor' batches could produce negative results. Production of Mab
raised in mice or rats changed the quality control aspect of serotherapy since the Mab
have the potential to be as pure as a chemical compound. Most of the Mab of murine or
rat origin, however, proved to be ineffective clinically because of the short duration of
their use in patients. Usually, human antimonoclonal antibody (HAMA) responses
meant that only 2 weeks of therapy was possible before the Mab were eliminated or
neutralized. Genetically engineered Mab produced chimeric or humanized antibodies
that kept the murine variable or antigen-binding region (Fig. 2.8) but replaced the
murine constant regions by human constant regions. Since the murine or rat constant
regions were the main immunogenic component of murine or rat Mab, their elimination
has enabled prolonged use of genetically engineered Mab and this has been associated
with successful clinical use.

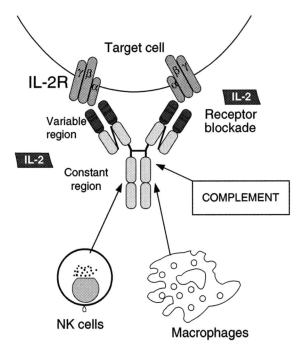

Fig. 2.8 Antibody-mediated immunosuppression. The variable region of the antibody is shown
in dark shading and constitutes the antigen binding site. The constant region is shown in
light shading. Abbreviations: IL-2=interleukin 2; IL-2R=interleukin 2 receptor complex;
NK=natural killer.

Serotherapy with polyclonal antibodies or Mab has its pharmacological effects by either destroying the target cell, blocking an important ligand–receptor binding site, or causing the cell not to migrate to its normal site of action. The means by which cells to which antibodies are attached become destroyed include complement fixation and lysis. There are, however, very potent protective molecules on the surfaces of nucleated cells which prevent our own complement initiating damage (e.g. homologous restriction factor), and it probably plays only a minor role in cell destruction mediated by most antibodies. The predominant mode of cell destruction is antibody-dependent cellular cytotoxicity (Fig. 2.8). Antibody attached to a target cell provides a point to which macrophages or NK cells can bind and under the appropriate conditions lead to death of the target cell. Blocking access of a ligand to its receptor is another important mechanism by which antibodies have an immunosuppressive effect. The example given in Fig. 2.8 is of IL-2 binding to the IL-2R. Lastly, antibodies that bind to adhesion or selectin molecules on the surface of a T cell can interfere with cell binding to endothelial surfaces and lead to inappropriate migration of the cell through the body.

These functions as well as their implications for immunosuppression and infection will be summarized for the commonly used antibodies in renal transplantation.

Antithymocyte or antilymphocyte antibodies

The exact mechanism of action of polyclonal ATG or ALG is unknown. Most preparations used today are T-cell specific and contain a wide range of lymphocyte specificities (e.g. CD4 or T helper, CD8 or cytotoxic T cell, CD45 or leucocyte common antigen). A combination of cell destruction, receptor blockade, and defective migration of the lymphocytes is thought to account for the immunosuppressive effect. Rabbits are the most effective species for raising polyclonal antibodies and the rabbit immunoglobulin constant region binds very well to human Fc receptors (IgG binding receptors on macrophages and NK cells). This suggests that cell killing may play an important part in the immunosuppression. The immunosuppression is not selective and all T cells will be affected including 'memory' T cells for common pathogens. The recommended dosage of most ATG or ALG preparations leads to a prolonged lymphocytopenia. Careful titration of the dose of ATG can avoid this, but in most cases of standard therapy the lymphocytopenia (almost entirely T cells) will last for several months. The consequence is a susceptibility to viral and intracellular infections, and an increase in CMV and PTLD has been described for patients treated with ATG.

Campath-1

Campath-1 is a rat Mab recognizing CD52, a molecule highly expressed on lymphocytes and monocytes. It is a glycoprotein bearing a glycosyl-phosphatidylinositol (GPI) anchor. The function of CD52 is unknown, but its high expression on lymphoid cells (5×10^5 molecules per cell) and its close proximity to the cell membrane have made it a good target for immunosuppression. The original campath-1 was a rat IgM, but selection of mutants allowed several rat IgG forms to be made and subsequently it has been humanized as an human IgG1-bearing Mab. It is one of the very few Mab capable of causing complement-mediated lysis of lymphocytes. The disadvantage of campath-1 is that it is not selectively expressed on lymphocytes but will bind to T cells, B cells, and monocytes. The widespread lysis of lymphocytes is associated with severe systemic symptoms, including fever, rigors, diarrhoea, back pain, and headaches.

Campath-1 has been used extensively in bone marrow transplantation and for a limited number of patients with autoimmune and vasculitic diseases. When it was originally used for solid organ transplantation, it reduced acute rejection episodes but the incidence of infections was so severe that any benefit was lost (Friend *et al.* 1989). Recently, a very short exposure to campath-1 is being assessed with the aim of inducing transplantation tolerance (Calne *et al.* 1998) and it has been used in autoimmune diseases together with a CD4 Mab to try and restore tolerance to autoantigens.

Anti-CD3

OKT3 is a murine Mab that binds the CD3ε chain and causes down-regulation of the T-cell receptor associated with CD3 (Fig. 2.6). This 'blinding' of T cells may contribute to the therapeutic effect of the Mab. OKT3 was the first Mab to be used in human treatment and is effective in reversing transplant rejection. It is similar in efficacy to high-dose methyl prednisolone and can work where glucocorticoids have failed. Unfortunately, its administration is associated with the rapid onset of the 'first-dose effect'. This includes the same symptoms as those described above for campath-1. The excessive use of OKT3 has been blamed for an undue increase in EBV and PTLD (Swinnen *et al.* 1990). However, it is difficult to blame OKT3 alone and once more it is likely to be the total intensity of immunosuppression that contributes to the risk. In series where a very high incidence of PTLD occurred, OKT3 was given together with CSA, while groups that suspended treatment with CSA during OKT3 therapy did not see an increase in PTLD (Cosimi and Rubin 1998).

Anti-CD25

Two genetically engineered Mab that block binding of IL-2 to the IL-2Rα chain have recently been introduced into clinical transplantation. They have both been proven to decrease the risk of transplant rejection episodes during the first year post-transplant (Amlot *et al.* 1995; Vincenti *et al.* 1998; Yabe *et al.* 1994). Figure 2.6 shows the mode of action of these Mab, similar to sirolimus, except that there is no effect upon other signalling pathways not associated with the IL-2/IL-2R pathway. The reduction of acute rejection episodes seen with the use of these Mab given for the first 4 days (basiliximab) and 28 days (daclizumab) with a duration of action lasting from 1 to 3 months was similar to that seen when MMF was given for a year (Mathew *et al.* for the Tricontinental Mycophenolate Mofetil Renal Transplantation Study Group1998). What has been remarkable with these CD25 Mabs is that for an increase in immunosuppression there has not been an increase in infection. For a comparable increase in freedom from rejection, patients treated with MMF had an increase in tissue-invasive CMV. This is the first time that an increase in immunosuppressive effect has not had to pay the price of an increase in infection.

References

Amlot PL, Rawlings E, Fernando ON, Griffin PJ, Heinrich G, Schreier MH, Castaigne JP, Moore R, and Sweny P (1995). Prolonged action of a chimeric IL-2 receptor (CD25) monoclonal antibody used in cadaveric renal transplantation. *Transplantation*, 60: 748–56.

Barnes PJ (1998). Anti-inflammatory actions of glucocorticoids: molecular mechanisms. *Clin Sci*, 94: 557–72.

Berlyne GM and Danovitch GM (1971). Cyclophosphamide for immunosuppression in renal transplantation. *The Lancet*, 2: 924–5.

Butler WT and Rossen RD (1973a). Effects of corticosteroids on immunity in man. I. Decreased serum IgG concentration caused by 3 or 5 days of high doses of methylprednisolone. *J Clin Invest*, 52: 2629–40.

Butler WT and Rossen RD (1973b). Effects of corticosteroids on immunity in man. II. Alterations in serum protein components after methylprednisolone. *Transplant Proc*, 5: 1215–19.

Calne R, Friend P, Moffatt S, Bradley A, Hale G, Firth J, Bradley J, Smith K, and Waldmann H (1998). Prope tolerance, perioperative campath 1H, and low-dose cyclosporin monotherapy in renal allograft recipients [letter]. *The Lancet* 351: 1701–2. (Erratum (1998). *The Lancet*, 352: 408.)

Cosimi AB and Rubin RH (1998). Post-transplantation lymphoproliferative disorder and OKT3. *New Engl J Med*, 324: 1438.

Faulds D, Goa KL, and Benfield P (1993). Cyclosporin. A review of its pharmacodynamic and pharmacokinetic properties, and therapeutic use in immunoregulatory disorders. *Drugs*, 45: 953–1040.

Franklin T.J. and Cook J.M. (1969). The inhibition of nucleic acid synthesis by mycophenolic acid. *Biochem J*, 113: 515–24.

Friend PJ, Hale G, Waldmann H, Gore S, Thiru S, Joysey V, Evans DB, and Calne RY (1989). Campath 1-M—prophylactic use after kidney transplantation. A randomised controlled trial. *Transplantation*, 48: 248–53.

Gaya SB, Rees AJ, Lechler RI, Williams G, and Mason PD (1995). Malignant disease in patients with long-term renal transplants. *Transplantation*, 59: 1705–9.

Giblett ER, Anderson JE, Cohen F, Pollara B, and Meuwissen HJ (1972). Adenosine-deaminase deficiency in two patients with severely impaired cellular immunity. *The Lancet*, 2: 1067–9.

Giordano A and Avantaggiata ML (1999). p300 and CBP: partners for life and death. *J Cell Physiol*, 181: 218–30.

Groth CG, Backman L, Morales JM, Calne R, Kreis H, Lang P, Touraine JL, Claesson K, Campistol JM, Durand D, Wramner L, Brattstrom C, and Charpentier B (1999). Sirolimus (rapamycin)-based therapy in human renal transplantation: similar efficacy and different toxicity compared with cyclosporine. Sirolimus European Renal Transplant Study Group. *Transplantation*, 67: 1036–42.

Haesslein HC, Pierce JC, Lee HM, and Hume DM (1972). Leukopenia and azathioprine management in renal homotransplantation. *Surgery*, 71: 598–604.

Hojo M, Morimoto T, Maluccio M, Asano T, Morimoto K, Lagman M, Shimbo T, and Suthanthiran M (1999). Cyclosporine induces cancer progression by a cell-autonomous mechanism. *Nature*, 397: 530–4.

Kimball JA, Pescovitz MD Book BK, and Norman DJ (1995). Reduced human IgG anti-ATGAM antibody formation in renal transplant recipients receiving mycophenolate mofetil. *Transplantation*, 60: 1379–83.

Leo C and Chen JD (2000). The SRC family of nuclear receptor coactivators. *Gene* **245**: 1–11.

Lynch WS and Roenigk HH, Jr (1977). Mycophenolic acid for psoriasis. *Arch Dermatol*, **113**: 1203–8.

Mathew TH *et al.* for the Tricontinental Mycophenolate Mofetil Renal Transplantation Study Group (1998). A blinded, long-term, randomized multicenter study of mycophenolate mofetil in cadaveric renal transplantation: results at three years. *Transplantation* **65**: 1450–4.

Nagai M, Natsumeda Y, and Weber G (1992). Proliferation-linked regulation of type II IMP dehydrogenase gene in human normal lymphocytes and HL-60 leukemic cells. *Cancer Res*, **52**: 258–61.

Ohlman S, Albertioni F, and Peterson C (1994). Day-to-day variability in azathioprine pharmacokinetics in renal transplant recipients. *Clin Transplant*, **8**: 217–23.

Opelz G and Dohler B (2000). Critical threshold of azathioprine dosage for maintenance immuno-suppression in kidney graft recipients. Collaborative Transplant Study. *Transplantation*, **69**: 818–21.

Plosker GL and Foster RH (2000). Tacrolimus: a further update of its pharmacology and therapeutic use in the management of organ transplantation. *Drugs*, **59**: 323–89.

Rubin R.H. (1993). Infectious disease complications of renal transplantation. *Kidney Int*, **44**: 221–36.

Sehgal SN (1998). Rapamune (RAPA, rapamycin, sirolimus): mechanism of action immuno-suppressive effect results from blockade of signal transduction and inhibition of cell cycle progression. *Clin. Biochem*, **31**: 335–40.

Smith KG, Isbel NM, Catton MG, Leydon JA, Becker GJ, and Walker RG (1998). Suppression of the humoral immune response by mycophenolate mofetil. *Nephrol Dial Transplant*, **13**: 160–4.

Spencer CM, Goa KL, and Gillis JC (1997). Tacrolimus. An update of its pharmacology and clinical efficacy in the management of organ transplantation. *Drugs*, **54**: 925–75.

Swinnen LJ, Costanzo-Nordin MR, Fisher SG, O'Sullivan EJ, Johnson MR, Heroux AL, Dizikes GJ, Pifarre R, and Fisher RI (1990). Increased incidence of lympho-proliferative disorder after immunosuppression with the monoclonal antibody OKT3 in cardiac-transplant patients. *New Engl J Med*, **323**: 1723–8.

Vincenti F, Kirkman R, Light S, Bumgardner G, Pescovitz M, Halloran P, Neylan J, Wilkinson A, Ekberg H, Gaston R, Backman L, and Burdick J (1998). Interleukin-2-receptor blockade with daclizumab to prevent acute rejection in renal transplantation. Daclizumab Triple Therapy Study Group. *New Engl J Med*, **338**: 161–5.

Wassner SJ, Malekzadeh MH, Pennisi AJ, Ettenger RB, Uittenbogaart CH, and Fine RN (1977). Allograft survival in patients receiving anticonvulsant medications. *Clin Nephrol*, **8**: 293–7.

Yabe M, Yabe H, Hattori K, Hinohara T, Morimoto T, Kato S, and Kusunoki A (1994). Transition of T cell receptor gamma/delta expressing double negative (CD4-/CD8-) lymphocytes after allogeneic bone marrow transplantation. *Bone Marrow Transplant*, **14**: 741–6.

3

Peritoneal host defence in patients with end-stage renal failure treated by peritoneal dialysis

Andrew Davenport

Introduction

Peritoneal dialysis, in the form of continuous ambulatory peritoneal dialysis (CAPD), was introduced in 1976 (Popovich *et al.* 1976). In those days CAPD had two major complications: firstly the original dialysis solutions came in glass jars, which made the exchanges time-consuming and difficult to complete, and secondly there was a high rate of peritoneal infection, due to the frequency of exchanges with the consequent disconnection and reconnection of the dialysis circuit. The introduction of plastic bags for the dialysate reduced the frequency of changes in connections, with a resultant decrease in the rate of peritonitis, down to around one episode per patient year (Oreopoulos *et al.* 1978). Infection rates were further reduced with the introduction of the 'Y set' disconnection system, designed by Buoncristiani, during which additional fresh dialysate was used to flush the connecting system (Buoncristiani 1989). These improvements led to the widespread increase in the number of patients with end-stage renal failure (ESRF) treated by CAPD. However, when compared with haemodialysis technique survival is less, and depending upon the centre, most patients fail peritoneal dialysis either due to peritonitis or due to failure to achieve adequate solute and/or water clearance. It may well be that those patients who develop so-called peritoneal membrane failure do so as a consequence of changes in peritoneal host defence.

Normal host defence mechanisms

The normal peritoneal membrane surface comprises a single layer of peritoneal mesothelial cells which have microvilli on their apical surface and lie on a basement membrane. The apical surface is coated by a matrix comprising glycosaminoglycans, such as laminin, vitronectin, and hyaluronan (Fig. 3.1). Underneath the mesothelial cells is a matrix containing type III collagen and glycosaminoglycans, interspersed with fibroblasts, and a network of capillary and lymphatic vessels. In addition there are resident reticuloendothelial cells within the peritoneal membrane. Typically mature macrophages (MØ) and mast cells reside in the submesothelial space (Suassuna *et al.* 1994).

In health the peritoneal cavity contains less than 50 ml of clear fluid with cell yields varying between 7×10^6 and 12×10^6 in 3–15 ml of fluid taken during gynaecological laparoscopy. The typical white blood cell differential comprises some 90% MØ, 5–10%

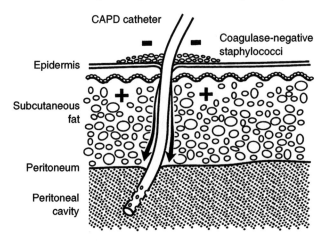

Fig. 3.1 Insertion of a peritoneal dialysis catheter breaks the integrity of the epidermis and sets up an electrical gradient. Negatively charged bacteria which colonize the skin, such as coagulase-negative staphylococci, spread periluminally down alongside the catheter and can create a biofilm on the catheter.

lymphocytes, and less than 5% polymorphonuclear neutrophils (PMN) (Bos *et al*. 1988). In addition to these migrating cells within the peritoneal cavity there are also mature MØ adherent to the peritoneal surface of the peritoneal membrane. The concentration of immunoglobulin G (IgG) and complement protein 3 (C3) in the peritoneal fluid from healthy patients is similar to that found in the plasma. These proteins are important in opsonizing bacteria, so aiding MØ phagocytosis. Patients with chronic liver disease and ascites are reported to have decreased peritoneal protein concentrations. As C3 is important in opsonizing Gram-negative bacteria, this may explain the increased incidence of spontaneous bacterial peritontis observed in patients with ascites due to chronic liver disease (Such *et al*. 1988).

Inflammation is localized, if at all possible, due to the production of fibrinogen, thromboplastin, and other coagulation proteins. Trapping of bacteria prevents dissemination of infection and allows easier MØ phagocytosis. As peritoneal mesothelial cells have a similar embryological derivation to endothelial cells, from mesenchyme, then activation of mesothelial cells, directly by bacterial products or by adherent or migratory intraperitoneal MØ, results in the production of coagulation proteins (Sitter *et al*. 1995).

Inflammation within the peritoneal cavity usually arises due to sepsis of the large bowel or female urogenital tract. If inflammation cannot be localized and controlled by resident MØ and the omentum, then recruitment and transmigration of other proinflammatory cells, typically PMN, occurs. Although MØ can be directly activated by bacteria and bacterial products, cell recruitment and amplification of the inflammatory response usually depends upon T-lymphocyte activation. Both bacteria and MØ are cleared from the peritoneal cavity through the lymphatic system. In animal experiments, bacteria can be recovered from the lymphatics within minutes of intraperitoneal innoculation (Hau *et al*. 1979). Similarly bacteraemia has been reported in up to 30% of cases of bacterial peritonitis.

Host defence during peritoneal dialysis

General effects of uraemia

Patients with ESRF treated by peritoneal dialysis may have underlying defects of both humoral and cellular immunity (Girndt *et al.* 2001). These may be due to the effects of previous or currently prescribed immunosuppressant therapy for those patients with a history of vasculitis, such as Wegener's granulomatosis and systemic lupus erythematosus, bone marrow disorders including myeloma and lymphoma, solid organ malignancy, and those with solid organ transplantation (renal, liver, bone-marrow, and cardiac). This may result in an increased risk of peritonitis (Andrews *et al.* 1998). In addition malnutrition is a well recognized problem in CAPD patients, and is a known risk factor for infection. The immune response is decreased in the elderly, and when CAPD was first introduced it was targeted at the older patient. The combination of poor nutrition and inadequate dialysis, in terms of urea and creatinine clearance (Lemaire *et al.* 2001), is more prevalent in the older patient group, and this will increase the risk of infection (Table 3.1).

As a group, humoral responses, in terms of antibody production following immunization with hepatitis B or tetanus toxoid or the recall response to pneumococcal antigen, is depressed in CAPD patients compared with healthy controls (Beaman *et al.* 1989). Similarly cell-mediated immunity, including lymphocyte (Bonomini *et al.* 1993), MØ, and PMN function is depressed in ESRF (Table 3.2), possibly due to iron overload, zinc deficiency, and increased intracellular calcium concentration (Haag-Weber and Hörl 1993; Massry and Smogorzewski 2001). The general effects of uraemia are discussed in Chapter 1.

Table 3.1 The effect of uraemia and treatment with peritoneal dialysis on general immune function

Chronic renal failure	Malnutrition
	Hyperparathyroidism
	Previous treatment with immunosuppression
Inadequate dialysis	Retention of uraemic toxins (e.g. granulocyte inhibitory protein)
	Increased lymphocyte/leucocyte apoptosis
	Reduced T-lymphocyte costimulatory factors
	Reduced response to non-polysaccharide vaccines
General effects of peritoneal dialysate	Reduced concentration of intraperitoneal opsonins (complement, fibrinogen, fibronectin, and immunoglobulins)
	Immature intraperitoneal macrophages
Potential toxic effects of dialysates	Low pH impairs leucocyte and macrophage function
	Additive effect of low pH and high lactate
	Effect of hypertonic glucose solutions
	Glucose degradation products
	Plasticizers

Table 3.2   The effect of peritoneal dialysis on peripheral blood white blood cells

Blood cell type	Effect of peritoneal dialysis
Polymorphonuclear leucocyte	Increased apoptosis
	Reduced respiratory burst
	Reduced chemotaxis
	Reduced bactericidal killing
Peripheral blood lymphocyte	Increased apoptosis
	Normal CD4/CD8 ratio
	Reduced INF-γ and IL-2 following stimulation
	Increased T_{H1} phenotype rather than T_{H2}
	Reduced B-cell response due to decreased T_{H2}
	Normal total Igs and subclasses
	Non-specific low-titre increase in autoantibodies
Peripheral blood monocyte	Increased immature forms
	Increased T_{H1} activated phenotype

Catheter insertion

Bacterial invasion of the peritoneal cavity in CAPD patients occurs most commonly due to bacteria entering through the internal lumen of the peritoneal dialysis catheter and tubing or entering at the exit site and migrating along the external surface of the catheter (Keane and Vas 1994). To prevent contamination at the time of catheter insertion, prophylactic antibiotics and eradication of the nasal carriage of *Staphylococcus aureus* have been reported to decrease the incidence of exit site infections and secondary peritonitis (Swartz *et al.* 1991). As there is a correlation between exit site sepsis and subsequent peritonitis, it is important that the exit site is carefully made as small as possible and points caudally, so that sloughed cells within the catheter tunnel can pass downwards and out, thus not blocking the tunnel. In addition allowing the catheter wound to heal before using the catheter reduces the risk of leaks and infection.

The insertion of the peritoneal catheter disrupts the integrity of the epidermis, and creates an epidermoperitoneal electrical gradient (Davenport and Dealler 1992). The direction of the electrical gradient created encourages the migration of bacteria with negatively charged surface coats from the skin surface towards the peritoneum (Fig. 3.2). To try to prevent bacterial migration, different insertion techniques have been tried in an attempt to increase the length of the subcutaneous tunnel and so reduce bacterial colonization (Keane and Vas 1994). In recent years the presternal exit site and also burying the catheter for 2 weeks and then creating the exit site some 2 weeks later as a second procedure (Moncrieff and Popovitch 1995) have been advocated to reduce exit site infection. The cuffs around the catheter create areas of fibrosis which may reduce bacterial colonization. Although catheters with two cuffs appear to confer an advantage over those with one cuff, this may reflect the increased length of the subcutaneous tunnel, as three cuffs have not been shown to have any additional effect. In animal experiments the use of a silver-coated cuff was shown to reduce bacterial colonization. This was thought to be due to dissolution of silver which then may have had either a direct antibacterial effect or

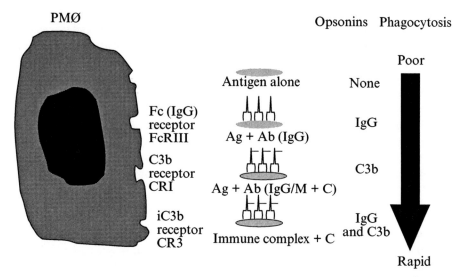

Fig. 3.2 Opsonization of bacteria increases the ability of peritoneal macrophages (PMØ) to phagocytose bacteria. Ag=antigen, Ab=antibody, C=complement, Ig=immunoglobulin.

reduced the electrical gradient. However, in a multicentre prospective trial silver-cuffed peritoneal dialysis catheters were not shown to confer any benefit compared with standard catheters (Pommer *et al.* 1998).

Catheter colonization

Bacteria can adhere to the peritoneal dialysis catheter either directly by forming a biofilm or by adhering to the protein coating formed as part of the host response to a foreign body. Coagulase-negative staphyloccoci and pseudomonads can both produce a biofilm and adhere to peritoneal dialysis catheters. It has been estimated that biofilm is present on 80 to 100% of catheters of non-disconnect CAPD systems (Marine *et al.* 1983), but may be much less in those treated with disconnect systems (Verger *et al.* 1987). Whereas coagulase-negative staphyloccoci are rapidly cleared from the peritoneum when injected directly into the peritoneal cavity of mice, if they are injected through a peritoneal catheter the catheter remains heavily colonized (Gallimore *et al.* 1988). In clinical practice catheters colonized with biofilm coagulase-negative staphyloccoci may result in the development of resistant or relapsing peritonitis, as the biofilm reduces bacterial opsonization by affecting the binding of complement protein (Holmes and Evans 1986).

Disruption or removal of the biofilm by using urokinase or the simultaneous removal of the colonized CAPD catheter and replacement with a new catheter have been advocated to treat both resistant and relapsing peritonitis (Paterson *et al.* 1985).

Bacterial virulence

Several prospective studies have reported that bacteria can be cultured from the spent peritoneal dialysate from healthy CAPD patients (Williams *et al.* 1987). These organisms tend to be of low virulence and often take 2 or more weeks of culture before they can be detected, suggesting that they are only present in very small numbers and therefore do not provoke a response from the host (Keane and Vas 1994). Coagulase-negative staphyloccoci that are sessile and produce a biofilm have a slower growth rate than planktonic organisms, and both grow much slower than *S. aureus* and *Pseudomonas* species. (Glancey *et al.* 1992). Thus simply carrying out three CAPD exchanges could remove as many sessile coagulase-negative staphyloccoci in a day as are produced, so preventing bacterial proliferation and the development of peritonitis. Three or four daily CAPD exchanges did not significantly reduce the number of planktonic coagulase-negative staphyloccoci (Rowe and Miller 1993) or *S. aureus* in the intraperitoneal catheter or cavity, so not inhibiting bacterial proliferation and allowing the development of peritonitis.

Lymphatic removal of bacteria

The lymphatic removal of both phagocytosed bacteria and free bacteria occurs rapidly in previously healthy patients who develop severe intraperitoneal inflammation. Whereas bacteraemia often occurs in these patients, bacteraemia is unusual during CAPD peritonitis. The large volume of dialysate could impair the normal movement of phagocytosed and free bacteria to the lymphatics (Khanna and Mactier 1992). However, it has been estimated that daily lymphatic fluid removal from the peritoneal cavity during peritoneal dialysis is only 5–10% of the total daily peritoneal volume. This may reflect that lymphatic removal does not play a significant role in preventing CAPD peritonitis. Compared with typical intra-abdominal Gram-negative sepsis, CAPD patients usually suffer Gram-positive infections. These have come from skin contamination or a break in technique. The numbers of bacteria and the rapidity of bacterial growth are different, and therefore lymphatic removal may not be as relevant (Holmes 1994). As the number of bacteria may be considerably less during CAPD peritonitis, those which do reach the lymphatics may be taken up in draining lymph nodes so preventing bacteraemia.

Humoral host defence

Opsonization in peritoneal dialysis patients

Compared with healthy patients intraperitoneal IgG concentrations in CAPD patients are reduced from around 12.5 g/litre down to less than 0.5 g/litre (Holmes and Lewis 1991), presumably due to the dilutional effect of the dialysate. The majority of IgG is of subclass 1, whereas IgG2 is the most important immunoglobulin in opsonizing polysaccharide-coated bacteria. In one study children who were deficient in IgG2 were reported to have an increased incidence of CAPD peritonitis (Schroeder *et al.* 1989). The levels of IgG2 in peritoneal dialysate effluent are below the level of detection of current assays. Other opsonins are similarly reduced in peritoneal dialysate effluent; C3 from 800 mg/litre down to less than 30 mg/litre, and dialysate fibronectin to less than 5 mg/litre compared with plasma concentrations of 245 mg/litre. Longitudinal studies have shown that this defect in opsonization remains, and that there is no detectable compensatory increase in immunoglobulin, fibronectin, or specific antistaphylococcal antibody level (Nielsen *et al.* 1992).

In addition, it is now recognized that uraemic patients have increased post-translational modification of plasma proteins, including glycation, carbamylation, and carbamoylation. Thus CAPD patients have been reported to have both increased glycated IgG in their serum and peritoneal dialysate effluent (Davin *et al.* 1997). This is thought to reflect increased glycation of serum IgG, rather than glycation within the peritoneum. However, structural alteration of IgG may affect its ability to opsonize bacteria due to changes in the binding of activated C3 components (Davin *et al.* 1997).

Thus the ability of peritoneal dialysate effluent to opsonize bacteria is reduced (Nielsen *et al.* 1992). However, there is variability both between patients and within individual patients. For example, the longer the exchange period, the greater the ability to opsonize bacteria, which may reflect increased concentrations of IgG, fibronectin, and C3 coupled with a higher pH (Davies *et al.* 1990).

Although opsonization is defective in CAPD patients, the results of studies which have tried to correlate the *in vitro* ability to opsonize bacteria and clinical susceptibility to bacterial peritonitis have produced varying results (Holmes 1994). The majority of studies have suggested an inverse correlation between the ability to opsonize bacteria and the risk of clinical peritonitis (Coles *et al.* 1994). Although the majority of patients who developed peritonitis in one prospective study had peritoneal dialysate effluent concentrations of less than 0.1 g/litre, not all patients with reduced peritoneal IgG developed peritonitis (Coles *et al.* 1987). This may reflect that IgG alone is not the best marker for bacterial opsonization in CAPD patients. Other studies have assessed total opsonization activity, but whereas IgG and fibronectin are important in opsonizing Gram-positive bacteria, activated C3 components are more important for Gram-negative bacteria, and fibrinogen may actively reduce opsonization (Davies *et al.* 1990). In the latter case *S. aureus* induces polymerization of fibrinogen to form fibrin. When organisms are sequestered by fibrin they are more resistant to phagocytosis. *In vitro* experiments have reported that the addition of urokinase, by breaking down fibrin, can increase *S. aureus* opsonization in peritoneal dialysate effluent. As C3 deposition is important for the oxidative burst response of MØ, then this would affect those studies which used optical chemiluminescence to assess bacterial phagocytosis. Thus the methodology used to assess opsonization may have affected the results of the study, and account for the discrepencies reported. In addition, not all phagocytosis requires opsonization. Peritoneal MØ (PMØ) can phagocytose *S. aureus* due to the interaction between MØ surface IgG, so-called cytophilic IgG, and *S. aureus* cell wall protein. Similarly MØ can phagocytose *Escherichia coli* with type I fimbriae due to a direct interaction between specific mannose lectins on the fimbriae and a manosyl/fucosyl receptor on the MØ surface. Other interactions, known as leptinophagocytosis (Boner *et al.* 1989), have been reported between bacterial lectins and MØ surface lectin receptors including CR3, p150,95, and LFA-1 and lipopolysaccharide and β-glucans present in bacterial outer cell walls. The fact that MØ bacterial phagocytosis can occur without conventional osponiza-tion, and that intraperitoneal concentrations of IgG, complement proteins, fibronectin, and antistaphyloccal antibodies vary markedly not only between patients but also within the same patient (Nielsen *et al.* 1992), probably accounts for the failure of prospective studies to demonstrate a relationship between peritoneal opsonization and clinical peritonitis (Anwar *et al.* 1996).

Two uncontrolled trials of administering immunoglobulin intraperitoneally, using different doses and frequency of administration, reported a reduction in the incidence of peritonitis in two groups of adult CAPD patients with a very high frequency of peritonitis (Lamperi and Carozzi 1986; Keane *et al.* 1988). Subsequent studies noted that the majority of intraperitoneal immunoglobulin was recovered in the subsequent peritoneal dialysis exchanges, and this has cast doubt on the success of administration of intraperitoneal immunoglobulin (Glancey *et al.* 1990). However, this may be of benefit in children, who have been reported to have reduced total intraperitoneal IgG and/or subclass IgG2 compared with adult CAPD patients (Bouts *et al.* 2000).

Cellular peritoneal defence mechanisms

Whereas peritoneal white blood cell populations are relatively constant in normal healthy patients, with MØ predominanting (90%), and smaller numbers of lymphocytes (5–10%), and less than 5% PMN, this is not the case for stable peritoneal dialysis patients (Table 3.3). There is a great variation between patients, with MØ ranging from 20 to 95%, lymphocytes 2 to 84% and PMN from 0 to 27% (Lewis and Holmes 1991). Others have reported up to 6% of the peritoneal dialysate effluent cell population to comprise dendritic cells (Betjes *et al.* 1993). Although there is marked interpatient variability in terms of peritoneal cell populations, in general for individual patients the cell counts remain relatively stable over time on peritoneal dialysis (Betjes *et al.* 1993).

Peritoneal macrophages (PMØ)

Resident PMØ account for 90% of PMØ in the normal unstimulated peritoneal cavity, whereas during peritoneal dialysis immature PMØ predominate (Betjes *et al.* 1993). These immature PMØ have transmigrated from the peritoneal capillaries across the peritoneal membrane into the peritoneal cavity. Transmigration of monocytes into the peritoneal cavity parallels the selective up-regulation of the functional receptors CD11b/CD18, CD11c/CD18, HLA-DR, and ICAM-1 (Scherberich and Nockher 2000). It must be remembered that peritoneal dialysis patients have an increased number

Table 3.3   Effect of peritoneal dialysis on intraperitoneal white blood cells

Blood cell type	Effect of peritoneal dialysis
Peritoneal macrophage	Increased immature forms Normal/reduced bactericidal activity Increased T_{H1} phenotype
Peritoneal lymphocytes	Normal/reduced cell population Increased activated cell phenotype T_{H2} preponderance Reduced NK cell population Increased B cells, but reduced responsiveness
Peritoneal polymorphonuclear leucocytes	Reduced chemotaxis Reduced respiratory burst Reduced bactericidal activity

of activated, proinflammatory peripheral blood monocytes bearing the CD16 phenotype compared with regular haemodialysis patients (Jedlicka *et al.* 1998). Unlike the resident macrophages, which having transformed from circulating monocytes remain within the peritoneum, these inflammatory macrophages are either removed during peritoneal exchanges or return through the peritoneal lymphatics to draining lymph nodes. It has been estimated that each day between 3 and 4×10^7 PMØ are lost in the dialysate effluent (Goldstein *et al.* 1984). This continued loss of PMØ is thought to stimulate the bone marrow to increase monocyte production with the release of immature monocytes into the circulation (McGregor *et al.* 1996). Although PMØ cell surface expression shows an immature cell with reduced CD11c and increased transferrin receptor expression, and loss of intracellular peroxidase staining, PMØ cell phenotypes are similar to those found in women undergoing laparoscopic sterilization and peripheral blood monocytes (Betjes *et al.* 1993). Thus there was no difference in HLA class I or II, CD22, CD2, CD14, or CD68 surface expression.

The *in vitro* phagocytic capacity of PMØ from CAPD patients recovered from the dialysate effluent of the overnight dwell is similar to that of normal PMØ and PMN (Goldstein *et al.* 1984). However, the number of PMØ in the overnight dialysate effluent is greatest, the PMØ having been exposed for many hours to a stable and normal dialysate pH with relatively low glucose and lactate concentrations. At other times, these osmotic, pH, and lactate conditions may not be as favourable and may affect PMØ function.

Similarly most studies have reported that the bactericidal ability of PMØ is normal compared with PMN, normal PMØ, and peripheral blood monocytes (Goldstein *et al.* 1984), although some investigators have reported a decreased bactericidal capacity (McGregor *et al.* 1987). Several groups have reported a difference in PMØ phagocytic and bactericidal activity in those patients with a high rate of CAPD peritonitis compared with those with no or infrequent peritonitis (Lamperi and Carozzi 1986b; Lin *et al.* 1988; Davies *et al.* 1989). Some studies have not been able to show any correlation between intracellular killing and the frequency of peritonitis (McGregor *et al.* 1987). These studies were cross sectional rather than prospective and longitudinal, and therefore it is difficult to be sure that these defects in PMØ bactericidal activity were the primary underlying cause of the increased incidence of peritonitis observed, or were a consequence of repeated episodes of peritonitis. Longitudinal studies which have prospectively assessed PMØ activity have recorded a progressive decrease in both phagocytic and bactericidal activity over the first year of CAPD (McGregor *et al.* 1992; Lin *et al.* 1990).

Oxidative metabolism of PMØ, assessed by luminol- or lucigenin–enhanced chemiluminescence or hydrogen peroxide generation, has been reported to be normal by most investigators (Goldstein *et al.* 1984), but others have reported it to be increased (Lewis and Norris 1990) or decreased (Lamperi and Carozzi 1986). Most groups noted that the chemiluminescent response of PMØ was intact, but the oxidative burst was similar to that of activated cells. Chemiluminescence was reported to be decreased in those CAPD patients with high a frequency of peritonitis (Davies *et al.* 1989), but whether this was the cause of increased susceptibility to frequent infection or a consequence of peritonitis could not be established.

PMØ surface receptor expression suggests increased cell activation with increased C5a (Lewis and Norris 1990) and Fc receptor expression (Lewis and Holmes 1991), but with normal complement receptors (CR1 and CR3). Constitutive cytokine secretion by PMØ, including TNF-α and IL-6, was reported to increase with time on CAPD, and was greater than that of peripheral monocytes (McGregor *et al.* 1996). However, when cells were stimulated, then the response to lipopolysaccharide was much greater from the peripheral blood monoctyes than the PMØ, but there was no apparent change in response to stimulation with time on CAPD. There was no significant change in constitutive prostanoid secretion by PMØ with time on CAPD (McGregor *et al.* 1996).

Clinical studies have shown that PMØ can be increased by the intraperitoneal administration of granulocyte–macrophage colony-stimulating factor. This effect is only short term, with the increase in intraperitoneal MØ lasting less than 3 days after the last injection (Selgas *et al.* 1996). However, the phagocytic index of the infiltrating PMØ was also increased, showing that these cells were functional. More importantly there were only minimal changes in inflammatory mediators, with an increase in spent peritoneal dialysate effluent interleukin 6 (IL-6) and monocyte chemotactic protein 1 (MCP-1), whereas there was no increase in TNF-α, IL-1, IL-8, monocyte inhibitory protein (MIP-1α), and regulated-upon-activation normal T-cell expressed and presumably secreted protein (RANTES).

Thus PMØ show increased immaturity yet up-regulation, suggesting increased cellular activation. The decrease in peritoneal cell number and chemotactic activity during the first year of CAPD implies adaptation to the chronic stimulus of the dialysate.

Peritoneal lymphocytes

Whereas the normal peritoneal lymphocyte population is approximately 5–10% of the white blood cells, the percentage varies in CAPD patients with a reported range of 2–84% (Goldstein *et al.* 1984), with mean ranges of 20–30% (Lewis *et al.* 1992). Lymphocytes can be subdivided into T and B cells, and then T cells subdivided into T helper cells (CD4), suppressor cells (CD8), and natural killer cells (NK). T helper cells can be further separated into the T_{H1} phenotype, which secrete IL-2 and interferon-γ, and the T_{H2} phenotype, which secrete IL-4, 5, and 10. The T_{H1} phenotype is associated with increased cytotoxic cell activation, leading to increased secretion of proinflammatory cytokines secretion such as TNF-α; the T_{H2} phenotype is associated with delayed type hypersensitivity reactions.

Previous studies on peritoneal lymphocyte populations in CAPD patients have suggested a normal or reduced total T-lymphocyte population, with a reduction in CD4 cells with an increase in CD8 (Lewis *et al.* 1993). Other investigators have reported an excess of CD4 compared with CD8, with in some cases a 10-fold excess (Betjes *et al.* 1993). An increase in NK cells has been observed in adults (Lewis *et al.* 1993), although a more recent study reported a decrease in NK cell populations in children (Bouts *et al.* 2000). Most investigators have reported an increase in activated T cells, with increased HLA class II expression (Davies 1990). As IL-2 production and IL-2 receptor expression appeared to be down-regulated (Davies 1990), this would suggest that in stable CAPD patients the balance of T_H phenotype had swung to the T_{H2} phenotype; this is supported by more recent work (Fricke *et al.* 1996). This would suggest adaptation to a chronic inflammatory stimulus. However, there does appear to be a marked interpatient variability, and this may reflect individual differences in terms of immunophenotyping, and the response to peritoneal dialysate (Fig. 3.3).

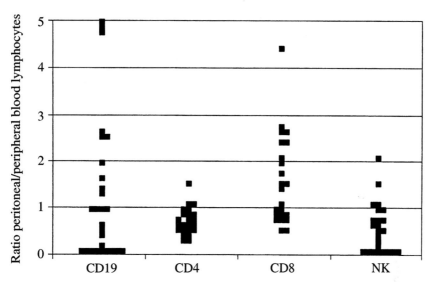

Fig. 3.3 Comparison of the peritoneal lymphocyte population, obtained from spent peritoneal dialysate, and peripheral blood lymphocytes, in a series of 24 adult CAPD patients who have never experienced peritonitis, to show marked interpatient variability. Key: CD19=B cells, CD4= T helper cells, CD8=T suppressor cells, NK=natural killer cells. Results are expressed as a percentage of the total lymphocyte population.

Intraperitoneal B-cell populations have been reported to be increased in the majority of adult studies (Davies *et al.* 1989; Betjes *et al.* 1993), or normal in the minority. However, there has be no observed increase in B-cell function, and when stimulated *in vitro* the response to mitogen was down-regulated (Davies 1990). B-cell populations have been reported to be reduced in children on peritoneal dialysis, in keeping with reports of reduced intraperitoneal Ig (Bouts 2000).

Longitudinal studies on peritoneal lymphocyte populations have suggested that although there is considerable variation for any individual patient, they are stable for any single individual (Betjes *et al.* 1993). As lymphocytes play a crucial response in orchestrating the immune response, it may be that imbalance in lymphocte T_H phenotypes could either lead to a predisposition to increased inflammation within the peritoneal cavity and consequent failure of CAPD due to damage to the peritoneal membrane, or conversely an increased risk of peritonitis. Most published studies to date were carried out before sophisticated T-lymphocyte typing was available. However, there are reports suggesting that an excess of the T_{H2} phenotype and a reduction in T_{H1} phenotype is associated with an increased risk of peritonitis (Lamperi and Carozzi 1988; Bouts *et al.* 2000).

Peritoneal neutrophils

The number of PMN in the peritoneal effluent in CAPD patients is usually very low, with estimates of 0–27% (Lewis and Holmes 1991), this compares with less than 5% in the normal healthy peritoneal cavity. During episodes of peritonitis, there is an early and marked influx of PMN into the peritoneal cavity. At times there are increases in numbers of peritoneal PMN, but not associated with clinical peritonitis. This may be due to a local influx due to a localized area of inflammation, with resolution. PMN are short-lived cells and either die or undergo apoptosis and are then removed by both PMØ and mesothelial cells.

In one study PMN taken from CAPD patients with peritonitis showed reduced phagocytosis when exposed to coagulase-negative staphylococci *in vitro* with spent peritoneal dialysate effluent (Harvey *et al.* 1988). This defect in phagocytosis was corrected following the addition of serum. In addition bacterial killing was normal for *Candida* spp., but impaired for coagulase-negative staphylococci. Although this may suggest impaired PMN function during an episode of peritonitis, it may equally reflect PMN activation and then the use of effete cells in the *in vitro* experiments.

Peritoneal mast cells

Mast cells are present in the submesothelial matrix. Their role in peritoneal host defence, in both the normal peritoneum and that of the CAPD patient, has yet to be elucidated.

Peritoneal mesothelial cells

Peritoneal mesothelial cells line the peritoneal cavity. In the healthy non-uraemic peritoneum these cells are involved in lubrication, allowing free movement of the intraperitoneal contents and preventing adhesions, by secreting phospholipids such as phosphatidylcholine (Betjes *et al.* 1991), and fibrinolytics (Sitter *et al.* 1995). In addition peritoneal mesothelial cells can produce vasodilatory prostanoids and thus may play a role in the local regulation of peritoneal capillary blood flow and capillary permeability (Stylianou *et al.* 1990). As inflammatory cells have to transmigrate from the peritoneal capillaries, pass through matrix, and then cross the peritoneal mesothelial monolayer (Topley *et al.* 1996), more recent studies have shown that when activated peritoneal mesothelial cells are capable of producing specific chemotactic factors, in both a direction- and time-dependent manner for PMN, peritoneal lymphocytes, and MØ (Li *et al.* 1998), designed to recruit inflammatory cells into the peritoneal cavity.

Studies of the effects of peritoneal dialysis on the peritoneal mesothelial cells have shown changes in cell structure and function with time on CAPD. The number of cell surface microvilli declines with time on CAPD and cell density increases, resulting in an increase in the length of the cellular junctions (Dobbie 1994). Similarly peritoneal mesothelial cells shed into the peritoneal dialysate show changes in terms of an increase in cell size with abnormal nuclear morphology. Phosphatidylcholine and other phospholipid secretion decreases during the first 6 months of CAPD and stabilizes at a lower level, and this correlates with decreased pinocytic vesicles and lamellar bodies within the peritoneal mesothelial cells (Betjes *et al.* 1991). Basement membrane reduplication occurs with time on CAPD, with loss of the superficial capillaries and the development of localized areas of inflammation within the deeper matrix (Dobbie 1994).

The normal peritoneal mesothelial cell is covered with a negatively charged glycocalyx. Although bacteria have both anionic and cationic sites in their outer walls, there is a net negative charge due to the glycoproteins. Thus a negatively charged surface glycocalyx would help prevent baceterial adherence and so help to prevent infection. For bacteria to proliferate and cause peritonitis they must adhere to a surface such as the peritoneal dialysis catheter or the peritoneal surface. Damage to the glycocalyx, or underlying peritoneal mesothelial cells, or a change in bacterial cationic charge would enhance bacterial adherence and colonization. *In vitro S. aureus* adheres to peritoneal mesothelial cells (Muijsken *et al.* 1991), whereas coagulase-negative staphylococci do not. This is due to specific interaction of the bacterial cell wall with the glycocalyx, due to both protein A and lipoteichoic acid (Teti *et al.* 1987). This difference in adherence may result in the difference in clinical severity of the subsequent peritonitis episode.

Peritoneal mesothelial cells are attached to their underlying basement membrane, a poorly defined basal lamina of type IV collagen and fibronectin (Topley and Williams 1994), through a series of receptors for extracellular matrix components (Leavesley *et al.* 1999). During episodes of peritonitis, areas of the peritoneum are denuded. Thus for successful repair to occur proliferation of peritoneal mesothelial cells and cell migration are both required. It is unknown whether all peritoneal mesothelial cells have the ability to proliferate, or whether there are a group of stem cells from which all new cells arise. The fact that peritoneal mesothelial cells can be successfully cultured from spent peritoneal dialysate effluent would suggest the former, as it would be unusual to shed stem cells into the peritoneal cavity. *In vitro* peritoneal mesothelial cells migrate towards extracellular components, fastest towards fibronectin, slower for vitronectin, collagen type IV, collagen type I, and slowest for laminin (Leavesley *et al.* 1999).

Peritoneal fibroblasts

Within the stroma of the peritoneal membrane are interspersed peritoneal fibroblasts. Fibroblasts contribute to extracellular matrix remodelling and thus may affect the long-term function of the peritoneal membrane by increasing matrix production. When stimulated *in vitro*, peritoneal fibroblasts are capable of producing proinflammatory cytokines (Topley and Williams 1994). Whether they play an active role in the inflammatory response remains to be determined.

The effect of peritoneal dialysis on peripheral blood cell–mediated and humoral immunity

The continued loss of MØ into the peritoneal dialysate effluent leads to increased marrow monocyte production and the release of immature monocytes into the peripheral blood. More recent studies have suggested that peripheral blood monocytes taken from healthy peritoneal dialysis patients show an activated phenotype (Libetta *et al.* 1996). Similarly *in vitro* experiments have reported that baseline proinflammatory cytokine synthesis is increased. However, depending upon the stimulus, MØ production of hydrogen peroxide or free oxygen radicals is reduced in CAPD patients (Coles *et al.* 1996). Phenotyping of peripheral blood lymphocytes has shown normal numbers of T helper and suppressor cells, but increased numbers of both NK cells, and activated T lymphocytes (Lewis *et al.* 1992). This implies that peritoneal dialysis causes a low-grade systemic inflammatory response (Libetta *et al.* 1996), similar to that reported in haemodialysis patients.

Despite continual losses of immunoglobulin and complement proteins in the peritoneal dialysate effluent, most patients maintain normal serum concentrations of IgG, C3, and C4 (Chan *et al.* 1988). Similarly, numbers of B lymphocytes in the peripheral blood are comparable with those in healthy controls (Lewis *et al.* 1993). T-lymphocyte subsets in terms of the number of peripheral CD4+ and CD8+ cells have been shown not to differ from healthy controls, and there is no change with time on CAPD. However, the number of activated T cells is increased, as are the proportion of NK cells. Lymphocyte IL-2 production is decreased (Lewis *et al.* 1993), suggesting a possible switch to a T_{H2} subtype, in keeping with adaptation to a chronic inflammatory condition.

Peripheral blood PMN from peritoneal dialysis patients have been reported to have decreased chemotactic response to the anaphylotoxin C5a, which may be due to a reduction in C5a receptors, and also to other potent chemoattractants such as the bacterial tripeptide f-Met–Leu–Phe (fMLP). Similarly, the observed oxidative response to C5a and fMLP was reduced compared with PMN from healthy subjects (Lewis *et al.* 1988). This is supported by other work which showed decreased peripheral blood PMN phagocytosis and bactericidal activity in uninfected healthy CAPD patients (Harvey *et al.* 1988). However, when the experiments were repeated using peripheral PMN from CAPD patients with peritonitis, then both phagocytosis and bactericidal activity had returned to normal.

The effect of dialysate on host defence

Fresh dialysate

Current commercially available dialysates are acidic (pH 5.2), hyperosmolar (1.5% dextrose solution has an osmolality of 326 mosmol/kg, and 4.25% an osmolality of 483 mosmol/kg), and hyperlactataemic (35–40 mmol/litre of either L-lactate or a racemic mixture of D- and L-lactate). The initial effects of instillation of dialysate are to dilute the normal host defence mechanisms of opsonins and intraperitoneal MØ. This initial dilutional effect decreases PMØ to concentrations between 10^4 and 10^5/ml. *In vitro* experiments have suggested that there is a critical concentration of PMØ needed to prevent the growth of Gram-positive bacteria in spent peritoneal dialysate effluent of more than 5×10^5/ml (Verbrugh *et al.* 1984), with greater numbers required to prevent the growth of Gram-negative bacteria (Sheth *et al.* 1986).

Not surprisingly, fresh dialysate is toxic to PMN, PMØ, lymphocytes, and peritoneal mesothelial cells. The effect on phagocytic cells is greater for PMN than PMØ, and with longer incubation times there is loss of cell viability (Liberek *et al.* 1993). Even short incubation times of as little as 15 min, result in significant loss of cell function, in terms of depressed phagocytosis, respiratory burst, and intracellular bactericidal activity (Holmes 1994). In addition PMN adhesion is decreased, and so is leucocyte adhesion receptor expression (Kaupke *et al.* 1996). When fresh peritoneal dialysis solution is drained into the peritoneum, the intraperitoneal pH increases rapidly and equilibrates to 7.0, within 30 min. However, clinical studies have shown that if PMØ are recovered 30 min after instillation they still exhibit decreased phagocytic and bactericidal capacity when compared with those recovered when a dialysate of pH 7.0 is used (DeFitjer *et al.*

1993). Thus the main adverse effect of fresh peritoneal dialysis fluid is the development of intracellular acidosis (Liberek *et al.* 1993), and this affects both phagocytic cells and peritoneal mesothelial cells.

Osmolality and glucose

Both the high osmolality and the increased glucose content of dialysate solutions have been independently shown to impair function of PMN and PMØ (Liberek *et al.* 1993). Whereas pH normalizes within 30 min, at the end of a standard 4-h dwell, the dialysate effluent, even if only a 1.5% dextrose solution was used, will be hypertonic compared with serum. Exposure of PMN and PMØ to hypertonic glucose solutions shows that PMN are more susceptible, as shown by greater apoptosis and decreased phagocytic index (Cendoroglo *et al.* 1997). In addition adhesion of PMN is reduced *in vitro*. This effect appears to be secondary to decreased expression of integrin receptor, with reduced PMN surface expression of CD11b, CD18, and CD14, and occurs with both high-glucose dialysates and also hyperosmolar dialysates (Kaupke *et al.* 1996). Exposure to peritoneal dialysis fluids also results in changes to the vascular endothelium with increased vascular permeability and local nitric oxide production (Combet *et al.* 2000).

Similarly, in *in vivo* animal experiments hypertonic glucose also results in changes in peritoneal mesothelial cells characterized by increased cell volume and reduced density (Wajsbrot *et al.* 1998). This is due to compensatory changes within the peritoneal mesothelial cell designed to increase intracellular osmolality by synthesizing the organic osmolytes myoinositol and sorbitol (Matsuoka *et al.* 1999).

More recently, alternative dialysis solutions, which are iso–osmolar or marginally hypertonic and based on glucose polymer and/or amino acids, have been developed. *In vitro* experiments have suggested that these newer fluids have either equal or improved bioincompatibility when compared with the standard lactate-based 1.5% dextrose dialysate (Plum *et al.* 1998). For example, PMØ cell metabolism was much improved when cultured with glucose polymer compared with standard 1.5% dextrose/lactate fluid, with a significant reduction in the number of necrotic cells (Plum *et al.* 1997).

Bicarbonate versus lactate as the anionic buffer

Initially peritoneal dialysates contained lactate or acetate as the anionic base. Acetate was withdrawn due to a possible link with the development of sclerosing peritonitis. Lactate was originally a racemic mixture of the D and L isomers. D–lactate metabolism is delayed in humans, and is metabolized by muscle. L–lactate, the natural form of lactate, is converted indirectly mainly in the liver through to bicarbonate. If the rate of lactate administration exceeds the metabolic rate then lactate accumulation, or hyperlactataemia, occurs. This is associated with an increase in intracellular lactate concentration. *In vitro* testing has shown that lactate-based dialysate, by increasing intracellular lactate concentrations, can decrease both PMN and PMØ function, especially when accompanied by intracellular acidosis (Liberek *et al.* 1993). With the development of bicarbonate-based dialysate solutions, *in vitro* testing has shown that intracellular PMØ metabolism is significantly better with bicarbonate-based fluids than lactate at pH 7.5, which is substantially better than lactate at pH 5.5 (Plum *et al.* 1998). Similarly, incubation with these fluids showed a stepwise increase in the number of apoptotic and necrotic cells when exposed to bicarbonate, pH neutralized lactate, and standard lactate-based glucose dialysate (Plum *et al.* 1988). Whether the improved phagocytic function observed in *in vitro* experiments, in terms of bacterial phagocytosis and intracellular killing (Topley *et al.* 1996), will further reduce the incidence of peritonitis in clinical practice has yet to be determined.

Calcium concentration

Macrophages have vitamin D receptors and respond to changes in the extracellular calcium concentration. Earlier studies reported that PMØ clearance of coagulase-negative staphylococci was reduced when PMØ were cultured in lower calcium concentrations. When lower calcium dialysate solutions (1.25 mmol/litre compared with 1.75 mmol/litre in standard solutions) were introduced, there was concern that this would lead to increased peritonitis rates due to impaired PMØ function, and early reports did suggest an increased frequency of peritonitis (Piraino *et al.* 1992). Although further studies have shown that the complement-mediated uptake of bacteria by PMØ is calcium dependent, antibody-dependent uptake of coagulase-negative staphylococci is not (deFitjer *et al.* 1996). However at the calcium concentrations used in the commercially available solutions there was no detrimental effect on either PMØ or peritoneal mesothelial cell responses (deFitjer *et al.* 1996). Later clinical studies have not confirmed that the calcium concentration of the dialysate affects peritonitis rates (Keane and Vas 1994).

Toxic compounds in the peritoneal dialysate

Heat sterilization of glucose-based dialysate solutions results in the formation of glucose degradation products, which include acetaldehyde, formaldehyde, methylglyoxal, 2-furaldehyde, and 5-hydroxymethylfurfural. These compounds are increased in the higher-glucose solutions. Laboratory experiments have shown that filter-sterilized dialysate solutions (free of glucose degradation products) are more biocompatible than standard solutions (Sundaram *et al.* 1997). Some of the earlier negative effects on PMN and PMØ function attributed to the combination of hyperosmolar glucose, lactate, and low pH, may in retrospect have been exacerbated by these glucose degradation products (Sundaram *et al.* 1997). These glucose degradation products also adversely affect mesothelial cell function *in vitro*, by reducing cell proliferation and IL-6 production following stimulation with IL-1β, and so could potentially affect the role of the mesothelial cell in response to intraperitoneal inflammation (Witowski *et al.* 2000). As yet, filter-sterilized dialysate is not universally available, and therefore there are no long-term clinical trials to determine whether improved host defence due to improved dialysate biocompatibility will result in a reduced frequency of peritonitis.

When plastics were first developed, a plasticizer was required to give the polymer flexibility. The plasticizer is not chemically bound to the polypropylene polymer and can therefore be leached out. During each peritoneal dialysis exchange some of the plasticizer is washed from the plastic bag and lines into the peritoneal cavity. 2-diethylhexylphthalate (2DEHP) is the commonest plasticizer used, and is taken up by PMØ. *In vitro* studies suggest that 2DEHP can have an adverse effect on both PMN and PMØ and also peritoneal mesothelial cells and fibroblasts (Stabellini *et al.* 1998). Several of the major manufacturers of peritoneal dialysate now make plasticizer-free bags and lines.

The effect of different peritoneal dialysis prescriptions

The introduction of overnight intermittent peritoneal dialysis was associated with a decreased incidence of peritonitis (Holley *et al.* 1990). This suggested that the effect of different dwell cycles and no daytime exchanges may have a significant effect on improving intraperitoneal host defence mechanisms. Studies in patients treated by standard Y-set CAPD and continuous cyclic peritoneal dialysis showed that when dwell-times were equal, then there were no differences in MØ function or effluent opsonic activity (deFitjer *et al.* 1992). However, when dwell-times were extended, then there was an increase in both MØ function and opsonic activity. MØ taken from peritoneal dialysate effluent from patients undergoing tidal peritoneal dialysis were more effective in phagocytosing *E. coli in vitro* than those taken from continuous cyclic peritoneal dialysis (deFitjer *et al.* 1994). However, there were no differences between the treatments in terms of the peritoneal concentrations of IgG and complement and peritoneal losses. Similarly opsonization, phagocytosis, and intracellular killing of coagulase-negative staphylococci were no different.

Response to inflammation within the peritoneum

Control and resolution of acute inflammation within the peritoneal cavity depends upon a series of linked events, from infection, activation of the resident cells, amplification of the inflammatory signal, recruitment of inflammatory cells, transmigration to the site of infection, followed by destruction of the infective agent and resolution of the inflammation.

Infection

The majority of peritoneal dialysis catheters are colonized by sessile coagulase-negative staphylococci which produce a biofilm around the catheter. Under normal conditions this does not lead to infection, as presumably there is a balance between bacterial virulence and host defence mechanisms and peritoneal lavage, which not only affects host defence but also removes bacteria and bacterial products (Glancey *et al.* 1992). For infection to occur there has to be either a breakdown of host defence mechanisms or an invasion of more virulent bacteria into the peritoneal cavity. Bacteria then have to adhere to the glycocalyx of peritoneal mesothelial cells and replicate.

Activation of peritoneal resident cells

The PMØ is the primary host defence cell. In the peritoneal cavity in CAPD patients the absolute concentration is reduced in the non-infected state to a level below that which can control Gram-positive bacteria *in vitro*. The number of free-floating PMØ and the low number of bacteria suggests that chance meeting and subsequent phagocytosis could not

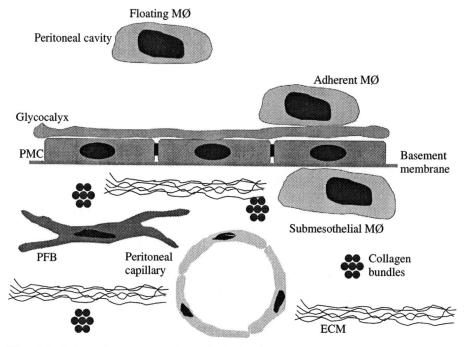

Fig. 3.4 Schematic representation of the peritoneal membrane. MØ=macrophage, PMC=peritoneal mesothelial cell, PFB=peritoneal fibroblast, ECM=extracellular matrix.

be a major defence mechanism. As staphylococci adhere to peritoneal mesothelial cells, it is more likely that PMØ adherent to the peritoneal mesothelium come into contact with adherent bacteria and so become activated (Topley and Williams 1996). Although electron microscopy studies have failed to identify such MØ, this is most likely due to difficulty in obtaining tissue samples, as the mesothelial layer is easily disrupted during biopsy procedures. Other MØ which could be involved in the initial inflammatory process are those in the submesothelial layer (Suassuna *et al.* 1994). PMØ in CAPD patients are less mature and in a state of activation compared with resident PMØ. When these PMØ come into contact with bacteria adherent to the peritoneal membrane, they become further activated, secreting a series of proinflammatory cytokines (including IL-1β, TNF-α, IL-6), and chemotactic factors (leukotriene B_4 and IL-8) (Fig. 3.4). Depending upon the particular bacteria, phagocytosis may occur depending or not on the presence of opsonins.

Amplification of the inflammatory signal

The number of PMØ is relatively low, and this raises the question as to whether other cell populations may be involved in the amplification of the inflammatory process. Peritoneal mesothelial cells cover the surface of the peritoneal cavity. These cells come into direct contact with both invading bacteria and PMØ. Both bacteria, by direct contact and by releasing bacterial products, and activated PMØ can cause direct activation of peritoneal mesothelial cells (Topley *et al.* 1996). Following activation of peritoneal mesothelial cells with IL-1β and TNF-α from PMØ, peritoneal mesothelial cells become capable of producing and secreting vasodilatory prostanoids and nitric oxide (Stylianou *et al.* 1990), which increase local capillary blood supply. This increases the number of leucocytes flowing through the local capillaries, and by increasing capillary permeability allows more plasma proteins, including immunoglobulins and other potential opsonins, to diffuse into the peritoneal cavity. Indeed the characteristic changes in peritoneal permeability to albumin and other large-molecular-weight proteins is related to the magnitude of the leucocyte infiltration (Luo *et al.* 2000). Peritoneal mesothelial cells also produce increased fibrinogen and vitronectin, which may both limit bacterial spread and aid engulfment by phagocytes (Sitter *et al.* 1995). In addition, peritoneal mesothelial cells play a key role in attracting inflammatory cells into the peritoneal cavity by secreting chemoattractant factors in a specific directional fashion, including IL-8 to recruit PMN, RANTES for lymphocytes, and MCP-1 for MØ (Li *et al.* 1998). Peritoneal mesothelial cells are also capable of expressing class II HLA-DR, and phagocytosing staphylococci. By up-regulating class II expression and secreting IL-6 and prostacyclin, this increases both adherent and free-floating peritoneal MØ. Thus the initial signal from the small number of PMØ is amplified by the large number of peritoneal mesothelial cells (Fig. 3.5).

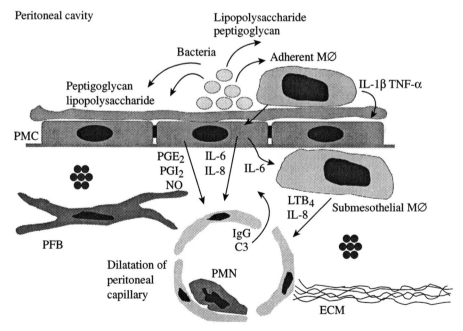

Fig. 3.5 Infection results in activation of macrophages (MØ), and peritoneal mesothelial cells (PMC), with the release of proinflammatory cytokines (IL-1β, TNF-α from MØ, and IL-6 from both PMC and MØ), prostanoids (prostaglandin E and prostacyclin), nitric oxide (NO) and chemoattractants (leukotriene B$_4$ and IL-8) which cause endothelial activation and increased local capillary blood flow and permeability.

Recruitment of inflammatory cells

During CAPD peritonitis there is an intial influx of PMN into the peritoneal cavity followed later by lymphocytes and MØ. Peritoneal mesothelial activation results in increased local capillary blood flow and endothelial activation. This leads to increased leucocyte rolling, changes in the actin cytoskeleton, and shedding of P selectin, thus allowing contact with the activated endothelium and starting the process of transmigration through the peritoneal capillary, with opening up of CD31 junctions between the endothelial cells (Adams and Shaw 1994). Once in the submesothelial matrix, PMN, lymphocytes, and MØ migrate towards the surface mesothelial monolayer, due to a chemoattractant concentration gradient (Li *et al.* 1988). PMN are recruited along an IL-8 gradient, and adhesion to peritoneal mesothelial cells is ICAM-1 dependent. PMN migrate across mesothelial monolayers readily, due to opening up of the intercellular tight junctions (Topley *et al.* 1996). Similarly lymphocytes are recruited along a RANTES gradient and MØ with MCP-1 (Li *et al.* 1988). As the gradients of these chemoattractants are present in both the submesothelial matrix and also in the glycocalyx of the outer peritoneal surface, there is a continued gradient driving these inflammatory cells into the peritoneal cavity (Fig. 3.6). For example MØ transmigration can be blocked by antibodies to MCP-1 added to the apical surface of peritoneal mesothelial cell monolayers (Li *et al.* 1988).

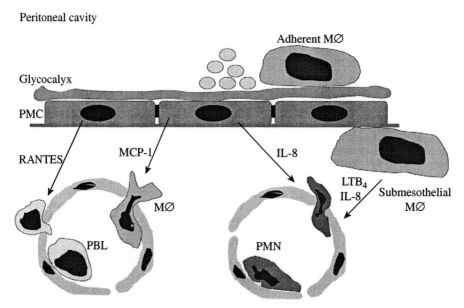

Fig. 3.6 Amplification of infection requires the recruitment of inflammatory cells by the secretion of chemoattractants, IL-8 (interleukin 8) and leukotriene B_4 for polymorphonuclear leucocytes (PMN), RANTES for lymphocytes, and monocyte chemoattractant protein (MCP-1) for monocytes.

Bacterial destruction

Opsonized bacteria are phagocytosed by infiltrating MØ and PMN (Holmes 1994). In some cases peritoneal MØ are capable of phagocytosing bacteria directly. Once phagocytosed, bacteria are lysed following respiratory burst and generation of hydrogen peroxide and free radical oxygen species (Goldstein *et al.* 1984).

Resolution

If uncontrolled inflammation persisted within the peritoneum this would lead to heavy protein losses in the dialysate effluent, continued activation of peritoneal mesothelial cells, and fibroblasts with increased matrix production and resulting fibrosis of the peritoneal membrane with consequent loss of function. Following transmigration, PMN are short-lived cells either dying by necrosis or apoptosis. Both MØ and peritoneal mesothelial cells can phagocytose apoptotic PMN. Infiltrated lymphocytes change their phenotype from predominantly T_{H1} to T_{H2}, so switching the balance from proinflammatory to one of resolution (Lamperi and Carozzi 1986). MØ leave the peritoneal cavity in the draining lymphatics and pass through to the local lymph nodes.

Peritoneal mesothelial cells replicate and migrate (Yung and Davies 1998), to repopulate areas which have been denuded of cells (Leavesley *et al.* 1999) and lyse fibrin (Sitter *et al.* 1995). Peritoneal fibroblasts decrease *de novo* matrix production and increase matrix degradation, so that normal submesothelial extracellular matrix is restored (Topley and Williams 1996).

Summary

Peritoneal dialysis is one of the major modes of therapy for the treatment of patients with end-stage renal failure. Peritonitis, however, remains a frequent complication despite improvements in technique and in particular delivery systems which have significantly reduced the frequency of infective episodes.

The majority of peritoneal dialysis catheters become colonized with bacteria, and therefore the balance between bacterial load and virulence on the one hand and host defence on the other determines whether infection develops. Prophylactic antibiotics at the time of catheter insertion, nasal eradication of staphylococci, and allowing the catheter track to heal properly before use may all reduce or delay catheter colonization. However, the actual technique of peritoneal dialysis, by lavaging the peritoneal cavity, reduces host defence by continually removing proteins, which are required in bacterial opsonization, and peritoneal MØ, so reducing the concentration of MØ. The continued addition of fresh peritoneal dialysate, which is an acidic, hyperosmolar glucose and lactate-based solution, causes adverse changes in peritoneal mesothelial cells and reduces the function of peritoneal phagocytic cells. Dialysate not only reduces host defence but also promotes changes within the peritoneal membrane, resulting in eventual failure of the membrane to function as a dialysing surface. Newer peritoneal dialysis solutions that will shortly become widely available are bicarbonate based at neutral pH, iso-osmolar or less hypertonic, and are free of glucose degradation products and plasticizers. These may further improve the balance towards host defence and reduce the incidence of CAPD peritonitis.

References

Adams DH, Shaw S (1994). Leucocyte endothelial interactions and regulation of leucocyte migration. *Lancet* 343: 831–6.

Andrews PA, Warr KJ, Hicks KJ, Cameron JS (1996). Impaired outcome of continuous ambulatory peritoneal dialysis in immunosuppressed patients. *Nephrol Dial Transplant* 11: 1104–8.

Anwar N, Hutchinson A, Manos J, Utley L, Brenchley P, Gokal R (1997). Peritoneal dialysate IgG/C3 levels do not predict peritonitis. *Peri Dial Int* 16: 154–7.

Beaman M, Michael J, Maclennan ICM, Adu D (1989). T-cell independent and T-cell dependent antibody responses in patients with chronic renal failure. *Nephrol. Dial. Transplant.* 4: 216–21.

Betjes MGH, Bos HJ, Krediet RT, Arisz L (1991). The mesothelial cells in CAPD effluent and their relation to peritonitis incidence. *Perit Dial Int* 11: 22–6.

Betjes MGH, Tuk CW, Struijk DG, Krediet RT, Arisz L, Hoefsmit ECM, Beelen RHJ (1993a). Immuno-effector characteristics of peritoneal cells during CAPD treatment: a longitudinal study. *Kidney Int* 43: 641–8.

Betjes MGH, Tuk CW, Struijk DG, Krediet RT, Arisz L, Beelen RHJ (1993b). Antigen present-ing capacity of macrophages and dendritic cells in the peritoneal cavity of patients treated with peritoneal dialysis. *Clin Exp Immunol* 94: 377–84.

Boner G, Mhashilkar AM, Rodriguez-Ortega M, Sharon N (1989). Lectin-mediated non-opsonic phagocytosis of type I Escherichia coli by human peritoneal macrophages of uraemic patients treated by peritoneal dialysis. *J Leukocyte Biol* 14: 239–45.

Bonomini M, Manfrini V, Capelli P, Albertazzi A (1993). Zinc and cell mediated immunity in chronic uremia. *Nephron* 65: 1–4.

Bos HJ, vanBronwijk H, Helmerhorst TJM, Oe PL, Hoefsmit ECM, Beelen RHJ (1988). Distinct subpopulations of elicited human macrophages in peritoneal dialysis patients and women under-going laparoscopy: a study of peroxidative activity. *J Leukocyte Biol* 43: 172–8.

Bouts AH, Out TA, Schroder CH, Monnens LA, Nauta J, Krediet RT, Davin JC (2000). Characteristics of peripheral and peritoneal white blood cells in children with chronic renal failure, dialyzed or not. *Perit Dial Int* 20: 748–56.

Buoncristiani U (1989). The Y set with disinfectant is here to stay. *Perit Dial Int* 9: 149.

Cendoroglo M, Sundaram S, Jaber BL, Pereiral BJ (1998). Effect of glucose concentration, osmo-lality and sterilization process of peritoneal dialysis fluids on cytokine production by peripheral blood mononuclear cells and polymorphonuclear cell functions *in vivo*. *Am J Kidney Dis* 31: 273–82.

Chan MK, Baillod RA, Varghese Z, Sweny P, Moorhead JF (1983). Immunoglobulins and complement components (C3, C4) in CAPD and haemodialysis patients. *Nephrol Dial Transplant* 12: 777–8.

Coles GA, Alobaidi H, Topley N, Davies M (1987). Osponic activity of dialysis effluent predicts those at risk of *Staphylococcus epidermidis* peritonitis. *Nephrol Dial Transplant* 2: 359–65.

Coles GA, Lewis SL, Williams JD (1994). Host defence and effects of solutions on peritoneal cells. In: Gokal R, Nolph KD (eds) *The Textbook of Peritoneal Dialysis* pp. 503–28. Kluwer Academic, Boston, MA.

Combet S, Miyata T, Moulin P, Pouthier D, Goffin E, Devuyst O (2000). Vascular proliferation and enhanced expression of endothelial nitric oxide synthase in human peritoneum exposed to long term peritoneal dialysis. *J Am Soc Nephrol* 11: 717–28.

Davenport A, Dealler SF (1993). The epidermo-peritoneal potential in patients treated with continuous ambulatory peritoneal dialysis. *Int J Artif Organs* 16: 71–4.

Davies SJ (1990). Peritoneal lymphocyte populations in CAPD patients. *Contrib Nephrol* 85: 16–23.

Davies SJ, Saussuna J, Ogg CS, Cameron JS (1989). Activation of immunocompetent cells in the peritoneum of patients treated with CAPD. *Kidney Int* 36: 661–8.

Davies SJ, Yewdall VMA, Ogg CS, Cameron JS (1990). Peritoneal defence mechanisms and Staphylococcus aureus in patients treated with continuous ambulatory peritoneal dialysis (CAPD). *Perit Dial Int* 10: 135–40.

Davin JC, Bouts AH, Krediet RT, van der Weel M, Weening RS, Groothoff J, Out TA (1997). IgG glycation and function during continuous ambulatory peritoneal dialysis. *Nephrol Dial Transplant* 12: 310–14.

DeFitjer CWH, Verbrugh HA, Oe LP, Peters EDJ, van der Meulen J, Donker AJM, Verhoef J (1992). Peritoneal defence in continuous ambulatory versus continuous cyclic peritoneal dialysis. *Kidney Int* 42: 947–50.

DeFitjer CWH, Verbrugh HA, Peters EDJ, Oe LP, Heezius ECJM, van der Meulen J, Verhoef J, Donker AJ (1993). *In vivo* exposure to currently available peritoneal dialysis fluids decreases the function of peritoneal macrophages in CAPD. *Clin Nephrol* 39: 75–80.

DeFitjer CWH, Verbrugh HA, Oe LP, Heezius ECJM, Verhoef J, Donker AJM (1994). Antibacterial peritoneal defence in automated peritoneal dialysis: advantages of tidal over continuous cyclic peritoneal dialysis? *Nephrol Dial Transplant* 9: 156–62.

DeFitjer CWH , Oe LP, Heezius ECJM, Verhoef J, Donker AJM, Verbrugh HA (1996). Low calcium peritoneal dialysis fluid should not impact peritonitis rates in continuous ambulatory peritoneal dialysis. *Am J Kidney Dis* 27: 409–15.

Dobbie JW (1994). Ultrastructure and pathology of the peritoneum in peritoneal dialysis. In: Gokal R, Nolph KD (eds) *The Textbook of Peritoneal Dialysis*, pp. 17–44. Kluwer Academic, Boston, MA.

Fricke H, Hartmann J, Sitter T, Steldinger R, Rieber P, Schiffl H (1996). Continuous ambulatory peritoneal dialysis impairs T lymphocyte selection in the peritoneum. *Kidney Int* 49: 1386–95.

Gallimore B, Gagnon RF, Richards GK (1988). Role of an intraperitoneal catheter implant in the pathogenesis of experimental peritoneal infection in renal failure mice. *Am J Nephrol* 36: 406–13.

Girndt M, Sester M, Sester U, Kaul H, Kohler H (2001). Molecular aspects of T- and B-cell function in uremia. *Kidney Int* 59 suppl. 78: S206–S211.

Glancey GR, Cameron JS, Ogg CS, DeFitjer CWH, van der Meulen J (1990). The washout kinetics of intraperitoneal IgG in CAPD patients. *Nephrol Dial Transplant* 5: 78.

Glancey GR, Cameron JS, Ogg CS (1992). Peritoneal drainage: an important element in host defence against staphylococcal peritonitis in patients on CAPD. *Nephrol Dial Transplant* 7: 627–31.

Goldstein CS, Bomalaski JS, Zurier RB, Neilson EG, Douglas SD (1984). Analysis of peritoneal macrophages in continuous ambulatory peritoneal dialysis patients. *Kidney Int* 26: 733–40.

Haag-Weber M, Hörl WH (1993). Uremia and infection: mechanisms of impaired cellular host defense. *Nephron* 63: 125–31.

Harvey DM, Shepard KJ, Morgan AG (1988). Neutrophil function in patients on CAPD. *Br J Haematol* 68: 273–8.

Hau T, Ahrenholz DH, Simmons RL (1979). Secondary bacterial peritonitis: the biological basis of treatment. In: Ravitch MM (ed.) *Current Problems in Surgery*, pp. 1–3. Year Book Medical Publishers, Boston, MA.

Holley JL, Bernardini J, Piraino B (1990). Continuous cyclic peritoneal dialysis is associated with lower rates of catheter infections than continuous ambulatory peritoneal dialysis. *Am J Kidney Dis* 16: 133–6.

Holmes CJ (1994). Peritoneal host defence mechanisms in peritoneal dialysis. *Kidney Int.* 46 suppl. 48: S58–S70.

Holmes CJ, Evans R (1986). Biofilm and foreign body infection—the significance to CAPD-associated peritonitis. *Perit Dial Bull* 6: 168–77.

Holmes CJ, Lewis S (1991). Host defence mechanisms in the peritoneal cavity of continuous ambulatory peritoneal dialysis patients: humoral defences. *Perit Dial Int* 11: 112–17.

Jedlicka J, Segerer W, Scherberich JE (1998). Comparative analysis of leucocyte endotoxin receptor expression in patients under CAPD or chronic hemodialysis treatment. *Kidney Blood Pressure Res* 21: 199–200.

Kaupke CJ, Zhang J, Rajpoot D, Wang J, Zhou XJ, Vaziri ND (1996). Effects of conventional peritoneal dialysates on leukocyte adhesion and CD11b, CD18 and CD14 expression. *Kidney Int* 50: 1676–83.

Keane WF, Bergerson B, Pence T, Peterson PK (1988). Challenges for continuous peritoneal ambulatory dialysis. In: Davison AM (ed.) *Proc Xth Int Congress of Nephrology*, pp. 1255–67. Balliere Tindall, London.

Keane WF, Vas SI (1994). Peritonitis. In: Gokal R, Nolph KD (eds) *The Textbook of Peritoneal Dialysis*, pp. 473–502. Kluwer Academic Publishers, Boston, MA.

Khanna R, Mactier R (1992). Role of lymphatics in peritoneal dialysis. *Blood Purif* 10: 163–72.

Lameire N, Vanholder R, De Smet R (2001). Uremic toxins and peritoneal dialysis. *Kidney Int* 59: S292–S297.

Lamperi S, Carozzi S (1986a). Defective opsonic activity of peritoneal effluent during continuous ambulatory peritoneal dialysis (CAPD). Importance and prevention. *Perit Dial Bull* 6: 87–92.

Lamperi S, Carozzi S (1986b). Suppressor resident macrophages and peritonitis incidence in CAPD. *Nephron* 44: 219–25.

Lamperi S, Carozzi S (1988). Interferon γ as an enhancing factor of peritoneal macrophage defective of bacterial activity during continuous ambulatory peritoneal dialysis (CAPD). *Am J Kidney Dis* 11: 225–30.

Leavesley DI, Stanley JM, Fault RJ (1999). Epidermal growth factor modifies the expression and function of extracellular matrix adhesion receptors expressed by peritoneal mesothelial cells from patients on CAPD. *Nephrol Dial Transplant* 14: 1208–16.

Lewis SL, Holmes CJ (1991). Host defence mechanisms in the peritoneal cavity of continuous ambulatory peritoneal dialysis patients. *Perit Dial Int* 11: 14–21.

Lewis SL, Norris PJ (1990). Monocyte/macrophage function in continuous ambulatory peritoneal dialysis patients. *Contrib Nephrol* 85: 1–9.

Lewis SL, van Epps DE, Chenoworth DE (1988). Alterations in chemotactic factor induced responses of neutrophils and monocytes from chronic dialysis patients. *Clin Nephrol* 30: 63–72.

Lewis SL, Bonner PN, Cooper CL, Holmes CJ (1992). Prospective comparison of blood and peritoneal lymphocytes from CAPD patients. *J Clin Lab Immunol* 37: 3–19.

Lewis SL, Kutvirt SG, Cooper CL, Bonner PN, Holmes CJ (1993). Characteristics of peripheral and peritoneal lymphocytes from CAPD patients. *Perit Dial Int* suppl 2, 13.

Li FK, Davenport A, Robson RL, Loetscher P, Rothlein R, Williams JD, Topley N (1998). Leukocyte migration across human peritoneal mesothelial cells (HPMC) is dependent on directed chemokine secretion and ICAM-1 expression. *Kidney Int* 54: 2170–83.

Libetta C, DeNicola L, Rampino T, DeSimone W, Memoli B (1996). Inflammatory effects of peritoneal dialysis: evidence of systemic monocyte activation. *Kidney Int* 49: 506–11.

Liberek T, Topley N, Jörres A, Petersen MM, Coles GA, Gahl GM, Williams JD (1993a). Peritoneal dialysis fluid inhibition of polmorphonuclear leukocyte respiratory burst activation is related to the lowering of intracellular pH. *Nephron* 65: 260–5.

Liberek T, Topley N, Jörres A, Coles GA, Gahl GM, Williams JD (1993b). Peritoneal dialysis fluid inhibition of phagocyte function: effects of osmolality and glucose concentration. *J Am Soc Nephrol* 3: 1508–15.

Lin CY, Ku WL, Huang TP (1990). Serial peritoneal macrophage function studies in new and established continuous ambulatory peritoneal dialysis patients. *Am J Nephrol* 10: 368–73.

Luo Q, Cheung AK, Kamerath CD, Reimer LG, Leypoldt JK (2000). Increased protein loss during peritonitis with peritoneal dialysis is neutrophil dependent. *Kidney Int* 57: 1736–42.

Marine TJ, Bobel MA, Costerton JW (1983). Examination of the morphology of bacteria adhering to peritoneal dialysis catheters by scanning and transmission electron microscopy. *J Clin Microsc* 18: 1388–98.

Massry S, Smogorzewski M (2001). Dysfunction of polymorphonuclear leukocytes in uremia: role of parathyroid hormone. *Kidney Int* 59 suppl. 78: S195–S196.

Matsuoka Y, Yamaauchi A, Nakanishi T, Sugiura T, Kitamura H, Horio M, Takamitsu Y, Ando A, Imai E, Hori M (1999). Response to hypertonicity in mesothelial cells: role of Na+/myo-inositol co-transporter. *Nephrol Dial Transplant* 14: 1217–23.

McGregor SJ, Brock JH, Briggs JD, Junor BJR (1987). Bactericidal activity of peritoneal macrophages from CAPD patients. *Nephrol Dial Transplant* 2: 104–8.

McGregor SJ, Topley N, Jörres A, Speekenbrink ABJ, Gordon A, Gahl GM, Junor BJR, Briggs JD, Brock JH (1996). Longitudinal evaluation of peritoneal macrophage function and activation during CAPD: maturity, cytokine synthesis and arachidonic acid metabolism. *Kidney Int* 49: 525–33.

Muijsken MA, Heezius HCM, Verhoef J, Verbrugh HA (1991). Role of mesothelial cells in peritoneal antibacterial defence. *J Clin Pathol* 44: 600–4.

Nielsen H, Espersen F, Kharazmi A, Antonsen S, Ejlersen E, Joffe P, Pedersen FB (1992). Specific opsonic activity for staphylococci in peritoneal dialysis effluent during continuous ambulatory peritoneal dialysis. *Am J Kidney Dis* 20: 372–5.

Oreopoulos DG, Robson M, Izatt S, Clayton S, deVeber GA (1978). A simple and safe technique for continuous ambulatory peritoneal dialysis. *Trans Am Soc Artif Intern Organs* 24: 484.

Paterson AD, Bishop MC, Morgan AG, Burden RP (1986). Removal and replacement of Tenckhoff catheter at a single operation: successful treatment of resistant peritonitis in continuous ambulatory peritoneal dialysis. *Lancet* ii: 1245–7.

Piraino B, Bernardini J, Holley JL, Perlmutter JA (1992). Increased risk of *Staphylococcus epidermidis* peritonitis in patients on dialysate containing 1.25 mmol/l calcium. *Am J Kidney Dis* 19: 371–4.

Plum J, Schoenicke, Grabensee B (1997). Osmotic agents and buffers in peritoneal dialysis solution: monocyte cytokine release and *in vitro* toxicity. *Am J Kidney Dis.* 30: 413–22.

Plum J, Schoenicke, Grabensee B (1998). Effect of alternative peritoneal dialysis solutions on cell viability apoptosis/necrosis and cytokine expression in human monocytes. *Kidney Int* 54: 224–35.

Pommer W, Brauner M, Westphale HJ, Brunkhorst R, Kramer R, Bundschu D, Hoffken B, Steinhauer HB, Schumann E, Luttgen FM, Schillinger-Pokorny E, Schaefer F, Wende R, Offner G, Nather S, Osten B, Zimmering M, Ehrich JH, Kehn M, Mansmann U, Grosse-Siestrup C (1998). Effect of a silver device in preventing catheter-related infections in peritoneal dialysis patients: silver ring prophylaxis at the catheter exit study. *Am J Kidney Dis* 32: 752–60.

Popovich RP, Moncrieff JW (1996). Peritoneal dialysis access technology: the Austin diagnostic clinic experience. *Perit Dial Int* 16 suppl. 1, S327–S329.

Popovich RP, Moncrieff JW, Decherd JB, Bomar JB, Pyle WF (1976). The definition of a novel portable/wearable equilibrium peritoneal dialysis technique. *Trans Am Soc Artif Intern Organs* 5: 64.

Rowe L, Miller TE (1993). Effect of dialysis on the clearance of *Staphylococcus epidermidis* from the peritoneal cavity: an experimental evaluation. *Clin Nephrol* 40: 106–13.

Scherberich JE, Nockher WA (2000). Blood monocyte phenotypes and soluble endotoxin receptor CD14 in systemic inflammatory diseases and patients with chronic renal failure. *Nephrol Dial Transplant* 15: 574–8.

Schroeder CH, Bakkeren JAJM, Weemaes CMR (1989). IgG2 deficiency in young children treated with continuous ambulatory peritoneal dialysis. *Perit Dial Int* 9: 201–5.

Selgas R, deCastro MF, Jiménez C, Cárcamo C, Contreras T, Bajo MA, Vara F, Corbí A (1996). Immunomodulation by peritoneal macrophages by granulocyte macrophage colony stimulating factor in humans. *Kidney Int* 50: 2070–8.

Sheth NK, Bartell CA, Roth DA (1986). *In vitro* study of bacterial growth in continuous ambulatory peritoneal dialysis fluids. *J Clin Microbiol* 23: 1096–8.

Sitter T, Spannagl M, Schiffl H, Held E, vanHinsbergh VWM, Kooistra T (1995). Imbalance between intraperitoneal coagulation and fibrinolysis during peritonitis of CAPD patients: the role of mesothelial cells. *Nephrol Dial Transplant* 10: 677–83.

Stabellini G, Bedani PL, Fiocchi O, Calsatrini C, Pagliarini A, Lunghi M, Carinci F, Pellati A, Giuliani A, Berti G (1998). DEHP induced alterations in the lining tissue of the rat air pouch. *Int J Artif Organs* 21: 87–94.

Stylianou E, Mackenzie R, Davies M, Coles GA, Williams JD (1990). The interaction of organism, phagocyte and mesothelial cell. *Contrib Nephrol* 85: 30–8.

Suassuna JHR, DasNeves FC, Hartley RB, Ogg CS, Cameron JS (1994). Immunohistological studies of the peritoneal membrane and infiltrating cells in normal subjects and patients on CAPD. *Kidney Int* 46: 443–54.

Such J, Guarner G, Enriquez J, Rodriguez JL, Seres I, Vilandell F (1988). Low C3 cirrhotic ascites predisposes to spontaneous bacterial peritonitis. *J Hepatol* 6: 80–4.

Sundaram S, Cendoroglo M, Cooker LA, Jaber BL, Faict D, Holmes CJ, Pereira BJ (1997). Effect of two-chambered bicarbonate lactate peritoneal dialysis fluids on peripheral blood mononuclear cell and polymorphonuclear cell function *in vitro*. *Am J Kidney Dis* 30: 680–9.

Swartz R, Messana J, Starman B, Weber M, Reynolds J (1991). Preventing *Staphylococcus aureus* infection during chronic peritoneal dialysis. *J Am Soc Nephrol* 2: 1085–8.

Teti G, Chiofalo MS, Tamasello F, Fava C, Mastroeni P (1987). Mediation of *Staphylococcus saprophyticus* adherence to uroepithelial cells by lipoteichoic acid. *Infect Immun* 55: 839–42.

Topley N, Williams JD (1994). The role of the peritoneal membrane in the control of inflammation in the peritoneal cavity. *Kidney Int* 46 suppl. 48: S71–S78.

Topley N, Davenport A, Li FK, Fear H, Williams JD (1996). Activation of inflammation and leukocyte recruitment into the peritoneal cavity. *Kidney Int* 50: S17–S21.

Verbrugh HA, Keane WF, Conroy WE, Petersen PK (1984). Bacterial growth and killing in CAPD fluids. *J Clin Microbiol* 20: 199–203.

Verger C, Chesneau AM, Thibault M, Bataille N (1987). Biofilm on Tenckoff catheters: a negligible source of contamination. *Perit Dial Bull* 7: 174–8.

Wajsbrot V, Shostak A, Gotloib L, Kushnier R (1988). Biocompatibility of a glucose free, acidic lactated solution for peritoneal dialysis evaluated by population analysis of mesothelium. *Nephron* 79: 322–32.

Williams PS, Hendy MS, Ackrill P (1987). Routine daily surveillance cultures in the management of CAPD patients. *Perit Dial Bull* 7: 183–6.

Witowski J, Korybalska K, Wisiewska J, Breborowicz A, Gahl G, Frei U, Passlick-Deetjen J, Jörres A (2000). Effect of glucose degradation products on human peritoneal mesothelial cell function. *J Am Soc Nephrol* 11: 729–39.

Yung S, Davies M (1998). Response of the human peritoneal mesothelial cell to injury: an in-vitro model of peritoneal wound healing. *Kidney Int* 54: 2160–9.

4

Infection in renal transplantation

Robert H. Rubin

Over the past three decades renal transplantation has been established as the best possible means of rehabilitating patients with end-stage renal disease of virtually any aetiology. Recently published data from the United States have documented that the 1-year survival rate now stands at 94% (with a subsequent half-life of 22 years) for allografts from living related donors and 88% for cadaveric donor allografts (with a subsequent half-life of 14 years).[1] Indeed, the attention of transplant medicine has shifted from acute rejection processes to chronic allograft nephropathy, a process in which many factors, including infection, appear to play an important role. Despite this gratifying success story, infection continues to be an important factor in shaping the post-transplant course, with evidence of microbial replication and invasion being found in more than 75% of transplant recipients. The clinical effects of infection are diverse, and can be grouped into two general categories: the direct and the indirect. The direct manifestations of infection include all the clinical manifestations caused by microbial invasion, including fever, mononucleosis, pneumonia, bloodstream infection, hepatitis, gastroenteritis, meningitis, etc., in which microbial invasion and the inflammatory response to such invasion are directly responsible for the clinical syndrome of infectious disease. The indirect manifestations of infection are due to the elaboration of cytokines, chemokines, and growth factors by the host as a consequence of microbial replication and invasion. Once these pluripotent mediators are elaborated, the microbe's sole role is providing a continuing stimulus for the elaboration of these mediators. These indirect effects can be grouped into three general categories:[2,3]

1. Certain infections, most notably systemic viral infections, can produce a global depression in host defences, thus predisposing to serious opportunistic infections due to a variety of pathogens: *Pneumocystis carinii*, *Aspergillus* spp., *Cryptococcus neoformans*, *Listeria monocytogenes*, *Candida* spp., and others (see Chapter 16).
2. Certain viruses contribute significantly to the pathogenesis of those malignancies that are particularly common in the transplant recipient, e.g. post-transplant lymphoproliferative disease (primarily Epstein–Barr virus, but also cytomegalovirus), hepatocellular carcinoma (hepatitis B and C viruses), squamous cell carcinoma of mucocutaneous surfaces (papovaviruses), and Kaposi's sarcoma (human herpesvirus 8) (see Chapter 14).
3. The modulation of the expression of major histocompatibility antigens and the level of activation of both vascular endothelium and inflammatory cells can play an important role in the pathogenesis of acute and chronic allograft injury.

What is particularly notable about these indirect effects is that they are bidirectional; that is, not only can cytokines and other mediators liberated in the course of infection modulate the processes listed, but mediators liberated in the course of such conditions as rejection, trauma, and other stresses can modulate the course of infection. The bidirectionality of these relationships is perhaps best illustrated by the answer to a question that has been a subject of intense controversy for the past two decades: 'Which comes first, rejection or infection?' The answer is clearly 'Either!'—the events described can proceed in either direction.[2,3]

Risk of infection

The first factor to be considered in the pathogenesis of infection following renal transplantation is whether or not technically impeccable surgery (and perioperative care) was accomplished. Any technical mishap that results in devitalized tissue, a urine leak, or the continuing need for drains, catheters, endotracheal tubes, and/or vascular access devices will result in an increased risk of infection. Fortunately, the present state of the technical aspects of renal transplantation is such that such considerations play a role in fewer than 5% of renal allograft recipients. For the others, the risk of infection is largely determined by the interaction between two factors—the epidemiological exposures the patient encounters and the patient's net state of immunosuppression. The relationship between these two factors is a semiquantitative one; that is, if the exposure is great enough, even patients who are minimally immunosuppressed can develop life-threatening infection, while if the net state of immunosuppression is great enough, even trivial exposures can result in significant infection.[2,3]

The epidemiological exposures of importance for the transplant patient can be divided into two general categories: those occurring in the community and those occurring within the hospital (Table 4.1). In the community the primary considerations are recent and remote exposures to *Mycobacterium tuberculosis* and the geographically restricted systemic mycoses (blastomycosis, coccidioidomycosis, histoplasmosis, and paracoccidioidomycosis), *Strongyloides stercoralis*, and community-acquired respiratory viruses and enteric pathogens. In addition, we have observed an increased incidence of nocardiosis and aspergillosis among renal transplant recipients who have engaged in active gardening and farming that results in the aerosolization and inhalation of dust from the soil.[2,3]

When considering tuberculosis and the endemic mycoses both recent and remote exposures must be considered, as three patterns of disease can be observed post-transplant: progressive primary infection with primary dissemination; reactivation disease with secondary dissemination; and reinfection disease, in which previous immunity is attenuated by post-transplant immunosuppression and new exposure results in active infection, again with a high risk of systemic dissemination. Thus, the clinical presentation of these infections in the transplant patient can be quite diverse, including pulmonary disease with or without cavities, miliary disease, fever of unknown origin, or metastatic infection involving mucocutaneous structures, the kidneys, liver, or skeletal system.[2,3]

Strongyloides stercoralis, due to its unique autoinoculation cycle, is the one helminth that can remain asymptomatically in the gastrointestinal tract for decades after the

Table 4.1 Epidemiological exposures of importance to the renal transplant patient

Type of infection	Organism
Infections related to particular exposures in the community	
Geographically restricted systemic mycoses	*Blastomyces dermatitidis*
	Coccidioides immitis
	Histoplasma capsulatum
	Paracoccidioides brasilensis
Strongyloides stercoralis	
Community acquired opportunistic infection resulting from inhalation of aerosolized organisms	*Aspergillus* spp.
	Cryptococcus neoformans
	Nocardia species
Respiratory infections	Viruses: influenza, parainfluenza, respiratory syncytial virus, adenovirus
	Mycobacterium tuberculosis
Infections acquired by the consumption of contaminated food or water	*Salmonella* spp.
	Listeria spp.
	Campylobacter jejuni
	Escherichia coli
	Crytosporidium parvum
Infections related to particular exposures in the hospital	
Infections related to contaminated air or potable water	*Aspergillus* spp.
	Legionella spp.
	Pseudomonas aeruginosa and other Gram-negative bacilli
Infections related to person-to-person contact (often on the hands of medical personnel)	Methicillin-resistant *Staphylococcus aureus*
	Vancomycin-resistant enterococci
	Highly resistant Gram-negative bacilli
	Azole-resistant yeast
	Clostridium difficile

subject has taken up residence outside endemic regions of the world. With the initiation of immunosuppressive therapy symptomatic disease will occur that can take one of two forms—a hyperinfestation syndrome or a disseminated infection syndrome. The hyperinfestation syndrome results in haemorrhagic pneumonia and/or haemorrhagic enterocolitis, an exaggeration of the effects of this parasite in the normal host. In the disseminated syndrome, trophozoites actually leave the bowel and invade other tissues, including the central nervous system. Not uncommonly, bacterial gut flora will accompany the parasites resulting in a clinical syndrome of Gram-negative bacteraemia or meningitis unresponsive to appropriate antimicrobial therapy (unless the parasite is also treated). These post-transplant strongyloidiasis syndromes carry a mortality rate of 50% or higher, hence we advocate pretransplant screening of individuals with a history of residence in endemic areas (e.g. the southern United States, Central and South America,

Africa, and Southeast Asia). Routine examination of stools for ova and parasites has a sensitivity of less than 20%. Far better is sampling of duodenal contents or serological testing. Our practice is to screen serologically, and to treat those who are serologically positive pre-emptively with ivermectin or thiobendazole.[2–6]

The most common community-acquired infections occurring in the transplant patient are those caused by respiratory viruses, most notably influenza, parainfluenza, respiratory syncytial virus, and adenoviruses. The consequences of infection with these viruses in the transplant patient are several: in the context of a community-wide outbreak, the incidence, severity, and duration of symptomatic disease is greater among transplant patients, the attack rate for viral pneumonia is higher, and the risk of secondary bacterial or fungal pneumonia is great. Unfortunately, neither vaccination (as for influenza) nor available antiviral strategies (amantadine, rimantidine, or the new neuraminidase inhibitors for influenza or ribavirin for respiratory syncytial virus) are of proven value in this patient population, so avoidance of exposure is of primary importance. Influenza immunization has been shown to be safe in the transplant patient, but its efficacy is far less than in the normal host.[2,3,7,8]

The enteric pathogens *Salmonella* and *Campylobacter* have a greater impact on the transplant patient, with more prolonged diarrhoea, higher rates of bacteraemia, and, in the case of *Salmonella*, a greater risk of metastatic infection than that observed in the normal host. Although prompt antimicrobial therapy is indicated for gastroenteritis due to these organisms in this patient population, avoidance of dubious food establishments and inadequately cooked food bears particular emphasis. Two additional enteric pathogens merit comment here. *Listeria monocytogenes*, a not uncommon cause of bacteraemia and central nervous system infection in this patient population, can present with a febrile gastroenteritis syndrome as the first clinical manifestation of infection. Rotavirus can cause a prolonged diarrhoeal syndrome, particularly among paediatric renal transplant recipients.[2]

Even more important to the well-being of transplant patients are epidemiological exposures encountered in the hospital. Contamination of air (often associated with construction) or potable water with *Aspergillus* spp., *Legionella* spp., *Pseudomonas aeruginosa*, and other Gram-negative bacilli has resulted in epidemic disease among transplant patients, with two patterns of outbreak observed: a domiciliary pattern, in which the exposure occurs on the ward where the patient is housed, with clustering of cases in time and space; and a non-domiciliary pattern, in which exposure occurs in the patient's travels within the hospital for essential procedures (e.g. to the operating theatre, the radiology suite, the endoscopy facility, etc.), and there is thus no clustering of cases in time or space. Domiciliary cases are far easier to detect, but non-domiciliary hazards are more common. The most useful clue to the presence of an unsuspected environmental hazard is the occurrence of opportunistic infection with one of these organisms at a time when the patient's net state of immunosuppression would not normally be great enough for such an infection to occur.[2,3,9]

In recent years, transplant patients have been at particularly high risk of person-to-person spread, especially on the hands of medical personnel, of infection with methicillin-resistant *Staphylococcus aureus*, vancomycin-resistant enterococci, azole-resistant *Candida* spp., and highly resistant Gram-negative bacilli and *Clostridium difficile*. Following colonization with these organisms, the attack rate for symptomatic

Table 4.2 Factors contributing to the net state of immunosuppression

Host defence defects engendered by the underlying disease process

Dose, duration, nature, and temporal sequence of immunosuppressive therapy

Technical factors that damage tissue, abridge the primary mucocutaneous barrier to infection, or result in the need for an indwelling foreign body

Neutropenia

Such metabolic factors as protein-calorie malnutrition, uraemia, and perhaps diabetes mellitus

Infection with an immunomodulating virus (e.g. cytomegalovirus, Epstein–Barr virus, hepatitis B and C virus, and the human immunodeficiency virus)

disease and the gravity of the illness is far higher in transplant patients than in the non-immunosuppressed patient population. Strict isolation with barrier nursing and assiduous handwashing procedures are essential for protecting these susceptible hosts against the acquisition of these organisms.[2,3]

The net state of immunosuppression is a complex function determined by the inter-action of a number of factors (Table 4.2). The major determinant is the nature of the immunosuppressive therapy being administered—the dose, duration, and even temporal sequence in which the drugs are deployed. However, other factors such as metabolic abnormalities and concomitant viral infection can contribute significantly to the net state of immunosuppression, as demonstrated by the following observations. At the Massachusetts General Hospital it has been found that those transplant patients with a serum albumin of less than 2.5 g/dl had a more than 10-fold increase in life-threatening infection when compared with transplant patients with higher albumin levels. Even more compelling is the observation that around 90% of the opportunistic infection occurring in transplant recipients occurs in individuals with concomitant infection with one or more of the immunomodulating viruses: cytomegalovirus (CMV), Epstein–Barr virus (EBV), hepatitis B and C (HBV and HCV), the human immunodeficiency virus (HIV), and, probably, human herpesvirus 6 (HHV-6). Indeed, the 10% of exceptions to this observa-tion were almost invariably traced to a previously unsuspected environmental exposure.[2,3]

Timetable of infection post-transplant

There is a temporal pattern, a timetable, as to when different infections occur post-transplant; that is, although infectious disease syndromes such as pneumonia can occur at any time post-transplant, the microbial aetiology of the syndrome is very different at different points in the post-transplant course (Fig. 4.1). This timetable is useful in three different ways: in formulating the differential diagnosis in the individual patient who presents with an infectious disease syndrome; as an epidemiological tool, for exceptions to the timetable are usually due to excessive environmental exposures that need correction; and as a guide to the design and deployment of focused cost-effective strategies for preventing infection post-transplant. The post-transplant course for the renal transplant recipient can be usefully divided into three time periods: the first month, the period 1–6 months post-transplant, and the late period more than 6 months post-transplant.[2,3,10]

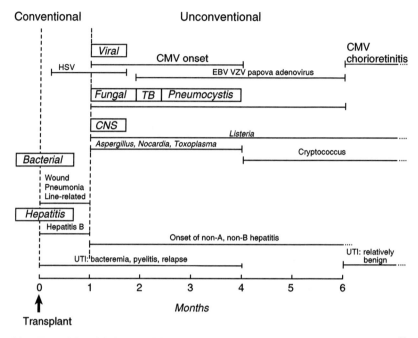

Conventional   Unconventional

Fig. 4.1 Timetable of infection following renal transplantation (from Rubin *et al*.[10] with permission). Abbreviations: HSV, herpes simplex virus; CMV, cytomegalovirus; EBV, Epstein–Barr virus; VZV, varicella zoster virus; TB, tuberculosis; CNS, central nervous sytem; UTI, urinary tract infection.

The first month post-transplant

In this time period there are three categories of infection:

1. Infection that was present pretransplant and was not eradicated prior to surgery and may, indeed, be exacerbated by surgery, anaesthesia, and post-transplant immuno-suppression.

The first rule of transplant infectious disease practice is that all treatable infection should be eradicated prior to transplant. Ongoing bacteraemia or fungaemia threatens vascular suture lines; recent lung injury, whether this is due to infection, chemical injury following aspiration, or infarction due to pulmonary emboli, is at high risk for post-transplant Gram-negative and/or fungal superinfection; and active urinary tract infection is likely to result in pyelonephritis of the allograft.

2. Infection conveyed with the allograft.
3. More than 90% of the infections that occur in the first month post-transplant are the same bacterial and candidal infections of the wound, the lungs, the urinary tract, or of vascular access catheters that occur in non-immunosuppressed patients undergoing comparable forms of surgery; that is, the aetiology and pathogenesis are the same, although the impact can be far greater in the transplant patient.

The major determinant of the incidence of infection in this time period is the technical skill with which the surgery is performed, the endotracheal tube is managed, and vascular access and drains and catheters are managed. In this patient population a technical error that leads to devitalized tissue, fluid collection, or the need for indwelling lines and catheters that damage or traverse the primary mucocutaneous barriers to infection carry a high risk of infection. It is also of interest that such opportunistic infections as invasive aspergillosis, *Pneumocystis carinii* pneumonia, listeriosis, nocardiosis, and cryptococcosis are quite uncommon in this time period, unless an unusually intense environmental exposure occurs. Indeed, a single case of opportunistic infection occurring in this time period should be taken as *prima facie* evidence of an excessive environmental hazard that needs to be corrected. Since this is the time period in which the highest daily doses of immunosuppressive drugs are being administered, the virtual absence of opportunistic infection means that the major determinant of the net state of immunosuppression is sustained therapy (the 'area under the curve'), rather than the daily dose.[2,3,10]

One to 6 months post-transplant

Other than the lingering effects of infection related to technical mishaps, the major causes of infection in this time period can be divided into two major categories:

1. The major causes of symptomatic infection in this time period are the direct manifestations of the immunomodulating viruses, most notably CMV, EBV, and HHV-6. For example, approximately two-thirds of fevers occurring in this time period have been attributed to CMV.
2. The combined effects of sustained immunosuppression and viral infection create a net state of immunosuppression great enough to permit the occurrence of opportunistic infection with *Pneumocystis*, *Aspergillus*, *Nocardia*, and *Listeria* without a particularly intense environmental exposure.[2,3,10–15]

More than 6 months post-transplant

Patients who remain with a functioning allograft on chronic immunosuppression more 6 months post-transplant can be divided into three groups in terms of their infectious disease risks:

1. The great majority (~80%), who have had a good result from their transplant procedure—good renal function, minimal maintenance immunosuppression, freedom from chronic viral infection—are at low risk for opportunistic infection (unless a high-level environmental exposure occurs). Rather, their greatest risk is for community-acquired respiratory virus infection and bacterial urinary tract infection (with the pathogenesis of urinary tract infection being similar to that observed in the normal population).
2. Approximately 10% of the patients will have chronic viral infection, particularly with HBV and HCV. Unless effective antiviral therapy can be instituted, over time there will be progressive liver injury, cirrhosis, and/or the risk of hepatocellular carcinoma.

3. Approximately 10% of transplant recipients will have had a poor result from the procedure—poor allograft function, excessive amounts of acute and chronic immunosuppression, and a high prevalence of immunomodulating viral infection. These 'chronic ne'er-do-wells' are at particularly high risk for the development of life-threatening opportunistic infection with such organisms as *Pneumocystis carinii*, *Listeria monocytogenes*, *Aspergillus* spp., *Nocardia asteroides*, and *Cryptococcus neoformans*. If the epidemiological background is appropriate, this is the group of patients at particularly high risk for tuberculosis and systemic mycotic infection as well.[2,3,10]

Summary of infection timetable

As can be clearly seen from examination of the timetable, different infections occur at different points in time, and different antimicrobial strategies will be necessary to prevent the occurrence of these infections. In the first month post-transplant, the key preventative measures are technically impeccable surgery and postoperative care and perioperative antibacterial prophylaxis. In the period 1–6 months post-transplant, anti-viral strategies (particularly those aimed against CMV), anti-*Pneumocystis* prophylaxis (optimally with low-dose trimethoprim-sulfamethoxazole), and a clean air and water supply are the primary strategies for prevention of infection. Finally, in the late period, particular attention should be paid to the chronic ne'er-do-well population: long-term trimethoprim-sulfamethoxazole therapy, a consideration of fluconazole prophylaxis for invasive yeast infection (particularly cryptococcal), and avoidance of environmental hazards are the cornerstones of prevention efforts.[2,3]

Principles of antimicrobial management in the renal transplant patient

There are six general principles that underline the use of antimicrobial agents in the renal transplant patient:[2,3,16]

1. Prevention of infection, rather than the treatment of clinically overt disease, is the primary goal of the practitioner.
2. Because of the blunted inflammatory response caused by immunosuppressive therapy (particularly corticosteroids), signs and symptoms of infection will often be greatly muted until the infectious process is far advanced. Since the main prognostic factor in determining the outcome of therapy for most infections in this patient population is how early diagnosis is made and therapy instituted, there is a particular emphasis on an aggressive diagnostic approach for even subtle signs and symptoms of infection.
3. Microbial load (otherwise known as organism burden) is a key factor in determining the gravity of the infection, the dose, duration, and route of administration of the antimicrobial therapy required, and the risk of the development of antimicrobial resistance in the causative organisms.
4. The possibility of drug interactions with the two mainstays of modern immuno-suppression—cyclosporine and tacrolimus—particularly in terms of nephrotoxicity, are critically important considerations in the design of an antimicrobial programme.

5. When infection occurs in conjunction with or because of a technical/anatomical abnormality, optimal therapy requires the combination of optimal antimicrobial therapy with correction, often with surgery, of the abnormality that led to the infection in the first place. If antimicrobial therapy is given in the absence of correction of the anatomical abnormality, then treatment will probably fail, with the concomitant induction of antimicrobial resistance.

6. It is useful to think in terms of the therapeutic prescription for the renal transplant patient as having two components: an immunosuppressive component to prevent and treat rejection and an antimicrobial component to make it safe. These two components are closely linked, and any changes required in the immunosuppressive programme necessitate a modification of the antimicrobial programme—the two are inexorably linked, just as rejection and infection are closely linked.

In recognition of these principles, there are three different modes in which antimicrobial therapy can be prescribed for the renal transplant patient: therapeutic, prophylactic, and pre-emptive. The therapeutic mode describes the administration of antimicrobial agents to treat clinically symptomatic infection, with the goal of eradicating and curing the infection (although in some patients suppression of chronic infection may be all that can be obtained therapeutically). The prophylactic mode describes the administration of antimicrobial agents to an entire population before infection develops to prevent the development of infection that is common enough or important enough to merit this intervention. By far the most effective prophylactic strategy in renal transplant patients is the use of low-dose trimethoprim-sulfamethoxazole prophylaxis, which has had a major effect in decreasing the incidence of both urinary tract infection and urosepsis and in essentially eliminating the risk of *Pneumocystis carinii*, *Listeria monocytogenes*, *Nocardia asteroides*, and, probably, *Toxoplasma gondii* infection from patients receiving this therapy. The pre-emptive mode describes the administration of antimicrobial agents to a subset of patients identified as being at particularly high risk of clinically important infection on the basis of a clinical epidemiological characteristic or a laboratory marker.[2,3,16] For example, asymptomatic individuals shown to have CMV in the blood by culture, antigenaemia, or polymerase chain reaction (PCR) assay can be pre-emptively treated to prevent the development of symptomatic disease.[17–19] Alternatively, it has been shown that the administration of antilymphocyte antibodies to CMV seropositive individuals in the treatment of rejection is associated with a risk of subsequent CMV disease of about 65%. The combination of intravenous followed by oral ganciclovir, initiated at the same time as the antilymphocyte antibody therapy, has reduced this risk to less than 5%.[20–22]

As previously mentioned, drug interactions between antimicrobial agents and cyclosporine and tacrolimus are the rule, not the exception. There are three categories of drug interaction that can occur, the first two of which are due to effects of antimicrobial drugs on the metabolism of the immunosuppressive drugs by hepatic cytochrome P-450 enzymes:[2,3,16]

1. Certain antimicrobial agents will up-regulate the metabolism of cyclosporine and tacrolimus, resulting in a fall in blood levels of the immunosuppressive drugs and an increased risk of rejection. The antimicrobial agents most commonly associated with this effect are rifampin, nafcillin, and isoniazid.

2. Certain antimicrobial agents will down-regulate the metabolism of cyclosporine and tacrolimus, resulting in a rise in blood levels of the immunosuppressive drugs and an increased risk of nephrotoxicity and overimmunosuppression (with its attendant risk of opportunistic infection). The antimicrobial agents most commonly associated with this effect are the azole antifungal drugs (ketoconazole > itraconazole = voriconazole > fluconazole) and the macrolide antibiotics (erythromycin > clarithromycin > azithromycin).

3. Certain antimicrobial agents when utilized in patients with therapeutic blood levels of cyclosporine and tacrolimus will produce synergistic nephrotoxicity. Although the pathogenetic mechanisms for this are not well understood, there are three clinical forms of nephrotoxicity observed:

    (i)   Accelerated nephrotoxicity—drugs such as amphotericin, aminoglycosides, and vancomycin, which can produce renal injury in normal individuals after a given drug exposure, will now produce injury with far less exposure to these agents.

    (ii) Idiosyncratic nephrotoxicity—acute oliguric renal failure has been produced by single doses of amphotericin (as little as 10 mg), gentamicin (80 mg), vancomycin (500 mg), and trimethoprim-sulfamethoxazole (an intravenous dose containing trimethoprim 80 mg and sulfamethoxazole 400 mg) in the presence of therapeutic blood levels of cyclosporine and tacrolimus.

    (iii) Dose-related nephrotoxicity—whereas 250 mg of ciprofloxacin twice daily (and comparable doses of other fluoroquinolones) is well tolerated, higher doses are not. Similarly, although prophylactic doses of trimethoprim-sulfamethoxazole are well tolerated, the doses required to treat *Pneumocystis* pneumonia carry a high risk of nephrotoxicity. More recent is the suggestion that sirolimus increases the nephrotoxic potential of cyclosporine.

The end result of these various factors is the avoidance of amphotericin and amino-glycosides, the preferential use of advanced spectrum β-lactam drugs, azithromycin, moderate dose fluoroquinolone, and fluconazole in the treatment of infection in renal transplant patients, and a particular emphasis on prevention of infection, utilizing prophylactic and pre-emptive strategies.[2,3,16]

Infections of particular importance in the renal transplant recipient

Herpesviruses

The common viruses that cause the major clinical problems following solid organ transplantation are those of the herpes group. The major pathogen is CMV. Both EBV and Kaposi sarcoma virus (KSV) have oncogenic potential and are the most important causes of post-transplant malignancy once human papillomavirus (HPV) related squamous cell carcinoma has been excluded. Viral-related post-transplant tumours are discussed in Chapter 14 and CMV in Chapter 13.

Hepatitis viruses

Both HBV (Chapter 11) and HCV (Chapter 10) are important in transplant biology. Both can be transferred with the graft, both (particularly HBV) can cause progressive post-transplant liver disease, and both have oncogenic potential.

Fungal and parasitic infection

The immunocompromised transplant recipient is at risk both from certain geographically limited fungal infections (blastomycosis, coccidioidomycosis, etc.) and more widely distributed species including *Candida*, *Aspergillus*, *Cryptococcus*, and *Pneumocystis carinii*. Late diagnosis and inadequate therapy are associated with a high morbidity and mortality (see Chapter 16).

Bacterial infections of particular importance in the renal transplant recipient

Urinary tract infections

Urinary tract infections (UTI) are very common (30–60%) and are not infrequently complicated by bacteraemia (10%).[2,23,24] Spread to the transplanted kidney can mimic acute rejection. Inflammatory processes associated with infection may play a role in the reactivation of latent viruses (Chapter 15). *Candida* as well as bacteria may colonize the urinary tract. Obstructing fungal balls can develop. Such patients are at risk of haematogenous spread. Pre-emptive therapy with fluconazole or low-dose amphotericin (5–10 mg/day) should be instigated to prevent systemic spread.

Other bacterial infections

Mycobacterium tuberculosis is particularly common in certain at-risk ethnic groups, with reactivation an ever-present problem. Increasingly, atypical mycobacterial species are being identified. Other bacterial infections which need special consideration in the transplant period include *Listeria*, *Nocardia*, and non-typhoid salmonellae (Chapter 15).

Summary and conclusions

A wide range of organisms can cause clinically important infection in the renal transplant recipient. The risk of such infection is determined by the interaction of three factors: the occurrence of technical/anatomical abnormalities, the patient's net state of immunosuppression, and the epidemiological exposures encountered. The clinical impact of the infections can be of two types—the direct causation of infectious disease syndromes and the indirect effects, in which cytokines, chemokines, and growth factors elaborated in response to microbial invasion can cause a broad array of clinical abnormalities:

(1) they add to the net state of immunosuppression, thus predisposing to opportunistic superinfection;

(2) they play a role in causing allograft injury; and

(3) in some cases they contribute to the pathogenesis of certain malignancies.

Given the protean manifestations of infection in this patient population, there is a particular emphasis on preventative strategies that for maximal efficacy are linked to the nature of the immunosuppressive therapy required (the 'therapeutic prescription'). Early diagnosis and institution of effective therapy are the keys to success in the treatment of clinical infection. Great care is needed in treating infections in this patient population to avoid or manage drug interactions with the key components of the immunosuppressive regimen, namely cyclosporine and tacrolimus. Finally, it should be emphasized that because of the impaired inflammatory response created by immunosuppressive therapy signs and symptoms of infection are often greatly attenuated until late in the clinical course, requiring great skill and attention on the part of the clinician—an investment in time and energy that will be amply repaid by the well-being of these patients.

References

1. Hariharan S, Johnson CP, Bresnahan BA, *et al.* (2000). Improved graft survival after renal transplantation in the United States, 1988 to 1996. *New Engl J Med* **342**: 605–612.
2. Rubin RH (2000). Infection in the organ transplant recipient. In: Rubin RH and Young LS (eds) *Clinical approach to infection in the compromised host*, 4th edn. Plenum, New York.
3. Fishman JA, Rubin RH (1998). Infection in the organ transplant recipients. *New Engl J Med* **338**: 1741–1751.
4. Scowden EB, Schaffner W, Stone WJ (1978). Overwhelming strongyloidiasis: an unappreciated opportunistic infection. *Medicine (Baltimore)* **57**: 527–544.
5. Purtilo DT, Meyers WM, Commor DH (1974). Fatal strongyloidiasis in immunosuppressed patients. *Am J Med* **56**: 488–493.
6. DeVault GA Jr, King JW, Rohr MS, *et al.* (1990). Opportunistic infections with *Strongyloides stercoralis* in renal transplantatiom. *Rev Infect Dis* **12**: 653–671.
7. Dengler TJ, Strand N, Buhring I, *et al.* (1998). Differential immune response to influenza and pneumococcal vaccination in immunosuppressed patients after heart transplantation. *Transplantation* **66**: 1340–1347.
8. Huzly D, Neifer S, Reinke P, *et al.* (1997). Routine immunization in adult renal transplant recipients. *Transplantation* **63**: 839–845.
9. Hopkins C, Weber DJ, Rubin RH (1989). Invasive aspergillus infection: possible non-ward common source within the hospital environment. *J Hosp Infect* **12**: 19–25.
10. Rubin RH, Wolfson JS, Cosimi AB, *et al.* (1981). Infection in the renal transplant recipient. *Am J Med* **70**: 405–411.
11. Rubin RH, Cosimi AB, Tolkoff-Rubin NE, *et al.* (1977). Infectious disease syndromes attributable to cytomegalovirus and their significance among renal transplant recipients. *Transplantation* **24**: 458–464.
12. Marker SC, Howard RJ, Simmons RL, *et al.* (1981). Cytomegalovirus infection: a quantitative prospective study of 320 consecutive renal transplants. *Surgery* **89**: 660–671.
13. Simmons RL, Lopez C, Balfour HH Jr, *et al.* (1974). Cytomegalovirus: clinical virological correlations in renal transplant recipients. *Ann Surg* **180**: 623–634.
14. Simmons RL, Matas AJ, Rattazzi LC, *et al.* (1977). Clinical characteristics of the lethal cytomegalovirus infection following renal transplantation. *Surgery* **82**: 537–546.

15. Hibberd PL, Snydman DR (1995). Cytomegalovirus infection in organ transplant recipients. *Infect Dis Clin N Am* **9**: 863–877.
16. Rubin RH, Tolkoff-Rubin NE (1993). Antimicrobial strategies in the care of organ transplant recipients. *Antimicrob Agents Chemother* **37**: 619–624.
17. Grossi P, Kusne S, Rinaldo C, *et al.* (1996). Guidance of ganciclovir therapy with pp65 antigenemia in cytomegalovirus-free recipients of livers from seropositive donors. *Transplantation* **61**: 1659–1660.
18. Rubin RH (1991). Preemptive therapy in immunocompromised hosts. *New Engl J Med* **324**: 1057–1059.
19. Singh N, Yu VL, Mieles L, *et al.* (1994). High dose acyclovir compared with short course preemptive ganciclovir therapy to prevent cytomegalovirus disease in liver transplant recipients. *Ann Intern Med* **120**: 375–381.
20. Hibberd PL, Tolkoff-Rubin NE, Cosimi AB, *et al.* (1992). Symptomatic cytomegalovirus disease in the cytomegalovirus antibody seropositive renal transplant recipient treated with OKT3. *Transplantation* **53**: 68–72.
21. Hibberd PL, Tolkoff-Rubin NE, Conti D, *et al.* (1995). Preemptive ganciclovir therapy to prevent cytomegalovirus disease in cytomegalovirus antibody positive renal transplant recipients: a randomized controlled trial. *Ann Intern Med* **123**: 18–25.
22. Turgeon N, Fishman JA, Basgoz N, *et al.* (1998). Effect of oral acyclovir or ganciclovir therapy after preemptive intravenous ganciclovir therapy to prevent cytomegalovirus disease in cytomegalovirus seropositive renal and liver transplant recipients receiving antilymphocyte antibody therapy. *Transplantation* **66**: 1780–1786.
23. Tolkoff-Rubin NE, Rubin RH (1997). Urinary tract infection in the immunocompromised host. Lessons from kidney transplantation and the AIDS epidemic. *Infect Dis Clin N Am* **11**: 707–717.
24. Tolkoff-Rubin NE, Rubin RH (1998). Urinary tract infection in the compromised host. In: Brumfitt W, Hamilton-Miller JMT, Bailey RR (eds) *Urinary tract infections*, pp. 211–216. Chapman and Hall Medical, London.

PART II

INFECTIOUS COMPLICATIONS OF COMMON RENAL CONDITIONS, RENAL FAILURE, AND TRANSPLANTATION

5

Infectious complications of vasculitis, glomerulonephritis, and the nephrotic syndrome

Gill Gaskin

Introduction

Infection is an important cause of morbidity, and even mortality, in vasculitis and glomerular disease.[1,2] The predisposing factors include immunological abnormalities, structural damage directly attributable to the diseases, and the wide range of drug regimens used to treat them (summarized in Table 5.1). The breadth of the resulting immunosuppression contributes to the wide range of infections seen, and some patients may be infected with multiple pathogens. Immunosuppressed patients with infection may deteriorate rapidly, and urgent investigation is required. Distinguishing infection from active inflammatory disease can be difficult in multisystem diseases such as vasculitis and systemic lupus erythematosus (SLE).

Immunosuppressive treatments and the risk of infection

First-line treatment for vasculitis, rapidly progressive glomerulonephritis, and lupus nephritis includes corticosteroids, often at high dose. Many regimens contain pulsed methylprednisolone, while the starting dose of oral prednisolone dose is typically 1 mg/kg daily. A study in 75 patients with immunologically mediated renal disease suggested that steroid dose was the treatment factor most closely associated with severe infection, while the National Institutes of Health experience in Wegener's granulomatosis pointed to a greater risk of infection in patients on high doses of daily steroids than those treated on alternate days.[3,4] The risk of major infection was increased 20-fold in the month following a course of pulsed methylprednisolone in one study of patients with SLE.[5]

The alkylating agents cyclophosphamide and chlorambucil may predispose to infection by the induction of neutropenia, and to opportunistic organisms such as *Pneumocystis carinii* by the induction of lymphopenia when used in conjunction with corticosteroids.[6,7] Regimens involving intermittent pulses of cyclophosphamide appear to be safer than continuous oral dosing.[8,9] Pulsed therapy has been widely adopted in lupus nephritis, but in antineutrophil cytoplasmic antibody (ANCA) associated vasculitis doubts remain over its efficacy and clinical trials continue. Regimens avoiding cyclophosphamide are not themselves free of risk, as demonstrated by a study of prednisolone and methotrexate in Wegener's granulomatosis in which *Pneumocystis carinii* proved fatal in two patients.[10]

Table 5.1   Immunosuppression regimens in vasculitis and other causes of glomerular disease

Disease	First-line treatment	Alternatives
ANCA-associated vasculitis	Prednisolone + cyclophosphamide ± methylprednisolone pulses or plasma exchange	Prednisolone + methotrexate. Prednisolone + azathioprine or mycophenolate (remission treatment). Anti-T-cell antibodies (refractory disease)
Anti-GBM disease	Prednisolone + cyclophosphamide + plasma exchange	
SLE	Prednisolone + cyclophosphamide (usually as intermittent pulses) ± methylprednisolone pulses	Prednisolone + azathioprine or mycophenolate
Other forms of crescentic glomerulonephritis	Prednisolone + cyclophosphamide ± methylprednisolone pulses ± plasma exchange	
Membranous nephropathy	Prednisolone + chlorambucil (or no treatment)	Cyclosporine
Minimal change nephrotic syndrome	Prednisolone	Cyclophosphamide, cyclosporine
Focal segmental glomerulosclerosis	Prednisolone	Cyclophosphamide, cyclosporine

Abbreviations: ANCA, antineutrophil cytoplasmic antibodies; GBM, glomerular basement membrane; SLE, systemic lupus erythematosus.

Anti-T-cell agents such as cyclosporine A, used in certain types of nephrotic syndrome, increase the risk of viral infections, though it is worth noting that treatment doses are often lower than those used in organ transplantation. Treatment-associated infections are infrequent, as exemplified by a recent study of cyclosporine A in focal segmental glomerulosclerosis.[11] Plasma exchange is used in certain diseases, but despite immunoglobulin depletion, and concerns from early studies there is no evidence that this contributes substantially to the risk of infection when the contribution of concurrent immunosuppressive drugs is excluded.[12,13] Infections of vascular access sites may be problematic, but these also occur in dialysed patients not treated with plasma exchange (see Chapter 18).[14]

Many studies have pointed to the particular susceptibility of elderly patients to infectious complications of immunosuppression, particularly in the presence of renal failure.[15–17] Experience suggests that doses of alkylating agents should be reduced and combinations of multiple immunosuppressive strategies avoided. Continued immunosuppression after the onset of end-stage renal failure increases the risk of infection in patients established on continuous ambulatory peritoneal dialysis, in comparison with non-immunosuppressed patients, but the relative merits of haemodialysis and peritoneal dialysis in this setting have not been tested.[18]

This chapter focuses principally on the infections which have commonly been reported using current approaches to treatment. Future therapeutic developments may alter the spectrum of organisms encountered, and will further strengthen the arguments for thorough investigation of any infection in an immunocompromised patient with renal disease.

Infection in vasculitis

The primary vasculitic diseases are now commonly classified according to the Chapel Hill consensus nomenclature, which categorizes syndromes according to the smallest vessel affected, together with other characteristic features.[19] The primary small vessel vasculitides, affecting arterioles, capillaries, and venules, are commonly managed by the nephrologist due to their propensity to cause necrotizing and crescentic glomerulonephritis. They include Wegener's granulomatosis which is characterized by granulomatous inflammation in the respiratory tract. The resulting structural damage to the nasal cavity, sinuses, and airways predisposes to infection. The other small vessel vasculitides are microscopic polyangiitis and the Churg–Strauss syndrome (with characteristic asthma and eosinophilia). All three conditions, together with renal-limited vasculitis (isolated pauci-immune necrotizing glomerulonephritis) are associated with ANCA directed against one of two neutrophil granule enzymes: proteinase 3 and myeloperoxidase. Using standardized assays, the specificity of these autoantibodies for small vessel vasculitis exceeds 95% and the sensitivity in the presence of renal involvement exceeds 80%. These conditions run a relapsing course in up to 50% of patients, and prolonged or repeated courses of immunosuppressive drugs are often required.[20]

Other vasculitides (including polyarteritis nodosa affecting medium-sized arteries, and temporal arteritis and Takayasu's arteritis affecting large arteries) are more commonly treated by rheumatologists and will not be discussed in detail here, but share some of the infectious complications of ANCA-associated vasculitis due to similarities in treatment.

The number of cases of vasculitis referred for treatment is increasing, and the median age at presentation is rising. A recent study in a well-defined United Kingdom population estimated that the incidence of primary systemic vasculitis peaked in the 65–74 year age group, at 60.1 per million.[21] This is important in view of the susceptibility of older patients to infectious complications.[15–17] It is unclear whether the increased referral rate is due to a genuine increase in incidence or to improved recognition, but the net effect is that vasculitis is now an important cause of opportunistic infection, accounting for 22% of cases of *Pneumocystis carinii* in patients without AIDS in one series.[22]

There are few recent data on the precise incidence of infection with current approaches to immunosuppressive therapy, though older data give an indication of its importance. In an assiduous study of the induction therapy period in 75 patients with immune-mediated renal disease treated in the late 1970s, Cohen *et al.* reported 3.69 infections per patient, or 0.74 infections per week of induction immunosuppression; the majority were caused by 'ordinary' bacteria.[3] The study was designed to pick up all infections however trivial and some infections related to interventions which are now rarely used, including acute peritoneal dialysis and arteriovenous shunts for temporary vascular access. Nonetheless, 70% of the infections identified were 'clinically significant' and overall 11.3% of the patients with vasculitis experienced a serious opportunistic infection. More recently, Adu *et al.* reporting a randomized controlled trial in which two immunosuppression regimens were compared noted 1.7 infections per patient over a median follow-up period of around 40 months, while Hoffman *et al.* in a long-term follow-up series (follow-up 6 months to 24 years) noted that 46% of the patients had one or more serious infections, amounting to 0.11 per patient year.[4,23] Investigation and treatment of infection has significant resource implications; Aasarod and colleagues reported that 32% of patients treated in Norway for Wegener's granulomatosis with renal involvement required hospitalization for infection during a median follow-up period of 41.5 months.[17]

Immunosuppressive regimens for vasculitis typically follow a tapering schedule. Serious and fatal infections occur most commonly in the first 3 months of treatment and account for half to two-thirds of the early deaths.[24] Most of the remainder are due to active vasculitis, illustrating the difficult balance between undertreatment and over-treatment. Table 5.2 lists the most common fatal infections in published series.

Infection in other glomerular diseases

Many of the factors predisposing to infection are common to a variety of diseases, including the immunosuppressive effect of renal impairment (if present) and the effects of immunosuppressive treatment (see Table 5.1). However, it is worth noting that most regimens used for the more chronic glomerulonephritides are associated with lower infection rates than the intensive regimens used for rapidly progressive glomerulonephritis and diffuse proliferative lupus nephritis. For example, the alternating methylprednisolone and chlorambucil regimen advocated for nephrotic syndrome due to membranous nephropathy has been associated with surprisingly few serious infections when used in patients with normal renal function.

Some specific predisposing factors relating to the renal diseases themselves merit comment: the hypocomplementaemia which may be associated with SLE and with some cases of mesangiocapillary glomerulonephritis, the particular susceptibility to encapsulated organisms in the nephrotic syndrome (predisposing to the same range of infectious agents), and the culture medium provided by the tissue oedema and ascites of the nephrotic patient.

In Cohen's series the infection rate was higher in SLE than in vasculitis or antiglomerular basement membrane-mediated nephritis. There is no doubt that SLE patients are predisposed to an extended range of pathogens, including *Salmonella*, a susceptibility which is not fully explained.[3,25] However, recent data suggest a much lower incidence of infection in SLE, at 0.14 major infections and 0.29 minor infections per patient year, and this may reflect the trend towards use of pulsed cyclophosphamide therapy with a lower cumulative dose.[5]

Infection in the nephrotic syndrome has been studied most comprehensively in children. Historically, the nephrotic syndrome carried a significant mortality and this was largely due to sepsis. The overall death rate is now much lower, but infection remains an important cause, particularly in less developed countries. The International Study of Kidney Disease in Children reported 10 deaths in 389 children with minimal change nephrotic syndrome, of which six were due to sepsis.[26] Although there are fewer

Table 5.2 Fatal infections in treatment of vasculitis (series containing at least 20 patients)

Author	Diagnosis	Incidence	Nature of infection
Coward et al.[46] (1986)	WG or MP with nephritis	6/36 (17%)	Pneumonia (6)
Adu et al.[24] (1987)	Vasculitis with nephritis	8/43 (19%)	'Generalised infection' (3), respiratory infection (5)
Fuiano et al.[47] (1988)	WG or MP with nephritis	2/20 (10%)	Pneumonia (1), septicaemia (1)
Falk et al.[48] (1990)	AASV with nephritis	4/70 (6%)	Peritonitis after perforated viscus (1), not specified (3)
Andrassy et al.[49] (1991)	WG with nephritis	0/25 (0%)	
Haubitz et al.[50] (1991)	WG	0/23 (0%)	
Hoffman et al.[4] (1992)	WG (Rx cyclophosphamide)	5/158 (3%)	Not specified
Hoffman et al.[10] (1992)	WG (Rx methotrexate)	2/29 (7%)	PCP (2)
Guillevin et al.[51] (1992)	PAN and CSS	1/78 (1%)	Septicaemia
Bindi et al.[28] (1993)	AASV with nephritis	4/40 (10%)	Septic shock (1), varicella zoster encephalitis (1), pulmonary aspergillus (1), post-transfusion AIDS (1)
Gordon et al.[20] (1993)	SV	13/150 (9%)	Early deaths; nature of infection not specified
Adu et al.[23] (1997)	ANCA-associated vasculitis	2/54 (4%)	Septicaemia (2)
Gayraud et al.[52] (1997)	Good prognosis CSS and PAN	1/25 (4%)	Multiple respiratory pathogens (*Pseudomonas, Aspergillus, S. aureus*)
Guillevin et al.[8] (1997)	WG	9/50 (18%)	Bacterial pneumonia (1), PCP (6), encephalitis (1), septic shock (1)
Haubitz et al.[9] (1998)	WG	3/47 (6%)	Not specified
McLaughlin et al.[53] (1998)	Pauci-immune nephritis	4/47 (9%)	Bacterial pneumonia (2), PCP (2)
Aasarod et al.[17] (2000)	WG	5/108 (5%)	Pneumonia (3), PCP (2)

Abbreviations: SV = systemic vasculitis; AASV = ANCA-associated vasculitis (ANCA = antineutrophil cytoplasmic antibodies); WG = Wegener's granulomatosis; MP = microscopic polyangiitis; PAN = polyarteritis nodosa; CSS = Churg–Strauss syndrome; PCP = *Pneumocystis carinii* pneumonia.

systematic studies in adults, the combination of hypoglobulinaemia and renal impairment has been associated with an increased risk of bacterial infections, which may prove fatal.[27]

Patterns of infection in vasculitis and glomerular disease

Respiratory infections

The most common fatal infections in immune-mediated renal disease are respiratory. A variety of pathogens can be responsible, singly or in combination, and the symptoms and radiological findings are rarely specific. In Cohen's series Gram-negative bacteria were the largest single category, accounting for 40% of the respiratory infections.[3] Table 5.3 illustrates some of the infections which may present with fever and pulmonary infiltrates, together with non-infectious differential diagnoses. The range of organisms illustrates the difficulty of empirical therapy and the need for swift investigation.

Bacterial infection

Bacterial pneumonias are common in the debilitated hospitalized patient when Gram-negative organisms often predominate. They may also arise distal to obstructing

Table 5.3   Causes of fever and pulmonary infiltrates in patients treated for immune-mediated renal disease (this list is not exhaustive)

Infective causes	
Bacteria	Conventional respiratory pathogens including Gram-negative bacteria and *S. aureus* Mycobacteria *Nocardia* *Legionella* *Mycoplasma*
Fungi	*Pneumocystis carinii* *Aspergillus fumigatus* *Histoplasma* *Coccidioides*
Parasites	*Strongyloides stercoralis* *Toxoplasma* spp.
Viruses	Cytomegalovirus Herpes simplex Varicella zoster Respiratory syncytial virus Adenovirus
Non-infective causes	Pulmonary oedema Pulmonary haemorrhage Pulmonary granulomas Pulmonary emboli Tumour Drug-induced pneumonitis (e.g. methotrexate)

airway lesions in Wegener's granulomatosis, and late in the disease course where vasculitic damage has led to focal areas of bronchiectasis. Hypocomplementaemic and nephrotic patients are at risk of pneumonia due to encapsulated bacteria, even in the absence of specific immunosuppressive therapy.

Atypical pneumonias due to *Legionella* and *Mycoplasma* are also reported in immune-mediated disease, though less commonly.

Reactivated tuberculosis

Reactivated tuberculosis is a recognized complication of vasculitis treatment, and can present with similar respiratory symptoms and radiological appearances to the underlying disease.[28,29] The presentation of reactivated disease may often be extrapulmonary and atypical. To prevent these clinical dilemmas, patients with clinical or radiological evidence of previous tuberculous infection who are to commence intensive immunosuppression (comprising, for example, more than 15 mg prednisolone/day) should be treated with prophylactic isoniazid 300 mg/day, together with pyridoxine 10 mg/day, for 1 year.

Fungal infection

Aspergillus fumigatus infection may be acquired through inhalation of spores, and may colonize damaged lung, including residual cavities from resolved granulomas. Secondary infection should always be excluded in patients with apparently non-resolving Wegener's granulomas before escalating their immunosuppressive therapy. Invasive disease is confined to the immunosuppressed and may become generalized; it often coexists with other infections and carries a significant mortality. Following acute treatment of *Aspergillus* with amphotericin, patients requiring continuing immunosuppression should receive prophylactic itraconazole.[2]

Pneumocystis carinii

Pneumocystis carinii is the most commonly reported opportunistic respiratory pathogen, affecting 6–20% of patients in series reported prior to the use of cotrimoxazole prophylaxis. In two detailed reports of *Pneumocystis carinii* pneumonia in patients treated for Wegener's granulomatosis infection tended to occur during the period of intensive immunosuppression for induction of remission of newly diagnosed or recurrent disease, typically at 2–4 months from commencement of therapy.[7,30] The highest incidence (6/23 patients) was reported by Jarrousse *et al.* in recruits to a randomized controlled trial; the completed trial was reported by Guillevin *et al.* with a final incidence of *Pneumocystis carinii* pneumonia of 20%.[8,30] The six patients described in detail by Jarrousse *et al.* had impaired renal function, and had received intensive induction immunosuppression (three pulses of methylprednisolone, oral prednisolone at 1 mg/kg, and a pulse of intravenous cyclophosphamide followed by further oral or intravenous therapy, with doses adjusted to suppress the nadir neutrophil count to less than 3000/mm^3.[30] Mean prednisolone dose at diagnosis of *Pneumocystis carinii* pneumonia was 56.6 mg/day, while the mean daily oral dose of cyclophosphamide was 117 mg/day, and the mean pulse dose was 1.3 g. The mean lymphocyte count at diagnosis of *Pneumocystis carinii* pneumonia was 495/mm^3. The findings of Ognibene *et al.* were similar: mean lymphocyte count was 303/mm^3 and immunosuppression invariably comprised a combination of moderate to high dose steroids, together with a second immunosuppressive agent.[7]

Godeau *et al.* compared 12 patients with Wegener's granulomatosis who developed *Pneumocystis carinii* pneumonia with 32 patients treated in the same four hospitals during the same period (1984–92) who did not experience the infection, and who had not received prophylactic cotrimoxazole.[6] Both groups developed lymphopenia during treatment, with a similar absolute fall in lymphocyte numbers. The resulting lymphopenia was more marked in the infected group in terms of mean lymphocyte count (1060/mm^3 versus 1426/mm^3), lowest absolute lymphocyte count (244/mm^3 versus 738/mm^3), and number of patients with lymphocyte counts of less than 600/mm^3 in the first 3 months (10/12 versus 11/32); a multivariate analysis demonstrated that the infected group had a lower count prior to immunosuppressive treatment. The infected group had a higher mean cumulative cyclophosphamide dose at the end of the second and third months of treatment, but did not differ in cumulative steroid dose or in the proportion of patients treated with cyclophosphamide pulses.

Since the appreciation of *Pneumocystis carinii* as an important opportunistic pathogen in patients treated for ANCA-associated vasculitis, it has become common practice to use low-dose cotrimoxazole prophylaxis. It seems particularly prudent to use it in patients with a marked fall in lymphocyte count.

The clinical presentation of *Pneumocystis carinii* pneumonia in vasculitis is comparable to that in other immunosuppressed patients, with a combination of cough, fever, and dyspnoea. Infiltrates are seen on the chest radiograph in most cases, but must be compared with previous imaging to distinguish new infective changes with pre-existing vasculitic or granulomatous disease. Diagnosis was made in most of the published cases by bronchoalveolar lavage. Ten of the 11 patients reported by Ognibene *et al.* and three of the six reported by Jarrousse *et al.* responded to high-dose cotrimoxazole.[7,30] The recommended dose is 15–20 mg trimethoprim and 75–100 mg sulphamethoxazole/kg/day, divided into two or four doses, given intravenously or orally for 2 weeks. The dose should be reduced in the presence of moderate or severe renal impairment.

Pneumocystis carinii may also complicate other immune-mediated diseases treated with immunosuppression, but it is a less common problem than in ANCA-associated vasculitis. A Californian study, in which hospital admissions for *Pneumocystis carinii* pneumonia in patients with connective tissue diseases were identified from a State database, demonstrated that patients with Wegener's granulomatosis and polyarteritis nodosa had the highest frequency of infection, with a five-fold higher incidence than in SLE.[31]

Other opportunistic respiratory infections

Cytomegalovirus (CMV) is an important cause of pneumonitis in the immunosuppressed patient, and may coexist with *Pneumocystis carinii*. Clinical clues to its presence include cytopenias and evidence of extrapulmonary disease such as hepatitis and enteritis. Treatment with ganciclovir (with appropriate dose adjustments for renal function) is usually successful. Other causes of viral pneumonitis include influenza, respiratory syncytial virus, and adenovirus.

Nocardia asteroides is a soil-living Gram-positive branching bacterium that is acquired by inhalation. The primary respiratory infection often, but not invariably, produces focal or even nodular infiltrates, and may spread haematogenously to the central nervous system. It is an unusual infection in immune-mediated renal disease.

Strongyloides stercoralis hyperinfection (see below) may rarely present with respiratory symptoms, and should be considered in patients from endemic areas.

Management of the patient with suspected respiratory infection

There are several important principles:

1. Deterioration may occur rapidly in immunosuppressed patients, and there may be a brief window of opportunity for investigation.
2. There may be multiple pathogens.
3. Not all pulmonary shadowing is infective.

For these reasons urgent investigations directed towards confirming or excluding specific diagnoses are to be preferred to blind therapy. All patients should undergo routine blood count and culture of blood and sputum, though some care is needed in interpreting the result of sputum culture: some organisms detected may derive from the nasopharynx (e.g. *Candida*) while other important pulmonary pathogens (e.g. *Pneumocystis carinii*) may not appear in the sputum at all. Serological tests for *Legionella* and *Mycoplasma* should also be performed. Investigation should also include a chest radiograph and analysis of blood gases, to assess the extent and severity of the suspected infection. In patients with normal oxygenation at rest, desaturation after exercise (a 6-min walk) may reveal early evidence of a pneumonitis. Where pulmonary haemorrhage due to active alveolar capillaritis is an alternative diagnosis (and it is rare for this to develop once other indices of the disease are under control) measurement of the transfer factor for carbon monoxide (K_{CO}) is a useful investigation; uptake of carbon monoxide by blood in the alveolar space increases the K_{CO}, while pneumonitis reduces it. Supplementary oxygen, or even assisted ventilation, may be required to support the patient while awaiting a response to specific therapy.

Empirical broad-spectrum antibacterial therapy may be appropriate if an opportunistic pathogen is unlikely, for example when the doses of immunosuppressive drugs are low, gas exchange is normal, the radiological changes are not widespread, and the patient is clinically stable. In other circumstances it is wise to proceed to bronchoscopy and bronchoalveolar lavage to obtain samples for microbiological analysis. If a diagnosis is not secured by the combination of these approaches, open lung biopsy may be required after weighing the significant risks of the procedure against the risks of failing to make a diagnosis and institute appropriate therapy.

Gastrointestinal and liver infections

This group of infections includes those which affect the gut (at any level from the mouth to the rectum) those which cause peritonitis and those which cause a hepatitis.

Mucosal and oesophageal Candida

Cohen's series contained nine cases of *Candida* infection of either the mouth or vagina, complicated by fungaemia in one case and gastro-oesophageal invasion in another.[3] Oral candidiasis, which causes characteristic creamy-white patches on the buccal mucosa, was also a common minor infection in patients treated for SLE.[5] Topical antifungal agents (nystatin solution, amphotericin lozenges) are often sufficient to treat oral *Candida* and are widely used for prevention of mucosal colonization in patients on high–dose steroids. Patients on immunosuppression who develop retrosternal burning pain or dysphagia should undergo endoscopy to look for *Candida* oesophagitis, which can then be treated with fluconazaole. The differential diagnosis includes herpes simplex infection, peptic ulceration due to steroid therapy, and CMV oesophagitis and gastritis.

Herpes simplex stomatitis

Labial or oral herpes simplex is a common complication in patients treated with immuno-suppression, and may occasionally be complicated by a systemic febrile illness. In Cohen's series, two patients had a probable hepatitis due to the virus, and one developed an ocular infection.[3] However, recurrent oral ulceration may also be part of a vasculitic illness, and virus culture from the base of the ulcer may assist in the differential diagnosis. The choice of route of treatment with aciclovir or similar agents will depend on the severity and extent of the infection.

Cytomegalovirus

Cytomegalovirus is a common asymptomatic infection in healthy individuals. Infection in immunosuppressed patients usually represents reactivation of latent disease. The infection does not invariably cause tissue invasive disease, and its manifestations are sometimes limited to a high spiking fever and reductions in the leucocyte and platelet count. Rises in transaminases are common. Gut involvement is a feature of invasive disease, and may occur at any level in the alimentary tract. It may mimic gut vasculitis or gastrointestinal complications of steroid therapy—presenting with pain, bleeding, or even perforation. In the presence of diarrhoea, there is a wide differential diagnosis as discussed below. While CMV enteritis generally develops after an apparent response to vasculitis therapy, the infection has been diagnosed as early as 10 days into treatment.

Cytomegalovirus infection is usually accompanied by detectable virus in throat washings and/or urine (for example by detection of early antigens in infected cell cultures), and by detection of antigenaemia or DNA by PCR; gastric or intestinal biopsies may reveal typical inclusion bodies. Viral culture and changes in CMV IgG titre are too slow to be clinically valuable. Tissue-invasive disease should be treated with ganciclovir, with dose modification in the presence of renal failure.

Strongyloidiasis

Infection with *Strongyloides stercoralis* which has been asymptomatic for many years may be transformed into hyperinfection by corticosteroid therapy. This may present with non-specific intestinal symptoms or clinical features consequent upon the haematogenous spread of the larvae after entry through the skin, including polymicrobial bacteraemia, pulmonary infiltrates, or meninigitis. This is uncommon; one case of disseminated *Strongyloides* was reported in a patient treated for rapidly progressive glomerulonephritis by Rondeau *et al.*[15] A careful past medical and travel history is important for identifying patients at risk. The diagnosis may be confirmed by the detection of larvae in the stool or duodenal aspirates; treatment is thiabendazole or mebendazole.

Differential diagnosis of enteric symptoms

In addition to the opportunistic infections which are described above, immunosuppressed patients are also susceptible to hospital-acquired *Clostridium difficile* pseudomembranous colitis, to common food-borne infections such as *Campylobacter* and *Salmonella* and to drug-associated pancreatitis (corticosteroids and azathioprine have been implicated). Patients with SLE appear to be at particular risk of a more severe systemic illness when infected with non-typhoid *Salmonella*.[25] Older patients, representing the majority of those with ANCA-associated vasculitis, may also present with complications of diverticular disease, which is common in this age group.

Thorough investigation is therefore required in the patient presenting with enteric symptoms: blood and stool cultures should be obtained. The stool should be tested for *Clostridium difficile* toxin and examined for parasites. If these tests proved negative endoscopies should be considered to obtain aspirates (from the stomach) or biopsies for the presence of CMV. Where enteric symptoms are accompanied by extraintestinal evidence of CMV, immediate ganciclovir therapy is appropriate.

To complicate matters further, gastrointestinal vasculitis may itself present with abdominal pain, diarrhoea, or gastrointestinal bleeding, though this is rare in the absence of other evidence of active disease. The diagnosis is supported by the finding of mucosal purpura at endoscopy and by areas of neutrophil uptake on indium-labelled leucocyte scanning. Biopsies, though rarely undertaken, may be diagnostic and in Churg–Strauss syndrome they may show intense eosinophil infiltration. Involvement of larger vessels, more characteristic of polyarteritis nodosa, may lead to symptomatic gut ischaemia. Perforation of gut affected by small or medium vessel vasculitis may lead to peritonitis and secondary bacterial infection.

Primary bacterial peritonitis

This is a particular complication of the nephrotic syndrome and has been most commonly reported in children with minimal change disease. The oldest patient reported by Cameron from the Guy's Hospital experience was 21.[32] In one study of 351 American children with nephrotic syndrome, 5.5% of those diagnosed between 1970 and 1980 developed peritonitis, with approximately a quarter experiencing more than one episode.[33] *Streptococcus pneumoniae* accounted for 50% of cases, and *Escherischia coli* 25% (including two cases with underlying gut pathology). Importantly, all children had peritonism even in the face of corticosteroid therapy. In another American study there had been little change in the incidence (17%) or spectrum of infecting organisms over a 20-year period; around 50% were proven pneumococcal infections or were culture negative but responded to penicillin.[34] More recent data confirm that peritonitis remains a significant problem in less developed countries and that penicillin-resistant pneumococcal infections are beginning to be recognized in nephrotic children.[35,36] The differential diagnosis includes abdominal pain related to intravascular depletion and primary gut pathology; in two cases in Krensky's series this was the cause of *Escherischia coli*-positive peritonitis.[33]

When primary bacterial peritonitis is suspected blood culture and diagnostic aspirate of ascitic fluid should be performed, and empirical antibiotics commenced. The chosen antibiotics should have broad-spectrum activity, unless diplococci have been identified on Gram stain. Local pneumococcal resistance patterns should be taken into account.

Continuous ambulatory peritoneal dialysis peritonitis

Andrews *et al.* identified immunosuppressive treatment for immune-mediated renal disease as a risk factor for the development of peritonitis in patients on continuous ambulatory peritoneal dialysis (CAPD).[18] Patients treated with immunosuppression at any point in the preceding 12 months had more episodes of peritonitis than other patients treated simultaneously on the same CAPD programme (1.8 versus 0.68 episodes per patient year), and the rate was highest in the small subgroup with vasculitis, at three episodes per patient year. Immunosuppression was also associated with a higher incidence of infection with *Staphylococcus aureus*, and with fungi, although the latter often followed treatment for recurrent episodes of bacterial infection. Acute peritoneal dialysis is now rarely used for acute renal failure due to immune-mediated disease, but may equally be associated with an increased risk of infection. Cohen's series, based on clinical experience in the late 1970s when acute peritoneal dialysis with non-tunnelled catheters was common, contained 19 episodes of peritoneal infection in 23 patients treated using the technique; 85% were clinically significant.[3] The differential diagnosis of dialysis-related peritonitis includes direct trauma to the bowel during catheter insertion and perforation of the gut due to active vasculitis or steroid-related peptic ulceration; we have seen both.

In immunosuppressed patients reporting cloudy dialysis effluent, microscopy and culture must be performed promptly and empirical antibiotics commenced using a standard first-line regimen (e.g. intraperitoneal vancomycin and gentamicin), pending culture. If mixed cultures, gut flora or anaerobes are cultured, serious consideration should be given to laparotomy to look for intestinal pathology.

Viral hepatitis

Transmission of viral hepatitis is a potential risk in a group of patients who commonly require blood products during their initial illness, but should be infrequent with current screening methods. Bindi *et al.* reported one patient who acquired HIV through transfusion during treatment for vasculitis.[28] Ponticelli *et al.* reported one case of fulminant viral hepatitis 40 months after completion of combined steroid/chlorambucil therapy, but the relationship to the treatment is unknown.[37] Hepatitis B and C are more commonly appreciated as causes rather than consequences of vasculitis illnesses (polyarteritis nodosa and cryoglobulinaemia respectively) and both may be associated with isolated glomerulonephritis.

Central nervous system infections

Central nervous system (CNS) infections generally occur as opportunistic events in patients who, due to difficult disease, have received particularly heavy immunosuppression, and are not common in vasculitis or nephritis. No cerebral infections were seen in the patients with immune-mediated renal disease studied during their induction therapy by Cohen *et al.* although there are a few episodes in other reported series.[3] There were

Table 5.4 Patterns of cerebral infection in immune-mediated renal disease

Type of infection	Cause
Meningitis	*Streptococcus pneumoniae, Haemophilus influenzae, Neisseria meningitidis* *Listeria monocytogenes* Echovirus *Cryptococcus* *Mycobacterium tuberculosis**
Focal lesions/abscesses	*Aspergillus* *Toxoplasma gondii* *Nocardia* *Mycobacterium tuberculosis* *Cryptococcus* Pyogenic and anaerobic bacteria
Encephalitis	*Toxoplasma gondii* *Listeria* Progressive multifocal leucoencephalopathy Varicella zoster Herpes simplex Cytomegalovirus

*Subacute course.

two cases of *Cryptococcus* in the series by Krafcik *et al.* in which the rate of fatal infectious complications was generally high in an older group of patients requiring intensive treatment.[16] Where CNS infections occur, they may present with meningitis, following either an acute or more indolent course, an encephalitic picture or with focal signs due to abscess. Investigation should occur early without waiting for 'classical' symptoms to develop. Table 5.4 indicates the most common causative organisms for different patterns of disease. Impairment of cell-mediated immunity due to high-dose steroids is associated particularly with *Listeria* and *Cryptococcus*, while neutropenia induced by cytotoxic agents is more likely to be associated with pyogenic infections or *Aspergillus*.

Meningitis

While patients on immunosuppressive treatment may develop acute meningitis due to the usual pyogenic infections (*Streptococcus pneumoniae, Haemophilus influenzae*, and *Neisseria meningitidis*) their susceptibility to these is only significantly increased if they are hypocomplementaemic (for example in association with SLE or mesangiocapillary glomerulonephritis), nephrotic or have impaired splenic function. Rarely, meningococcal disease may be the first indicator of a systemic disease causing hypocomplementaemia. Otherwise *Listeria monocytogenes* is the major concern. The clinical presentation typically comprises 2 to 10 days of fever and headache, although focal signs due to a cerebritis or a septicaemic presentation are also possible. In spite of the name, the organism usually causes a neutrophil leucocytosis in the cerebrospinal fluid (CSF), which is indistinguishable from the pattern in other bacterial infections. *Listeria* does not respond to treatment with third-generation cephalosporins, which might otherwise be used as blind treatment for meningitis pending CT scan and culture results. The addition of high-dose ampicillin, with or without gentamicin, is advisable.

Cryptococcus neoformans is an important CNS pathogen in chronically immunosuppressed patients. The typical presentation is subacute, with fever and headache, often with rather subtle signs of meningism; altered level of consciousness, focal signs, and seizures are also possible. The presence of pulmonary or skin lesions may point to the diagnosis; the rarer *Nocardia* is an important differential diagnosis in such circumstances and biopsy is required to make the distinction. Definitive diagnosis of cryptococcal meningitis requires identification of the organism in the CSF by India ink staining or detection of cryptococcal antigen; assay of serum for cryptococcal antigen is insufficient. Treatment is with amphotericin B.

Focal cerebral lesions

Cerebral abscesses are commonly fungal. *Aspergillus* is an important organism, particularly in neutropenic patients with evidence of disseminated fungal infection. *Nocardia asteroides* has been reported as an opportunistic infection in several cases of immune-mediated renal disease, classically causing multifocal abnormalities. The infection is spread haematogenously, and associated pulmonary and cutaneous lesions may be found. Toxoplasmosis is uncommon in immune-mediated renal disease. Empirical treatment for this organism alone is not to be preferred to seeking a tissue diagnosis.

Patients with Wegener's granulomatosis with unusually destructive sinus abnormalities are at risk of dural defects through which the CSF can be infected although this degree of tissue destruction is very rare. We have seen one patient who developed a *Staphylococcus aureus* meningitis and later a jugular foramen abscess responding to antistaphylococcal antibiotics.

Encephalitis

This a rare infectious complication of immune-mediated renal disease, although deaths from varicella zoster encephalitis and from a papovavirus multifocal encephalitis have been reported.[8,28] *Listeria* and *Toxoplasma* can present with an encephalitic picture; herpes simplex and CMV do so rarely in immunocompromised patients.

Differential diagnosis

The differential diagnosis includes manifestations of the underlying disease or noninfectious complications of therapy.

A minority of patients with ANCA-associated vasculitis have CNS involvement in the initial illness which may manifest in a variety of ways—as impaired consciousness, focal signs or seizures. The signs may result from intracerebral vascular lesions or rarely from granulomatous lesions: Wegener's granulomatosis may directly involve the meninges. Neuropsychiatric involvement is more common in SLE but in all of these syndromes the neurological abnormalities usually improve quickly with therapy and rarely recur in isolation. Where neurological abnormalities emerge during therapy, an infectious cause must therefore be sought. In patients with the nephrotic syndrome, thrombotic complications such as cortical vein thrombosis must be considered as an alternative explanation.

The treatment itself may cause neurological symptoms and signs. Aseptic meningitis is a recognized complication of intravenous immunoglobulin therapy, and high-dose corticosteroids are a potent cause of psychiatric disturbance. Finally, cerebral lymphoma should be considered in patients who have had prolonged exposure to immunosuppressive agents.

Investigation of CNS infections

The initial assessment should include a detailed history including contacts with infection, travel history (malaria should not be forgotten) and previous neurological manifestations of the underlying disease. It is critical to gauge the speed of progression. Clinical examination should include a thorough search for skin lesions which can be biopsied for microscopy and culture. Immediate investigations should include a blood count, blood and urine cultures, and a chest radiograph. An urgent CT scan should be arranged followed by CSF examination if there are no contraindications. Where focal lesions are identified, consideration should be given to biopsy.

Bacteraemia and line-related sepsis

Cohen *et al.* reported bacterial infections in 22 of 50 patients with an arteriovenous shunt for renal support or plasma exchange; 60% of the infections were with Gram-positive organisms.[3] Thirteen of the patients had an episode of septicaemia, but with a different causative organism, implying that the risk factor was access to the circulation rather than the presence of a local infection. Septicaemia was unusual in the absence of a shunt. Shunts are now used only rarely, but dual-lumen venous lines used in their place predispose to similar infections.

Investigation and treatment of suspected line-related sepsis follows the conventions in dialysis patients (see Chapter 18): empirical therapy should cover *Staphylococcus aureus*, including MRSA in units with a high prevalence, and temporary lines should be removed.

Empirical therapy for septicaemia where the primary focus is not certain will depend on the nature of the underlying disease and immunodeficiency. It should include cover for Gram-negative organisms in all cases, cover for *Staphylococcus aureus* in patients with in-dwelling lines or with Wegener's granulomatosis, cover for encapsulated bacteria in patients with nephrotic syndrome or hypocomplementaemia and cover for *Pseudomonas* in the presence of neutropenia. Local patterns of antibiotic resistance (including the prevalence of penicillin-resistant pneumococci) should be borne in mind when selecting antibiotics.

Skin and soft tissue infections

Cellulitis

Risk factors for bacterial infections of the skin and soft tissues include tissue ischaemia or necrosis due to vasculitis, tissue oedema due to the nephrotic state, portals for entry of infection at venepuncture sites and areas of skin breakdown, and defects of humoral immunity. Patients with the nephrotic syndrome are therefore at particular risk. Cellulitis in nephrotic syndrome is not confined to 'conventional' Gram-positive organisms and there are numerous reports of *Escherischia coli* and other Gram-negative organisms causing cellulitis (and even Fournier's gangrene developing in an oedematous scrotum) in nephrotic children. Investigation should therefore include blood cultures and aspirates of cellulitic tissue if possible prior to starting broad-spectrum antibiotics.

Herpes zoster

Herpes zoster is a common complication of steroid therapy and combined immunosuppressive regimens. It has been reported in 10–20% of patients treated for vasculitis and lupus nephritis, and also in patients treated with combined regimens for membranous nephropathy.[4,38–41] It may occasionally become a generalized infection and prove fatal and requires prompt treatment with high-dose aciclovir, with dose adjusted for renal function.[28] Primary varicella zoster infection can be a very severe infection in immunocompromised patients, and postexposure prophylaxis with zoster-immune globulin should be considered in any patient exposed to chickenpox who does not have a clear prior history of chickenpox, and in whom urgent serology does not demonstrate immunity.

Skin involvement in systemic opportunistic infections

Skin lesions may be early manifestations of certain opportunistic infections, including *Cryptococcus* and *Nocardia*. Unexplained lesions should be biopsied, smears performed on the biopsy sample, and the biopsy cultured. Confirmation of cutaneous infection with these organisms should be accompanied by screening for pulmonary and CSF infection, and should be fully treated, as systemic spread may follow.

Urinary infections

The typical pattern in published series of vasculitis and immune-mediated renal disease is that urinary infections are common but rarely serious or life-threatening.[3,23] Urinary infections were the most common bacterial infection in patients studied during the induction phase of their immunosuppression in Cohen's series and were more common in females than males.[3] However, only 60% of the proven infections were considered clinically significant and urine infection only contributed to one death—in a neutropenic patient with *Pseudomonas* in the blood, urine, and sputum. Most infections were caused by enterobacteria and the most common single isolate was *Klebsiella*. Urinary infection was the most common cause of minor infection in a large cohort of patients treated in Malaysia for SLE of whom 93% were female. Urinary tract infection is perhaps more common than generally appreciated in nephrotic children with urinary infections accounting for 40% of infections in one series in the absence of urinary tract malformation in the majority of cases.[42]

Predisposing factors in hospitalized patients include urinary catheterization and this should be avoided wherever possible. Hourly monitoring of urine output is not required in the oliguric patient with rapidly progressive glomerulonephritis since the primary problem is not renal perfusion amenable to hour-by-hour manipulations of the patient's fluid balance and haemodynamics. Obstruction to the urinary tract by prostatic granuloma in Wegener's granulomatosis is a rare but recognized cause of urinary sepsis.

Where urinary symptoms develop in patients who are established on treatment regimens containing cyclophosphamide, haemorrhagic cystitis due to a toxic metabolite of the drug, acrolein, is an important differential diagnosis. Cystoscopy should be arranged if the urine is culture negative or there is persistent microscopic haematuria not attributable to the underlying renal disease. Cyclophosphamide should be permanently withdrawn if haemorrhagic cystitis is confirmed. If urinary symptoms develop during or after prolonged treatment with cyclophosphamide, whether or not infection is proven, the possibility of a transitional cell carcinoma of the bladder must also be considered; experience in Wegener's granulomatosis indicates a 33-fold increase in risk in such patients.

Treatment of urinary infection should be guided by culture and sensitivity results but initial therapy may follow conventional practice in non-immunosuppressed patients.

Ear, nose, and throat infections

Ear, nose, and throat (ENT) infections are a major problem in Wegener's granulomatosis and stem largely from the impaired drainage and mucosal atrophy which follow active inflammation. Fauci *et al.* reported that nearly all patients with residual structural damage had secondary infection.[43] Hoffman *et al.* noted that *Staphylococcus aureus* was the most common cause of sinusitis and also described cases of suppurative otitis media and mastoiditis.[4] Management of recurrent infections requires a combined medical and surgical approach with sinus irrigation, surgical drainage, antibiotics, and regular saline irrigations to reduce the accumulation of nasal crusts.

Stegeman *et al.* have reported a high prevalence of *Staphylococcus aureus* carriage in patients with Wegener's granulomatosis, even in the absence of macroscopic nasal damage.[44] Carriage of the organism identified patients at a seven-fold higher risk of disease relapse, with the majority of relapses affecting the nose and sinuses. Recent work has demonstrated an association between the detection of staphylococcal superantigens and tendency to relapse. It is speculated that activation of T lymphocytes is relevant to the recurrence of active disease. Stegeman *et al.* went on to demonstrate that cotrimoxazole treatment (at full therapeutic doses) is effective in reducing the rate of relapse in Wegener's granulomatosis; a significant reduction was seen in respiratory relapses, although 20% of patients discontinued the drug due to adverse effects.[45] Both respiratory and non-respiratory infections were significantly less frequent in the cotrimoxazole group. Cotrimoxazole was not selected for its antimicrobial profile, but on the basis of anecdotes of benefit in controlling disease activity in Wegener's granulomatosis. Whether a therapy specifically directed against *Staphylococcus aureus* will achieve the same results remains to be proven.

It is often difficult to distinguish active Wegener's lesions in the nose from super-imposed infection, and the picture must be put into the context of the disease activity as a whole, and expert ENT advice sought. Even biopsies may not give the answer, as they are often small, and frequently demonstrate non-specific inflammatory changes.

Ear, nose, and throat infections are not a characteristic feature of any other immune-mediated disease but it is worth noting that sinus infection is common in the population as a whole. The sinuses may be important reservoirs of infection in drug-induced neutropenia in any disease.

Infection or inflammation?

This distinction can be particularly difficult in diseases characterized by multiorgan inflammation and the plan of investigation usually encompasses tests for both disease activity and infection. Some common dilemmas are illustrated in Table 5.5. There are, however, some clues which may give a lead as to whether infection or inflammation is more likely:

Timing

Conventional therapy induces remission of vasculitis in 75–90% of cases within 3 months in the majority. Equally, lupus activity usually responds to the institution of therapy within weeks. Furthermore, infectious complications are most likely when doses of immunosuppressive agents are high and in particular when the patient is taking high-dose daily corticosteroids. Infectious causes must, therefore, be vigorously pursued in the patient with fever or respiratory symptoms 2 to 3 months into treatment.

Context

Relapse of systemic vasculitis affects around 15–20% of patients in the first 2 years of therapy and 30–50% overall. It is two to four times more likely in patients with proteinase 3-specific ANCA and is more likely in patients with persistent ANCA positivity. In patients at low risk of relapse, consideration of an infectious explanation for new or atypical symptoms is particularly important.

Serological features

Trends in serological markers of disease may make relapse of disease a more or less likely option though they are not absolute predictors. Relapse of vasculitis may be preceded by a rise in ANCA concentration but the interval is highly variable; ANCA may persist without clinically evident disease activity. In SLE, antidouble-stranded DNA antibodies

Table 5.5   Infection or inflammation—common dilemmas in follow-up of vasculitis and SLE

Clinical picture	Differential diagnosis
Pancytopenia and fever	CMV or active SLE?
Patchy pulmonary infiltrates	Infection or active Wegener's granulomatosis?
Diffuse pulmonary shadowing	Opportunistic pneumonitis or pulmonary haemorrhage?
Sinus pain and epistaxis	Infection or active Wegener's granulomatosis?
Fever and night sweats	Occult infection or early vasculitis or SLE relapse?

Abbreviations: CMV = cytomegalovirus; SLE = systemic lupus erythematosus.

may rise and complement levels may fall with impending relapse in some patients but remain persistently abnormal in others. Anti-C1q antibodies may indicate active lupus nephritis. C-reactive protein is usually raised in active bacterial or fungal infection but may reach similar levels in active ANCA-associated vasculitis. A markedly raised C-reactive protein is not, however, a feature of active SLE and if detected in SLE, is likely to reflect infection.

Conclusions

There are several common themes which recur throughout this discussion. The first is the range of infections to which patients with glomerular disease and systemic inflammation are susceptible. The second theme is the frequent difficulty in distinguishing infection from active inflammatory disease or non-infectious complications. The third theme is the urgency of investigation (and the risk of rapid deterioration) particularly in respiratory infections. These factors together mandate thorough but speedy investigation in any patient presenting with a fever or organ dysfunction suggestive of infection.

References

1. Sneller MC (1998). Evaluation, treatment, and prophylaxis of infections complicating systemic vasculitis. *Curr Opin Rheumatol* **10**: 38–44.
2. Cohen J, Armstrong D, Cohen J (ed.) (2000). Immunologically mediated diseases. In: *Infectious Diseases*, section 4, p. 6. Mosby, London.
3. Cohen J, Pinching AJ, Rees AJ, Peters DK (1982). Infection and immunosuppression. A study of the infective complications of 75 patients with immunologically-mediated renal disease. *Q J Med* **51**: 1–15.
4. Hoffman GS, Kerr GS, Leavitt RY, Hallahan CW, Lebovics RS, Travis WD, Rottem M, Fauci AS (1992). Wegener granulomatosis: an analysis of 158 patients. *Ann Intern Med* **116**: 488–98.
5. Paton NIJ, Cheong IKS, Kong NCT, Segasothy M (1996). Risk factors for infection in Malaysian patients with systemic lupus erythematosus. *Q J Med* **89**: 531–8.
6. Godeau B, Mainardi J-L, Roudot-Thoraval F, Hachulla E, Guillevin L, Huong Du LT, Jarrousse B, Remy P, Schaeffer A, Piette J-C (2000). Factors associated with *Pneumocystis carinii* pneumonia in Wegener's granulomatosis. *Annals of the Rheumatic Diseases* **54**: 991–4.
7. Ognibene FP, Shelhamer JH, Hoffman GS, Kerr GS, Reda D, Fauci AS, Leavitt RY (1995). *Pneumocystis carinii* pneumonia: a major complication of immunosuppressive therapy in patients with Wegener's granulomatosis. *Am J Respir Crit Care Med* **151**: 795–9.
8. Guillevin L, Cordier J-F, Lhote F, Cohen P, Jarrousse B, Royer I, Lesavre P, Jacquot C, Bindi P, Bielefeld P, *et al.* (1997). A prospective, multicenter, randomized trial comparing steroids and pulse cyclophosphamide versus steroids and oral cyclophosphamide in the treatment of generalized Wegener's granulomatosis. *Arthritis and Rheumatism* **40**: 2187–98.
9. Haubitz M, Schellong S, Gobel U, Schurek HJ, Schaumann D, Koch KM, Brunkhorst R (1998). Intravenous pulse administration of cyclophosphamide versus daily oral treatment in patients with anti-neutrophil cytoplasmic antibody-associated vasculitis and renal involvement: a prospective, randomized study. *Arthritis and Rheumatism* **41**: 1835–44.
10. Hoffman GS, Leavitt RY, Kerr GS, Fauci AS (1992). The treatment of Wegener's granulomatosis with glucocorticoids and methotrexate. *Arthritis and Rheumatism* **35**: 1322–9.

11. Cattran DC, Appel GB, Hebert LA, Hunsicker LG, Pohl MA, Hoy WE, Maxwell DR, Kunis CL (1999). A randomized trial of cyclosporine in patients with steroid-resistant focal segmental glomerulosclerosis. *Kidney International* 56: 2220–6.

12. Wing EJ, Bruns FJ, Fraley DS, Segel DP, Adler S (1980). Infectious complications with plasmapheresis in rapidly progressive glomerulonephritis. *Journal of the American Medical Association* 244: 2423–6.

13. Pohl M, Lan S, Berl T, and the Lupus Nephritis collaborative study group (1991). Plasmapheresis does not increase the risk for infection in immunosuppressed patients with severe lupus nephritis. *Ann Intern Med* 114: 924–9.

14. Singer DRJ, Roberts B, Cohen J (1987). Infective complications of plasma exchange: a prospective study. *Arthritis and Rheumatism* 30: 443–7.

15. Rondeau E, Levy M, Dosquet P, Ruedin P, Mougenot B, Kanfer A, Sraer JD (1989). Plasma exchange and immunosuppression for rapidly progressive glomerulonephritis: prognosis and complications. *Nephrol Dial Transplant* 4: 196–200.

16. Krafcik SS, Covin RB, Lynch JP III, Sitrin RG (1996). Wegener's granulomatosis in the elderly. *Chest* 109: 430–7.

17. Aasarod K, Iversen BM, Hammerstrom J, Bostad L, Vatten L, Joseph M (2000). Wegener's granulomatosis: clinical course in 108 patients with renal involvement. *Nephrol Dial Transplant* 15: 611–18.

18. Andrews PA, Warr KJ, Hicks JA, Cameron JS (1996). Impaired outcome of continuous ambulatory peritoneal dialysis in immunocompromised patients. *Nephrol. Dial. Transplant.* 11: 1104–8.

19. Jennette JC, Falk RJ, Andrassy K, Bacon PA, Churg J, Gross WL, Hagen EC, Hoffman GS, Hunder GG, Kallenberg CGM, *et al.* (1994). Nomenclature of systemic vasculitides. Proposal of an international consensus conference. *Arthritis and Rheumatism* 37: 187–92.

20. Gordon M, Luqmani RA, Adu D, Greaves I, Richards N, Michael J, Emery P, Howie AJ, Bacon PA (1993). Relapses in patients with a systemic vasculitis. *Q J Med* 86: 779–89.

21. Watts RA, Lane SE, Bentham G, Scott DGI (2000). Epidemiology of systemic vasculitis. *Arthritis and Rheumatism* 43: 414–19.

22. Arend SM, Kroon FP, van't Wout JW (1995). *Pneumocystis carinii* pneumonia in patients without AIDS, 1980 through 1993. An analysis of 78 cases. *Arch Intern Med* 155: 2436–341.

23. Adu D, Pall A, Luqmani RA, Richards NT, Howie AJ, Emery P, Michael J, Savage CO, Bacon PA (1997). Controlled trial of pulse versus continuous prednisolone and cyclophosphamide in the treatment of systemic vasculitis. *Q J Med* 90: 401–9.

24. Adu D, Howie AJ, Scott DGI, Bacon PA, McGonigle RJS, Michael J (1987). Polyarteritis and the kidney. *Q J Med* 62: 221–37.

25. Pablos JL, Aragon A, Gomez-Reino JJ (1994). Salmonellosis and systemic lupus erythematosus. Report of ten cases. *British Journal of Rheumatology* 33: 129–32.

26. International Study of Kidney Disease in Children (2000). Minimal change nephrotic syndrome in children: deaths during the first 5 to 15 years' observation. *Pediatrics* 73: 497–501.

27. Ogi M, Yokoyama H, Tomosugi N, Hisada Y, Ohta S, Takaeda M, Wada T, Naito T, Ikeda T, Goshima S, *et al.* (1994). Risk factors for infection and immunglobulin replacement therapy in adult nephrotic syndrome. *Am J Kidney Dis* 24: 427–36.

28. Bindi P, Mougenot B, Mentre F, Noel L-H, Peraldi M-N, Vanhille P, Lesavre P, Mignon F, Ronco PM (1993). Necrotizing crescentic glomerulonephritis without significant immune deposits: a clinical and serological study. *Q J Med* 86: 55–68.

29. Bolton WK, Sturgill BC (1989). Methylprednisolone therapy for acute crescentic rapidly progressive glomerulonephritis. *Am J Nephrol* 9: 368–75.

30. Jarrousse B, Guillevin L, Bindi P, Hachulla E, Leclerc P, Gilson B, Remy P, Rossert J, Jacquot C (1993). Increased risk of *Pneumocystis carinii* pneumonia in patients with Wegener's granulomatosis. *Clinical and Experimental Rheumatology* **11**: 615–21.

31. Ward MM, Donald F (1999). *Pneumocystis carinii* pneumonia in patients with connective tissue diseases: the role of hospital experience in diagnosis and mortality. *Arthritis and Rheumatism* **42**: 780–9.

32. Cameron JS, Davison AM, Cameron JS, Grunfeld J-P, Kerr DNS, Ritz E, Winearls CG (ed.) (1998). The nephrotic syndrome: management, complications and pathophysiology. In: *Oxford Textbook of Clinical Nephrology*, 2nd edn, chapter 3.5, pp. 461–92. Oxford University Press, Oxford.

33. Krensky AM, Ingelfinger JR, Grupe WE (1982). Peritonitis in childhood nephrotic syndrome: 1970–1980. *American Journal of Diseases of Children* **136**: 732–6.

34. Gorensek MJ, Lebel MH, Nelson JD (1988). Peritonitis in children with nephrotic syndrome. *Pediatrics* **81**: 849–56.

35. Gulati S, Kher V, Gupta A, Arora P, Rai PK, Sharma SD (1995). Spectrum of infections in Indian children with nephrotic syndrome. *Pediatric Nephrology* **9**: 431–4.

36. Tain YL, Lin G, Cher TW (1999). Microbiological spectrum of septicemia and peritonitis in nephrotic children. *Pediatr Nephrol* **13**: 835–7.

37. Ponticelli C, Zuchelli P, Passerini P (1989). A randomized trial of methylprednisolone and chlorambucil in idiopathic membranous nephropathy. *New Engl J Med* **320**: 8–13.

38. Gourley MF, Austin HA III, Scott D, Yarboro CH, Vaughan EM, Muir J, Boumpas DT, Klippel JH, Balow JE, Steinberg AD (1996). Methylprednisolone and cyclophosphamide, alone or in combination, in patients with lupus nephritis. A randomized, controlled trial. *Ann Intern Med* **125**: 549–57.

39. Moroni G, Maccario M, Banfi G, Quaglini S, Ponticelli C (1998). Treatment of membranous lupus nephritis. *Am J Kidney Dis* **31**: 681–6.

40. Ponticelli C, Zuchelli P, Passerini P, Cesana B (1992). Methylprednisolone plus chlorambucil as compared with methylprednisolone alone for the treatment of idiopathic membranous nephropathy. *New Engl J Med* **327**: 638–9.

41. Branten AJ, Reichert LJ, Koene RA, Wetzels JF (1998). Oral cyclophosphamide versus chlorambucil in the treatment of patients with membranous nephropathy and renal insufficiency. *Q J Med* **91**: 359–66.

42. Gulati S, Kher V, Arora P, Gupta S, Kale S (1996). Urinary tract infection in nephrotic syndrome. *Pediatric Infectious Disease Journal* **15**: 237–40.

43. Fauci AS, Haynes BF, Katz P, Wolff S (1983). Wegener's granulomatosis: prospective clinical and therapeutic experience with 85 patients over 21 years. *Ann Intern Med* **98**: 76–85.

44. Stegeman CA, Tervaert JW, Sluiter WJ, Manson WL, de Jong PE, Kallenberg CG (1994). Association of chronic nasal carriage of *Staphylococcus aureus* and higher relapse rates in Wegener's granulomatosis [see comments]. *Ann Intern Med* **120**: 12–17.

45. Stegeman CA, Cohen Tervaert JW, de Jong PE, Kallenberg CGM (1996). Trimethoprim-sulphamethoxazole (co-trimoxazole) for the prevention of relapses of Wegener's granulomatosis. Dutch Co-Trimoxazole Wegener study group. *New Engl J Med* **335**: 16–20.

46. Coward RA, Hamdy NAT, Shortland JS, Brown CB (1986). Renal micropolyarteritis: a treatable condition. *Nephrology, Dialysis, Transplantation* **1**: 31–7.

47. Fuiano G, Cameron JS, Raftery M, Hartley BH, Williams DG, Ogg CS (1988). Improved prognosis of renal microscopic polyarteritis in recent years. *Nephrol Dial Transplant* **3**: 383–91.

48. Falk RJ, Hogan S, Carey TS, Jennette JC (1990). Clinical course of anti-neutrophil cytoplasmic autoantibody-associated glomerulonephritis and systemic vasculitis. *Ann Intern Med* **113**: 656–63.

49.   Andrassy K, Erb A, Koderisch J, Waldherr R, Ritz E (1991). Wegener's granulomatosis with renal involvement: patient survival and correlations between initial renal function, renal histology, therapy and renal outcome. *Clin Nephrol* **35**: 139–47.
50.   Haubitz M, Frei U, Rother U, Brunkhorst R, Koch KM (1991). Cyclophosphamide pulse therapy in Wegener's granulomatosis. *Nephrol Dial Transplant* **6**: 531–5.
51.   Guillevin L, Fain O, Lhote F, Jarrousse B, Le THD, Bussel A, Leon A (1992). Lack of superiority of steroids plus plasma exchange to steroids alone in the treatment of polyarteritis nodosa and Churg–Strauss syndrome. A prospective randomised trial in 78 patients. *Arthritis and Rheumatism* **35**: 208–15.
52.   Gayraud M, Guillevin L, Cohen P, Lhote F, Cacoub P, Deblois P, Godeau P, Ruel M, Vidal E, Pointud M, *et al.* (1997). Treatment of good-prognosis polyarteritis nodosa and Churg–Strauss syndrome: comparison of steroids and oral or pulse cyclophosphamide in 25 patients. *Br J Rheumatol.* **36**: 1290–7.
53.   McLaughlin K, Jerimiah P, Fox JG, Mactier RA, Simpson K, Boulton-Jones JM (1998). Has the prognosis for patients with pauci-immune necrotizing glomerulonephritis improved? *Nephrol Dial Transplant* **13**: 1696–701.

6

Infectious complications of the diabetic patient with renal disease

Phoung-Chi T. Pham, Phuong-Thu T. Pham, and Glenn Mathisen

Diabetic patients are predisposed to infectious complications due to variable impairment of their host defence mechanisms and diabetes-associated complications. Patients with renal disease, especially those with advanced renal impairment, are also at increased risks due to their depressed immune system (Chapter 1) and complications associated with renal failure. Diabetic patients with concomitant renal disease, whether due to diabetic or non-diabetic nephropathy, may be at particularly increased risks due to the potential combined adverse effects of depressed host defence mechanisms, malnutrition, vascular insufficiency, neuropathy, and urinary tract abnormalities. Although there is ample literature on the infectious complications of either diabetic or renal failure patients alone, similar documentation for patients affected by both diseases is lacking. In this chapter common infectious complications among patients with diabetes and renal failure will be discussed. In addition, the effect of the combined conditions on the infectious complications will be emphasized.

Factors contributing to the increased risks for infectious complications in patients with diabetes mellitus and renal disease (Table 6.1)

Defects in host defence mechanisms

As immunodeficiency in renal patients is discussed elsewhere (Chapter 1), only diabetes-associated immune dysfunction is discussed here.

In many diabetic patients, the first line of the host defence mechanism is affected when they are subject to multiple daily insulin injections, finger-pricks for glucose monitoring, and skin breaks associated with neuropathy. Moreover, the second line of host defence, involving both cellular and humoral mechanisms, can be altered.

Several alterations in cell-mediated immune defence may occur. Chemotactic activities of granulocytes and monocytes have been shown to be depressed. The adherence of phagocytes and phagocytosis have been demonstrated to be defective in the presence of hyperglycaemia, hyperosmolality, and acidaemia. Polymorphonuclear granulocytes may have intrinsic defects, with alterations in specific membrane components necessary for target recognition and phagocytosis. Bactericidal activities of polymorphonuclear

Table 6.1 Factors influencing the increased risks for infectious complications among patients with diabetes mellitus and renal disease

	Diabetes mellitus	Renal insufficiency
Immunosuppression		
First line:		
Skin, mucosal barrier, secretory IgA	+	+
Second line:		
Cellular mechanisms	+	+
Humoral mechanisms	+	+
Malnutrition	+	+
Metabolic disturbances		
Hyperglycaemia/glucosuria	+	−
Hyperosmolality	+	−
Acidaemia	+	+
Organ-specific abnormalities		
Pulmonary	+?	+
Cardiovascular	+	+
Genitourinary	+	+
Neurological	+	±

granulocytes may be reduced in association with hyperglycaemia, a phenomenon thought to be related to the production of sorbitol.[1] In addition, several studies have shown an imbalance of T-cell subsets in association with insulin deficiency.[2–5]

In the humorally mediated immune defence the immunoglobulin response appears to be normal, but the complement system may be affected by non-enzymatic glycosylation. The binding of glucose to the biochemically active site of the third component of complement C3 may inhibit its attachment to the surface of the micro-organism and lead to impairment of opsonization. The latter event is an antigen-coating process necessary for recognition and binding of micro-organisms by receptors in the membrane of phagocytic cells.[1,6,7]

Malnutrition

Among patients with coexisting diabetes mellitus and renal disease, malnutrition commonly results from poor oral intake, inappropriate protein restriction, excessive catabolism, and/or excessive urinary protein loss. Malnutrition has been demonstrated to affect several lines of the host defence mechanism and to correlate with the extent of impairment of host defence. The first line of defence can be impaired as the skin and mucous membrane barriers are thinned. Although circulating immunoglobulins are not affected, secretory IgA has been shown to be depressed.[8,9] Monocytes and polymorphonuclear granulocytes may have impaired chemotaxis, adherence, phagocytosis, and intracellular bactericidal activities.[1,10] T-lymphocyte count and helper–suppressor ratios may be reduced. The maturation and antigenic responsiveness of lymphocytes may be variably impaired. Similar impairment of the immune system has also been reported for deficiencies of trace elements and vitamins such as zinc, iron, selenium, vitamins A, B_6, C, and E.[1,6,10–12] In addition, significant proteinuria associated with either diabetic nephropathy or other renal disease may result in a significant loss of circulating immunoglobulins.

Metabolic abnormalities

Hyperglycaemia/glucosuria

Diminished bactericidal activity, and other macrophage functions, as well as impaired proliferation of lymphocytes in diabetic patients have long been attributed to systemic hyperglycaemia.[7,13–16] Similarly, a high degree of glucosuria has been shown to impair the phagocytic function of granulocytes in the urinary tract and, in addition, to enhance bacterial growth. Glucosuria *per se*, however, has not been shown clinically to correlate with the incidence of bacterial infections of the urinary tract. The addition of glucose to urine allows it to support a much higher bacterial growth. High concentrations of glucose in the urine and mucosal secretions, however, have been linked to the increased incidence of oral, genitourinary, and vaginal candidiasis.[13] The mechanism whereby *Candida albicans* may prosper in the hyperglycaemic milieu is its possession of a glucose-inducible protein that promotes adhesion to the host yet inhibits phagocytosis by the host.[7] The higher prevalence of candidiasis in diabetic patients may in turn be responsible for further infectious complications in the host. For example, in females, recurrent vaginitis has been implicated to be a significant contributing factor to genitourinary infectious complications.[13]

Acidaemia

The role of acidaemia on the susceptibility of the host to infectious complications in both diabetic and renal patients is unclear. The well-known association between acidaemia and infection is diabetic ketoacidosis (DKA) and mucormycosis. Although less common, mucormycosis has also been reported in uraemic patients (Chapter 9). The exact cause and effect of DKA/renal failure and mucormycosis are not well understood. In DKA, it is felt that acidaemia or hyperglycaemia *per se* is insufficient to promote fungal replication within macrophages. Nevertheless, mucormycosis has been reported in patients with only acidaemia.[6,17] The altered availability of iron in association with acidaemia is a possible mechanism that may explain the propensity for mucormycosis to occur in patients with DKA and possibly also in patients with uraemia. The availability of iron for the growth of micro-organisms may be enhanced in acidaemia due to the reduced iron binding capacity of transferrin.[18] In the lungs of patients with renal failure, acidaemia has been proposed to play a role in suppressing clearance of micro-organisms, hence promoting bacterial colonization and infection of the respiratory tract.[19]

Pulmonary abnormalities

Although structural and functional abnormalities within the lungs have been implicated in predisposing diabetic patients to pulmonary infections, diabetes mellitus itself has not been shown to be associated with an increased risk of respiratory tract infection.[19,20]

However, there is some evidence suggesting that Gram-negative bacillary pneumonias may be more prevalent in diabetic patients, presumably due to the increased colonization with Gram-negative bacteria and defective polymorphonuclear granulocyte function.[19] More recently, infections due to *Staphylococcus aureus* and *Mycobacterium tuberculosis* have also been reported to occur with increased frequency in diabetic patients.[21]

The association of respiratory tract infection with renal failure is stronger than that with diabetes mellitus. In a literature review, Montgomerie *et al.* reported the incidence of pneumonia in patients with acute renal failure to range from 40 to 80%, and in their own retrospective study pneumonia developed in 51% of hospitalized patients with chronic renal failure and 29% of patients with acute renal failure.[22] Important factors influencing the increased rate of respiratory tract infection in renal failure are felt to include immunosuppression, colonization with gram-negative bacilli and staphylococci, pulmonary edema, and possibly impaired mucocilliary clearance.[19,22]

Urinary tract abnormalities

Patients with both diabetes mellitus and renal disease may suffer from anatomical or functional problems in the urinary tract that can lead to infectious complications. Typical problems include neurogenic bladder, poor urinary flow, and urinary obstruction. Diabetic patients in particular are known to develop complications such as neurogenic bladder and papillary necrosis that may cause urinary stasis, obstruction, and recurrent urinary tract infections. Contrary to previous beliefs, urinary instrumentation is suspected to contribute only a minor infectious risk.[13]

Microangiopathy and polyneuropathy

Accelerated atherosclerosis and/or microangiopathy, a systemic state of vascular compromise among diabetic patients, may independently accentuate the risk of infectious complications. The associated vascular compromise among diabetics has been suggested to significantly contribute to the development of urinary tract infections. Diabetic microvascular disease may exacerbate the relative ischaemia of the normal renal medulla and potentiate parenchymal infection leading to necrotizing papillitis. With the exception of diabetic nephropathy and the requirement for insulin use, the presence of diabetic retinopathy, neuropathy, coronary artery disease, and peripheral vascular disease have all been documented to correlate with an increased incidence of urinary tract infections.[23] Poor peripheral circulation may deliver inadequate host defence components and appropriate antimicrobial agents to the site of micro-organism invasion or periulcerous tissues.[24,25] Concomitant polyneuropathy may suppress painful sensations and hence delay recognition of infections, thus allowing time for microbial spread and invasion.

In summary, patients who suffer from both diabetes mellitus and renal disease suffer from multiple disadvantages in terms of acquiring as well as controlling infections. Infectious complications among these patients range from common infections, such as diabetic foot cellulitis and urinary tract infections, to the more life-threatening infections such as mucormycosis. The rest of this chapter focuses on specific morbid and potentially fatal infections frequently associated with this patient population (Table 6.2).

Table 6.2 Common diabetic infectious complications that may be exacerbated by renal insufficiency

Ear, nose, throat	Mucormycosis
	Aspergillosis
	Malignant otitis media?
Pulmonary	Bacterial pneumonia
	Tuberculosis
Gastroenterological	Emphysematous cholecystitis?
Genitourinary	Urinary tract infections
	Pyelonephritis
	Intrarenal abscesses
Soft tissues, bones, joints	Foot ulcerations
	Necrotizing fasciitis
	Infectious arthritis

Specific infections among patients with diabetes mellitus and renal insufficiency

Diabetic foot infections

Despite advanced medical technologies, diabetic foot infections are still responsible for a significant percentage (50% in the United States) of all non-traumatic lower extremity amputations.[26] Over 24% of diabetic patients with severe lower limb infections present with a serum creatinine greater than 1.3 mg/dl.[27] The two major contributory factors in the development of an initial foot injury in diabetic patients with renal failure include polyneuropathy and vascular insufficiency. Negligence in regular foot care may exacerbate the situation by allowing entry of bacteria into the initial site of injury, spreading to adjacent soft tissues and bones, and potential haematogenous spread.[28,29]

Polyneuropathy plays a dual role in the formation of foot ulcerations. The foot is a complex apparatus which requires a high degree of environmental feedback for maintenance of balance as well as gait while exerting minimal stress upon itself. In patients with diabetic polyneuropathy, this protective mechanism is diminished. The resulting unchecked stress or pressure on the foot can lead to pressure ulcerations. This type of neuropathic ulceration typically occurs in the plantar forefoot where the force of body weight and the shear force produced by rotations of the metatarsal heads maximally summate. Apart from neuropathic ulceration, sensory mechanisms required for the patient to recognize any foot injury may also be diminished. The lack of awareness of even a benign skin break may allow time for unchecked bacterial entry and invasion.[29]

Vascular insufficiency exerts its damaging effect by the initial development of ischaemic tissues, followed by skin breakdown and bacterial invasion. Poor tissue perfusion also permits suboptimal delivery of host defences to the site of injury. The resulting unattended ulceration invites a host of polymicrobial invasions.

Therapy

The ultimate goal in the management of a diabetic foot ulcer is prevention. Screening programs for the presence of neuropathy, ischaemia, joint deformity, and oedema have been shown to be effective in reducing the need for amputations.[30,31] Treatment of diabetic foot ulcers should be done on an individual basis to optimize responses. Factors including the severity and extent of infection, the micro-organisms responsible, and the medical condition of the patient are used to dictate the choice of therapy.[28,29]

In general, diabetic foot infections can be classified as mild, moderate, or severe. Mild foot infections include superficial ulceration with or without surrounding cellulitis; moderate conditions include ulcerations with widespread cellulitis and local tissue necrosis with or without associated osteomyelitis; and severe conditions include advanced cases with potentially fatal bacteraemia and clinical evidence of septic shock. In mild cases oral antibiotics (1–2 weeks), local wet to dry dressing changes with normal saline, and elevation of the involved extremity, are sufficient. In moderate cases hospitalization is required for administration of intravenous antibiotics and surgical intervention. Local debridement to amputation of the infected bone may be required depending on the degree of involvement. The duration of antibiotic administration is typically 6 weeks, but may be longer in more severe or resistant cases. In severe cases with systemic shock intravenous antibiotics and fluid administration followed by prompt resection of the gangrenous tissues are required to prevent rapid haemodynamic deterioration and collapse.[28,32]

Identification of the pathogen is key to the success of therapy. In cases of diabetic foot ulceration cultures are often unreliable due to contamination by non-pathogenic organisms. The best site for isolation of pathogens is from central deep tissues or fresh purulent drainage. Cultures of superficial ulcerations often yield a broad flora which often includes non-pathogenic organisms. The spectrum of organisms involved in diabetic foot ulcerations is wide given the often delayed presentation and allowance for involvement of multiple organisms. Polymicrobial involvement has been reported to occur in more than 50% of cases in many studies. Commonly isolated organisms include staphylococci, streptococci, *Proteus* spp., *Klebsiella* spp., *Escherichia coli*, *Pseudomonas* spp., and anaerobes. Empirical therapy for diabetic foot ulceration, therefore, often requires broad antimicrobial coverage.[28,29] Antibiotic-naive patients who present with mild infections, however, may only have one or two different aerobic Gram-positive cocci with *Staphylococcus aureus* or β-haemolytic streptococci, and do not necessarily require broad antimicrobial coverage.[32] Other clinical considerations for empirical antimicrobial therapy include: Gram-negative bacilli, specifically Enterobacteriaceae, in chronic or previously treated infections; *Pseudomonas* spp. in wounds previously soaked or treated with wet dressings; enterococci among patients previously treated with cephalosporin therapy; anaerobes in necrotic, foul-smelling wounds; and methicillin-resistant *S. aureus* (MRSA) among previously hospitalized or institutionalized patients.[32–34]

Diabetic foot ulcerations may occasionally be resistant to therapy due to associated severe vascular insufficiency and inadequate delivery of antibiotic to the affected site. Vascular insufficiency should be routinely evaluated in this population. Poor peripheral pulses have to be evaluated with ankle brachial blood pressure indices, followed by angiography of the lower extremities as dictated by the findings of the former. Revascularization should be performed as necessary.

Urinary tract infections

Diabetic patients with renal disease are at increased risk of developing urinary tract infections due to functional complications of the urinary tract, impaired host defence mechanisms, and poor urinary flow. Interestingly, the frequency of urinary tract infections has been shown to be increased only in diabetic women compared with non-diabetic women, but not in diabetic men compared with non-diabetic men. This difference may be secondary to the increased incidence of vaginitis among women with diabetes mellitus. Urinary tract infections in these patients may be further complicated by pyelonephritis, intrarenal or perinephric abscesses, papillary necrosis, and sepsis. In addition, the widespread use of broad-spectrum antibiotics in recent years has selectively caused an increased incidence of fungal infections in the urinary tract.[13,35]

Pathogenesis

Micro-organisms may infect the urinary tract by ascending through the urethra into the bladder or by haematogenous or lymphatic spread. The first mechanism is by far most common and can explain the association of the increased incidence of urinary tract infections in patients with frequent vaginitis and lower urinary tract abnormalities. Reported antibacterial host factors include the urea, organic acid, and salt content of the urine, and a high osmolality in the presence of a low pH. Other factors protecting the host include urinary inhibitors to bacterial adherence such as Tamm–Horsfall protein, bladder mucopolysaccharide, low-molecular-weight oligosaccharides, secretory IgA, and lactoferrin. In addition, proper urine flow, micturition, and emptying of the bladder are crucial in inhibiting bacterial proliferation and extension to the upper urinary tract.[36]

Clinical manifestations

Clinical presentation and the therapy of urinary tract infections depend on the degree of infection and associated complications.

Asymptomatic bacteriuria. The incidence of asymptomatic bacteriuria in diabetic patients is estimated from several studies to range between 7 and 32%.[36–41] Despite its high incidence in diabetic patients, asymptomatic bacteriuria is not affected by hyperglycaemic control or the degree of renal failure.[42] Empirical treatment of asymptomatic bacteriuria still remains a clinical challenge. Undertreatment of asymptomatic bacturia may theoretically predispose to pyelonephritis, renal papillary necrosis, and renal insufficiency, whereas overtreatment may give rise to multiple complications including poor tolerance to the side-effects of antimicrobial agents, development of antibiotic-resistant organisms, fungal superinfection, and antimicrobial-induced renal failure. The latter complication may be irreversible in patients with underlying renal insufficiency. In diabetic patients, the presence of asymptomatic bacteriuria may be more problematic, especially in those with associated diabetic neurogenic bladders and urinary retention.

Significant asymptomatic bacteriuria is defined as the presence of bacteriuria greater than or equal to 10^5 colony-forming units (cfu)/ml of one or more organisms in the absence of symptoms associated with urinary tract infection. Among patients requiring in-dwelling catheterization, a culture obtained directly from the catheter with more than 100 cfu/ml should be considered positive for infection, since these counts have been reported to persist or increase within 48 h.[43] The major concern with in-dwelling catheters is based on previous studies showing that bacteria may be protected by the build-up of biofilms composed of Tamm–Horsfall protein and urinary salts on the catheter's surface.[44] The organism most commonly isolated in different studies is *Escherichia coli* (40%). Gram-negative bacilli occur in 60–70% of cases. Other organisms reported include Gram-positive cocci, for example *S. aureus*, *S. epidermidis*, and enterococci. The disturbing finding is the poor sensitivity (33%) of these organisms to the commonly used antibiotics including ampicillin and cotrimoxazole. Other antimicrobials tested as empirical agents with over 80% sensitivity include nitrofurantoin, gentamicin, ceftazidime, augmentin, cefuroxime, and norfloxacin.[38]

   Treatment of asymptomatic bacteriuria requires careful clinical judgment. In general, the prognosis for asymptomatic bacteriuria is excellent. Although an earlier study revealed that as many as 50% of diabetic patients with asymptomatic bacteriuria had upper urinary tract involvement, a subsequent 14–year follow-up study of untreated asymptomatic bacteriuria in diabetic patients revealed similar frequencies of acute pyelonephritis, deterioration of kidney function, and systemic hypertension compared with control subjects.[40,41] Currently, treatment of asymptomatic bacteriuria is recommended for patients with frequent episodes of symptomatic urinary tract infections, pregnancy, after renal transplantation, and prior to urological interventions.[42]

Recurrent urinary tract infections. Recurrent urinary tract infections generally benefit from antimicrobial suppressive therapy except in the subset of patients requiring chronic in-dwelling catheters. The choice of prophylactic antibiotic is dictated by drug safety, the bactericidal activity of the antibiotic against common aetiological agents in urinary tract infections, the low risk of development of resistance, and the ability to achieve adequate active drug concentrations in the urine. Some of the commonly used antibiotics for prophylaxis against recurrent urinary tract infections include trimethoprim, nitrofurantoin (patients receiving long-term prophylaxis with nitrofurantoin are at risk of developing interstitial pneumonitis and hepatitis), sulphonamides, quinolones, fluoroquinolones, methenamine hippurate, and methenamine mandelate.[45]

Fungal infections of the urinary tract

Fungal species most commonly observed in urinary tract infections are *Candida* spp. Involvement of *Candida* may occur as simple cystitis or more complex renal invasion. Predisposing factors for the development of complex infections and systemic involvement include obstructive uropathy, malnutrition, neoplasia, renal failure, and prolonged use of antibiotics. More complex renal infections may occur as an ascending infection or haematogenous spread.[46]

Diagnosis. The diagnosis of candiduria is difficult because contamination is frequent, especially in patients with in-dwelling catheters. In a patient without an in-dwelling catheter, an accepted diagnostic measure is the documentation of a titre greater than 10^4 cfu/ml obtained from a midstream urine specimen. Although absent in most cases, a positive blood culture may be helpful in diagnosing renal invasion. Persistent candiduria following amphotericin bladder irrigation for simple cystitis (25 mg/500 ml at 42 ml/h for 3 days) may also indicate renal involvement.[35,46]

Therapy. Treatment of *Candida* in the urinary tract depends on the degree of involvement. Current treatment options include irrigation of the bladder with amphotericin or systemic antifungal therapy. Effective systemic therapies include the use of 5-fluorocytosine, oral ketoconazole, itraconazole, and amphotericin. In our opinion, diabetic patients with renal disease and poor urinary output may benefit from bladder irrigation as they may not respond well to systemic therapy alone. Patients with invasive *Candida* pyelonephritis may require surgical intervention. Imaging studies including intravenous or retrograde pyelography should be performed to rule out obstruction or the presence of fungus ball if candiduria persists despite treatment.[35,46]

Pyelonephritis and emphysematous pyelonephritis

Patients with pyelonephritis typically present with flank pain, fevers, nausea, vomiting, and urinary symptoms such as dysuria and urgency. Renal function usually remains stable. A rapid worsening of renal function should alert the clinician to volume depletion, formation of intrarenal microabscesses, antibiotic-induced acute renal failure, erroneous antimicrobial therapy, or urinary obstruction (i.e. papillary necrosis, blood clots, or an obstructed/non-functioning in-dwelling Foley catheter).

A subset of patients with pyelonephritis develops a serious entity known as emphysematous pyelonephritis. Although the majority (80%) of these cases have been reported in diabetic patients, they may also be seen in patients with functional or structural abnormalities such as reflux uropathy and obstruction. Emphysematous pyelonephritis is an uncommon radiological and clinical diagnosis. Plain abdominal radiographs may reveal air pockets within the involved kidneys. Although renal ultrasound may detect the presence of emphysematous pyelonephritis, erroneous reading as hydronephrosis may occur. CT or MRI are felt to be the preferred diagnostic imaging modalities. The presence of air within the renal parenchyma may be due to several mechanisms: the presence of gas-producing organisms, direct fistulas between the gastrointestinal tract and the urinary tract, and/or poor local blood perfusion necessary for gas absorption. Most causative agents are of the enterobacter and enterococcus type, but cases of non-enterococcal streptococcal infections have also been reported.[47]

Uncomplicated pyelonephritis may be treated with oral or intravenous antibiotics for 2 weeks depending on the overall condition of the patient and their ability to tolerate oral intake. Conservative empirical therapy, such as intravenous ampicillin and gentamicin or oral fluoroquinolone such as ciprofloxacin, may be adequate for compliant patients. For more severe cases requiring hospitalization, triple therapy using a fluoroquinolone, ampicillin, and gentamicin, a third-generation cephalosporin, or an antipseudomonal β-lactamase-resistant penicillin may be necessary. At present therapy for emphy-sematous pyelonephritis involves surgical removal of the involved kidney due to its aggressive and potentially fatal nature. There are, however, reports of successful medical therapy when surgery was not an option. The duration of the medical therapy however, is not well established, and should be decided on the basis of the clinical course in individual cases.[47,48]

Intrarenal abscess

Intrarenal abscesses are classified according to their location and extent of involvement. Intrarenal abscesses can present in the cortex or the corticomedullary regions. Patients at risk include those with diabetes mellitus, chronic renal failure requiring haemodialysis, and drug abusers.

Renal cortical abscesses. Although up to one-third of renal cortical abscesses have no apparent source, the majority are thought to result from haematogenous spread of bacteria from a distant source such as the skin to the cortical parenchyma. Not surprisingly, the most common organism isolated is *S. aureus*. The time lapse from an initial distant infection to the development of the renal cortical abscess may range from a few days to months, with an average interval of 7 weeks. Clinically, affected patients present with symptoms typical of pyelonephritis such as flank pain, fevers, and chills. However, since the cortical abscesses often do not extend into the urinary excretory system, lower urinary symptoms are typically absent. Laboratory findings may reveal leucocytosis, but urinalysis can be normal and sterile. Definitive diagnosis requires imaging studies such as ultrasound or CT. Renal cortical abscesses infected by *S. aureus* respond well to antibiotics alone. Surgical drainage, either percutaneous or open drainage, is only required when the patient does not respond to antibiotics within 48 h. Empirical therapy with a semisynthetic penicillin (oxacillin or nafcillin) against *S. aureus* is generally recommended. Alternative therapy with a first-generation cephalosporin or vancomycin may be used in cases of penicillin allergy. The duration of therapy should be 10 to 14 days of parenteral antibiotics followed by oral antibiotics for a total course of 4 to 6 weeks.[48]

Corticomedullary abscesses. Corticomedullary abscesses are classified according to the chronicity of the infection and the extent of involvement. Corticomedullary abscesses can present as acute or chronic and focal or multifocal. Biopsies of the involved parenchyma reveal interstitial inflammation associated with infiltration of polymorphonuclear leucocytes. The development of corticomedullary abscesses predominantly occurs as a result of ascending urinary tract infections associated with vesicoureteral reflux, urinary tract obstruction or neurogenic urinary tract abnormalities. Commonly involved organisms are those associated with lower urinary tract infections including *Escherichia coli*, *Klebsiella* and *Proteus* spp. Two uncommon clinical entities of corticomedullary abscesses include emphysematous pyelonephritis, which has been discussed previously, and xanthogranulomatous pyelonephritis.[48]

The aetiology of xanthogranulomatous pyelonephritis is thought to be due to urinary tract abnormalities with or without renal calculi in association with chronic urinary tract infection. Radiologically, xanthogranulomatous pyelonephritis can present as an enlarged non-functioning kidney (80%) or a focal mass in association with renal calculi (70%). Pathological examination of the involved tissue shows replacement of normal tissue by granulomatous tissue containing foam cells.[48,49]

Therapy. Corticomedullary abscesses may respond to antimicrobial agents alone. Empirical therapy should be directed towards the commonly involved Gram-negative bacilli. Antibiotics should be administered parenterally until the patient defervesces for at least 24 to 48 h followed by oral antibiotics for at least 2 weeks. Surgical drainage or nephrectomy is reserved for severe cases or those resistant to medical therapy alone.[48] In the case of xanthogranulomatous pyelonephritis, however, surgical resection or total nephrectomy is generally required due to a high associated mortality rate.[51] Although cases of xanthogranulomatous pyelonephritis successfully treated with antibiotics alone have been reported, non-surgical management should only be recommended for focal disease in patients younger than 50 years due to the possible coexistence of early renal malignancy.[49]

Perinephric abscess

A perinephric abscess may arise from haematogenous/lymphatic spread, or direct extension from adjacent structures/abscesses (cortical/corticomedullary abscess).[48,50] As a perinephric abscess may arise from a wide variety of sources, the micro-organisms involved range from the common Gram-negative bacilli *E. coli*, *Proteus* spp., and *Klebsiella* to *S. aureus*, anaerobes such as *Clostridium* and *Bacteroides* spp., fungi including *Candida* spp., and *Mycobacterium tuberculosis*. Diagnosis of a perinephric abscess requires imaging studies such as CT scan or MRI. Although ultrasound may detect perinephric abscesses, its sensitivity is suboptimal. A study of 47 cases reported a false negative rate of 36%.[52] Treatment of perinephric abscesses requires both drainage (surgical or percutaneous) and administration of antimicrobials directed against the causative agent.[48,51]

Malignant otitis externa

Although *Pseudomonas aeruginosa* may play a pathogenic role in otitis externa in patients with trauma, inflammation or just excess moisture in the auditory canal, it is usually non-invasive and benign. However, in elderly patients with diabetes mellitus and those with chronic illnesses associated with microangiopathy, the infection may become aggressive and is referred to as malignant otitis externa. The percentage of adults affected with malignant otitis externa who also have glucose intolerance was reported in one study to be over 90%. Other predisposing factors for malignant otitis externa include other immunosuppressive states, malnourishment, skin breaks in the external ear, and aural exposure to water contaminated with *P. aeruginosa*.[53]

Pathogenesis

Necrotizing otitis externa begins with bacterial invasion and penetration into the bony–cartilaginous junction of the external ear canal. The infection then spreads into the mastoid bone and progresses medially along the skull base. Although *P. aeruginosa* is the causative organism in over 95% of cases of necrotizing otitis externa, there are reports of other causative organisms including fungal species such as *Aspergillus*.[53]

Clinical manifestations

Otalgia and otorrhoea are common presenting features. Otalgia has been described to be severe and worse at night. In the early phase, a purulent aural discharge may be observed. Other associated symptoms include headache and temporomandibular joint pain. In advanced cases, spread to cranial nerves, especially the facial nerve, and the central nervous system can occur. On physical examination, the external auditory canal typically appears inflamed and erythematous. Granulation tissue or ulceration with associated soft tissue inflammation over the bony–cartilaginous external auditory canal may be found. The pinna, periauricular, and adjacent areas may also be inflamed and tender. Trismus may suggest temporomandibular involvement. Neurological deficits may be present in association with cranial nerve involvement. Diagnostic laboratory findings are limited. An elevated sedimendation rate is non-specific, but a high level may suggest malignant rather than benign otitis externa. Cultures of deep tissue specimens obtained from the external auditory canal can confirm the diagnosis. Imaging studies should be done to evaluate the extent of involvement of soft tissue and bone.[53] While MRI with gadolinium and gallium-67 single-photon emission CT have both been reported to be useful for early diagnosis, the latter has also been suggested to be useful during follow-up.[22]

Therapy

The first line of therapy is administration of antimicrobial agents. Systemic antipseudomonal antibiotics include an intravenous combination of an antipseudomonal penicillin and an aminoglycoside, a third-generation cephalosporin, or oral quinolones. The quinolones offer the advantage of shorter hospitalization. The duration of therapy should be 4–8 weeks.[22,53] Recurrence of disease requires prolonged treatment for 8–12 weeks. In more extensive cases, surgical debridement may be necessary. Routine exploratory surgery is not advocated. To prevent occurrence of the disease, efforts should be made to promote patient awareness to only use sterile water when aural irrigation is required.[53]

Necrotizing fasciitis

Necrotizing fasciitis is an aggressive form of soft tissue infection that typically presents as a rapid progression of necrosis of subcutaneous fat and fascia. Associated mortality has been documented to be approximately 40%.[22] Commonly recognized predisposing factors include systemic diseases such as diabetes mellitus, renal failure, malignancy, and other immunosuppressed states. Mortality risk factors have been reported to include age, female gender, degree of involvement, time to initiation of debridement, elevated serum creatinine, elevated blood lactate, and the presence of multiorgan dysfunction. Diabetes mellitus alone does not alter the mortality rate unless it is associated with renal failure or peripheral vascular disease.[54,55]

Pathogenesis

Although the aetiology of necrotizing fasciitis is unknown in some cases a traumatic event responsible for a break in the integrity of the skin can usually be readily identified prior to its development. Introduction of micro-organisms into the relatively poorly vascularized fascia in the immunocompromised host can facilitate proliferation of the micro-organisms followed by subcutaneous and fascial plane spread. Causative micro-organisms can be both aerobic and anaerobic. Commonly reported organisms include streptococci, staphylococci, *E. coli*, *Klebsiella*, *Pseudomonas*, and *Bacteroides fragilis* or *Clostridium* spp.[22,54,55]

Clinical manifestations

Necrotizing fasciitis frequently occurs in the extremities, the abdomen, and the perineum. The associated pain is characteristically disproportionate to the severity of physical findings. At early onset, the involved area can present as an intense cellulitis characterized by oedema, erythema, and tenderness. Unlike cellulitis, necrotizing fasciitis is rapidly progressive despite antimicrobial therapy. Within 72 h the involved tissue may change from red and erythematous to bluish gray. Bullae may also be present. They are initially filled with a serosanguinous fluid that is later replaced by a haemorrhagic fluid. By the fifth day, the skin may become gangrenous and slough off when it is deprived of its nutrient support from the underlying necrotic tissues. Underlying muscles, however, are typically spared, presumably because of a better vascular support. Constitutional symptoms such as fevers, chills, and leucocytosis are common. Crepitus may be present, but its absence does not rule out the condition. Routine radiographs typically reveal marked soft tissue swelling with or without subcutaneous gas.[22,54,55] Gadolinium-enhanced MRI may help distinguish viable from non-viable tissue.

Therapy

Necrotizing fasciitis is potentially fatal if not promptly recognized and treated. Broad antimicrobial therapy should be immediately administered when the diagnosis is suspected. Accepted empirical regimens include penicillin with clindamycin and an aminoglycoside, or timentin and clindamycin. Both penicillin and clindamycin are recommended in the empirical regimen due to the possibility of clindamycin resistance and decreased efficacy of penicillin. Every effort should be made to culture swabs from the necrotic centre for both aerobes and anaerobes. Concomitant extensive surgical debridement should be promptly performed to halt the progression of the infection. Adjunctive therapies, including topical platelet-derived wound healing factors and hyperbaric oxygen, have also been advocated but their utility remains ill-defined due to the lack of well-controlled human clinical trials. Proper nutritional support should also be integrated into the complete treatment programme.[22,54,55]

Mucormycosis and related fungal infections

Although rare, mucormycosis is a highly feared complication observed in immuno-compromised patients including those with diabetes mellitus or serious trauma. Mucormycosis is a generic term widely used to refer to infections caused by any fungus in the order Mucorales. Mucorales is one of two orders of fungi in the class of zygomycetes that are known to be pathogenic in humans: Mucorales and Entomophthorales. Commonly isolated pathogens in the order Mucorales include *Mucor*, *Rhizopus*, and *Absidia*. Entomophthoramycosis refers to diseases caused by any fungus of the order Entomophthorales. Reported pathogens from the order Entomophthorales include *Conidiobolus* and *Basidiobolus*. Both Mucorales and Entomophthorales are ubiquitous in nature, yet associated diseases are uncommon due to their low virulence.[17]

Pathogenesis

The fungus gains entry visa the respiratory tract or skin, whereupon the spores germinate. The factors that predispose to spread include diabetes mellitus *per se* (imparied macrophage activity) and acidaemia.[56] As discussed in Chapter 9, the use of iron or aluminium chelating agents (desferrioxamine) increases the risk of infection.[6,17]

Clinical features

Infection can be localized to many different sites (nasal mucosa, lungs, central nervous system, gut, kidney, or liver).[17,58] Widespread dissemination can occur. Harril *et al.* described 16 cases of chronic rhinocerebral mucormycosis, 12 of which had diabetes mellitus and seven had also given a history of diabetic ketoacidosis. Diagnosis was often delayed, with a median time of 7 months.[17,57] Skin involvement is also seen in the diabetic in association with local trauma and poorly healing diabetic ulcers. Local invasion and dissemination may occur.[17] Renal involvement may occur in the diabetic and may be suggested by the finding of diffuse enlargement of the kidneys and multiple low-density areas in the renal parenchyma representing fungal abscessess.[17,59,60]

Therapy

Treatment requires both local surgical debridement, which should be as complete as possible, and antifungal therapy. Mucor is poorly susceptible to antifungal agents and high-dose amphotericin (1–1.5 mg/kg/day) is required.[17,22,57]

Aspergillosis

Aspergillosis is a fungal infection more commonly observed in cancer patients, but it may also be seen in patients with diabetes mellitus. *Aspergillus* species are ubiquitous fungi that grow in a wide variety of conditions including soil, dung, decaying vegetation, hay, or grain. Common species known to be pathogenic in humans include *A. fumigatus*, *A. flavus*, *A. niger*, and *A. terreus*.[35] Other known risks for the development of severe disease include neutropenia, major organ transplantation, chronic steroid use, chronic granulomatous disease, and other chronic diseases including both diabetes mellitus and renal failure. Hospital renovation and adjacent building construction have been implicated as a potential source for cases ranging from allergic bronchopulmonary aspergillosis to fatal invasive pulmonary aspergillosis among immunosuppressed patients in oncology, transplantation, and renal units.[61,62]

Clinical manifestations

As with mucormycosis, patients with aspergillosis may present with local symptoms secondary to vascular invasion, thrombosis, haemorrhagic infarction, and necrosis of specific organs. Focal neurological deficits such as isolated sixth nerve palsy resembling diabetic-associated sixth nerve palsy have been reported.[35,61,63]

Pathogenesis

Aspergillus species can gain entry into the host via airborne spores through the airways, nasal or paranasal sinuses or injured skin and cornea. When spores are inhaled and attached to alveolar macrophages or to any injured epithelial surfaces, activation of the alternative complement pathway and recruitment of monocytes and neutrophils occur. Following the initial invasion, spores germinate into hyphae, a form more susceptible to killing by the host's cellular immune system. Depending on the integrity of the host's immune system, the hyphae may grow and extend along blood vessels leading to haemorrhagic infarction and necrosis.[35,61]

Diagnosis

Microscopic examination and culture of the involved tissue are the best diagnostic tools. Although isolated contamination of a cultured specimen may occur, the demonstration of *Aspergillus* in any immunocompromised host generally warrants further investigation.[61]

Therapy

Intravenous amphotericin is advocated as first-line therapy for invasive disease. Lipid complex amphotericin B has been suggested in some studies to be effective without having the same nephrotoxic profile observed with the conventional preparation. In localized disease with poor prognosis for recovery (i.e. severe neutropenia) or symptomatic cases (severe haemoptysis), surgical excision may be necessary. In some indolent non-meningeal cases, itraconazole has been shown to be adequate.[35,61]

Tuberculosis

The immunocompromised state of patients with diabetes mellitus and/or renal failure has been repeatedly presented in the literature to be a risk factor for tuberculosis. In fact, the incidence of tuberculosis in dialysis patients has been estimated to be six to 16 times that in the general population.[64] Other studies have similarly shown a significantly higher prevalence of tuberculosis in patients with diabetes mellitus than in the general population. Diabetes mellitus has been noted to be a risk factor for tuberculosis since 1945. The prevalence of tuberculosis in diabetic patients reported during that time was approximately four times that in the general population and the risk was observed to be highest in those with poorly controlled diabetes.[65] More recently, however, tuberculosis appears to show no increased prevalence in diabetic patients in developed countries. The severity and the rate of active disease, however, have been found to correlate with insulin use.[65]

Tuberculosis is an infection that can be caused by two major species of mycobacteria, *Mycobacterium tuberculosis* and *Mycobacterium bovis*. Since tuberculosis caused by the latter is rare compared with *M. tuberculosis*, clinically tuberculosis is often used to refer to the disease caused by *M. tuberculosis*.

Mycobacterium tuberculi are aerobic acid-fast bacilli which resemble slightly bent rods when visualized under $100\times$ magnification with an oil-immersion objective. Growth and reproduction of these organisms is considerably slower than in other bacteria (the generation time is 15–20 h compared with 1 h). Available culture methods therefore require 3–6 weeks for visualization of colonies.[66]

Pathogenesis

The mode of spread is most commonly through the upper airways. Almost all infections are caused by inhalation of infectious droplets aerosolized by coughing, sneezing, or talking. Less frequently, the spread of tuberculosis may result from aerosolization of organisms during surgical dressing of cutaneous lesions. In the first few weeks, while the cellular defence system of the host requires time to mount an immune response, the organisms grow freely and multiply in the alveolar space or within alveolar macrophages. Poor host defence may allow uncontrolled growth and lymphatic and haematogenous spread.[66]

Clinical manifestations

At early onset of the disease patients may be asymptomatic. Constitutional symptoms such as fever, chills, night sweats, and weight loss usually manifest when the bacillary growth becomes significantly large. With progression of disease, symptoms may become localized, reflecting the areas or organs involved. Given that the upper airways are the most common route of inoculation, pulmonary involvement occurs in over 80% of all tuberculous cases. Of all extrapulmonary cases, lymphatics, pleura, genitourinary, and bones and joints follow in order of decreasing frequency. Pleuritic chest pain and haemoptysis signify local inflammation of the parietal pleura and erosions into endobronchial tissues or blood vessels respectively. Patients with advanced pulmonary disease may present with gastrointestinal symptoms that occur as a result of swallowing infected sputum. These include painful pharyngeal or oral ulcers, hoarseness secondary to laryngeal involvement, and dysphagia and diarrhoea with gastroenteric involvement. Direct extension from a pulmonary focus may result in tuberculous pericarditis, in which case, the patient may present with signs and symptoms associated with chronic constrictive pericarditis.[66]

Symptoms are often lacking for those with genitourinary involvement. Patients may present with non-specific signs and symptoms including epididymitis/orchitis, recurrent aseptic pyuria, microscopic haematuria, dysuria, frequency, flank pain, and gross haematuria. In more involved cases, papillary necrosis and nephrolithiasis (calcium stones) may occur.[66]

Skeletal involvement may occur as a result of direct extension or haematogenous or lymphatic spread. Skeletal tuberculosis has been shown to have a predilection for the spine, where involvement of the lower thoracic spine is most frequent. Associated symptoms such as back pain or stiffness may be minimal. Other less frequently seen conditions include peritoneal, meningeal, and otic tuberculosis.[66]

Tuberculosis, especially miliary disease, has to be considered in patients with diabetes mellitus and/or end-stage renal failure who present with fever of unknown origin. Affected patients who only presented with non-specific signs and symptoms such as high fevers and haematological abnormalities such as anaemia and leucopenia have been reported. In such cases, tuberculin skin testing may be negative and a chest radiograph may reveal atypical findings such as no infiltration, diffuse mottling or bilateral alveolar infiltrates.[67]

Diagnosis

Diagnosis of tuberculosis depends on the reactivity of the tuberculin test and a high clinical suspicion. The absence of a tuberculin skin test in high-risk patients, however, does not rule out the possibility of tuberculosis, particularly in the presence of renal failure or concomitant immunosuppression. Additional findings on the chest radiograph of apical cavitary lesions associated with a patchy or nodular infiltrate, pericardial calcifications, or spinal findings of anterior wedging of involved adjacent vertebral bodies and destruction of the intervertebral disc may aid in making the diagnosis. Although non-specific, a significantly elevated sedimentation rate may accompany active disease. Other laboratory findings may include hyponatraemia and hypercalcaemia. Depending on the clinical presentation, evaluations including sputum induction, gastric lavage, cerebral spinal fluid, joint fluid, and ascitic fluid examination may be required. Historically, definitive diagnosis requires the presence of the organism by acid-fast stain and cultures. Cultures, however, require 3–6 weeks, and may delay therapy. Techniques using polymerase chain reaction and molecular 'DNA fingerprinting' using restriction fragment length polymorphisms can give a diagnosis much more rapidly, but their use is not yet feasible in most clinical situations.[66,67]

Therapy

The Centers for Disease Control and Prevention and the American Thoracic Society currently recommend a standard 6-month therapy with isoniazid (INH 5 mg/kg/day not to exceed 300 mg/day) and rifampin (RMP 10 mg/kg/day not to exceed 600 mg/day), with pyrazinamide (PZA 15–30 mg/kg/day not to exceed 2000 mg/day) given for the first 2 months to compliant patients with susceptible organisms. Ethambutol (15–25 mg/kg/day) or streptomycin (15 mg/kg/day not to exceed 1000 mg/day) may be added if resistance is a concern. Conditions favouring a low possibility for resistance include: less than 4% resistance to INH in the given community; the patient has no previous exposure to antituberculosis medications; the patient has no known exposure to a drug-resistant case; the patient is not from a country with a high prevalence of drug resistance.

An alternative 9-month therapy with INH and RMP can be given to patients who cannot take PZA. Ethambutol or streptomycin should be added to the regimen if INH resistance is a concern while awaiting drug susceptibility studies. If resistance is present, both RMP and ethambutol must be continued for at least 12 months.

For extrapulmonary tuberculosis, the same regimen as pulmonary tuberculosis can be used but it is recommended that the duration of therapy should be at least 12 months.

The dosages for INH and RMP need to be halved for patients with creatinine clearance below 10 ml/min. For ethambutol, the dosing frequency should be decreased to every 36–48 h depending on the degree of renal failure. For those requiring haemo-dialysis, these drugs should be given following each treatment. In general, the use of streptomycin, kanamycin, and capreomycin should be avoided in patients with impaired renal function. As peripheral neuropathy is common in patients with diabetes mellitus and end-stage renal disease, pyridoxine should be given routinely.[68]

In general, therapy may have to be prolonged as dictated by clinical response.

In addition, preventive therapy should be considered for diabetics as well as patients with end-stage renal disease when the tuberculin skin test results in an induration greater than or equal to 10 mm regardless of age.[68] It is recommended that prophylactic therapy should continue for 6 months unless there are abnormal findings on the chest radiograph. In the latter case, 12-month therapy is recommended. Unfortunately, this group of patients is often anergic to tuberculin skin testing. Guidelines for immunosuppressed patients have suggested the use of purified protein derivative tuberculin and two companion delayed-type hypersensitivity antigens to assess anergy.[65]

Emphysematous cholecystitis

Emphysematous cholecystitis is a rare form of acute cholecystitis in which progression to gangrene, perforation, and potentially fatal sepsis may occur. Previous studies revealed that more than one-third of patients with emphysematous cholecystitis have diabetes mellitus. Vascular insufficiency is also reported to be a risk factor for the disease. Causative organisms include predominantly gas-forming *Clostridium* species, *C. welchii*, and less commonly *E. coli*.[69,70]

Clinical manifestations

Affected patients present with diffuse to localized right upper quadrant or epigastric pain associated with nausea and vomiting, and fevers. These signs and symptoms, however, may be relatively benign despite a grave clinical prognosis. In fact, one study reported that one-third of affected patients were afebrile and half had a white blood cell count of less than $16\,000/mm^3$.[70,71]

Pathogenesis

The development of emphysematous cholecystitis occurs with bacterial invasion of the gallbladder wall. Local ischaemia due to arterial occlusion is felt to be the predisposing factor. Hypoperfusion-induced ischaemia promotes local inflammatory changes and an undisturbed environment for bacterial growth. Inflammatory changes increase biliary pH and provide a more favourable medium for bacterial growth. Subsequent bacterial proliferation and gas formation result in air collections within the gallbladder wall. If the diagnosis is delayed, the infection may progress to cause perforation of the gallbladder and potentially fatal sepsis.[70,71]

Diagnosis

Diagnosis is based on the clinical presentation, radiographic findings, and biliary/blood cultures. Plain radiography or abdominal CT may reveal air within the gallbladder lumen, gallbladder wall or pericholecystic tissues. The last two findings may be more specific for emphysematous cholecystitis.[22,70,71]

Therapy

Treatment of emphysematous cholecystitis requires early surgical intervention. Empirical antibiotic coverage should cover clostridia, Gram-negative, and anaerobic organisms. Penicillin G should be part of the initial antimicrobial therapy when there is a concern for the disease. Clindamycin may be a substitute for penicillin G in penicillin-allergic patients. Clindamycin resistance of some clostridia species, however, may be high. Optimal therapy relies on cultures and sensitivity obtained from biliary samples.[70,71]

Infectious arthritis

Infectious arthritis is a serious condition that can lead to permanent loss of joint function (in 25–50% of cases) and death (in 5–15% of cases). In adults, infectious arthritis usually results from haematogenous inoculation of pathogenic organisms. Risks for the development of septic arthritis include patient's age, presence of rheumatoid arthritis, prostheses, skin infections, invasive surgical procedures, diabetes mellitus, and other underlying chronic medical conditions.[72,73] The presence of underlying osteodystrophy in chronic renal patients has been suggested to result in a worse outcome.[74]

Clinical manifestations

Common clinical manifestations include fevers (60–80% of cases) and monoarticular involvement (90% of cases). Commonly affected joints include the larger joints such as knees, hips, ankles, shoulders, elbows, and wrists. Joint tenderness associated with a limited range of motion and swelling secondary to synovial effusion is the typical presentation.[72,73]

Pathogenesis

Bacterial arthritis of native joints typically occurs via haematogenous seeding or direct invasion following trauma. With bacterial entry into the joint space, an acute inflammatory reaction takes place within the synovium. This is followed by a proliferative lining-cell hyperplasia, influx of inflammatory cells, cartilage degradation, and subchondral bone loss if intervention is delayed.[72,73]

Diagnosis

Although laboratory findings such as elevated sedimentation rates and peripheral leucocytosis are helpful clues for diagnosing infectious arthritis, examination of the synovial fluid from the affected joint is required for accurate diagnosis. The synovial fluid may appear serosanguinous or turbid and purulent. The leucocyte count is typically in the range of $(50–150)\times10^6$/ml with a predominance (>75%) for polymorphonuclear leucocytes. Non-specific inflammatory synovial fluid findings include depressed glucose and elevated lactic acid and lactate dehydrogenase levels. Definitive diagnosis is based on the demonstration of the pathogen on a stained smear of joint fluid and/or culture of the pathogen. Synovial fluid and blood cultures for the pathogen should be done both aerobically and anaerobically. If there is suspicion of mycobaterial or fungal involvement, cultures of the synovial tissue may be more sensitive (94% versus 80–90% for blood culture).[72,73]

Besides the most common pathogen *Staphylococcus aureus*, other reported causative micro-organisms in diabetic infectious arthritis include β-haemolytic streptococci, *Haemophilus influenzae*, *Enterococcus faecalis*, *Escherichia coli*, *Pseudomonas pseudomallei*, *Klebsiella pneumoniae*, *Nocardia*, and *Cryptococcus*. Other rare infections reported in patients with renal failure include *Candida parpsilosis*, *Pasteurella multocida*, and mycobacteria. Infectious arthritis involving Gram-negative bacilli may be more prevalent in diabetic patients with renal disease because it has been reported to occur more frequently in older patients with chronic debilitating systemic conditions, chronic arthritis, and in those who suffer from recurrent urinary tract infections with Gram-negative bacteraemia.

Therapy

Prompt empirical antimicrobial therapy should be initiated after the initial examination of the joint fluid and blood samples. If a Gram stain reveals clusters of Gram-positive organisms suspicious for *Staphylococcus aureus*, administration of an intravenous penicillinase-resistant penicillin such as nafcillin or oxacillin is recommended. Teicoplanin with flucloxocillin or fucidin is an alternative. If Gram-positive organisms in chains suggesting streptococci are present, penicillin G would be an appropriate initial therapy. For negative staining, empirical therapy should cover *S. aureus* and streptococci. For Gram-negative bacilli, combinations of a β-lactam and an aminoglycoside or second-generation quinolone may be appropriate. The typical duration of treatment is 2 weeks but may have to be extended to 3–4 weeks in the case of involvement of staphylococci or Gram-negative bacilli. Recurrent joint effusions may be alleviated with repeated needle aspiration. However, persistent effusion beyond 7 days generally requires surgical drainage. Following drainage, antimicrobial therapy is usually continued for up to a week and the wound is allowed to close by secondary intention. Early gentle physical therapy for the involved joint should be integrated into the overall treatment plan to ensure appropriate functional recovery.[72,73]

Prevention and management options for all infectious complications in patients with diabetes mellitus and renal disease

Prevention of infectious complications is targeted at correctable predisposing factors. Optimizing metabolic control including normalization of serum glucose and minimizing insulin deficiency/resistance are valuable tools for early interventions. Uncontrolled diabetes predisposes to intercurrent infection and intercurrent infections invariably make diabetic control difficult. Such patients may initially require a continuous infusion of insulin to regain control. For patients with renal disease, renoprotective measures including tight control of blood pressure and proteinuria are essential. Patient education about self-care and early wound detection should be emphasized. Appropriate nutritional advice should be incorporated into the patient's routine evaluation. The importance of specialized diabetic foot care cannot be overstated (see Chapter 19).

Conventional management in patients with infectious complications has always depended heavily on the acute or chronic suppressive use of antimicrobials. More recently, the use of biological response modifier substances (BRMS) has been advocated as second-line treatment in patients with chronic recurrent infections. These include natural or synthetic substances that can directly or indirectly modulate the activities of immune cells. Reported substances include synthetic thymic hormones, zinc, and myelopoietic stimulating factors.[19] A precise microbiological diagnosis is essential. This may necessitate invasive procedures which should not be delayed.

References

1. Pozzilli P, Leslie RG (1994). Infections and diabetes: mechanisms and prospects for prevention. *Diab Med* 11: 935–41.
2. Al-Kassab AS, Raziuddin S (1990). Immune activation and T cell subset abnormalities in circulation of patients with recently diagnosed type I diabetes mellitus. *Clin Exp Immunol* 81: 267–71.

3. Galluzzo A, Giordano C, Rubino G, Bompiani GD (1984). Immunoregulatory T-lymphocyte subset deficiency in newly diagnosed type 1 (insulin-dependent) diabetes mellitus. *Diabetologia* **26**: 426–30.

4. Gupta S, Fikrig SM, Khanna S, Orti E (1982). Deficiency of suppressor T-cells in insulin-dependent diabetes mellitus: an analysis with monoclonal antibodies. *Immunol Lett* **4**: 289–94.

5. Cattaneo R, Saibene V, Margonato A, Pozza G (1977). *In vitro* effect of insulin on peripheral T-lymphocyte E-rosette function from normal and diabetic subjects. *Boll Ist Sieroter Milan* **56**: 139–43.

6. Jos WM Van Der Meer (1994). Defects in host defense mechanisms. In: RH Rubin and LS Young (eds) *Clinical Approach to Infection in the Compromised Host* 3rd edn, pp. 33–65. Plenum Medical Book Company, New York.

7. Hostetter MK (1990). Handicaps to host defense. Effects of hyperglycemia on C3 and *Candida albicans Diabetes* **39**: 271–5.

8. Ha CL, Woodward B (1998). Depression in the quantity of intestinal secretory IgA and in the expression of the polymeric immunoglobulin receptor in caloric deficiency of the weanling mouse. *Lab Invest* **78**: 1255–66.

9. Amesty-Valbuena A, Diez-Ewald M, de Villarroel M, Montiel N, Granados A, Diaz S, Salas D, Rivero M (1996). Immunologic characteristics of undernutrition. I. The undernourished patient in nutritional recovery. *Invest Clin* **37**: 95–111.

10. Chandra RK (1999). Nutrition and immunology: from the clinic to cellular biology and back again. *Proc Nutr Soc* **58**: 681–3.

11. Fraser DA, Thoen J, Reseland JE, Forre O, Kjeldsen-Kragh J (1999). Decreased CD4+ lymphocyte activation and increased interleukin-4 production in peripheral blood of rheumatoid arthritis patients after acute starvation. *Clin Rheumatol* **18**: 394–401.

12. Hirsch S, de la Maza MP, Gattas V, Barrera G, Petermann M, Gotteland M, Munoz C, Lopez M, Bunout D (1999). Nutritional support in alcoholic cirrhotic patients improves host defenses. *J Am Coll Nutr* **18**: 434–41.

13. Patterson JE and Andriole VT (1997). Bacterial urinary tract infections in diabetes. *Infectious Disease Clinics of North America* **11**: 735–50.

14. Hill JR, Kwon G, Marshall CA, McDaniel ML (1998). Hyperglycemic levels of glucose inhibit interleukin 1 release from RAW 264.7 murine macrophages by activation of protein kinase C. *J Biol Chem* **273**: 3308–13.

15. Bagdade JD, Stewart M, Walters E (1978). Impaired granulocyte adherence. A reversible defect in patients with poorly controlled diabetes. *Diabetes* **27**: 677–81.

16. Alexiewicz JM, Kumar D, Smogorzewski M, Massry SG (1997). Elevated cytosolic calcium and impaired proliferation of B lymphocytes in type II diabetes mellitus. *Am J Kidney Dis.* **30**: 98–104.

17. Sugar AM (1995). Agents of mucormycosis and related species. In: GL Mandell, JE Bennett, R Dolin (eds) *Principles and Practice of Infectious Diseases* 4th edn, pp. 2311–21. John Wiley, New York.

18. Artis WM, Fountain JA, Delcher HK, Jones HE (1982). A mechanism of susceptibility to mucormycosis in diabetic ketoacidosis: transferrin and iron availability. *Diabetes* **31**: 1109–14.

19. Skerrett SJ, Niederman MS, Fein AM (1989). Respiratory infections and acute lung injury in systemic illness. *Clinics in Chest Med* **10**: 469–502.

20. Marvisi M, Marani G, Brianti M, Della Porta R (1996). Pulmonary complications in diabetes mellitus. *Recent Prog Med* **87**: 623–7.

21. Joshi N, Caputo GM, Weitekamp MR, Karchmer AW (1999). Infections in patients with diabetes mellitus. *New Engl J Med* **341**: 1906–12.

22. Montgomerie JZ, Kalmanson GM, Guze LB (1968). Renal failure and infection. *Medicine* **47**: 1–32.

23. Vejlsgaard R (1966). Studies on urinary infection in diabetes: II. Significant bacteriuria in relation to long-term diabetic manifestations. *Acta Med Scand* **179**: 183–188.

24. Seabrook GR, Edmiston CE, Schmitt DD, Krepel C, Bandyk DF, Towne JB (1991). Comparison of serum tissue antibiotic levels in diabetes-related foot infections. *Surgery* **110**: 671–76.

25. Duckworth C, Fisher JF, Carter SA, Newman CL, Cogburn C, Nesbit RR, Wray CH (1993). Tissue penetration of clindamycin in diabetic foot infections. *J Antimicrob Chemother* **31**: 581–4.

26. Centers for Disease Control (1991). Lower extremity amputations among persons with diabetes mellitus—Washington, 1988. *MMWR* **40**: 737.

27. Grayson ML, Gibbons GW, Habershaw GM, Freeman DV, Pomposelli FB, Rosenblum BI, Levin E, Karchmer AW (1994). Use of ampicillin/sulbactam versus imipenem/cilastatin in the treatment of limb-threatening foot infections in diabetic patients. *Clin Infect Dis* **18**: 683–93.

28. Grayson ML (1995). Diabetic foot infections: antimicrobial therapy. *Infect Dis Clin of North Am* **9**: 143–61.

29. Laing P (1994). Diabetic foot ulcers. *Am J Surg* **167** (1A): 31S–36S.

30. Edmonds ME (1999). Progress in care of the diabetic foot. *Lancet* **354**: 270–72.

31. ZMcCabe CJ, Stevenson RC, Dolan AM (1998). Evaluation of a diabetic foot screening and protection programme. *Diabet Med* **15**: 80–84.

32. Lipsky BA (1999). Evidence-based antibiotic therapy of diabetic foot infections. *FEMS Immunol Med Microbiol* **26**: 267–76.

33. Lipsky BA, Pecoraro RE, Wheat JL (1990). The diabetic foot: soft tissue and bone infection. *Infect Dis Clin North Am* **4**: 409–32.

34. Day MR and Armstrong DG (1997). Factors associated with methicillin resistance in diabetic foot infections. *J Foot Ankle Surg* **36**: 322–27.

35. Jose A, Vazquez MD, and Sobel JD (1995). Fungal infections in diabetes. *Infectious Dis Clin of North Am* **9**: 97–116.

36. Sobel JD (1997). Pathogenesis of urinary tract infection. *Infect Dis Clin North Am* **11**: 531–549.

37. Batalla MA, Balodimos MC, Bradley RF (1971). Bacteriuria in diabetes mellitus. *Diabetologia* **7**: 297–99.

38. Kayima JK, Otieno LS, Twahir A, Njenga E (1996). Asymptomatic bacteriuria among diabetics attending Kenyatta National Hospital. *East African Med J* **73**: 524–526.

39. Zhanel GG, Nicolle LE, Harding GKM *et al.* (1995). Prevalence of asymptomatic bacteriuria and associated host factors in women with diabetes mellitus. *Clin Infect Dis* **21**: 316–22.

40. Zhanel GG, Harding GK, Nicolle LE (1991). Asymptomatic bacteriuria in patients with diabetes mellitus. *Rev Infect Dis* **13**: 150–154.

41. Semetkowska-Jurkiewicz E, Horoszek-Maziarz S, Galinski J, Manitius A, Krupa-Wojciechowska B. (1995). The clinical course of untreated asymptomatic bacteriuria in diabetic patients—14-year follow-up. *Mater Med Pol* **27**: 91–95.

42. Stein G and Funfstuck R (1999). Asymptomatic bacteriuria—what to do. *Nephrol Dial Transplant* **14**: 1618–21.

43. Nicolle LE (1997). Asymptomatic bacteriuria in the elderly. *Infectious Dis Clin North Am* **11**: 647–63.

44. Stamm WE and Hooton TM (1993). Management of urinary tract infections in adults. *New Engl J Med* **329**: 1328–34.
45. Kunin CM (1994). Chemoprophylaxis and suppressive therapy in the management of urinary tract infections. *J Antimicrobial Chemother* **33** (suppl A): 51–62.
46. Wainstein MA, Graham RC, Resnick MI (1995). Predisposing factors of systemic fungal infections of the genitourinary tract. *J Urol* **154**: 160–163.
47. Shokeir AA, El-Azab M, Mohsen T, El-Diasty T (1997). Emphysematous pyelonephritis: a 15-year experience with 20 cases. *Urology* **49**: 343–346.
48. Dembry LM and Andriole VT (1997). Renal and perirenal abscesses. *Infect Dis Clin North Am* **11**: 663–679.
49. Brown PS Jr, Dodson M, Weintrub PS (1996). Xanthogranulomatous pyelonephritis: report of nonsurgical management of a case and review of the literature. *Clin Infect Dis* **22**: 308–314.
50. McCoy RI, Kurtz AB, Rifkin MD, Kodroff MB, Bidula MM (1985). Ultrasound detection of focal bacterial nephritis (lobar nephronia) and its evolution into a renal abscess. *Urol Radiol* **7**: 109–11.
51. Roberts JA (1999). Management of pyelonephritis and upper urinary tract infections. *Urol Clin North Am* **26**: 753–763.
52. Edelstein H, McCabe RE (1988). Perinephric abscess: modern diagnosis and treatment in 47 cases. *Medicine (Baltimore)* **67**: 118–31.
53. Graandis JR, Yu VL (1997). Necrotizing (malignant) external otitis. In: JT Johnson, VL Yu (eds) *Infectious Diseases and Antimicrobial Therapy of the Ears, Nose and Throat*, pp. 314–320. W.B. Saunders, Philadelphia, PA.
54. Elliott DC, Kufera JA, Myers RA (1996). Necrotizing soft tissue infections: risks factors for mortality and strategies for management. *Ann Surg* **224**: 672–83.
55. Cha JY, Releford BJ Jr, Marcarelli P (1994). Necrotizing fasciitis: a classification of necrotizing soft tissue infections. *J Foot Ankle Surg* **33**: 148–55.
56. Utas C, Unluhizarci K, Oken T, Unlu Y, Doganay M, Kelestimur F (1995). Acute renal failure associated with rhinosinuso-orbital mucormycosis infection in a patient with diabetic nephropathy. *Nephron* **71**: 235.
57. Lee FY, Mossad SB, Adal KA (199). Pulmonary mucormycosis: the last 30 years. *Arch Intern Med* **159**: 1301–1309.
58. Harrill WC, Stewart MG, Lee AG, Cernoch P (1996). Chronic rhinocerebral mucormycosis. *Laryngoscope* **106**: 1292–1297.
59. Davila RM, Moser SA, Grosso LE (1991). Renal mucormycosis: a case report and review of the literature. *J Urol* **145**: 1242–1244.
60. Chugh KS, Sakhuja V, Gupta KL, Jha V, Chakravarty A, Malik N, Kathuria P, Pahwa N, Kalra OP (1993). Renal mucormycosis: computerized tomographic findings and their diagnostic significance. *Am J Kid Disease* **22**: 393–397.
61. Bennet JE (1995). *Aspergillus* species. In: GL Mandell, JE Bennett, R Dolin (eds) *Principles and Practice of Infectious Diseases*, 4th edn, pp. 2306–2311. John Wiley, New York.
62. Sessa A, Meroni M, Battini G, Pitingolo F, Giordano F, Marks M, Casella P (1996). Nosocomial outbreak of *Aspergillus fumigatus* infection among patients in a renal unit? *Nephrol Dial Transplant* **11**: 1322–1324.
63. Lana-Peixoto MI, Lana-Peixoto MA (1992). Invasive aspergillosis of the sphenoid sinus and paralysis of the 6th nerve. *Arq Neuropsiquiatr* **50**: 110–115.
64. Cohen G, Haag-Weber M, Horl WH (1997). Immune dysfunction in uremia. *Kidney Int* **52** (S52): S79–S82.

65. Reichman LB, Hershfield ES (ed.) (1997). *Tuberculosis: a comprehensive international approach*. W.B. Saunders, Philadelphia. PA.

66. Haas DW, Des Prez RM (1995). *Mycobacterium tuberculosis*. In: GL Mandell, JE Bennett, R Dolin (eds) *Principles and Practice of Infectious Diseases*, 4th edn, pp.2213–2243. John Wiley, New York.

67. Bobrowitz D (1982). Active tuberculosis undiagnosed until autopsy. *Am J Med* 72: 650–658.

68. Bass JB Jr, Farer LS, Hopewell PC, O'Brien R, Jacobs RF, Ruben F, Snider DE Jr, Thornton G (1994). Treatment of tuberculosis and tuberculosis infection in adults and children. *Am J Respir Crit Care Med* 49: 1359–1374.

69. Abengowe CU, McManamon PJM (1974). Acute emphysematous cholecystitis. *CMAJ* 111: 1112–1114.

70. Mentzer RM Jr, Golden GT, Chandler JG, Horsley JS III (1975). A comparative appraisal of emphysematous cholecystitis. *Am J Surg* 129: 10–15.

71. Jolly TM and Love JN (1993). Emphysematous cholecystitis in an elderly woman: case report and review of the literature. *J Emerg Med* 11: 593–697.

72. Goldenberg DL (1998). Septic arthritis. *Lancet* 351: 197–202.

73. Kaandorp CJ, van Schaardenburg D, Krijnen P, Habbema JD, van de Laar MA (1995). Risk factors for septic arthritis in patients with joint disease. *Arthritis Rheumatism* 38: 1819–1825.

74. Ciernik IF, Gerster JC, Burckhardt P (1997). Destructive pneumococcal septic arthritis in end-stage renal disease. *Clin Rheumatol* 16: 477–9.

7

Sepsis syndrome and infective complications of acute renal failure

Jane Goddard and Allan Cumming

The connection between sepsis and acute renal failure is a 'two-way street'. Sepsis is a dominant cause of acute renal failure and renal dysfunction is a common and important component of the sepsis syndrome and consequent multiorgan failure. In turn, patients with acute renal failure are at increased risk of infective complications which at best prolong their illness and at worst may contribute to mortality. This chapter deals with both sides of this relationship in turn, beginning with the pathophysiology of the sepsis syndrome and the role of sepsis in the causation of acute renal failure.

Sepsis syndrome

The importance of sepsis syndrome and septic shock is apparent in the mortality associated with these conditions. In one prospective study of 191 patients admitted to an intensive care facility there was a 13% mortality associated with a diagnosis of sepsis syndrome, rising to 43% in patients with septic shock supervening after admission.[1] Mortality in septic shock with three or more organs failed is in excess of 70%.[2] While many new therapies have been proposed for the treatment of sepsis and have yielded promising results in animal studies, trials in humans have been generally disappointing. The heterogeneous nature of the population under study and confusion regarding definitions in sepsis, and thus exclusion and inclusion criteria for such trials, account, at least in part, for the discrepancies between animal and human studies.

In an attempt to overcome this, in 1992 the ACCP/SCCM consensus conference attempted to define standard criteria for the recognition of sepsis.[3] From this meeting, sepsis syndrome is defined as the systemic response to infection manifested by two or more of the following as a result of infection: hypo- or hyperthermia ($<36°C$ or $>38°C$), tachypnoea (>20 breaths/min or $PaCO_2 <32$ mmHg), tachycardia (>90 beats/min), and a white blood cell count below $4000/mm^3$ or above $12\,000/mm^3$. Sepsis is one cause of the systemic inflammatory response syndrome (SIRS). The progression to septic shock is characterized by hypotension or the need for inotropes despite adequate fluid resuscitation and evidence of compromised organ perfusion, as may be indicated by increased plasma lactate, oliguria, or altered cognition.[3]

The clinical features we recognize as sepsis syndrome are the result not of the direct action of infective agents or their products, but the consequence of the activation of a complex cascade of events within the patient in response to infection. For example, bacteria or their products, such as endotoxins, will be recognized and bound by proteins on immune-competent cells, particularly polymorphs and macrophages. These cells, thus activated, release a series of cytokines such as tumour necrosis factor-α (TNF-α), interferon-γ (IFN-γ, and interleukin 1 (IL-1) and activate the plasma cascades of the complement, coagulation, and contact systems. This, in turn, results in further cell recruitment and mediator release. Endothelial cells, activated by cell injury either directly or via the release of inflammatory mediators, will also participate in this inflammatory response. It is now well recognized that the vascular endothelium, far from being an inert conduit for blood, has an integral role in regulating vascular tone and structure, platelet adhesion, coagulation, and immunological reactivity. Many of the cytokine cascades activated by sepsis will be modulated by, or cause their effects via, the vascular endothelium, with endothelium-derived compounds such as endothelin 1 (ET-1), prostacyclin (PGI_2), nitric oxide (NO), and platelet activating factor (PAF) playing a major role in the alterations resulting from sepsis. Though these mechanisms initially act locally to cause vasodilatation, increased vascular permeability, egress of leucocytes from the blood stream, oedema, and microthrombi—all designed to limit infection in that area—occasionally the process will escape local control and systemic activation will result in the sepsis syndrome.

In its early stages or in a well-resuscitated patient, the hypotension of septic shock is associated with a low systemic vascular resistance (SVR) and an increased cardiac output—a hyperdynamic picture. In the presence of inadequate fluids or impaired cardiac function, a hypodynamic picture of low cardiac output and vasoconstriction may accompany the low blood pressure. As blood pressure drops, so perfusion to end organs will fall. The kidney will, in normal circumstances, preserve renal perfusion pressure, and thus glomerular filtration, by efferent arteriolar vasoconstriction within the limits of its capacity to autoregulate (as low as a mean arterial pressure of 75 mmHg).[4] However, this capacity may eventually be exceeded, with consequent ischaemia and tubular necrosis. Also, there is evidence that this ability to autoregulate is impaired in acute renal failure.[5] Though evidence in animals and humans regarding renal alterations in RBF in sepsis is conflicting, there is evidence to suggest that, particularly in the hypodynamic state, but also, in some circumstances, in the hyperdynamic state with maintenance of blood pressure, the renal circulation will vasoconstrict disproportionately relative to the systemic circulation.[6–8] Additionally, there may be deleterious alterations in intrarenal blood flow specific to septic as opposed to other forms of shock that exacerbate ischaemic tubular damage.[8,9] Consequently, acute renal failure is a common concomitant of sepsis. Sepsis can be implicated, at least in part, as a causal agent in at least half of hospital cases of acute renal failure, and a similar proportion of septic patients will go on to develop acute renal failure in isolation or as part of multiorgan failure.[10–12]

Acute renal failure in sepsis

Endotoxin administered to an isolated perfused kidney does not reduce perfusate flow except at high concentrations.[13] The alterations in renal haemodynamics in sepsis are therefore more likely to be a consequence of secondary mediators activated by endotoxin.

It has been proposed that renal injury in sepsis is the result of ischaemia, occurring via activation of vasoconstricting compounds such as angiotensin II, ET-1, PAF, and thromboxane (TxA_2) and formation of intrarenal microthrombi. Endothelial damage with a local reduction in vasodilators such as NO and PGI_2 will also contribute to the overall reduction in RBF.[14] We will explore some of these mechanisms below and question why the renal response differs from that of the systemic circulation.

Nitric oxide

Nitric oxide is an inorganic short-lived free radical synthesized from L-arginine by a series of nitric oxide synthases (NOS). In the blood vessels it will cause direct relaxation of vascular smooth muscle cells and hence vasodilatation. Blockade of NOS in healthy volunteers increases SVR, indicating a role for basal NO generation in the maintenance of normal vascular tone.[15,16] NO also inhibits platelet aggregation and adhesion to the vessel wall. Activation of macrophage inducible nitric oxide synthase (iNOS) in sepsis results in massive generation of NO that, as a superoxide anion, acts as a killing mechanism for the macrophage by causing oxidative injury to the target cell. Once expressed, iNOS remains maximally active for several hours, and there is evidence for a positive feedback loop involving IL-1 that augments NO production further.[17,18] Overproduction of NO, from endothelial as well as immune competent cells, as a consequence of iNOS activation by endotoxins and inflammatory cytokines has been implicated as a major cause of the vasodilatation, hypotension, and hyporesponsiveness to pressor agents seen in sepsis.

The evidence for the importance of NO in sepsis comes from several sources. Firstly, plasma concentrations of NO products, nitrites and nitrates, are elevated in sepsis correlating with the degree of vasodilatation.[19–23] Secondly, transgenic mice with no iNOS gene do not become hypotensive when given endotoxin.[24,25] Thirdly, in both animals and humans, a series of studies have demonstrated the effectiveness of specific inhibitors of NO synthesis in reversing the vasodilatation of sepsis and restoring the vascular response to pressor agents.[19–23,26] Glucocorticoids, which have been used with varying success to combat the haemodynamic response to sepsis, could be acting at this point in the sepsis cascade as they can inhibit the induction of iNOS by cytokines.[27]

However, despite the haemodynamic success of NOS inhibitors in sepsis, the immune function and antiplatelet effects of NO must be remembered.[28] Blockade of NOS might increase formation of microthrombi and reduce the efficiency of the immune system. NOS inhibitors have also been associated, in animal models, with adverse events such as increasing pulmonary artery pressures and pulmonary vascular resistance, already elevated by lipopolysaccharide administration and, worryingly, increased mortality, though this may be a dose-related effect.[29–31] One option is to block NOS activity and replace the beneficial effects of NO by the administration of titrated amounts of exogenous NO donors. Compounds that scavenge NO in biological systems such as free haemoglobin or ruthenium complexes have also produced systemic haemodynamic benefits in animal models of sepsis with less effect on pulmonary artery pressure.[17,32] Their use in humans has yet to be explored.

While the systemic vasculature dilates, the renal vasculature is constricting. Within the renal circulation, NO may, therefore, function to preserve RBF in sepsis; thus inhibition of NOS for systemic benefits may be deleterious to the kidney. Certainly, inhibition of NOS has been shown to aggravate experimental sepsis-induced renal hypoperfusion and increase the formation of microthrombi within the glomerulus, thus compromising function.[28,33,34]

In terms of why the renal circulation should differ from the systemic, there is evidence that ischaemia impairs endothelial NO-dependent vascular relaxation.[35,36] Thus, while NO will cause systemic dilatation and hypotension, overwhelming compensatory constrictor mechanisms, the consequent renal hypoperfusion and ischaemia may, in fact, impair renal NO production and alter the endothelial balance of constrictors and dilators in the kidney in favour of vasoconstrictors. NO can also cause direct cell damage in conjunction with reactive oxygen species (see below) and this endothelial injury will further impair the ability of the renal circulation to dilate.[37]

Endothelin

Endothelins are a family of 21-amino-acid peptides that have vasoactive, mitogenic, and inotropic properties and interact with neuroendocrine systems. Endothelin 1 is the predominant vascular isoform, being produced by vascular endothelial cells, and is the most powerful vasoconstrictor yet discovered.[38] It mediates vasoconstriction via ET-A receptors on vascular smooth muscle cells but will also cause release of the vasodilatory compounds NO and PGI_2 via activation of endothelial ET-B receptors. Studies with ET receptor antagonists have demonstrated the importance of endothelin in the maintenance of normal vascular tone.[39] The inhibition of production of ET-1 production by NO, and the ability of ET receptor antagonism to counteract the haemodynamic changes induced by NOS inhibition, underscores the importance of the interaction between these two systems in this respect.[40-42] However, the precise balance of NO and ET in sepsis, both systemic and local, is, as yet, unclear.

As with NO, plasma ET-1 concentrations are increased in sepsis.[23,43,44] This may relate, in part, to decreased renal clearance consequent upon sepsis-associated renal dysfunction or it may represent endothelial cell synthesis and secretion in response to bacterial toxins or cytokines.[45] Sequential measurements of ET and nitrite/nitrate in the plasma of septic rats have shown that the time courses of these changes in concentration are different, with the plasma NO concentration rising later than ET but remaining elevated for longer, producing an imbalance between NO and ET.[46]

It has been suggested that these high plasma ET-1 concentrations represent an attempt by the body to counteract the vasodilatation produced by the excess NO. In one study of septic patients, the increase in blood pressure and SVR in response to L-NAME (an NOS inhibitor) correlated not with plasma nitrite/nitrate concentrations, but with ET.[23] Plasma concentrations of an essentially paracrine compound may be misleading but if ET is attempting to restore normal vascular tone, then blockade of this system must be viewed, in systemic terms, as deleterious.[47]

However, while ET may be a counter-regulatory response to NO-induced vasodilatation, it is also possible that ET participates in regional vasoconstrictor responses resulting in ischaemic organ failure. In respect of the kidney, exogenous administration of ET-1 produces profound reductions in RBF and glomerular filtration rate (GFR) and mesangial cells will also contract in response to ET-1 reducing the filtration coefficient.[48] Additionally, the renal circulation is more sensitive to the vasoconstricting effects of ET-1 than other regional vascular beds.[49]

TNF, an early cytokine in the sepsis cascade, will stimulate ET-1 synthesis by glomerular endothelial and mesangial cells and endotoxin has been shown to increase renal endothelin receptor density in the rat.[50–52] Combined with reduced renal production of NO, this local ET activity will promote renal vasoconstriction.

Though blockade of the ET system has been effective in attenuating renovascular changes in non-septic ischaemic models of acute renal failure, the picture in sepsis is less clear but local administration of anti-ET antibody can block endotoxin-induced renal vasoconstriction.[53–55] In rats with experimental abdominal sepsis with a hypodynamic picture, systemic ET-A receptor antagonism increased CO and reduced SVR.[56] While such antagonism may also be useful in ameliorating renal dysfunction, it is likely, however, to be a counterproductive manoeuvre in hyperdynamic sepsis as far as the systemic circulation is concerned. It may be that, as a therapeutic manoeuvre, ET antagonism will only be relevant if it can be locally administered. The role of ET-B receptor blockade, thus inhibiting ET-induced release of NO and PGI_2, has also yet to be defined.

Platelet activating factor

Platelet activating factor is a phospholipid derivative produced by phospholipase A_2 (PLA_2) in a variety of cell types including neutrophils, platelets, and endothelial cells and is a major mediator of inflammatory reactions. It is a chemoattractant for immune competent cells, promotes platelet and leucocyte aggregation and activation, and increases vascular permeability with consequent oedema and reduced cardiac output and blood pressure. It is not stored but is synthesized and immediately released in response to specific triggers.[57,58] Exogenous PAF can mimic the cardiovascular features of endotoxin administration. It is notable that while low doses produce vasodilatation in the circulation as a whole (higher doses constrict), the renal circulation constricts.[7,58,59]

Plasma PAF concentrations are increased in sepsis and the kidneys appear to be major site of production.[7] Thrombin, a product of the activated clotting cascade, triggers mesangial and endothelial cells to synthesize PAF and up-regulates basal PAF expression in glomerular endothelial cells.[60,61] TNF, an early mediator in the sepsis cascade, also stimulates PAF production by human mesangial cells.[62] ET-1 will stimulate the production of PAF by mesangial and endothelial cells and may be the mechanism by which ET induces mesangial cell contraction and reduction of filtration coefficient.[63] Experimentally, PAF inhibitors have been shown to improve renal function in endotoxaemic acute renal failure.[7]

Ecosanoids

Ecosanoids are a family of compounds derived from arachidonic acid, which is formed from the hydrolysis of membrane phospholipids by PLA_2. Arachidonic acid is then converted by cyclo-oxygenases (COX) to form PGH_2 which is subsequently metabolized to

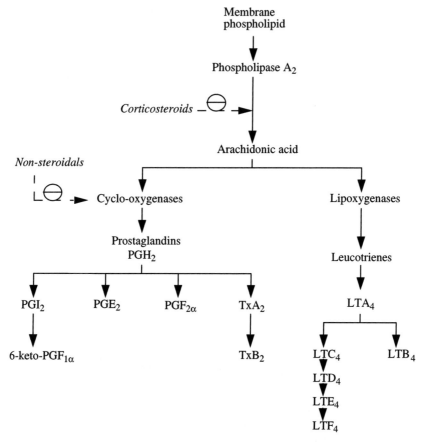

Fig. 7.1 Ecosanoid synthesis: PGE_2=prostaglandin E_2, PGF=prostaglandin F, PGH_2= prostaglandin H2, PGI_2=prostacyclin, Tx=thromboxane, LT=leucotriene.

form various prostaglandins such as PGE_2, PGI_2, or TxA_2. Arachidonic acid can also be metabolized by lipoxygenases to form leucotrienes (LTs) (Fig. 7.1). Prostaglandins are not stored in cells but are synthesized and released immediately, and their half-life is short, with rapid uptake by cells and subsequent inactivation.[57]

These ecosanoids have a wide variety of functions; in particular they are involved in the maintenance of vascular tone and platelet aggregation and adherence. PGI_2 is vasodilatory and inhibits platelet aggregation and adherence to endothelium; PGE_2 is a vasodilator that promotes clotting; TxA_2 and leucotrienes cause smooth muscle and glomerular mesangial cell contraction, increasing vascular tone and reducing the glomerular filtration coefficient. TxA_2 is abundant in platelets where it promotes aggregation.[57] Glomerular alterations will depend on the local balance between the vasodilators and constrictors.

As well as the pathways mentioned above, in sepsis, arachidonic acid can be converted via free radical lipid peroxidation to 8–epi-$PGF_{2\alpha}$ which is a powerful vasoconstrictor.[64]

Additionally, it must be remembered that while PGE_2 and PGI_2 will provide a protective vasodilatory mechanism within the renal circulation, they may be a factor in the detrimental systemic vasodilatation of the sepsis syndrome.

High circulating levels of the secretory form of phospholipase A_2 ($sPLA_2$) have been documented in human sepsis, correlating with endotoxaemia.[65] Experimentally, endotoxin or cytokine exposure will increase the expression of $sPLA_2$ in glomerular mesangial cells which can then act locally on endothelial and epithelial cells to increase production of arachidonic acid.[66,67] Cyclo-oxygenases are also induced in mesangial cells by endotoxin, interleukin-1 and TNF-α suggesting a mechanism whereby regulation of ecosanoids in the kidney may differ from the systemic circulation.[68] Certainly, experimental administration of endotoxin in animal models which show reduction in RBF and GFR in the face of maintained mean arterial pressures, is associated with an increase in intrarenal production of PGE_2, PGI_2 and TxA_2 metabolites as measured directly in cortical tissue, or in the urine.[69,70] Similar urinary findings have been noted in severe human sepsis.[71,72] Given that the observed renal haemodynamic response is vasoconstriction, one must assume that the local balance is altered in favour of TxA_2, though the precise renal mechanism for this is not yet clear.

Non-steroidal anti-inflammatory drugs have been associated with reports of clinical improvement in some studies of sepsis, but their use is difficult as they will inhibit production of PGI_2 and PGE_2 as well as TxA_2 and, by their inhibition of renal vasodilators, worsen renal function.[72] Specific blockade of TxA_2 with thromboxane synthase inhibitors will abolish the endotoxin-induced fall in RBF and GFR without altering renal production of vasodilatory prostaglandins or adversely affecting systemic haemodynamics, and may be a more promising therapeutic option for the kidney.[69,70]

Free radicals

Free radicals are molecules or atoms with unpaired electrons. This electrical imbalance means that they are highly reactive species, combining in the body with lipids, proteins, carbohydrates, and nucleic acids, destroying their structural and functional integrity. Oxygen and nitric oxide species are free radicals and are thus powerful mediators of oxidant injury. They are produced within the body as a consequence of normal metabolism. In cell-mediated immunity, the generation of free radicals is necessary to the cellular killing mechanism. As discussed, in sepsis induction of macrophage and neutrophil NO generation is one source of the excess NO associated with this condition.

In addition to ischaemic renal injury in sepsis, it is now recognized that these free radical species can also mediate renal damage. In human sepsis increased concentrations of free radicals, evidence of free radical damage, and reduced concentrations of anti-oxidants have been documented.[73,74] Free radical damage to the kidney in sepsis is a consequence of inflammation and ischaemia/reperfusion injury. Additionally, nephrotoxins such as gentamicin may also cause renal damage via free radical generation.[75]

Neutrophils are one source of free radicals and have been demonstrated to mediate tubular damage in ischaemic renal injury.[76] *In vitro*, neutrophils perfusing an ischaemic kidney accumulate and become activated. Pretreatment of mice *in vivo* with anti-neutrophil antibodies will protect against ischaemic renal failure.[77-79] Intercellular adhesion molecule-1 (ICAM-1) appears to be at least partially mediating this effect, in that anti-ICAM-1 antibodies will prevent accumulation of neutrophils and consequent renal damage.[78–80] Additionally, mice deficient in ICAM-1 do not show neutrophil accumulation and are protected from renal injury in ischaemia.[79] Endotoxin upregulates endothelial cell expression of ICAM-1; thus sepsis and ischaemia may synergistically increase neutrophil adhesion.[81] Free radical species are also implicated in that free radical scavengers can prevent this ischaemia-induced neutrophil retention and activation.[78] The local loss of endothelial NO production, with its antiaggregant properties, as a consequence of endothelial cell damage exacerbates immune cell adhesion.

However, ischaemia also promotes the formation of free radicals within other cells and oxidative damage has been demonstrated *in vitro* in the absence of neutrophils.[82] Renal tubular epithelial cells produce oxygen free radicals in response to hypoxia and sustain damage from these species, preventable by antioxidants.[83] Interaction of renal mesangial cells with an activated complement system can also result in their production of oxygen free radicals.[84]

Thus in sepsis, ischaemia of end organs such as the kidney, neutrophil priming and adherence (which can occur as a consequence of sepsis or ischaemia) and generation of free radicals within activated neutrophils or renal cells provide a mechanism for oxidative renal injury. Damage to tubular cells will exacerbate tubular necrosis; damage to endothelial cells by this mechanism may further impair the production of endothelium-derived vasodilators. Added to this in sepsis, as discussed, free radical lipid peroxidation of arachidonic acid produces the vasoconstrictor 8-epi-PGF$_{2\alpha}$ (see Fig. 7.2).

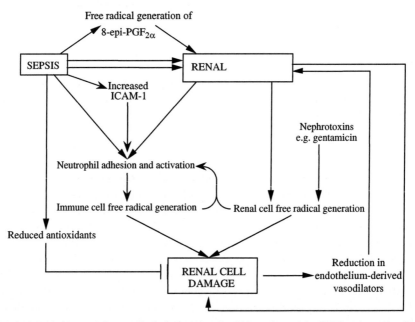

Fig. 7.2 Mechanism of free radical damage to the kidney in sepsis: PGF = prostaglandin F, ICAM-1 = intercellular adhesion molecule-1.

Arginine vasopressin and angiotensin II

Endotoxin increases plasma concentrations of other vasoconstrictors such as angiotensin II, arginine vasopressin (AVP), and noradrenaline in animal models.[85–87] This is, however, coupled with a decrease in responsiveness to exogenous administration of noradrenaline, angiotensin II, and AVP that has been attributed to the overriding dilating effects of NO.[87]

AVP is released from the posterior pituitary into the circulation as a baroreflex response to decreases in blood pressure. As noted, plasma concentrations are high in experimental sepsis coupled with a decreased vessel responsiveness.[87] However, in one study in patients, plasma AVP was found to be inappropriately low in patients with advanced circulatory failure, and correcting plasma concentrations with exogenous AVP to achieve the levels predicted for the degree of hypotension was able to restore blood pressure.[88] Endotoxin does stimulate rapid secretion of AVP in animal models of septic shock.[89] The plasma concentrations peak at 1–2 h after endotoxin administration and subsequently decline.[86] It is possible that AVP stores in the patients investigated had been depleted earlier in the course of their disease as AVP attempted to maintain blood pressure, and lack of this constrictor in advanced shock aggravates the vasodilatation.

In vascular smooth muscle cells exposed to endotoxin there is a significant increase in angiotensin II binding corresponding to an increase the expression of angiotensin I receptors responsible for vasoconstriction. This may represent an attempt by cells to compensate for the decrease in vascular responsiveness, or it may simply be that there is a non-specific induction of genes by endotoxin, though the lack of effect of endotoxin in the same study on AVP binding favours some specificity of gene induction.[90]

While production of these pressor agents may be an attempt by the body to counter NO vasodilatation, if NO production in the renal circulation is impaired, then excess concentrations of these constrictors, either systemic or local, are likely to promote renal vasoconstriction. This local detrimental effect needs to be balanced against the benefits of improved renal perfusion if exogenous administration of these compounds as pressor agents is considered.

Summary

The body's response to infection is characterized at a cellular level by the activation of a cascade of inflammatory mediators designed to isolate any infective agent. For reasons that are unclear, in some cases there is loss of local control of this inflammation resulting in systemic activation of these cascades. There is a complex interplay of mediators, in particular between constrictor and dilator substances, but, in the systemic circulation, the balance is usually in favour of dilators and the net haemodynamic effect is, ultimately, a clinical picture that we recognize as septic shock with reduced systemic vascular resistance and hypotension. There appear, however, to be differing responses in the regional circulation. In the kidney there is local up-regulation of constrictor mechanisms and impairment of vasodilator mechanisms that alters the balance of vasoactive mediators in favour of constriction, contributing to ischaemic acute renal

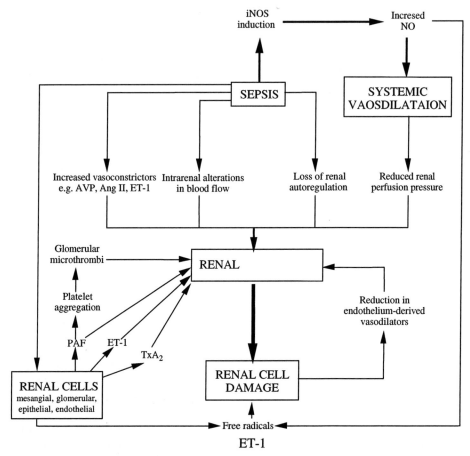

Fig. 7.3 Renal injury in sepsis: NO = nitric oxide, iNOS = inducible nitric oxide synthase, AVP = arginine vasopressin, Ang II = angiotensin II, ET-1 = endothelin 1, PAF = platelet activating factor, TxA$_2$ = thromboxane A$_2$.

failure. Thus, while compounds that increase systemic vascular tone, by enhancing constriction or blocking dilatation, may restore blood pressure, the altered renal response in sepsis could render such systemic treatments hazardous, as they might exacerbate renal vasoconstriction and worsen ischaemic acute renal failure.

Infectious complications of acute renal failure

A recent large multicentre trial showed that in patients with acute renal failure treated in intensive care units the presence of infection was an independent predictor of in-hospital mortality.[91] It is recognized that patients with renal failure exhibit abnormalities of immune function which predispose them to infection, as reviewed by Haag-Weber and Horl and elsewhere in this volume (Chapter 1).[92] It has been estimated that 50% of patients with acute renal failure have positive blood cultures at some point in their admission, and the combined rate of local and systemic infection is obviously even higher.[93] Thus, patients with acute renal failure are unusually susceptible to a common complication which has an important influence on their prognosis. The overall mortality of acute renal failure remains in the region of 50% and is much higher for those with multiorgan failure. Infection is an important contributor to the development of multi-organ failure, as outlined above. Clearly, one of the key challenges to those involved in the management of patients with acute renal failure is to reduce the rates of secondary infection and to improve the treatment of septic complications, with a view to reducing the overall mortality of acute renal failure.

Predisposition of acute renal failure patients to infection

The predisposition of uraemic patients to infection involves abnormal phagocytosis by neutrophils and monocytes, defective T-cell function, impaired antibody responses, and abnormalities of the cytokine network.[94] In addition, treatment of acute renal failure by extracorporeal circuits and artificial membranes may further modulate the activity of the immune system, for example through complement activation and consumption of complement components.[92]

In addition to these generalized abnormalities, patients with acute renal failure are at risk of infection related to other aspects of their treatment. Most specifically, they are exposed to the use of invasive treatments, including intravascular and other in-dwelling catheters and infusion devices. They are frequently relatively immobile for long periods, and unless care is taken to avoid it, may suffer from periods of inadequate nutrition and tissue catabolism. Cross-infection is a particular risk in high-dependency units and intensive care units with high concentrations of unwell septic patients. Multiresistant organisms are common in this setting due to the widespread use of potent broad-spectrum antibiotics. Acute renal failure is increasingly common in the elderly and in patients with other comorbid conditions such as diabetes or liver disease; again, the risk of secondary infectious complications is higher in this group than in, for example, a young man with post-traumatic acute renal failure.

Consequences of infection in acute renal failure

The pathophysiology of the sepsis syndrome and its relationship to multiorgan failure has been reviewed above. Severe or recurrent infection can obviously set in train the sequence of events leading to this usually fatal syndrome. However, complicating infection may have other adverse effects on patients with acute renal failure. It is known that patients with prolonged acute renal failure, if biopsied late in the course of their illness, show areas of tubular necrosis which are obviously of recent onset.[95] This has been ascribed to circulatory instability induced by haemodialysis and a failure of the kidney to autoregulate its blood flow during the course of acute renal failure. However, it seems likely that recurrent infection, and particularly the kind of systemic sepsis described by Frost *et al.* in 50% of patients, could have similar effects.[93] It is known that sepsis has potent effects on renal function even in the absence of systemic hypotension.[96] The clinical pattern of the patient with protracted acute renal failure who moves from one infectious complication to the next, and only recovers renal function after a period free of infection, is well know to all nephrologists. Others may not recover renal function and survive to require chronic renal replacement therapy.[97]

Infectious complications have other adverse consequences for patients with acute renal failure. They are exposed to antibiotics, some of which are nephrotoxic and which have the potential to induce resistant organisms or secondary fungal infection. There is a risk of inducing allergic interstitial nephritis with further renal damage. The nutritional and metabolic effects of renal failure are enhanced and prolonged by infection, with increased tissue catabolism, insulin resistance, and enhanced neuroendocrine activity.[98]

Types of infection

Patients with acute renal failure are exposed to any of the standard nosocomial infections to which ill patients are prone during hospital admissions. However, the majority of acute renal failure is now treated in the context of intensive care units. In this setting the risk of hospital-acquired infection is five to ten times higher than in other hospital wards, again related to the presence of concomitant severe disease, use of invasive devices and procedures, and prolonged use of broad-spectrum antibiotics.[99] It has been estimated that about a third of these infections should be preventable by appropriate surveillance and effective institutional policies.[100]

Intravascular catheter-related infection

Catheter-related sepsis, infective endocarditis, and suppurative phlebitis of major veins are all potential complications of intravascular catheters. In acute renal failure, catheters may be placed for peripheral or central fluid therapy, central pressure monitoring, nutritional support or vascular access for renal replacement therapy. Nosocomial catheter-related bacteraemia or candidaemia is associated with a two to three-fold increase in mortality rate.[101] In most series, the most common organisms are coagulase-negative staphylococci (30%) and *Staphylococcus aureus* (25%). Enterococci, *Acinetobacter*, and *Pseudomonas* species (1–4% each) and *Candida* species (around 5%) are also encountered.[102] Methicillin-resistant *S. aureus* (MRSA) and, to a lesser extent, vancomycin-resistant enterococci (VRE), are an increasing concern both in renal wards and in intensive care units; many intensive care units have been obliged to abandon attempts to isolate MRSA-colonized patients.

Treatment of such infections consists of removal of the infected catheter and appropriate antibiotic therapy. Unlike in chronic renal failure, there is seldom if ever a requirement to leave lines *in situ*. Routine replacement of central or peripheral catheters at intervals of 1–2 weeks has been advocated as prophylaxis, but has not been proved to be effective; changing catheters over a guidewire is associated with a high rate of contamination of the new catheter.[103] However, use of maximal sterile precautions at the time of insertion has been shown to favourably influence the rate of subsequent infection.[104]

Urinary infection

Urinary infection is the commonest nosocomial infection in hospitals, and accounts for about 40% of cases in intensive care units.[105] Most cases are related directly or indirectly to instrumentation or catheterization of the urinary tract and urethral catheterization is performed in the vast majority of cases of acute renal failure at some point. The majority of these infections are due to a single organism. *E. coli* accounts for about 50%, with *Klebsiella, Enterobacter, Proteus, Serratia, Pseudomonas*, staphylococci and enterococci as other important organisms. *Corynebacterium* group D2 has been recently recognized as a nosocomial urinary pathogen and is frequently resistant to most antibiotics.

The rate of catheter-associated urinary tract infection is six to ten per 1000 device days. Two to four per cent of patients who develop catheter-associated urinary tract infection will also develop Gram-negative bacteraemia, which is known to adversely affect prognosis. One recent study of patients in intensive case units suggested that at least 60% of patient days with a urinary catheter were unnecessary in relation to patient care.[106] The practice of maintaining urinary catheters *in situ* in anuric or very oliguric patients with acute renal failure should be abandoned. There is also little logic in performing residual urine catheterizations every few days, as practised in many intensive care units. Return of renal function in anuric patients is virtually always heralded by spontaneous voiding of urine, either voluntarily or otherwise.

Treatment of these infections again involves removal of the catheter wherever possible, and appropriate antibiotic therapy. Antibiotic prophylaxis is ineffective in prevention of catheter-associated urinary sepsis, but urinary tract instrumentation in patients with artificial heart valves should be covered with an appropriate antibiotic, such as a single dose of an aminoglycoside.

Respiratory infection

Infection of the respiratory tract is the second most common nosocomial infection in hospitals, accounting for about 15% of nosocomial infections, and is the most significant in terms of increased mortality.[107] Overall, the mortality attributable to hospital-acquired pneumonia has been reported to be of the order of 33%.[108] Patients with acute renal failure are at particular risk because of pre-existing comorbid conditions, relative immobility, and, in the intensive care setting, possible requirement for artificial ventilation and instrumentation of the respiratory tract.

A shift in the pattern of oropharyngeal colonization from Gram-positive to Gram-negative organisms is a well-recognized feature of critical illness, including acute renal failure. If this occurs, the risk of subsequent pneumonia increases from 3% to 23%.[109] Bacterial colonization of the stomach may also predispose to nosocomial pneumonia; use of H_2 antagonists, as commonly practised in acute renal failure and prolonged enteral tube feeding may contribute to this.[99] In patients with a decreased level of consciousness, aspiration of endogenous or hospital-acquired organisms is a further risk factor.

As one would expect from the above, Gram-negative organisms predominate in hospital-acquired pneumonia—*Klebsiella, Enterobacter, E. coli, Serratia*, and *Proteus* are important. Mixed infections are not uncommon. *Haemophilus* and *Neisseria* organisms are also recognized. *S. aureus*, including MRSA, accounts for about 20% of cases. The predominant organisms vary between units, depending on antibiotic policy, patterns of resistance, and infection control practices.

Diagnosis may not be straightforward. The classic features of fever, purulent sputum or secretions, leucocytosis, positive bacteriology, and radiological abnormalities may either be absent, masked by treatment or be explainable by other pathology, such as pulmonary oedema in acute renal failure. A high index of suspicion and careful monitoring, including cultures of blood and secretions, is necessary in predisposed patients. Bronchoalveolar lavage and, in a few cases, bronchoscopy, may be necessary to establish a bacteriological diagnosis in difficult cases.

Treatment consists of appropriate antibiotic therapy based on culture and sensitivities, physiotherapy to assist drainage of secretions, and avoidance of invasive procedures as far as possible. The use of selective gut decontamination to reduce the incidence of secondary pneumonia has been advocated, but most studies show no consistent effect on infection rates and no influence on overall mortality.[110,111]

Gastrointestinal infection

The most common secondary gastrointestinal infection is that due to *Clostridium difficile*. This is related to the use of broad-spectrum antibiotics for primary or secondary infection, and in some cases to contamination of the hospital environment with clostridial spores. Epidemics in renal units affecting patients with acute and chronic renal failure have been described, with demonstrable cross-infection shown by phage-typing.[112] Even in the absence of frank pseudomembranous colitis, this infection is a major cause of morbidity and mortality, particularly in the elderly and those with debilitating comorbid conditions. Treatment consists of withdrawal of the precipitating antibiotic wherever possible, administration of oral metronidazole or vancomycin, and careful attention to fluid and electrolyte balance and nutrition. While oral vancomycin (125 mg, 6-hourly) is widely considered as first-line treatment, use of vancomycin for this purpose should be limited because of the risk of inducing a strain of vancomycin-resistant enterococci—other enteric organisms which may cause outbreaks of diarrhoea and systemic sepsis in units treating renal patients. For *Clostridium difficile* infection, oral metronidazole (500 mg, 8-hourly) is cheaper than vancomycin, and several studies suggest it is just as effective.[113]

Bacterial peritonitis is a complication of peritoneal dialysis when used to treat either acute or chronic renal failure. In both cases, cloudy effluent dialysis fluid indicates the diagnosis, and the organism can usually be grown from the dialysate effluent. Skin organisms predominate, including coagulase-negative staphylocci and diphtheroids. Gram-negative or mixed infection should raise the possibility of an underlying bowel perforation. In acute renal failure, treatment should include removal or replacement of the temporary intraperitoneal catheter and an appropriate antibiotic given systemically or intraperitoneally. Meticulous asepsis during catheter insertion and when breaking the dialysate circuit is the key to prevention. Fungal peritonitis is a rare complication and always follows the use of antibiotics for a bacterial infection. Removal of the intraperitoneal catheter and treatment with systemic antifungals is mandatory in these infections.

Cutaneous infections

Various types of skin infections may occur in acute renal failure. They include cellulitis related to intravascular catheters or wounds; infection of pressure areas due to prolonged immobility; necrotizing fasciitis due to multiresistant staphylococci or streptococci; and occasionally, necrotizing myositis due to clostridial infection. Prevention depends on meticulous nursing practice and a high index of suspicion.

Fungal infection

The frequent debility of patients with acute renal failure and their exposure to multiple antibiotics creates a relatively high risk of both local and systemic fungal infection. Oral candidiasis is common and may impair nutritional intake as well as leading to systemic candidiasis in some patients. Pulmonary or systemic aspergillosis may complicate prolonged artificial ventilation. Specific cultures for fungal organisms should be performed routinely in critically ill patients with renal failure.

Viral infection

Cytomegalovirus is common in adult patients and reactivation may occur in the context of sepsis and ARF. Most units are also treating patients carrying hepatitis B and C also. Apart from the risk of cross-infection, there are no specific considerations with respect to viral infection in patients with acute renal failure. Disturbance of liver transaminases may be seen late in the course of acute renal failure due to transmission of viruses in blood or plasma used in resuscitation.

The immunosuppressed acute renal failure patient

Patients with acute renal failure secondary to immunological diseases such as vasculitis or antiglomerular basement membrane disease are usually treated with intensive immunosuppression often including plasmapheresis. They are at risk of all the recognized opportunist infections, bacterial, viral, and others which affect other immunosuppressed patients. This topic is reviewed elsewhere in this volume (Chapter 5).

Treatment of infection in acute renal failure

The principles of treatment are as follows:

1. Avoid further nephrotoxicity. Agents such as gentamicin and amphotericin should be used only if there is no acceptable alternative. If they must be used the duration of therapy should be kept as short as possible and appropriate monitoring of blood levels should be undertaken.
2. Be aware of altered pharmacokinetics in renal failure. This is reviewed elsewhere in this volume (Chapter 21). In most cases of acute renal failure, intravenous rather than oral administration of antibiotics will be mandatory, at least in the initial phase of treatment. The effect of renal replacement therapy on drug levels should be known and recognized in planning dosage regimes.
3. Avoid drug allergy. The possibility of drug allergy leading to an allergic interstitial nephritis must be remembered. This will delay or even prevent recovery of renal function in acute renal failure. Not all cases are accompanied by a cutaneous rash; eosinophilia in peripheral blood may be a more subtle marker. Drugs with a propensity to cause allergic responses, such as trimethoprim/sulphamethoxazole and early-generation cephalosporins, should be used sparingly if at all. The incidence of both

Table 7.1   Modes of excretion of commonly used antibiotics

Mode of excretion	Antibiotic
Renal	Aminoglycosides
	Cephalosporins
	Penicillins
	Tetracycline
	Vancomycin
	Teicoplanin
	Fluconazole
Hepatic	Clindamycin
	Erythromycin
	Clarythromycin
	Metronidazole
	Rifampicin
	Isoniazid
	Itraconazole
Renal and hepatic	Cefotaxime
	Ciprofloxacin and other quinolones
	Azlocillin
	Piperacillin

allergy and nephrotoxicity is greater with drugs which are primarily excreted by the kidney (Table 7.1).

4. Maintain a narrow spectrum of activity. As described above, patients with acute renal failure are peculiarly open to bacterial or fungal overgrowth and infection with resistant organisms. A narrow-spectrum agent chosen on the basis of culture and sensitivities should be used whenever possible. Routine bacteriological monitoring of patients with acute renal failure will often facilitate this process by making culture and sensitivity results available earlier in the course of an infectious episode. Awareness of local patterns of nosocomial infection and sensitivity of organisms is essential.

Prevention of infectious complications of acute renal failure

Strategies for prevention have been referred to above in relation to particular types of infection. In general terms, prevention requires an informed and meticulous approach, with close collaboration between medical staff, nursing staff, microbiologists, and others involved in patient care. Well-designed unit and institutional guidelines and protocols are important. These should be regularly reviewed in the light of audit data. The challenge of nosocomial infection has not been met—indeed data suggest that these infections are becoming more common and more severe.[99,100,103] A cooperative, multidisciplinary approach to the problem is essential if this trend is to be reversed.

References

1. Bone RC, Fisher CJ, Clemmer TP, *et al.* Sepsis syndrome: a valid clinical entity. *Crit Care Med* 1989;**17**:389–393.

2. Herbert PC, Drummond AJ, Singer J, *et al.* A simple multiple system organ failure scoring system predicts mortality of patients who have sepsis syndrome. *Chest* 1993;**104**:230–235.

3. Bone RC, Balk BA, Cerra FB, *et al.* ACCP/SCCM consensus conference: definitions for sepsis and organ failure and guidelines for the use of innovative therapies in sepsis. *Chest* 1992;**101**:1644–1655.

4. Guyton AC. Formation of urine by the kidney. In: Guyton AC (ed.) *Textbook of medical physiology*, 1991. W. B. Saunders, Philadelphia, PA.

5. Adams PL, Adams FF, Navar LG. Impaired renal blood flow autoregulation in ischaemic acute renal failure. *Kidney Int* 1980;**18**:68–76.

6. Cumming AD, Driedger AA, McDonald JW, *et al.* Vasoactive hormones in the renal response to systemic sepsis. *Am J Kid Dis* 1988;**11**:23–32.

7. Tolins JP, Vercelloti GM, Wilkowske M, *et al.* Role of platelet activating factor in endotoxaemic acute renal failure in the male rat. *J Lab Clin Med* 1989;**113**:316–324.

8. Goddard J, Cumming AD. Renal alterations in the septic patient. In: Ronco C, Bellomo R, (eds) *Critical care nephrology*, 1998:517–526. Kluwer Accademic, Dordrecht.

9. Hellberg POA, Kallskog O, Wolgast M. Red cell trapping and postischaemic renal blood flow. Differences between the cortex, outer and inner medulla. *Kidney Int* 1991;**40**:325–631.

10. Wiecek A, Zeier M, Ritz E. Role of infection in the genesis of acute renal failure. *Nephrol Dial Transplant* 1994;**9** (suppl. 4):40–44.

11. Hou SH, Bushinsky DA, Wish JB, *et al.* Hospital-acquired renal insufficiency: a prospective study. *Am J Med* 1983;**72**:243–248.

12. Karnik AM, Bashir R, Khan FA, *et al.* Renal involvement in the systemic inflammatory reaction syndrome. *Renal Failure* 1998;**20**:103–116.

13. Cohen JJ, Black AJ, Wertheim SJ. Direct effects of endotoxin on the function of the isolated perfused rat kidney. *Kidney Int* 1990;**37**:1219–1226.

14. Wardle NE. Acute renal failure and multiorgan failure. *Nephrol Dial Transplant* 1994;**9** (suppl. 4):104–107.

15. Calver H, Collier J, Vallance P. Nitric oxide and cardiovascular control. *Exp Physiol* 1993;**78**:303–326.

16. Haynes WG, Boon NB, Walker BR, *et al.* L-NMMA increases blood pressure in man. *Lancet* 1993;**342**:931–932.

17. Fricker SP, Slade E, Powell NA, *et al.* Ruthenium complexes as nitric oxide scavengers: a potential therapeutic approach to nitric oxide mediated diseases. *Br J Pharmacol* 1997;**122**:1441–1449.

18. Muhl H, Pfeilschifter J. Amplification of nitric oxide synthase expression by nitric oxide in interleukin-1 beta-stimulated rat mesangial cells. *J Clin Invest* 1995;**95**:1941–1946.

19. Petros A, Bennet D, Vallance P. Effect of nitric oxide synthase inhibitors on hypotension in patients with septic shock. *Lancet* 1991;**338**:1557–1558.

20. Meyer J, Traber LD, Nelson S, *et al.* Reversal of hyperdynamic response to continuous endotoxin administraton by inhibition of NO synthesis. *J Appl Physiol* 1992;**73**:324–328.

21. Meyer J, Hinder F, Stothert JJ, *et al.* Increased organ blood flow in chronic endotoxaemia is reversed by nitric oxide synthase inhibition. *J Appl Physiol* 1994;**76**:2785–2793.

22. Petros A, Lamb G, Leone A, *et al.* Effects of nitric oxide synthase inhibitor in humans with septic shock. *Cardiovasc Res* 1994;**28**:34–39.

23. Avontuur JA, Boomsma F, van den Meiracker AH, *et al.* Endothelin-1 and blood pressure after inhibition of nitric oxide synthesis in human septic shock. *Circulation* 1999;**99**: 271–275.

24. MacMicking JD, Nathan C, Hom G, *et al.* Altered response to bacterial infection and endotoxic shock in mice lacking inducible nitric oxide synthase. *Cell* 1995;**81**:641–650.

25. Wei X-Q, Charles IG, Smith A, *et al.* Altered immune responses in mice lacking inducible nitric oxide synthase. *Nature* 1995;**375**:408–411.

26. Meyer J, Booke M, Waurick R, *et al.* Nitric oxide synthesis restores vasopressor effects of norepinephrine in ovine hyperdynamic sepsis. *Anesth Analg* 1996;**83**:1009–1013.

27. Abraham E. Why immunomodulatory therapies have not worked in sepsis. *Intensive Care Med* 1999;**25**:556–566.

28. Schultz PJ, Raij L. Endogenously synthesised nitric oxide prevents endotoxin induced glomerular thrombosis. *J Clin Invest* 1992;**90**:1718–1725.

29. Robertson FM, Offner PJ, Ciceri DP, *et al.* Detrimental hemodynamic effects of nitric oxide synthase inhibition in septic shock. *Arch Surg* 1994;**129**:149–156.

30. Minnard EA, Shou J, Naama H, *et al.* Inhibition of nitric oxide synthesis is detrimental during endotoxaemia. *Arch Surg* 1994;**129**:142–148.

31. Wright CE, Rees DD, Moncada S. Protective and pathological mechanisms of nitric oxide in endotoxin shock. *Cardiovasc Res* 1992;**26**:48–57.

32. Bone HG, Waurick R, Van Aken H, *et al.* Comparison of the haemodynamic effects of nitric oxide synthase inhibition and nitric oxide scavenging in endotoxaemic sheep. *Intensive Care Med* 1998;**24**:48–54.

33. Mulder MF, Van Lambalgen AA, Huisman E, *et al.* Protective role of NO in the regional haemodynamic changes during endotoxaemia in rats. *Am J Physiol* 1994;**226**:H1558–H1564.

34. Spain DA, Wilson MA, Garrison RN. Nitric oxide synthase inhibition exacerbates sepsis-induced renal hypoperfusion. *Surgery* 1994;**116** (suppl. 2):322–330.

35. Conger JD, Robinette JB, Schrier RW. Smooth muscle calcium and endothelium derived relaxing factor in the abnormal vascular responses of acute renal failure. *J Clin Invest* 1988;**1988**:82.

36. Lieberthal W, Wolf EF, Rennke HG, *et al.* Renal ischaemia and reperfusion impair endothelium-dependent vascular relaxation. *Am J Physiol* 1989;**256**:F894–F900.

37. Volk T, Ioannidis I, Hansel M, *et al.* Endothelial damage induced by nitric oxide: synergism with reactive oxygen species. *Biochem Biophys Res Commun* 1995;**123**:196–203.

38. Yanagisawa M, Kurihara H, Kimura S, *et al.* A novel potent vasoconstrictor peptide produced by vascular endothelial cells. *Nature* 1988;**332**:411–415.

39. Haynes WG, Webb DJ. Endothelin as a regulator of cardiovascular function in health and disease. *J Hypertens* 1998;**16**:1081–98.

40. ZBoulanger C, Luscher TF. Release of endothelin from the porcine aorta. *J Clin Invest* 1990;**85**:587–590.

41. Richard V, Hogie M, Clozel M, *et al.* *In vivo* evidence of an endothelin-induced vasopressor tone after inhibition of nitric oxide synthesis in rats. *Circulation* 1995;**91**:771–775.

42. Filep JG. Endogenous endothelin modulates blood pressure, plasma volume, and albumin escape after systemic nitric oxide blockade. *Hypertension* 1997;**30**:22–28.

43. Weitzberg E, Lundberg JM, Rudehill A. Elevated plasma levels of endothelin in patients with sepsis syndrome. *Circ Shock* 1991;**33**:222–227.

44. Nambi P, Pullen M, Slivjak, *et al.* Endotoxin-mediated changes in plasma endothelin concentrations, kidney endothelin receptor density and renal function in the rat (abstract). *Circ Shock* 1991;**34**:48.

45. Sugiura M, Inagami T, Kon V. Endotoxin stimulates endothelin release *in vivo* and *in vitro* as determined by radioimmunoassay. *Biochem Biophys Res Commun* 1989;**161**:1220–1227.

46. Sharma AC, Motew SJ, Farias S, *et al.* Sepsis alters myocardial and plasma concentrations of endothelin and nitric oxide in rats. *J Mol Cell Cardiol* 1997;**29**:1469–1477.

47. Goddard J, Webb DJ. Plasma endothelin concentrations in hypertension. *J Cardiovasc Pharmacol* 1999; In press.

48. Rabelink TJ, Kaasjager KAH, Boer P, *et al.* Effects of endothelin-1 on renal function in humans: implications for physiology and pathophysiology. *Kidney Int* 1994;**46**:376–381.

49. Pernow J, Franco-Cereceda A, Matran R, *et al.* Effect of endothelin-1 on regional vascular resistance in the pig. *J Cardiovasc Pharmacol* 1989;**13** (suppl. 16):S205–S206.

50. Marsden PA, Dorfmen DM, Collins T, *et al.* Regulated expression of endothelin-1 by glomerular capillary endothelial cells. *Am J Physiol* 1991;**261**:F117–F125.

51. Kohan DE. Production of endothelin-1 by rat mesangial cells: regulation by tumour necrosis factor. *J Lab Clin Med* 1992;**119**:477–484.

52. Nambi P, Pullen M, Jugus M, *et al.* Rat kidney endothelin receptors in ischaemia-induced acute renal failure. *J Pharm Exp Ther* 1993;**264**:345–348.

53. Conger JD, Kim GE, Robinette JB. Effects of ANG II, ETA, and TxA2 receptor antagonists on cyclosporin A renal vasoconstriciton. *Am J Physiol* 1994;**59**:F443–F449.

54. Krause SM, Walsh TF, Greenlee WJ, *et al.* Renal protection by dual ETA/ETB endothelin antagonists L-754,142, after aortic cross-clamping in the dog. *J Am Soc Nephrol* 1997;**8**:1061–71.

55. Kon V, Badr KF. Biological actions and pathophysiological significance of endothelin in the kidney. *Kidney Int* 1991;**40**:1–12.

56. Szalay L, Kaszaki J, Nagy S, *et al.* The role of endothelin-1 in circulatory changes during hypodynamic sepsis in the rat. *Shock* 1998;**10**:123–128.

57. Glew RH. Lipid metabolism II; Pathways of metabolism of special lipids. In: Devlin TM (ed.) *Textbook of biochemistry* 1992:423–473. Wiley-Liss, New York.

58. Schlondorff D, Neuwirth R. Platelet activating factor and the kidney. *Am J Physiol* 1986;**251**:F1–F11.

59. Camussi G. Potential role of platelet activating factor in renal pathophysiology. *Kidney Int* 1986;**29**:469–477.

60. Zimmerman GA, Prescott SM, McIntyre TM. Endothelial cell interactions with granulocytes: tethering and signalling molecules. *Immunol Today* 1992;**13**:93–100.

61. Kester M, Nowinski RJ, Holthofer H, *et al.* Characterization of platelet activating factor synthesis in glomerular endothelial cell lines. *Kidney Int* 1994;**46**:1404–1412.

62. Camussi G, Turello E, Tetta C, *et al.* Tumour necrosis factor induces contraction of mesangial cells and alters their cytoskeletons. *Kidney Int* 1990;**38**:795–802.

63. Lopez-Farre A, Gomez-Garre D, Bernabeu M, *et al.* Renal effects and mesangial cell contraction induced by endothelin are mediated by PAF. *Kidney Int* 1991;**39**:624–630.

64. Morrow JD, Hill KE, Burk RF, *et al.* A series of prostaglandin-F2 like compounds are produced *in vivo* in humans by a non-cyclooxygenase, free radical-catalyzed mechanism. *Proc Natl Acad Sci USA* 1990;**87**:9383–9387.

65. Vadas P, Pruzanski W, Farewell V. A predictive model for the clearance of soluble phospholiase A2 duing septic shock. *J Lab Clin Med* 1991;**118**:471–475.

66. Pfeilschifter J, Muhl H. Interleukin 1 and tumour necrosis factor potentiate angiotensin II- and calcium ionophore stimulated prostaglandin E2 synthesis in rat renal mesangial cells. *Biochem Biophys Res Commun* 1990;**169**:585–595.

67. Pfeilschifter J, Schalkwijik C, Briner VA, *et al.* Cytokine-stimulated secretion of group II phospholipase A2 by rat mesangial cells. Its contribution to arachidonic acid release

and prostaglandin synthesis by cultured rat glomerular cells. *J Clin Invest* 1993; 92:2516–2523.

68. Coyne DW, Nikols M, Bertrand W, *et al*. Regulation of mesangial cell cyclooxygenase synthesis by cytokines and glucocorticoids. *Am J Physiol* 1992;263:F97–F102.

69. Badr KF, Kelley VE, Rennke HG, *et al*. Roles for thromboxane A2 and leukotrienes in endotoxin-induced acute renal failure. *Kidney Int* 1986;30:474–480.

70. Cumming AD, McDonald JW, Lindsay RM, *et al*. The protective effect of thomboxane synthetase inhibition on renal function in systemic sepsis. *Am J Kidney Dis* 1989; 13:114–119.

71. Reines HD, Halushka PV, Cook JA, *et al*. Plasma thromboxane concentrations are raised in patients dying with septic shock. *Lancet* 1982;1:175–5.

72. Bernard GR, Reins HD, Halushka PV, *et al*. Prostacyclin and thromboxane A2 formation is increased in human sepsis syndrome. Effect of cyclooxygenase inhibition. *Am Rev Resp Dis* 1991;144:1095–2101.

73. Tanjoh K, Shima A, Aida M, *et al*. Nitric oxide and active oxygen species in severe sepsis and surgically stressed patients. *Surg Today* 1995;25:774–777.

74. Galley HF, Davies MJ, Webster NR. Xanthine oxidase activity and free radical generation in patients with sepsis syndrome. *Crit Care Med* 1996;24:1649–1653.

75. Walker PD, Shah SV. Gentamicin enhanced production of hydrogen peroxide by renal cortical mitochondria. *Am J Physiol* 1987;253:C495–C499.

76. Hellberg PO, Kallskog TO. Neutrophil-mediated post-ischaemic tubular leakage in the rat kidney. *Kidney Int* 1989;36:555–561.

77. Linas SL, Whittenburg D, Parsons PE, *et al*. Mild renal ischemia activates primed neutrophils to cause acute renal failure. *Kidney Int* 1992;42:610–616.

78. Linas SL, Whittenburg D, Parsons PE, *et al*. Ischemia increases neutrophil retention and worsens acute renal failure. *Kidney Int* 1995;45:1584–1591.

79. Kelly KJ, Williams WWJ, Colvin RB, *et al*. Intercellular adhesion molecule-1-deficient mice are protected against renal ischemic injury. *J Clin Invest* 1996;97:1056–1063.

80. Kelly KJ, Williams WWJ, Colvin RB, *et al*. Antibody to intercellular adhesion molecule 1 protects the kidney against ischemic injury. *Proc Natl Acad Sci USA* 1994;91:812–816.

81. Essani NA, McGuire GM, Manning AM, *et al*. Differential induction of mRNA for ICAM-1 and selectins in hepatocytes, Kupffer cells and endothelial cells during endo-toxaemia. *Biochem Biophys Res Commun* 1995;211:74–82.

82. Ratych RE, Chuknyiska RS, Bulkley GB. The primary localization of free radical generation after anoxia/reoxygenation in isolated endothelial cells. *Surgery* 1987;102:122–131.

83. Paller MS, Neumann TV. Reactive oxygen species and rat renal epithelial cells during hypoxia and reoxygenation. *Kidney Int* 1991;40:1041–1049.

84. Alder S, Baker PJ, Johnson RJ, *et al*. Complement membrane attack complex stimulates the production of reactive oxygen metabolites by cultured rat mesangial cells. *J Clin Invest* 1986;77:762–767.

85. Jones SB, Kotsonis P, Majewski H. Endotoxin enhances norepinephrine release in the rat by peripheral mechanisms. *Shock* 1994;2:370–375.

86. Brackett DJ, Schaefer CF, Tompkins P, *et al*. Evaluation of cardiac output, total peripheral vascular resistance, and plasma concentrations of vasopressin release in the conscious, unrestrained rat during endotoxaemia. *Circ Shock* 1985;17:273–284.

87. Schaller MD, Waeber B, Nussburger J, *et al*. Angiotensin II, vasopressin and sympa-thetic nervous activity in conscious rats with endotoxaemia. *Am J Physiol* 1985;249: H1086–H1092.

88. Landry DW, Levin HR, Gallant EM, *et al.* Vasopressin deficiency contributes to the vasodilatation of septic shock. *Circulation* 1997;**95**:1122–1125.

89. Wilson MF, Brackett DJ, Tompkins P, *et al.* Elevated plasma vasopressin concentrations during endotoxin and *E.coli* shock. *Adv Shock Res* 1981;**6**:15–26.

90. Burnier M, Centeno G, Waeber G, *et al.* Effect of endotoxin on the angiotensin II receptor in cultured vascular smooth muscle cells. *Br J Pharmacol* 1995;**116**:2524–2530.

91. Brivet FG, Kleinknecht DJ, Loirat P, *et al.* Acute renal failure in intensive care units— causes, outcome, and prognostic factors of hospital mortality; a prospective, multicentre study. French Study Group on Acute Renal Failure. *Crit Care Med* 1996;**24**:192–198.

92. Haag-Weber M, Horl WH. Uraemia and infection: mechanisms of impaired cellular host defense. *Nephron* 1993;**63**:125–131.

93. Frost L, Pedersen RS, Hansen HE. Prognosis in septicaemia complicated by acute renal failure requiring dialysis. *Scan J Urol Nephrol* 1991;**25**:307–310.

94. Descamps-Latscha B, Jungers P. Elements of applied immunology for the intensive care unit and chronic uraemia-related disorders. In: Ronco C, Bellomo R (eds) *Critical care nephrology*, 1998:85–101. Kluwer Academic, Dordrecht.

95. Conger JD, Hammond WS. Renal vasculature and ischemic injury. *Renal Failure* 1992;**14**:307–310.

96. Walker JF, Cumming AD, Lindsay RM, *et al.* The renal response produced by non-hypotensive sepsis in a large animal model. *Am J Kidney Dis* 1986;**8**:88–97.

97. Firth JD, Acute irreversible renal failure. *Q J Med* 1996;**89**:397–399.

98. Cumming AD, Kline R, Linton AL. Association between renal and sympathetic responses to non-hypotensive systemic sepsis. *Crit Care Med* 1988;**16**:1132–1137.

99. Weinstein RA. Epidemiology and control of nosocomial infections in adult intensive care units. *Am J Med* 1991;**91**(3B):S179–S184.

100. Haley RW, Culver DH, White JW, *et al.* The efficacy of infection surveillance and control programs in preventing nosocomial infections in US hospitals. *Am J Epidemiol* 1985;**121**:182–205.

101. Raad II, Bodey GP. Infectious complications of indwelling vascular catheters. *Clin Infect Dis* 1992;**15**:197–208.

102. Elliott TS, Faroqui MH, Armstrong RF, *et al.* Guidelines for good practice in central venous catheterisation. Hospital Infections Society and the Research Unit of the Royal College of Physicians. *J Hosp Infect* 1994;**28**:163–176.

103. Pellizer G, de Lalla F. Intravascular catheter infections in the intensive care unit. In: Ronco C, Bellomo R (eds) *Critical care nephrology*, 1998:469–477. Kluwer Academic, Dordrecht.

104. Raad II, Hohn DC, Gilbreath BJ, *et al.* Prevention of central venous catheter-related infections by using maximal sterile barrier precautions during insertion. *Infect Cont Hosp Epidemiol* 1994;**15**(4 pt 1):231–238.

105. Garibaldi RA. Hospital-acquired urinary tract infection. In: Wenzel RP (ed.) *Prevention and control of nosocomial infections*, 1993:600–613. Williams and Wilkins, Baltimore, MD.

106. Jain P, Parada JP, David A, *et al.* Overuse of the indwelling urinary tract catheter in hospitalized medical patients. *Arch Int Med* 1995;**155**:1425–1429.

107. Craven DE, Steger KA, Barber TW. Preventing nosocomial pneumonia: state of the art and perpectives for the 1990's. *Am J Med* 1991;**91**(3B):S44–S53.

108. Leu HS, Kaiser DL, Mori M, *et al.* Hospital-acquired pneumonia: attributable mortality and morbidity. *Am J Epidemiol* 1989;**129**:1258–1267.

109. Johanson WGJ, Pierce AK, Sanford JP, *et al.* Nosocomial respiratory infections with Gram-negative bacilli; the significance of colonisation of the respiratory tract. *Ann Intern Med* 1972;**77**:701–706.

110. McClelland P, Murray AE, Williams PS, *et al.* Reducing sepsis in severe combined acute renal and respiratory failure by selective decontamination of the digestive tract. *Crit Care Med* 1990;**18**:935–939.

111. Selective Decontamination of the Digestive Tract Trialist's Collaboration Group. Meta-analysis of randomised controlled trials of selective decontamination of the digestive tract. *Br Med J* 1993;**307**:525–532.

112. Cumming AD, Thomson BJ, Sharp J, *et al.* Diarrhoea due to *Clostridium difficile* associated with antibiotic treatment in patients receiving dialysis: the role of cross-infection. *Br Med J* 1986;**292**:238–239.

113. Anglim AM, Farr BM. Nosocomial infection due to *Clostridium difficile*. *Curr Opin Infect Dis* 1994;**7**:602–608.

8

Infections in peritoneal dialysis

Nina E. Tolkoff-Rubin, Prem P. Varma, and Robert H. Rubin

Continuous ambulatory peritoneal dialysis (CAPD) is an established modality for the treatment of end-stage renal disease (ESRD). Today over 20% of ESRD patients in the United States, more than 50% of ESRD patients in the United Kingdom, and over 90% of dialysis patients in Mexico are receiving CAPD.[1,2] Several recent studies suggest that CAPD has survival rates comparable to haemodialysis, when adjusted for patient age and comorbid conditions.[3–8] However, despite improvements in the technology of peritoneal dialysis, infection remains the most common problem plaguing CAPD patients and represents the most frequent cause for removal of peritoneal dialysis catheters and discontinuation of this form of renal replacement therapy.[2,3,9,10]

Peritoneal catheters: design and placement

The peritoneal catheter is the peritoneal dialysis patient's lifeline, and is critical to the success of chronic peritoneal dialysis therapy. The catheter consists of an intraperitoneal portion and an extraperitoneal subcutaneous portion that has Dacron cuffs to anchor the catheter.[9] Variations in the catheter design include the number of cuffs (one versus two), the design of the subcutaneous pathway (permanently bent versus straight), and the design of the intra-abdominal portion (straight versus coiled).[9] The standard two–cuff, straight, Tenckhoff catheter, originally introduced in the 1960s, remains the most widely used device.[10,11] It contains multiple side-holes to allow easy inflow and outflow of dialysate. Recently, a number of new catheter designs have been introduced.[11,12] The new coiled catheter has gained increased popularity (Fig. 8.1). It is suggested this intraperitoneal design, with more side-holes, enables better flow, gives less inflow pain, and has a decreased likelihood of catheter migration and omental wrapping.[11,13]

A number of studies have demonstrated that a downward-directed exit site is associated with lower rates of peritonitis, as well as a lower risk of exit site and tunnel infections.[14,15] While the subcutaneous segment of the standard straight Tenckhoff catheter can be implanted in an arcuate tunnel to enable the catheter to exit caudally, implantation of the straight catheter in this configuration may increase catheter tip migration or external cuff extrusion, as the straight catheter tends to resume its straightened position because of its resilience.[11] Twardorski *et al.* have advocated the use of a 'swan-neck' catheter with an inverted U-shaped arc (170 to 180°) between the deep and superficial cuff (Fig. 8.1).[16] This bend allows the catheter to exit the skin pointing downward and

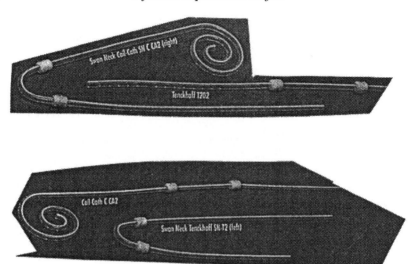

Fig. 8.1   Commonly used peritoneal dialysis catheters.

yet enter the peritoneum pointing towards the pelvis in an unstressed condition.[16]
It appears that curved catheters with a preformed bend have a lower probability of exit
site infections, cuff extrusions, and catheter migrations than straight Tenckhoff
catheters.[9,13,17,18] Prior to insertion, the exit site should be identified and marked, to avoid
irritation or pressure from the belt line which can lead to exit site infection.[9]

The Dacron cuffs on the peritoneal dialysis catheter function to anchor the catheter.
The question has been raised as to whether a single- or double-cuff catheter is preferable.
It now appears that the single-cuff catheters are associated with a shorter time until the
first peritonitis episode.[9,14] In addition, the single-cuff catheter is associated with more
exit site complications and shorter catheter survival than the double-cuffed catheter,
suggesting that the second cuff may act as a barrier to infections tracking down the exit
site or tunnel.[9,19] Consequently, the recent official report from the International Society
of Peritoneal Dialysis recommends that double-cuff catheters should be used rather than
single-cuff catheters.[9]

Prophylactic antibiotics should be administered at the time of catheter implantation,
as they appear to decrease the incidence of subsequent catheter infections, peritonitis,
and wound infection.[9,15,20] A first-generation cephalosporin has been most frequently
prescribed and is especially advocated in centres with a high incidence of perioperative
wound or exit site infections.[9] Vancomycin is not recommended for routine perioperative
prophylaxis, to avoid the development of resistant organisms, such as vancomycin-
resistant enterococci.[9,21]

After placement of a peritoneal dialysis catheter, the catheter should be anchored and
immobilized using a dressing or tape to minimize movement and reduce handling of the
catheter or exit site until healing of the wound and catheter tract is complete.[9] Generally,
ambulatory peritoneal dialysis is not initiated for at least 10 days to 2 weeks after catheter
insertion; the longer the period of healing, the fewer complications. If, however, dialysis

needs to be started immediately, then small exchanges of 500–1000 cm^3 should be performed in the supine position to decrease the risk of leakage.[9] The patient should avoid showering or submerging the exit site during healing, to avoid colonization with waterborne organisms. Once the catheter exit site is healed, it is critical that the patient perform daily exit site care utilizing strict hand washing and aseptic technique to prevent exit site infections.[22,23] This also entails monitoring of the exit site by visual inspection and palpation of the tunnel, and cleansing the exit site daily.[9,22,24]

Controversy exists as to the best cleansing agent. While one large multicentre study found significantly fewer infections with povidone-iodine as compared with pure soap, another study found similar rates of infection between povidone-iodine and soap.[24,25] In contrast, other studies found higher rates of infections in association with povidone than with antibacterial soap. Thus, while it appears that pure soap may be ineffective, an antibacterial soap or medical antiseptic appears appropriate for daily use during exit site care.[9] Liquid soap is recommended to avoid the potential of cross contamination from bar soap. It is of note that povidone-iodine solutions contaminated with *Pseudomonas* spp. have been implicated as a source of exit site infection and peritonitis in CAPD patients.[26]

While theoretically the use of dressings may help keep the exit site clean, in fact once the exit site is healed there are no data to document lower infection rates with the use of dressings in adults.[22] On the other hand, retrospective analysis does show significantly fewer exit site infections in children when the exit site is covered with sterile occlusive dressings.[9,25]

Exit site and tunnel infections

Prompt recognition and treatment of exit site and tunnel infections are critical, as these infections may lead to refractory or relapsing peritonitis, with the need for catheter removal to resolve the infection.[9,27–35]

An acute exit site infection is defined as purulent and/or bloody drainage from the exit site, which may be associated with erythema, tenderness, exuberant granulation tissue, and induration.[9,27,29] The extent of erythema needs to be twice the diameter of the catheter.[28] While pain and a scab may be present, the presence of crusting alone is not necessarily indicative of infection, but is more indicative of a traumatized exit site.[28] Purulent drainage must always be cultured. Positive cultures of a normal-appearing exit site reflect colonization rather than true infection.[9]

A tunnel infection is characterized by redness, swelling, and tenderness in the area over the subcutaneous pathway, as well as the presence of intermittent or chronic purulent or serosanguinous drainage, which discharges spontaneously or after pressure over the area.[9] Tunnel infections may be occult, and may require ultrasonography for detection.[36] Most tunnel infections occur in association with exit site infections, and increase the risk for peritonitis.[27,30]

Microbiology

Staphylococcus aureus is the organism responsible for the majority of exit site and tunnel infections.[9] In contrast, *S. epidermidis*, a frequent cause of peritonitis, is a less frequent cause of exit site and tunnel infections (less than 20%).[9] *Pseudomonas* is much less common, accounting for approximately 8% of exit site and tunnel infections.[9] Because *Pseudomonas* tends to form a biofilm, it is extremely difficult to eradicate, and *Pseudomonas* exit site infections frequently lead to relapsing peritonitis, often requiring removal of the peritoneal dialysis catheter.[9,10,37–42]

Therapy

Antibiotic therapy for exit site and tunnel infections should be initiated empirically on clinical grounds, pending culture results. Initial therapy should cover Gram-positive organisms, as these are the most frequent organisms isolated.[9,31] Oral penicillinase-resistant penicillins, fluoroquinolones, oral trimethoprim-sulfamethoxazole, or cephalosporins are recommended as convenient and cost-effective options.[9,43,44] Vancomycin should be avoided as first-line therapy, except in methicillin-resistant *S. aureus* infections, in view of the emergence of vancomycin-resistant enterococci.[9,21,45] Therapy can be adjusted once culture results are obtained. In severe or persistent *S. aureus* exit site infections, rifampin 300 mg twice daily may be added to antistaphylo-coccal penicillin or vancomycin therapy, 15–30 mg/kg daily in adults or 5–10 mg/kg twice daily in children. Rifampin provides good tissue penetration and acts synergisti-cally with vancomycin and antistaphylococcal penicillins. Contact lens wearers should be warned that rifampin enters tear secretions and may stain contact lenses orange.[9]

If Gram-negative infection is suspected, the patient should be treated with antipseudomonal antibiotics. Quinolones are generally used for *Pseudomonas aeruginosa* catheter infections, in combination with ceftazidime.[9,37–39,41] Ciprofloxacin can be given orally at 500 mg daily. Chelating interactions may occur between fluoroquinolones and concomitantly administered multivalent cations. This is of particular concern in patients with renal failure, who may be receiving calcium salts, oral iron supplements, zinc, sucralfate, magnesium- or aluminium-containing antacids, or milk, all of which may reduce quinolone absorption by 75% to 90%.[9] Therefore, staggering admini-stration of the antibiotics with these other agents is advised. In the paediatric patient, where quinolones are avoided because of potential effects on cartilage, or in the patient who cannot tolerate oral medications, intraperitoneal treatment with ceftazidime may be initiated.[9]

In chronic exit site infections, prolonged antimicrobial treatment may be necessary and repeated cultures required, as the bacteriology and antibiotic sensitivities may change during the course of therapy. In some cases, long-term suppressive doses of systemic antibiotic may be required.[29–31] There are few data documenting the optimal choice or length of antibiotic therapy or route of administration (oral, intraperitoneal, or intra-venous) for exit site or tunnel infections. It is generally advised to continue therapy until the exit site appears completely normal.[9,27–31] If 3–4 weeks of antibiotics fail to resolve the infection and patient compliance with this regimen has been assured, the catheter should be replaced.[9] On occasion, the presence of a cuff extruding from the exit site can cause repeated irritation of the area, and exteriorization of the cuff or shaving of the cuff may help to resolve the source of infection.[46] Unfortunately, the long-term outlook for catheters with chronically infected exits is not good.

Topical treatment may sometimes be used as an adjunct to systemic antibiotics in the treatment of low-grade or equivocal exit site infections. The topical antibiotics that have been successfully employed include mupirocin and neosporin.[22] Topical antibiotic therapy is not appropriate for patients with acute exit site infections, as previously defined.[9] Cauterization of exuberant granulation tissue may be necessary. Crusts can often be softened with hydrogen peroxide, saline, chlorhexidine, or soap and water. These crusts should not be forcefully removed. Any occlusive dressing should be avoided, since this will trap any drainage and create moisture, which may encourage bacterial growth.[9,22,29,31]

Prophylaxis

S. aureus nasal carriage is a recognized risk factor for *S. aureus* exit site and tunnel infections.[9,42,43,47–51] A number of protocols have been demonstrated to be effective in preventing *S. aureus* catheter infections by decreasing *S. aureus* nasal carriage.[43,51,52] The Mupirocin Study Group reported on a trial of 267 CAPD patients who were nasal carriers of *S. aureus*, as defined by two separate positive cultures.[43] Patients were randomized to treatment with mupirocin, an antibiotic active against Gram-positive organisms, versus placebo. Mupirocin was given as a nasal ointment twice daily for 5 days every 4 weeks. After a follow-up period of 18 months, there was a lower incidence of nasal *S. aureus* carriage (10% versus 48%) noted in the treatment group, as well as a lower incidence of exit site infections due to *S. aureus* (14 versus 44 episodes).[43] There was no difference in the rate of exit site infections due to other organisms nor in the incidence of tunnel infections or peritonitis. There was no development of resistance to mupirocin during the time period of this study.[43] In contrast, Perez-Fontan *et al.* noted a reduction in both *S. aureus* catheter infections and peritonitis with a course of intranasal mupirocin for positive nasal cultures.[44]

An alternative regimen to decrease nasal carriage includes cyclical rifampin 600 mg per day for 5 days every 12 weeks.[49] Unfortunately, prophylactic use of rifampin leads to side-effects in 12% of patients, as well as rifampin resistance, precluding the use of this drug for therapy.[49] Consequently, the use of rifampin for prophylaxis is not recommended.[9]

Another approach that has recently gained increasing favour is the use of mupirocin ointment applied to the exit site as part of routine daily exit site care.[50,51,53] One study randomized 82 patients to treatment with either topical mupirocin applied to the exit site daily or to cyclical rifampin (600 mg for 5 days every 3 months) for 1 year.[50] Both therapies provided equivalent protection from *S. aureus* catheter infections, with equivalent rates of *S. aureus* peritonitis and catheter loss due to *S. aureus*. However, more frequent side-effects were observed in the rifampin-treated patients.[50] Another prospective study evaluated the effectiveness of 2% mupirocin ointment applied to the exit site daily in 180 peritoneal dialysis patients followed for 1 year.[53] The patients were not screened for *S. aureus* nasal coverage. Infection rates during the study period were compared with the rates in the same patients during the previous year. Mupirocin therapy significantly reduced the incidence of exit site infections due to *S. aureus* (21 versus 3 episodes), as well as *S. aureus* peritonitis (35 versus 11 episodes). Overall rates of peritonitis were also significantly reduced (p value < 0.01). No adverse reactions were noted.[53]

Catheter removal

Peritoneal catheter removal is frequently required in patients with exit site and tunnel infections, in association with peritonitis.[9,29–35,38,40–42] The development of peritonitis reflects infection along the length of the catheter, which is generally refractory to treatment with antibiotics, particularly if the infection is caused by *S. aureus* or *Pseudomonas*.[9,37–41] The catheter should be removed if the infection does not respond or progresses after several weeks of appropriate therapy. As previously noted, cuff extrusion may be an important factor contributing to exit site infection. Cuff deroofing, a procedure in which an incision is made to the depth of the outer cuff, with removal of the cuff and surrounding tissues, or cuff shaving may be attempted as salvage therapy for exit site infections deemed unresponsive to prolonged therapy prior to removal.[46] Medical therapy of pseudomonal infections is particularly difficult because of the nature of the biofilm that is formed, and treatment of these infections generally requires catheter removal.[38–41]

Peritonitis

Peritonitis remains a significant problem for CAPD patients. It is the leading cause of technique failure and catheter loss as well as accounting for more than 20% of the hospitalizations.[54,55] In addition patients with frequent bouts of peritonitis are at increased risk of death.[56]

Clinical presentation

The diagnosis of peritonitis should be entertained when a patient presents with abdominal pain and cloudy dialysate. Patients may frequently have fever, nausea, vomiting, or diarrhoea. Abdominal tenderness is the most common finding on physical examination, often with rebound tenderness.[3,31,55] The major diagnostic criterion is the white blood cell count in the peritoneal fluid. Patients with peritonitis generally show more than 100 white blood cells/mm^3, the normal value being fewer than 8 white blood cells/mm^3.[3] Neutrophils usually predominate, although lymphocytes may predominate in patients with fungal or mycobacterial infections.[55,57] In about 6% of episodes of peritonitis, patients may demonstrate low white cell counts in the dialysate fluid, with positive cultures suggesting poor immunological response to infection. The organism most commonly isolated in these circumstances is *S. aureus*.[58] On occasion a low white cell count in the peritoneal fluid may be indicative of tunnel infection as opposed to peritonitis (see section on tunnel infection).[34]

Diagnosis

A patient presenting with abdominal pain and cloudy effluent should have the fluid examined for cell count, Gram stain, and culture. In order to maximize the yield of the cultures, large volumes of the effluent, i.e. $>10\,cm^3$, should be placed in each of two blood culture bottles.[3,59,60] If the appropriate culture technique is adhered to, more than

90% of cultures should be positive.[60] If the patient presents with rigors or hypotension, blood cultures should be obtained, although they are seldom positive. While the Gram stain of the peritoneal fluid is often negative, the presence and identification of any organisms may be helpful in guiding initial therapy, particularly the diagnosis of fungal peritonitis. Antibiotic therapy should be initiated while awaiting culture results.[3,55]

Pathophysiology of peritonitis

Peritonitis can occur in the peritoneal dialysis patient by various routes. The most frequent is contamination, i.e. introduction of skin bacteria by breaks in sterile technique during the performance of the multiple dialysis exchange procedures.[3,55,61–72] *S. epidermidis* and *S. aureus* account for more than 50% of these contamination episodes. A number of modifications in the peritoneal dialysis system have been aimed at decreasing the risk of peritonitis (Table 8.1).[3,55,67–72] The major modification of the standard technique has been the introduction of the Y-set.[61] Previously the patient would drain the peritoneal cavity, discard the old dialysate, spike a new bag of dialysate, and then infuse the new dialysate into the peritoneal cavity. Any microbial contamination in the course of the spiking procedure had the potential for being flushed into the abdomen. The Y system, based on the principle of 'flush before fill sequence', has significantly reduced the incidence of peritonitis due to touch contamination.[61–71] The system is designed so that one of the limbs of the Y has a preattached drain bag, so that after spiking the new dialysate bag, the patient drains a small volume of fresh dialysate into this attached drain bag, thereby flushing out microbes that may have contaminated the spike. The peritoneal cavity is subsequently drained before new dialysate is instilled into the abdomen. As a result of this 'flush before fill' manoeuvre, any possible contamination from the spiking procedure is flushed away from the peritoneal cavity into the drain bag, diminishing the risk of peritonitis.

The Y-set is most effective against *S. epidermidis*.[65,71] In one study, touch contamination was simulated by intentionally contaminating the spike with *S. epidermidis*, *S. aureus*, and *Pseudomonas aeruginosa* immediately prior to an exchange; the dialysate was then cultured after an exchange using the 'flush before fill' technique. The flush led to 100% removal of *S. epidermidis* and only partial removal of *S. aureus* or *Pseudomonas* if the exchanges were done immediately.[66]

Recently systems have been introduced which have pre-attached dialysate solution bags as well as drain bags—the 'twin-bag system'—to completely avoid the need for

Table 8.1 Prevention of peritonitis

Prophylactic antibiotics before catheter placements

Two-cuffed catheter

Downward-pointing exit site

Twin-bag system 'flush before fill'

Eradicate *Staphylococcus* aureus nasal carriage

---

spiking.[68,69] These closed systems have been demonstrated to further decrease the risk of possible contamination during attachment. A number of reports have confirmed a significant reduction in peritonitis rates with systems that incorporate both the twin-bag and the Y-set connections.[65–72] In one report of 147 patients randomized to twin-bag, Y-set, or conventional spiking, the average peritonitis-free interval was highest among the twin-bag group at 24.8 months versus 12 months and 6 months for the Y-set and conventional spike systems respectively.[67]

The importance of decreasing the number of connections is also underscored by the observation from most centres that the rate of peritonitis is lower in patients on continuous cycler peritoneal dialysis (CCPD), an automated system in which there is only one disconnection per day that incorporates the 'flush before fill' technology.[3,5,73] In one series the incidence of peritonitis was significantly lower with an automated system, compared with the Y-set or standard spike (0.5 versus 1.46 to 2.11 episodes per patient per year; i.e. one episode every 2–3 years).[73]

The second major route of acquiring bacterial peritonitis in CAPD patients is related to the catheter, with preceding exit site and tunnel infections being the major contributing factors in approximately 20% of these episodes (see previous section).[3,9,10,27–31] The impact of training in terms of appropriate hand washing and aseptic technique must continuously be underscored, as this is the key to decreasing the level of bacterial contamination associated with touch contamination of connections during the dialysis procedure.[23]

It is now well recognized that *S. aureus* carriers are at greatest risk for catheter-associated infections. Over 50% of peritoneal dialysis patients are nasal carriers of *S. aureus*. It has been demonstrated that 75% of dialysis patients with *S. aureus* in their nares have *S. aureus* on their hands; in contrast fewer than 10% of dialysis patients without nasal carriage have *Staphylococcus* on their skin.[52] This *S. aureus* can be easily spread from hands to exit site or connections during an exchange. As previously reviewed, several different approaches are available to prevent *S. aureus* carriage.[42,43,47,48,51–53] Patients need to be identified by nasal culture before catheter placement. Positive cultures should be treated with intranasal mupirocin. Once dialysis is initiated mupirocin can be applied to the exit site as part of the daily exit site care and/or monthly intranasal mupirocin can be employed.[42,43,50,51,53,55]

Biofilms on the catheter may be significant in leading to relapsing or recurrent infections and catheter loss.[40] The organisms most likely to form biofilms and also the most difficult to eradicate are staphylococci and *Pseudomonas*.[9,10,37–40] Efforts to prevent the formation of biofilms may be important future strategies in treating these forms of infection.

The third major source of CAPD peritonitis is intra-abdominal pathology that can occur secondary to processes such as diverticulitis, ruptured appendix, ischaemic bowel, incarcerated hernias, pancreatitis, or gynaecological pathology. Intra-abdominal pathology generally accounts for fewer than 6% of cases of peritonitis in CAPD patients.[3,55] The major clue to significant intra-abdominal disease is the presence of polymicrobial enteric organisms on culture, particularly the presence of anaerobes in the dialysate. A CT scan may be helpful in identifying the anatomical site of the lesion. Although free air may be seen in asymptomatic patients on peritoneal dialysis (because of leakage of air through the insertion site), the presence of free air is of greater concern in a patient with peritoneal signs and should raise the possibility of a perforated viscus. Peritoneal fluid amylase and lipase levels may be helpful in differentiating an intra-abdominal process from dialysis-associated bacterial peritonitis.[74–77] Levels above 50 International Units per litre are suggestive of a primary intra-abdominal process.[75] The outcome of patients with bacterial peritonitis due to underlying intra-abdominal pathology is generally poor. In one series, 11 out of 26 patents died.[78] The key is to establish the diagnosis rapidly and, where appropriate, proceed directly to surgery.[79]

Another major factor contributing to the increased risk of peritonitis in the CAPD population is the impact of the dialytic procedure itself on various aspects of host defences (see Chapter 3).[80–87] While peritoneal dialysis utilizes a uniquely biocompatible membrane—the peritoneal membrane—the dialysis solutions in contrast are unphysiological, in that they are hyperosmolar, acidic, employ lactate as a buffer, and contain high concentrations of glucose (1.5–4.25% solutions).[80–87] Not only does the frequent instillation of dialysate fluid dilute normal host defence mechanisms (such as the immunoglobulins, opsonins, and intraperitoneal macrophages) but dialysis solutions are toxic to the polymorphonuclear leucocytes, inhibiting phagocytosis and antibacterial killing.[82,84,85] Moreover, heat sterilization of the dialysate leads to the formation of glucose degradation products that impair white cell, mesothelial cell, and fibroblast function.[82] Efforts are currently under way to develop a bicarbonate-based dialysate and also to investigate such glucose polymers as icodextran, which might provide a more physiological environment for white cells and macrophages, and thus improve phagocytosis and intracellular killing.[83]

Aetiological agents

Gram-positive bacterial peritonitis

Staphylococcus epidermidis has been the most common organism causing peritonitis in CAPD patients, occurring as a result of touch contamination during the procedure or secondary to spread of exit site or tunnel infections. Generally this organism responds rapidly to therapy. The second most common Gram-positive infection has been due to *S. aureus* (see Table 8.2). This tends to be a more virulent pathogen and is frequently more resistant to therapy.[34,55] On occasion, patients with *S. aureus* peritonitis present with a toxic-shock like syndrome. As previously noted, the recent introduction of disconnect systems that employ the 'flush before fill' technique has led to a reduction in the overall rate of peritonitis (particularly the incidence of *S. epidermidis* peritonitis) with a relative increase in the incidence of peritonitis due to *S. aureus*.[62,71,72]

Several cases of group B streptococcal peritonitis have been reported.[88] The patients presented critically ill with septic shock within 24 h after the onset of symptoms; one patient died. Although rare, this reinforces the need for patients to report symptoms early and to monitor blood pressure. Hypotension is clearly indicative of more severe disease, necessitating hospitalization.

Patients whose gastrointestinal tracts are colonized with vancomycin-resistant enterococci are at risk for peritonitis with this organism. Impeccable hygiene and attention to detail in carrying out the dialysis procedure is especially important in individuals colonized with vancomycin-resistant enterococci, as therapy of this organism is so difficult.

Table 8.2 Microbiology of CAPD peritonitis

Bacterial	
Gram positive	> 50%
S. epidermidis	30–40%
S. aureus	20%
S. enterococci	5%
Gram negative	15%
Pseudomonas	5%
non-Pseudomonas	15%
Polymicrobial	4%
Fungal	2%
Sterile	20%

Gram-negative bacterial peritonitis

Gram-negative peritonitis can be due to organisms from the skin, bowel, urinary tract, contaminated water, or contact with animals.[55] Treatment of constipation with enemas and the use of gastric acid inhibitors appears to predispose to Gram-negative peritonitis.[89,90] Documentation of epidemiological exposures may be helpful in making a diagnosis. *Campylobacter* peritonitis has been associated with severe diarrhoea, while peritonitis due to polymicrobial infection or aerobic Gram-negative organisms is generally associated with pathology of the gastrointestinal tract (diverticulitis or ischaemic bowel).[78,90,91] *E. coli* is an unusual pathogen in CAPD peritonitis. This may be due to the fact that human peritoneal macrophages are capable of phagocytosing *E. coli* even in the absence of opsonins in the peritoneal fluid.[92]

Pseudomonas accounts for 5 to 8% of episodes of CAPD peritonitis.[38,39] These infections are often difficult to eradicate because of the development of a biofilm, and consequently pseudomonas infections are frequently associated with catheter loss, and may cause damage to the peritoneal membrane.[38,40–42]

While one series reported a 80% success rate in the treatment of pseudomonas infections with combination of ceftazidime and aminoglycosides, 20% of patients required removal of the peritoneal dialysis catheter.[38] The involvement of exit-site or catheter-related infection appears to be an important factor determining the response to therapy.[41] In those patients in whom there was a preceding *Pseudomonas* exit site or catheter infection, the response rate to antimicrobials was only 32%, as opposed to 73% in whom there was no evidence of catheter-related infection.[41]

Therapy of CAPD peritonitis

There is no 'gold standard' treatment of peritonitis in peritoneal dialysis patients. A number of regimens have been found to be effective. The 1993 International Society of Peritoneal Dialysis guidelines for the treatment of peritonitis recommended vancomycin and an aminoglycoside as initial empirical therapy—not only because of the increasing frequency of methicillin-resistant staphylococci, but also because data suggested a reduction in hospitalization rates and relapse rates with this regimen.[93] However, in the last few years the increasing prevalence of vancomycin-resistant organisms has led to increasing concern that the large-scale use of vancomycin selects for these organisms, with the potential of transfer of the resistance to other species, such as staphylococci, especially methicillin-resistant *S. aureus* (MRSA).[21,45] Consequently, the recommendation of using vancomycin together with another antibiotic has been modified in the 2000 report from the Advisory Committee on Peritonitis Management of the International Society of Peritoneal Dialysis.[3] At present these guidelines recommend a first-generation cephalosporin such as cefazolin or cephalothin together with ceftazidime. These antibiotics can be mixed and administered in the same bag. Routine use of aminoglycosides is to be avoided in order to preserve residual renal function (Fig. 8.2).[3,94]

The loading dose for either cefazolin or cephalothin is 500 mg/litre, and maintenance dose is 125 mg/litre in each bag. While once-daily dosing of cefazolin at 1.5 g has been suggested because of ease of administration, pharmacokinetic studies show that maintenance doses in each bag may maintain a higher bactericidal level.[94-96] With continuous intraperitoneal dosing of cefazolin, the tissue level generally will exceed the maximum inhibitory concentration of 64 mg/litre, which defines relative resistance. A once daily intraperitoneal dose of 1000 to 1500 mg may not achieve such levels at the peritoneum, except during the one exchange that contains the antibiotic dose. Consequently there is the possibility of inadequate treatment or relapse.[3] Unfortunately, prospective/randomized studies are not available that examine intermittent versus continuous dosing of cephalosporins.

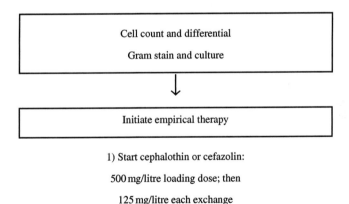

Fig. 8.2   Initial therapy for CAPD peritonitis.

Table 8.3 Antibiotic dosing guidelines for treatment of CAPD peritonitis

Antibiotic	Loading dose (mg/litre unless otherwise specified)	Intermittent dosing (1 bag/day unless otherwise specified)	Continuous dosing (mg/litre unless otherwise specified)
Aminoglycosides			
Amikacin	25	2 mg/kg	12
Gentamicin/tobramycin	8	0.6 mg/kg	4
Cephalosporins			
Cefazolin/cephalothin	500	15 mg/kg	125
Ceftazidime	250	1000 mg	125
Cefriaxone	250	1000 mg	125
Quinolones			
Ciprofloxacin		Avoid in children. 500 mg orally twice daily	Not recommended
Ofloxacin	400 orally	200 orally daily	Not recommended
Others			
Vancomycin	1000	15–30 mg/kg q 5–7 days	ND
Rifampin	NA	600 g orally, four times a day	NA
Ampicillin/sulbactam	1000 mg		100
Imipenem/cilistat	500		200

Possible alternatives to cefazolin and cephalothin to cover Gram-positive organisms include nafcillin, clindamycin, and quinolones.[3] Table 8.3 presents intraperitoneal antibiotic dosages for adults for some commonly used agents. This strategy has been consistent with the efforts to preserve vancomycin for true methicillin-resistant organisms.

Gentamicin, tobramycin, and netilmicin are dosed at 0.6 mg/kg body weight in only one exchange per day. Amikacin is dosed at 2.0 mg/kg body weight, also in one exchange per day. Recent pharmacokinetic data suggest that a single daily dose of aminoglycosides is as efficacious and may be less toxic than divided doses.[3,55,97,98] Increased bacterial killing rates associated with prolonged postantibiotic effect are obtained using once-daily dosing, while toxic drug accumulation in renal and cochlear tissue may be minimized.[3]

However, it is disturbing that a number of centres are beginning to note failures or relapses with first-generation cephalosporins for initial therapy, and are reporting an increase in the proportion of truly methicillin-resistant staphylococci (ranging from 33% to 77%, depending on the institution).[55,99] Vas et al. reported that cefazolin (1.5 g daily intraperitoneally for 3 weeks) led to resolution of only 45% of cases of peritonitis due to methicillin-resistant coagulase-negative staphylococci, compared with a 73% response during the time when vancomycin was employed (2 g intraperitoneally four times weekly for 3 weeks).[95] Van Diesen et al. noted that if the 1996 Advisory Committee recommendations had been utilized at their institution, only 76.5% of patients with Gram-positive infections, and 81% of patients with Gram-negative infections would have been effectively treated based on sensitivities.[100] Instead, they propose initiating therapy with intraperitoneal vancomycin plus intraperitoneal gentamicin. After 24 h, if the patient is an inpatient, intraperitoneal ceftazidime 250 mg per exchange and ciprofloxacin 50 mg per exchange are given. If the patient is an outpatient, ciprofloxacin is prescribed at 500 mg twice daily.[100] Within 2 to 3 days, the organism is generally identified and sensitivities obtained, at which point the antibiotic profile can be narrowed. This therapeutic algorithm would theoretically cover 100% of Gram-positive organisms and 87% of Gram-negative organisms.

The key point is that any therapeutic guidelines must be considered just that—guidelines; what is critical is that any antimicrobial programme must be tailored to the specific culture and sensitivity patterns documented at a given centre, and adjusted accordingly.

The optimal duration of treatment of bacterial peritonitis has not been clearly defined by controlled studies. At present, it is generally recommended that therapy should be 14 days for Gram-positive infections, except in the case of *S. aureus* where 21 days is suggested.[3,55] For culture-negative episodes, 14 days of therapy with a cephalosporin or vancomycin plus aminoglycoside is generally adequate. The same is true for single-organism Gram-negative peritonitis, except in the case of *Pseudomonas*, *Xanthomonas*, or polymicrobial peritonitis for which 21 days is recommended (Figs. 8.3 and 8.4).

If patients are not systemically ill, i.e. with nausea, vomiting, or severe abdominal pain, they can be treated successfully on an outpatient basis for an episode of peritonitis. Close follow-up is critical, however. Patients should be symptomatically improved and

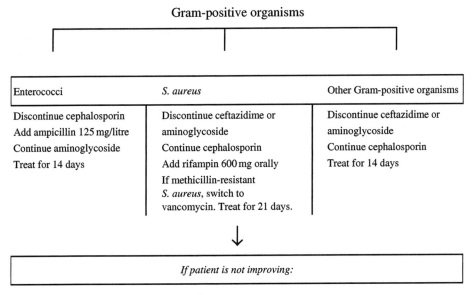

Fig. 8.3 Treatment of Gram-positive peritoneal dialysis infections (adapted from Keane *et al.*[3]).

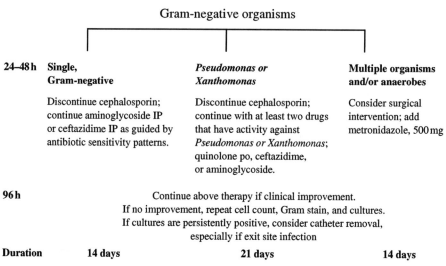

Fig. 8.4   Treatment of Gram-negative peritoneal dialysis infections (adapted from Keane *et al.* [3]) (po = orally; IP = intraperitoneally).

dialysate should start to clear within 48 h of beginning therapy. If there is no improvement within 96 h, despite the appropriate antibiotic as judged by cultures and sensitivity, then the fluid must be re-examined for cell count, Gram stain, and culture. In the case of a persistent *S. aureus* infection, an underlying tunnel infection should be excluded (see section on tunnel infection). Ultrasonography may be helpful in making the diagnosis. In all situations where there is failure to improve, serious consideration should be given to catheter removal.[3,34,55] The possibility of an intra-abdominal or gynaecological process, or the presence of unusual organisms such as *Mycobacterium*, *Nocardia*, or *Rhodococcus* should likewise be considered.

For patients on cycler dialysis, regimens similar to those outlined are recommended; however the dialysis itself should be modified to a regimen lasting a full 24 h, with 3–4-h dwells, to enable adequate antibiotic equilibration.[3] Once there is clinical resolution, the automated peritoneal dialysis regimen can be resumed, but with a daytime bag containing the antibiotics until completion of the treatment.

Relapsing peritonitis

In patients with relapsing peritonitis, defined as separate infective episodes caused by the same organism within 4 weeks of finishing the previous course of antibiotics, three major factors need to be considered.[3,55] First, has the patient complied with the antibiotic prescription, or has non-compliance led to inadequate therapy? If the latter can be ruled out, the two other concerns are the possibilities of persistent exit site or catheter-related problems contributing to recurrent peritonitis or the presence of biofilm adhering to the catheter, which could entrap organisms avoiding antibiotic penetration. There are reports suggesting that urokinase infusions may be beneficial in about 50% of patients with relapsing peritonitis, presumably by disrupting biofilms or fibrin thrombi, which may be harbouring bacteria.[101,102] In the absence of urokinase, streptokinase or tissue plasminogen activator have been utilized successfully (private communication).

Whatever the cause, it is crucial to recognize when a catheter needs to be removed in a patient with relapsing or refractory peritonitis as the mortality associated with peritonitis increases in those patients with delayed catheter removal.[3,34,55] Early catheter removal also avoids prolonged episodes of peritonitis that could potentially damage the peritoneal membrane.[34] It has been suggested that if the peritoneal cell count can be suppressed to less than 100 white blood cells/μl, then the catheter can be safely replaced at one setting, avoiding the need for interim haemodialysis.[102,103]

Tuberculous peritonitis

Although an extremely rare complication of peritoneal dialysis, the diagnosis of tuberculous peritonitis should be entertained in any patient who is not responding to antibiotic therapy. Tuberculous peritonitis is generally a reactivation disease of a latent peritoneal focus rather than primary infection introduced via the catheter.[3,55] Smears of the dialysis fluid may not reveal acid-fast organisms. Cultures are critical to establishing the diagnosis. New diagnostic techniques such as the detection of microbacterial DNA amplifed by polymerase chain reaction (PCR) offer the possibility of rapid detection of tuberculosis in the near future.[3]

The treatment for tuberculous peritonitis due to drug-sensitive organisms in a compliant patient is a 6-month regimen consisting of isoniazid (INH) 300 mg four times a day, rifampin 600 mg four times a day, and pyrazinamide 1.5 g orally four times a day for 2 months, followed by INH and rifampin for 4 months. A fourth drug, ethambutol or one of the fluoroquinolones, should be included in the initial regimen until the results of sensitivity testing are available. Streptomycin is usually avoided in patients with renal failure because of the increased risk of ototoxicity after prolonged use. Patients not tolerating pyrazinamide should be treated for 9 months with INH and rifampin. More prolonged courses of therapy are indicated for any patient slow to respond to one of the standard regimens, those with miliary or central nervous system disease, and children with multiple sites of involvement including the skeleton. The management of drug-resistant disease is determined by the results of *in vitro* susceptibility testing.[3]

Fungal peritonitis

Fungal peritonitis accounts for approximately 2% to 3% of the episodes of CAPD peritonitis, and may have a mortality rate as high as 17%.[3,55,104,105] Fungal peritonitis is difficult to distinguish from bacterial peritonitis on clinical grounds, with nausea, chills, abdominal pain, and distention being general features. On occasion, the patient can present acutely ill and appear to have a surgical abdomen.[104,105] Dialysate cell count may demonstrate a predominance of polymorphs; however, in some cases, up to 25% eosinophils have been reported.[104] Gram stain is positive in 30% to 50% of cases. The physician should have a high index of suspicion for fungal infection in a CAPD patient with classic symptoms of peritonitis and negative bacterial cultures, and the microbiology laboratory should be alerted. Positive fungal dialysate cultures should never be regarded as contaminants.[104,105]

Candida species account for more than 80% of episodes of fungal peritonitis, while other fungi such as *Mucor* and *Aspergillus* account for a minority of infections.[104,105] Several risk factors have been identified for the development of fungal peritonitis. Many investigators believe that preceding bacterial peritonitis and previous exposure to antibiotics are key risk factors for fungal peritonitis.[55,105–113] In one series of patients with fungal peritonitis, 90% of patients had a history of recent bacterial peritonitis and over 80% had been exposed to antibiotics in the preceding month.[104] Likewise immuno-suppressed patients, diabetics, and HIV-positive patients also appear to be at increased risk for fungal peritonitis.[105] One interesting report from Hong Kong noted an out-break of *C. tropicalis* peritonitis in CAPD patients secondary to contamination of the bath water used to warm dialysate. This method of warming dialysate should be discouraged.[114]

Several investigators have suggested that prophylactic nystatin, at 500 000 units orally three times a day, taken during the administration of antimicrobial agents and continued for 1 week after antibiotics have been discontinued allows the re-establishment of the normal bacterial flora and reduces the incidence of subsequent fungal peritonitis.[115–117] This prophylactic regimen may be particularly beneficial in high-risk patients, such as those with recurrent bouts of bacterial peritonitis requiring prolonged courses of anti-biotics, or those requiring immunosuppression.[55,106,115,117]

Treatment of fungal peritonitis

If fungi are identified on gram stain or culture antifungal therapy should be promptly instituted (see Fig. 8.5).[3,55,105] Before the availability of fluconazole, antifungal therapy usually consisted of amphotericin B (intravenously or intraperitoneally) and 5-flucytosine (orally, intravenously, or intraperitoneally). The overall cure rate without catheter removal was only about 10%; only 45% of cases could return to peritoneal dialysis and the mortality rate was 19%.[106] Recent experience with fluconazole (orally, intravenously, or intraperitoneally) suggests this agent is efficacious for those infections that are due to sensitive strains of *Candida* and is well tolerated.[55,104,105,111] As a general rule *C. albicans* and *C. tropicalis* (which account for over 80% of infections) are fluconazole-sensitive, while *C. glabrata* and *C. krusei* are resistant.

Yeast on Gram stain or culture of dialysate	
Flucytosine	Load 2000 mg po
and	Maintenance 1000 mg/day po
fluconazole	200 mg po/IP daily

If clinical improvement continue therapy for 4–6 weeks

If no clinical improvement by day 4, repeat cell count, Gram stain and culture, and remove catheter

If catheter removed, continue fluconazole for additional 10 days for sensitive yeast

Fig. 8.5 Fungal peritonitis (abbreviations as Fig. 8.4) (adapted from Keane *et al.*[3])

Fluconazole is a triazole with high oral and intraperitoneal bioavailability (87% for oral and 88% for intraperitoneal).[105] The drug has excellent penetration into the peritoneal fluid with a peritoneal level 60% that of serum.[105] If the patient is haemodynamically stable, fluconazole 200 mg orally or intraperitoneally is recommended. When used in combination with flucytosine these agents appear to have a synergistic effect, and retrospective analysis suggests similar cure rates to those reported historically with amphotericin B.[105] Whether a combination of fluconazole and 5-flucytosine is superior to fluconazole alone is still unclear, but the results of combined therapy appear no better than fluconazole alone in sensitive yeast.[104,105,111]

The key problem, however, is that fungal infections are extremely difficult to eradicate, despite appropriate antifungal therapy, due to blockage of the holes and lumen of the dialysis catheter with fungi embedded in an amorphous matrix.[118] Consequently if no clinical improvement is seen within 4 days, or if the patient becomes haemodynamically unstable, it is imperative that the dialysis catheter be removed.[3,104,105] Goldie *et al.* found that 15% of patients in whom the catheter was removed within 1 week of diagnosis died, compared to 50% mortality in patients in whom the catheter was left in place.[104] Several institutions, including our own, have a policy of removing the catheter as soon as the diagnosis is established (private communication).[55]

If the fungus is sensitive to the azoles, therapy with fluconazole should then be continued for at least an additional 10 days after catheter removal. Only about 50% of patients are able to return to CAPD after catheter removal and antifungal therapy.[105] A waiting period of 1–2 months on haemodialysis before attempting reinsertion of a catheter is recommended.[55]

Amphotericin remains the mainstay of therapy in patients who are critically ill and in whom the fungus is not sensitive to fluconazole. Amphotericin should be administered intravenously, as intraperitoneal amphotericin can cause severe pain and irritation of the peritoneum as well as potentially cause peritoneal adhesions and fibrosis.[105] The role of liposomal amphotericin preparations in patients with end-stage renal failure has not been determined.

References

1. Nolph KD. Registry results. In Gokal R, Nolph KD (eds): *The Textbook of Peritoneal Dialysis*. Kluwer Academic Publishers, Dordrecht 1994, pp. 735–750.
2. Pastan S, Bailey J. Dialysis therapy. *New Engl J Med* 1999; 338:1428–1437.
3. Keane WF, Bailie GR, Boeschoten E, Gokal R, Golper TA, Holmes CJ, et al. Adult peritoneal dialysis-related peritonitis treatment recommendations: 2000 update. *Perit Dial Int* 2000; 20(4):396–411.
4. Cancarini GC, Brunori G, Zani R et al. Long term outcomes of peritoneal dialysis. *Perit Dial Int* 1997; 17:S115–S119.
5. Maiorca R, Cancarini GC, Zubani R et al. CAPD viability: a long term comparison with hemodialysis. *Perit Dial Int* 1996; 16:276–287.
6. Fenton SSA, Schaubel DE, Desmeules, Morrison HI, Mao Y, Copleston P, et al. Hemodialysis versus peritoneal dialysis: A comparison of adjusted mortality rate. *Am J Kidney Dis* 1997; 30:334–342.

7. Vonesh EF, Moran J. Mortality in end-stage-renal-disease: a reassessment of differences between patients treated with hemodialysis and peritoneal dialysis. *J Am Soc Nephrol* 1999; 10:354–469.
8. Chatoth DK, Golper TA, Gokal R. Morbidity and mortality in redefining adequacy of peritoneal dialysis: a step beyond the National Kidney Foundation Quality Initiative. *Am J Kidney Dis* 1999; 33:617–632.
9. Gokal R, Alexander SR, Ash S, *et al.* Peritoneal catheters and exit site practices towards optimum peritoneal access: 1998 update, official report from the International Society for Peritoneal Dialysis. *Perit Dial Int* 1998; 18:11–33.
10. Keane WF, Vas SI. Peritonitis. In Gokal R, Nolph KD (eds): *The Textbook of Peritoneal Dialysis.* Kluwer Academic Publishers, Boston, MA, 1994:473–502.
11. Lupo A, Tarchini R, Carcarini G, Catizone L, Cocci R, DeVecchi A, *et al.* Long term outcome in CAPD: A 10-year-survey by the Italian Cooperative Peritoneal Dialysis Study Group. *Am J Kidney Dis* 1994; 24:826–837.
12. Ash SR. Chronic peritoneal dialysis catheters: effect of catheter design, materials, and location. *Semin Dial* 1990; 3:39–46.
13. Eklund BH, Honkanan EO, Kalen AR, Kyllonen LE. Catheter configurations and outcome in CAPD: a prospective comparison of two catheters. *Perit Dial Int* 1994; 14:70–74.
14. Warady BA, Sullivan EK, Alexander SR. Lessons from the peritoneal dialysis database: a report of the North American pediatric renal transplant cooperative study. *Kidney Int* 1996; 49:S68–S71.
15. Golper TA, Brier ME, Bunke M. Risk factors for peritonitis in long term peritoneal dialysis: The Network 9 peritoneal and catheter survival studies. *Am J Kidney Dis* 1996; 28:428–436.
16. Twardowski ZJ, Prowant BF, Nichols WK, Nolph KD, Khanna R. Six-year experience with swan neck catheters. *Perit Dial Int* 1992; 12:384–389.
17. Eklund BH, Honkanan EO, Kalen AR, Kyllonen LE. Peritoneal dialysis access: prospective randomized comparison of the swan neck and Tenckhoff catheters. *Perit Dial Int* 1995; 15:353–356.
18. Lye WC, Kour N-W, van der Straaten J, *et al.* A prospective randomized comparison of the swan neck, coiled, and straight Tenckhoff catheters in patients on CAPD. *Perit Dial Int* 1996; suppl. 1:S333–S335.
19. Lindblad AS, Hamilton RW, Nolph KD, Novak JW. A retrospective analysis of catheter configuration and cuff type: A National CAPD Registry report. *Perit Dial Int* 1988; 8:129–133.
20. Wickdahl AM, Engman V, Stegmayr B, Sorenson JB. One dose cefuroxime IV and IP reduces microbial growth in PD patients after catheter insertion. *Nephrol Dial Trans* 1997; 12:157–160.
21. Golper TA, Tranaeus A. Vancomycin revisited. *Perit Dial Int* 1996; 16:116–117.
22. Prowant BF, Twardowski ZJ. Recommendations for the exit care. *Perit Dial Int* 1996; 16 (suppl 3):S94–S99.
23. Miller TE, Findon G. Touch contamination of connection devices in peritoneal dialysis: a quantitative microbiologic analysis. *Perit Dial Int* 1997; 17:560–567.
24. Luzar MA, Brown C, Balt D, Hill L, Issad B, Monnier B, *et al.* Exit site care and exit site infections in continuous ambulatory peritoneal dialysis (CAPD): results of a randomized multicenter study. *Perit Dial Int* 1990; 10:25–29.
25. Warady BA, Jackson MA, Millspaugh J, Miller RM, Ford DM, Hellerstan M, *et al.* Prevention and treatment of catheter-related infections in children. *Perit Dial Bull* 1987; 7:34–36.

26. Parrott PL, Terry PM, Whitworth EN, *et al. Pseudomonas aeruginosa* peritonitis associated with contaminated poloxamer-iodine solution. *Lancet* 1982; 2:683–685.
27. Gupta B, Bernardini J, Piraino B. Peritonitis associated with exit site and tunnel infections. *Am J Kidney Dis* 1996; 28:415–419.
28. Twardowski ZJ, Prowant BF. Classification of normal and diseased exit sites. *Perit Dial Int* 1997; 16 (suppl 3): S32–S50.
29. Twardowski ZJ. Peritoneal dialysis catheter exit site infections: prevention, diagnosis, treatment, and future directions. *Semin Dial* 1992; 5:305–315.
30. Scalmogna A, Castelnovo C, De Veechi A, Ponticelli C. Exit site and tunnel infections in CAPD patients. *Am J Kidney Dis* 1991; 18:674–677.
31. Peritonitis and exit site infections. In Khanna R, Nolph KD, Oreopoulos DG (eds): *The Essentials of Peritoneal Dialysis*. Kluwer Academic Publishers, Dordrecht 1993:76–88.
32. Flanagan MJ, Hochstetter LA, Langholdt D, Win VS. CAPD catheter infections: diagnosis and management. *Perit Dial Int* 1994; 14:248–254.
33. Winchester JF. Recurrent peritoneal catheter exit-site infections: 1. *Semin Dial* 1993; 6:405–406.
34. Twardowski ZJ. Recurrent peritoneal catheter exit-site infections: II *Semin Dial* 1993; 6:406–408.
35. Twardowski ZJ, Porwant BF. Current approaches to exit site infections in patients on peritoneal dialysis. *Nephrol Dial Trans* 1997; 12:1284–1295.
36. Plum J, Sudkamp S, Grabenesse B. Results of ultrasound-assisted diagnosis of tunnel infections in CAPD. *Am J Kidney Dis* 1994; 23:99–104.
37. Lazmi HR, Rafone FD, Kliger AS, Fenkelstein FO. *Pseudomonas* exit site infections in CAPD patients. *J Am Soc Nephrol* 1992; 2:1498–1501.
38. Chan MK, Chan PCK, Cheng PK, *et al. Pseudomonas* peritonitis in CAPD patients. characteristics and outcome of treatment. *Nephrol Dial Transplant* 1989; 4:814–818.
39. Taber TE, Hegeman TF, York SM, Kinney RA, Webb DH. Treatment of *Pseudomonas* infections in peritoneal dialysis patients. *Perit Dial Int* 1991; 11:213–216.
40. Holmes CJ, Evans R. Biofilm and foreign body infection—the significance to CAPD associated peritonitis. *Perit Dial Bull* 1986; 6:168–177.
41. Millikan SP, Matzke GR, Keane WF. Antimicrobial treatment of peritonitis associated with continuous ambulatory peritoneal dialysis. *Perit Dial Int* 1991; 11:252–258.
42. Luzar MA, Coles GA, Faller B, *et al. Staphylococcus aureus* nasal carriage and infection in patients on continouous ambulatory peritoneal dialysis. *New Engl J Med* 1990; 322:505–507.
43. Mupirocin Study Group. Nasal mupirocin prevents *Staph. aureus* exit site infection during peritoneal dialysis. *J Am Soc Nephrol* 1996; 7:2403–2408.
44. Perez-Fontan M, Garcia-Falcon T, Rosales M. Treatment of *Staphylococcus aureus* nasal carriers in continuous ambulatory peritoneal dialysis with mupirocin: long-term results. *Am J Kidney Dis* 1993; 22:708–712.
45. Edmond MB, Wenzel RP, Pasculle W. Vancomycin-resistant *Staphylococcus aureus*: Perspectives on measures needed for control. *Ann Intern Med* 1996; 124:329–334.
46. Scalmogna A, De Vecchi A, Maccario M, *et al.* Cuff-shaving procedure. A rescue treatment for exit site infection unrepsonsive to medical therapy. *Nephrol Dial Transplant* 1995; 10:2325–2328.
47. Zimakoff J, Pederson FB, Bergen L. *Staphylococcus aureus* carriage and infections among patients in four haemo and peritoneal dialysis centres in Denmark. *J Hospital Infect* 1996; 33:289–300.
48. Turner K, Uttley L, Scrungzour A. Natural history of *Staphylococcus aureus* nasal carriage and its relationship to exit site infection. *Perit Dial Int* 1998; 18:271–273.

49. Zimmerman SW, Ahrens E, Johnson CA, Craig W, Leggett J, O'Brien M, *et al.* Randomized controlled trial of prophylactic rifampin for PD related infections. *Am J Kidney Dis* 1991; **18**:225–231.

50. Bernardini J, Piraino B, Holley JL, Johnstone JR, Lukes R. Randomized trial of *Staph. aureus* prophylaxis in PD patients: mupirocin calcium ointment 2% applied to the exit site versus oral rifampin. *Am J Kidney Dis* 1996; **26**:695–700.

51. Vychytil A, Lorenz M, Schneider B. New strategies to prevent *Staphyloccus aureus* infections in peritoneal dialysis patients. *J Am Soc Nephrol* 1998; **9**:669–672.

52. Boelaert JB, Van Landuyt HW, Gordts BZ. Nasal and cutaneous carriage of *Staphylococcous aureus* in hemodialysis patients: The effect of nasal mupirocin. *Infect Control Hospital Epidemiol* 1996; **17**:809–811.

53. Thodis E, Bhaskgram S, Pasadakis P, *et al.* Decrease in *Staphyloccus aureus* exit site infections and peritonitis in CAPD patients by local application of mupirocin ointment at the catheter exit site. *Perit Dial Int* 1998; **18**:261–266.

54. Woodrow G, Turney JH, Bownjohn AM. Technique failure in peritoneal dialysis and its impact on patient survival. *Perit Dial Int* 1997; **17**:360–364.

55. Piraino B. Peritonitis as a complication of peritoneal dialysis. *J Am Soc Nephrol* 1998; **9**:1956–1963.

56. Fried LF, Bernardini J, Johnston JR. Peritonitis influences mortality in peritoneal dialysis patients. *J Am Soc Nephrol* 1996; **7**:2176–2182.

57. Flanigan MJ, Freeman RM, Lim VS. Cellular response to peritonitis among peritoneal dialysis patients. *Am J Kidney Dis* 1985; **6**:420–424.

58. Koopmans JG, Boeschotein EW, Pannekect MM. Impaired initial cell reaction CAPD related peritonitis. *Perit Dial Int* 1996; suppl. 1:S362–S367.

59. Sewell DL, Golper TA, Hulman PB. Comparison of large volume culture to other methods of isolation of microorganisms from dialysate. *Perit Dial Int* 1990; **10**:49–52.

60. Holley JL, Moss AH. A prospective evaluation of blood culture vs. standard plate technique for diagnosing peritonitis in CAPD. *Am J Kidney Dis* 1989; **13**:184–189.

61. Buoncristiani U, Cozzari M, Quintaliani G. Abatement of exogenous peritonitis risk using the Perugia CAPD system. *Dial Transplant* 1983; **12**:14–16.

62. Burkart JM, Hylander B, Durnell-Figel T, *et al.* Comparison of peritonitis rates during long-term use of standard spike versus ultraset in continuous ambulatory peritoneal dialysis (CAPD). *Perit Dial Int* 1990; **10**:41–44.

63. Maiorca R, Cantaluppi A, Cancarini GC, *et al.* Prospective controlled tiral of a Y connector and disinfectant to prevent peritonitis in continuous ambulatory peritoneal dialysis. *Lancet* 1983; **2**:642–643.

64. Scalamogna A, De Vecchi A, Castelnovo C, *et al.* Long-term incidence of peritonitis in CAPD patients treated by the Y set technique: experience in a single center. *Nephron* 1990; **55**:24.

65. Port FK, Held PJ, Nolph KD, *et al.* Risk of peritonitis and technique failure by CAPD connection technique: a national study. *Kidney Int* 1992; **42**:967–971.

66. Luzar MA, Slingeneyer A, Cantaluppi A, *et al. In vitro* study of the flush effect in two reusable continuous ambulatory peritoneal dialysis (CAPD) disconnect systems. *Perit Dial Int* 1989; **9**:169–172.

67. Montcon F, Correa-Rotter R, Paniqqua R, *et al.* Prevention of peritonitis with disconnect systems in CAPD. An randomized controlled trial. *Kidney Int* 1998; **54**:2123–2126.

68. Kiernan L, Kliger A, Gorgan-Brennan N, *et al.* Comparison of continuous ambulatory peritoneal dialysis-related infections with different 'Y-tubing' exchange systems. *J Am Soc Nephrol* 1995; **5**:1835.

69. Harris DC, Yuill EJ, Byth K, *et al.* Twin- versus single-bag disconnect systems: infection rates and cost of continuous ambulatory peritoneal dialysis. *J Am Soc Nephrol* 1996; 11:2392–2397.

70. Canadian CAPD Clinical Trial Group. Peritonitis in continuous ambulatory peritoneal dialysis (CAPD): a multicenter randomized clinical trial comparing the Y connector disinfectant system to standard systems. *Perit Dial Int* 1989; 9:159.

71. Holley JL, Bernardini J, Piraino B. Infecting organisms in continuous ambulatory peritoneal dialysis patients on the Y-set. *Am J Kidney Dis* 1994; 23:569.

72. Grutzmacher P, Tsobanelis T, Bruns M, *et al.* Decrease in peritonitis rate by integrated disconnect system in patients on continuous ambulatory peritoneal dialysis. *Perit Dial Int* 1993; 13:S326.

73. Holley JL, Bernardini J, Piraino B. Continuous cycling peritoneal dialysis is associated with lower rates of catheter infections than continuous ambulatory peritoneal dialysis. *Am J Kidney Dis* 1990; 16:133.

74. Korbet SM, Vonesh EF, Firanek CA. Peritonitis in an urban peritoneal dialysis program: an analysis of infection pathogens. *Am J Kidney Dis* 1995; 26:47.

75. Caruana RJ, Burkhart JM, Segraves D, *et al.* Serum and peritoneal fluid amylase levels in CAPD. *Am J Nephrol* 1987; 7:169–171.

76. Twadorski ZJ, Schreiber MJ, Burkart JM. A 69-year-old male with elevated amylase in bloody and cloudy dialysate. *Perit Dial Int* 1993; 13:142–143.

77. Royse VL, Jensen DM, Corwin HL. Pancreatic enzymes in chronic renal failure. *Arch Intern Med* 1987; 147:537–539.

78. Tzamaloukas AH, Obermiller E, Gibel LJ. Peritonitis associated with intra-abdominal pathology in continuous ambulatory peritoneal dialysis patients. *Perit Dial Int* 1993; 13:S335–S341.

79. Harwell CM, Newman LN, Cacho CP. Abdominal catastrophe: visceral injury as a cause of peritonitis in patients treated by peritoneal dialysis. *Perit Dial Int* 1997; 17:586–594.

80. Sundaram S, Cendoroglo M, Cooker LA, Jaber BL, Faict D, Homes CJ, Pereira BJ. Effect of two chambered bicarbonate lactate-peritoneal dialysis fluids on peripheral blood mononuclear cell and polymorphonuclear cell function *in vitro*. *Am J Kidney Dis* 1997; 30:680–689.

81. Liberek T, Topley N, Jorres A, Coles GA, Gahl GM, Williams JD. Peritoneal dialysis fluid inhibition of phagocyte function: effects of osmolality and glucose concentration. *J Am Soc Nephrol* 1993; 3:1508–1515.

82. Cendoroglo M, Sundram S, Jaber BL, Pereira BJ. Effect of glucose concentration, osmolality and sterilization process of peritoneal dialysis fluids on cytokine production by peripheral blood mononuclear cells and polymorphonuclear cell functions *in vivo*. *Am J Kidney Dis* 1998; 31:273–282.

83. Thomas S, Schenk U, Fischer FP. *In vitro* effects of glucose polymer containing peritoneal fluids on phagocytic activity. *Am J Kidney Dis* 1997; 26:246–250.

84. Coles GA, Lewis SL, Williams JD. Host defense and effects of solution on peritoneal cells. In Gokal R, Nolph (eds): *The Textbook of Peritoneal Dialysis*. Kluwer Academic Publishers, Boston, MA, 1994:503–528.

85. Holmes CJ. Peritoneal host defense mechanisms in peritoneal dialysis. *Kidney Int* 1994; suppl. 48:S58–S70.

86. Plum J, Schrenicke G, Grabensee B. Osmotic agents and buffers in peritoneal dialysis solution: monocyte cytokine release and *in vitro* cytotoxicity. *Am J Kidney Dis* 1997; 30:413–422.

87. Plum J, Lordnejad MR, Grabensee B. Effect of alternative peritoneal dialysis solutions on cell viability, apoptosis/necrosis and cytokine expression in human monocytes. *Kidney Int* 1998; 54:224–235.

88. Borra SI, Chandarana J, Kleinfeld M. Fatal peritonitis due to group B beta-hemolytic streptococcus in a patient receiving chronic ambulatory peritoneal dialysis. *Am J Kidney Dis* 1992; **19**:257–259.

89. Singharetnam W, Holley JL. Acute treatment of constipation may lead to transmural migration of bacteria resulting in Gram negative, polymicrobial or fungal peritonitis. *Perit Dial Int* 1996; **16**:423–425.

90. Caravaca F, Ruz-Calero R, Dominguez C. Risk factors for developing peritonitis caused by micro-organisms of enteral origin in peritoneal dialysis patients. *Perit Dial Int* 1998; **18**:41–45.

91. Wood CJ, Fleming V, Turnidge J. *Campylobacter* peritonitis in continuous ambulatory peritoneal dialysis: report of 8 cases and a review of the literature. *Am J Kidney Dis* 1992; **16**:423–425.

92. Boner G, Mhashilkar AM, Rodriquez Ortega M, *et al.* Lectin-mediated, nonopsonic phago-cytosis of type I *Escherichia coli* by human peritoneal macrophages of uremic patients treated by peritoneal dialysis. *J Leukoc Biol* 1989; **46**:239–241.

93. Keane WF, Everett ED, Golpert T, *et al.* Peritoneal dialysis-related peritonitis: treatment recommendations, 1993 update. *Perit Dial Int* 1993; **13**:14–18.

94. Bunke CM, Aronoff GR, Brier ME, Sloan RS, Loft FC. Cefazolin-cephalexin kinetics in continuous ambulatory peritoneal dialysis. *Clin Pharm Ther* 1983; **33**:66–72.

95. Lai MN, Kao MT, Chen CC, Cheung SY, Chung WK. Intraperitoneal once daily dose of cefazolin and gentamicin for treating CAPD peritonitis. *Perit Dial Int* 1997; **17**:87–88.

96. Sandoe JAT, Gokal R, Struthers Y. Vancomycin-resistant enterococci and empirical vancomycin for CAPD peritonitis. *Perit Dial Int* 1997; **17**:617–618.

97. Vas S, Bargman J, Oreooules DG. Treatment in PD patients of peritonitis caused by Gram-positive organisms with single daily dose of antibiotics. *Perit Dial Int* 1997; **17**:91–94.

98. Lye WC, Wong PL, van der Straaten JC, Leong SO, Lee EJC. A prospective randomized comparison of single versus multidose gentamicin in the treatment of CAPD peritonitis. *Adv Perit Dial* 1995; **11**:179–1981.

99. Koo J, Tight R, Rajkumer V, Hang Z. Comparison of once daily versus pharmacokinetic dosing of aminoglycosides in elderly patients. *Am J Med* 1996; **101**:177–183.

100. Van Diesen W, Van Holder R, Vogelaers D. The need for a center tailored treatment protocol for peritonitis. *Perit Dial Int* 1998; **18**:274–281.

101. Innes A, Burden RP, Finoh RG. Treatment of resistant peritonitis in continuous ambu-latory peritoneal dialysis with intraperitoneal urokinase: a double blind clinical trial. *Nephrol Dial Transplant* 1994; **9**:797–799.

102. Williams AJ, Boletis I, Johnson BF. Tenchkhoff catheter replacement or intraperitoneal urokinase: a randomised trial in the management of recurrent continuous ambulatory peritoneal dialysis (CAPD) peritonitis. *Perit Dial Int* 1989; **9**:65–67.

103. Majkowski NL, Mendelay SR. Simultaneous removal and replacement of infected peritoneal dialysis catheters. *Am J Kidney Dis* 1997; **29**:706–711.

104. Goldie SJ, Kiernan-Troidle L, Torres C. Fungal peritonitis in a large chronic peritoneal dialysis population: a report of 55 episodes. *Am J Kidney Dis* 1996; **28**:86–91.

105. Lo WK, Chan TM, Lui SL, Li FK, Cheung IKP. Fungal peritonitis. Current status 1998. *Perit Dial Int* 1999; **19** (suppl. 2):286–290.

106. Cheung IKP, Fan GX, Chan TM, Chan CK, Chan MK. Fungal peritonitis complicating peritoneal dialysis: Report of 27 cases and review of treatment. *Q J Med* 1989; **71**:407–416.

107. Nagappan R, Collins JF, Lee WT. Fungal peritonitis in continuous ambulatory peritoneal dialysis—the Auckland experience. *Am J Kidney Dis* 1992; **5**:492–496.

108. Eisenberg ES, Leviton ES, Leviton S, Soeiro R. Fungal peritonitis in patients receiving peritoneal dialysis. Experience with 11 patients and review of the literature. *Rev Infect Dis* 1986; 8:309–321.

109. Bordes A, Campos-Herrero MI, Fernandez A, Vega N, Rodriquez JC, Palop L. Prediposing and prognostic factors of fungal peritonitis in peritoneal dialysis. *Perit Dial Int* 1995; 15:275–276.

110. Michel C, Courgault L, Alkhayat R, Viron B, Roux P, Mignon F. Fungal peritonitis on peritoneal dialysis. *Am J Nephrol* 1994; 14:113–120.

111. Chan TM, Chan CY, Cheung SW, Lo W, Lo CY, Cheung IKP. Treatment of fungal peritonitis with oral fluconazole: a series of 21 patients. *Nephrol Dial Transplant* 1994; 9:539–542.

112. Strvijk DG, Krediet RT, Boeschoten EW, Rictra PJM, Arisz L. Antifungal treatment of *Candida* peritonitis in continuous ambulatory peritoneal dialysis: a report of 17 cases. *Am J Kidney Dis* 1987; 9:66–70.

113. Rubin J, Kirchner K, Walsh D, Green M, Bower J. Fungal peritonitis during continuous ambulatory peritoneal dialysis. A report of 17 cases. *Am J Kidney Dis* 1987; 5:361–368.

114. Yuen KY, Seto WH, Ching TY, Cheun WC, Kwok Y, Chu YB. An outbreak of *Candida tropicalis* peritonitis in patients on intermittent peritoneal dialysis. *J Hosp Infect* 1992; 22:65–72.

115. Lo WK, Chan CY, Cheng SW. A prospective randomized control study of oral nystatin prophylaxis for *Candida* peritonitis complicating continuous ambulatory peritoneal dialysis. *Am J Kidney Dis* 1996; 28:549–552.

116. Wadhwa NK, Suh H, Thelma C. Antifungal prophylaxis for secondary fungal peritonitis in peritoneal dialysis patients. In Khanna R (ed): *Advances in Peritoneal Dialysis*, vol 12. Peritoneal Dialysis Publications, Toronto, 1996:189–191.

117. Zaruba K, Peters J, Jungbluth H. Successful prophylaxis for fungal peritonitis in patients on continuous ambulatory peritoneal dialysis: six years' experience. *Am J Kidney Dis* 1991; 17:43–46.

118. Marrie TJ, Noble MA, Costerton, JW. Examination of the morphology of bacteria adhering to peritoneal dialysis catheters by scanning electron microscopy. *J Clin Microbiology* 1983; 65:1388–1398.

9

Mucormycosis in dialysis patients

Jack W. Coburn and Hla M. Maung

Introduction

The term mucormycosis refers to the diseases produced by various fungi belonging to the order Mucorales. The terms phycomycosis and zygomycosis have also been used to describe such disorders; however, these terms are less familiar to the clinician. Several different species occur in association with clinical diseases. These fungi have a relatively low pathogenicity, and most episodes have occurred in patients with diabetes mellitus, diabetic ketoacidosis, and in those who are immunocompromised for one or more reasons. A substantial number have occurred in patients with renal failure and in those undergoing dialysis; this review focuses on the disorders that occur in dialysis patients. The occurrence of mucormycosis in association with immunosuppressive therapy for renal transplantation is considered in Chapter 16 while that seen in diabetic patient is reviewed in Chapter 6. The cases of mucormycosis developing in dialysis patients and those in patients with renal failure have had very high mortality, approaching 90%. The major role of desferrioxamine treatment in enhancing the susceptibility to mucormycosis is now well recognized. This review considers the microbiology of the responsible fungi, the pathogenesis of the clinical disorders, the diagnostic microbiology, and the various syndromes encountered. The methods for reaching a timely diagnosis, the effective treatment options, and the means for prevention are reviewed.

Microbiology and classification

The organisms isolated from patients with mucormycosis most often have been *Rhizopus*, *Rhizomucor*, and *Absidia* species; less commonly, *Mucor*, *Cunninghamella*, *Mortierella*, and *Saksenaea* have been identified as causative agents (Fig. 9.1). The Mucorales species, which grow naturally in decaying organic material, are ubiquitous in nature; thus, exposure to the spores of these fungi may be unavoidable (Sugar *et al.* 1992)[1]. They can be cultured aerobically after 2 to 3 days of incubation at 37 °C; because their growth is inhibited by cycloheximide, fungal culture media that contain cycloheximide, such as Mycosel or Mycobiotic agar, should not be used. Nonetheless, cultures are frequently negative. In the absence of evidence of tissue damage, a positive culture of a species of Mucorales may indicate contamination or colonization rather than the presence of a pathogenic organism. Light microscopy of a fresh sample, such as a specimen from bronchoscopy or

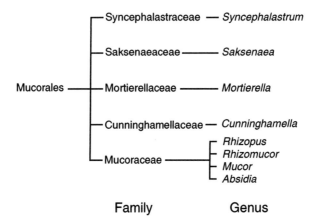

Family   Genus

Fig. 9.1   Genera of the order Mucorales that are considered medically important in causing clinical infection.

minced tissue, will reveal irregularly shaped hyphae, 10 to 20 μm in diameter, with branching at right angles. Various stains, such as haematoxylin and eosin, periodic acid–Schiff, and Grocott–Gomori methenamine–silver stains are useful for identifying the fungus.

In tissue samples Mucorales are commonly observed adjacent to blood vessels and are accompanied by neutrophilic infiltrates. A characteristic feature of mucormycosis is the invasion of blood vessels by the hyphae; such invasion leads to haemorrhage, thrombosis, infarction, and tissue necrosis. This fungal invasion of large vessels, depending on the location, can lead to sudden cerebral haemorrhage or massive and fatal pulmonary haemorrhage.

Pathogenesis

A consideration of the pathogenesis of mucormycosis must include both the potential route of entry of the micro–organism and the nature of altered host defence that renders an individual susceptible to the development of this infection.

Route of entry

The inhalation of spores of Mucorales results in their deposition on the nasal turbinates and/or direct passage into pulmonary alveoli. Cutaneous mucormycosis can arise from direct inoculation of the fungi onto abraded skin, with their subsequent invasion of subcutaneous tissue. It is known that patients who are intravenous drug abusers are susceptible to mucormycosis, an observation which suggests that the disease can arise by direct inoculation into the bloodstream. The haemodialysis procedure, with repeated needle punctures across the skin barrier, provides a potential route of entry for fungi into haemodialysis patients. In patients treated with peritoneal dialysis, the peritoneal dialysis catheter may offer an access for the intraperitoneal inoculation of fungi (Polo *et al.* 1989)[10].

Host factors

The risk factors from the standpoint of the host include:

(1) diabetes mellitus, particularly with ketoacidosis;
(2) various haematological malignancies, particularly with neutropenia;
(3) immunosuppressed states, including treatment with glucocorticoids and other immunosuppressive agents;
(4) desferrioxamine treatment for iron overload or aluminium toxicity;
(5) renal failure and uraemia treated with dialysis;
(6) sustained skin trauma, such as burns; and
(7) profound protein-energy malnutrition, including kwashiorkor.

Normal host factors can usually resist an opportunistic infection with species of Mucorales. Thus, the alveolar macrophages of normal mice can prevent the germination of *Rhizopus* spores following their inoculation into the lung; however, macrophages from mice with diabetes mellitus cannot inhibit the growth of spores of *Rhizopus*, and these mice develop progressive and fatal mucormycosis. The specific factors, such as hyperglycaemia or acidosis, that may account for the altered macrophage function are considered below (Artis *et al.* 1982)[3].

Role of renal failure

The mechanism whereby renal failure itself may increase the susceptibility to mucormycosis is uncertain. It is possible that abnormal function of granulocytes from patients undergoing haemodialysis may result in reduced chemotaxis that accounts for the migration and accumulation of macrophages; this could contribute to the increased susceptibility of dialysis patients to mucormycosis. Leucopenia, glucocorticoids, or other immunosuppressive agents can impair host response, and thereby increase the susceptibility to infection with *Rhizopus* spp. When added to the sera obtained from patients with uraemia or those with diabetes, the function of macrophages is impaired, as evaluated *in vitro*; dialysis of these sera reversed this inhibition of macrophage function. Such observations suggest that low-molecular-weight substances present in the sera of diabetics and uraemic patients are involved in inhibiting macrophage function (Jorens *et al.* 1995)[4].

Role of iron

It is well recognized that the availability of iron is a major limiting factor for the growth of various species of *Rhizopus*. During the years of dialysis before the availability of recombinant erythropoietin, multiple blood transfusions were given to many dialysis patients, and markedly elevated haemosiderin levels were observed in such patients. There is evidence that iron overload can impair phagocytosis and reduce the killing of certain micro-organisms by neutrophils.

In an *in vitro* study using sera from patients with diabetic ketoacidosis, there was no support for growth of *Rhizopus* by these sera after pH was normalized. Following the reduction of pH of these sera to acidotic levels, the fungal growth was no longer inhibited in most but not all of these samples. The acidotic serum samples that showed persistent inhibition each had a low level of serum iron, while the samples that promoted fungal growth all had normal or high serum iron levels. The effect of acidosis in decreasing the iron-binding capacity of transferrin is probably the mechanism for the augmented fungal growth that occurs as a result of greater access to free iron in acidotic patients with normal iron status.

Effect of desferrioxamine

It is now recognized that certain *Rhizopus* species generate their own endogenous siderophore, termed rhizoferrin, which facilitates the uptake of iron (Fig. 9.2). The transferrin (apotransferrin) present in normal serum can chelate and remove iron from rhizoferrin, and this effect probably accounts for the inhibition of fungal growth *in vitro* by normal plasma or serum. The exogenously administered siderophore desferrioxamine chelates iron independent of the affinity of transferrin for iron. The resulting desferrioxamine–iron complex, termed ferrioxamine, markedly augments the uptake of iron by *Rhizopus*; this stimulates fungal replication, enhances its pathogenicity, and blocks the antifungal action of amphotericin B (Boelaert *et al.* 1994)[2]. As noted below (van Cutsem *et al.* 1989)[5], nearly 75% of the cases of mucormycosis reported among dialysis patients have occurred in patients treated with desferrioxamine for aluminium toxicity or, less commonly, for iron overload. The kidney provides the major route for the excretion of ferrioxamine. The presence of renal failure, which markedly prolongs the circulating half-life of ferrioxamine, puts dialysis patients at a much greater risk for the development of mucormycosis than exists in haematological patients with normal renal function who have received desferrioxamine for the management of iron overload.

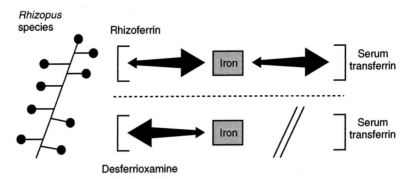

Fig. 9.2 Diagram illustrating the uptake of iron by Mucorales spp. and the influence of desferrioxamine. In the presence of serum containing transferrin, there is effective competition by transferrin for iron over the effect of the endogenous fungal siderophore, rhizoferrin. This results in reduced free iron with little uptake by the fungus, and fungal growth is inhibited (upper panel). In the presence of desferrioxamine, transferrin is unable to compete with desferrioxamine; the desferrioxamine-iron complex enhances the fungal uptake of iron, resulting in enhanced fungal growth. The serum transferrin is unable to prevent this action (lower panel). (Modified from Kulberg BJ and van der Meer JWM. Special population: chronic renal failure. In: D Armstrong and J Cohen (ed) *Infectious Diseases* Mosby, London, 1999, pp. 7–8.)

Clinical syndromes and their features

Mucormycosis presents with different clinical manifestations that are separated into several syndromes: disseminated, rhinocerebral (Yokei *et al.* 1994)[6] and including sinonasal, pulmonary (Tedder *et al.* 1994)[7], cutaneous, gastrointestinal, including peritoneal, and miscellaneous, including involvement of the central nervous system, kidney, heart, mediastinum, and arteries. All of these have been encountered in patients with renal failure and in those undergoing dialysis; and these will be reviewed before considering the syndromes that are more frequent in dialysis patients.

Rhinocerebral mucormycosis

The manifestations of rhinocerebral mucormycosis vary depending on the sinuses that are involved. The features include fever, headache, facial pain and swelling, sinusitis, and ulceration or necrosis of the nasal mucosa. When the infection extends superiorly from the nasal turbinates into the orbit, it can produce ptosis, proptosis, orbital cellulitis, visual loss, and ophthalmoplegia. The infection may affect nearby cranial nerves, including the third, fourth, fifth, sixth, and seventh cranial nerves, with clinical manifestations that depend on the cranial nerve affected. The extension of mucormycosis into the brain leads to the formation of abscess, infarction, and necrosis of the parenchyma of the brain, with the frontal lobes most commonly involved. A nasal infection can invade interiorly into the mouth causing a black discharge or eschar on the palate or nasal mucosa, with necrosis caused by the arterial invasion by the fungus that, in turn, leads to thrombosis. Because of vascular invasion, cavernous sinus thrombosis and thrombosis of the internal carotid artery are common with advancing rhinocerebral mucormycosis. Rhinocerebral mucormycosis is most often acute and rapidly progressive; however, rare cases of rhinocerebral mucormycosis have followed a chronic, indolent course that lasts for several months. Rhinocerebral mucormycosis is the most common form of mucormycosis in patients with diabetic acidosis, in diabetic patients without acidosis, and in patients with haematological malignancies.

Disseminated mucormycosis

Disseminated mucormycosis generally presents as a fulminant, rapidly progressive disease that is often fatal within a few days of the appearance of symptoms. It is believed to arise from direct invasion of blood vessels from the nose or paranasal sinuses, by haematogenous dissemination from another primary focus, or by direct fungal inoculation into the bloodstream, particularly in patients with intravenous drug abuse. The frequent needle insertions into the arteriovenous grafts or fistulas of haemodialysis patients may provide a route for inoculation of the fungus into the bloodstream. A common presenting symptom of disseminated mucormycosis is fever, a sudden or gradual alteration of mental status, features of meningitis or brain abscess, or hemiplegia. The involvement of intra-abdominal structures may lead to severe abdominal pain and features suggesting a surgical abdomen. Weakness of the lower extremities may arise due to infarction of the spinal cord, and a cauda equina syndrome may arise from infection of the vasculature of the cauda equina or lumbosacral nerve roots leading to focal demyeli-nation of these structures. Blood cultures are almost invariably negative; and the findings on examination of spinal fluid are non-specific. The diagnosis of disseminated mucormy-cosis can rarely be made during life but is discovered only at postmortem examination. Disseminated mucormycosis is quite rare other than in dialysis patients receiving desferrioxamine and in patients who abuse intravenous drugs.

Pulmonary mucormycosis

Fever, pleuritic chest pain, and cough, with or without sputum production, are the presenting symptoms in about 60% of patients with pulmonary mucormycosis. Others features include dyspnoea and haemoptysis. Pulmonary mucormycosis can present as pneumonia, a lung abscess, a pulmonary nodule, empyema, or mediastinitis. The disease is often rapidly progressive and can advance to fatal respiratory failure. Because of the angiocentric nature of fungal growth into and around blood vessels, erosion into a large pulmonary vessel commonly leads to massive and fatal haemoptysis. Erosion through the chest wall or the pleura can cause bronchocutaneous fistula or bronchopleural fistula. Rarely, granulomatous mediastinitis develops; this probably occurs due to fungal spread into the mediastinum via lymphatic channels from sites of pulmonary mucormycosis. Endobronchial mucormycosis usually presents as a subacute postobstructive pneumonia distal to an invasive mucormycotic bronchial plug. In patients with adult respiratory dis-tress syndrome (ARDS) and acute renal failure that necessitates dialysis, nosocomial mucormycosis has developed and progressed to fatal respiratory failure. In such cases, the high doses of glucocorticoids given for ARDS probably account for the increased sus-ceptibility to the fungus.

On occasion, a patient may appear and feel fairly well despite the presence of a large infiltrate observed on the chest radiograph. Pulmonary mucormycosis should be consid-ered in dialysis patients with progressive pneumonia that worsens or fails to improve with standard antibiotic therapy. The pulmonary form of mucormycosis is seen more com-monly in patients with haematological malignancies, in those receiving glucocorticoid therapy, and in patients with diabetes.

Gastrointestinal mucormycosis

Gastrointestinal mucormycosis has been most common in countries where extreme malnutrition is prevalent. It is rare in developed countries; however, gastrointestinal mucormycosis can occur in patients receiving immunosuppressive therapy for organ transplantation (Chapter 4) or for rapidly progressive glomerulonephritis (Chapter 5). All segments of the gastrointestinal tract can be involved, with the stomach, colon, and ileum most frequently affected. The most frequent symptom of gastrointestinal mucormycosis is epigastric discomfort; other symptoms include abdominal cramps, diarrhoea, haematemesis, and malaenic or bloody stools. Clinical symptoms may be non-specific or can mimic an intra-abdominal abscess. Gastric mucormycosis may present as a giant gastric ulcer, often with intestinal ulceration and the formation of multiple abscesses.

Peritonitis due to mucormycosis may be limited to uraemic patients being managed with peritoneal dialysis. In these patients, the features of peritoneal mucormycosis include the finding of cloudy peritoneal fluid with significant leucocytosis but with a negative culture and/or peritonitis that fails to respond to appropriate antibiotic therapy. Infection has been described in a CAPD patient after the patient had bathed in a farm cistern, an observation suggesting that the peritoneal catheter may be the route of infection. In such a patient, the level of suspicion for mucormycosis should be high, as the disease is commonly fatal; surgical removal of the peritoneal dialysis catheter may be urgently needed.

Cutaneous mucormycosis

Cutaneous mucormycosis can develop at the site of sustained trauma to the skin, usually a finger, toe, or at the site of a burn or wound. There is an enlarging black eschar with necrosis. Progressive amputation may be needed, and the diseases has progressed to fatal dissemination in desferrioxamine-treated dialysis patients. Cases have been reported in association with contaminated adhesive bandages and in acutely ill newborn infants at a site where a tongue depressor is taped to the skin to protect an intravenous catheter. Cutaneous mucormycosis can develop as a late manifestation of disseminated mucormycosis.

Renal mucormycosis

Renal mucormycosis has usually occurred as part of the spectrum of disseminated mucormycosis; however, isolated and bilateral renal involvement has occurred and led to acute renal failure that necessitated haemodialysis. Fever, loin pain, chills, urinary frequency, and frank haematuria are presenting symptoms of renal mucormycosis.

Mucormycosis in dialysis patients

In this chapter, the data on 71 dialysis patients identified to have mucormycosis have been analysed;.these include 58 patients previously reported in 1991 and 13 additional patients. The syndromes encountered in these patients, who are separated according to whether or not they had received desferrioxamine are shown in Table 9.1. More than half of the desferrioxamine-treated patients had disseminated mucormycosis, while the distribution of the syndromes of mucormycosis among the dialysis patients not receiving desferrioxamine does not differ greatly from the distribution reported in patients without renal failure (Boelaert *et al.* 1991)[9].

In many of the patients for whom data are available the desferrioxamine was given at the time of each dialysis, either during the last 2 h of dialysis or immediately after dialysis. In the 48 patients with data available, the dose of desferrioxamine with each dialysis was as high as 40 mg/kg; the dose was above 4.0 g/week in 25%, 1.0 to 4.0 g/week in 68%, and less than 1.0 g/kg in only 7%. The lowest doses were 300 mg/week in one patient and 500 mg/week in another. The shortest duration of desferrioxamine treatment before the appearance of mucormycosis was 2 to 3 weeks in two patients; most patients received the treatment for 12 weeks or longer.

Table 9.1   Syndromes of mucormycosis reported in dialysis patients separated according to desferrioxamine therapy

Syndrome	No desferrioxamine treatment (%) ($n=20$)	Desferrioxamine treated (%) ($n=51$)
Disseminated	3 (15)	26 (51)
Rhinocerebral	7 (35)	15 (29)
Pulmonary	5 (25)	3 (6)
Central nervous system	none	3 (6)
Miscellaneous*	5 (25)	4 (8)

* Includes gastrointestinal (4 no desferrioxamine, / 1 desferrioxamine), cutaneous (1 no desferrioxamine, / 2 desferrioxamine), and arterial (0 no desferrioxamine, /1 desferrioxamine).

Table 9.2   Risk factors for mucormycosis, other than renal failure and desferrioxamine treatment, among dialysis patients

Risk factor	No desferrioxamine treatment ($n=20$)*	Desferrioxamine treated ($n=51$)[†]
None	2	27
Diabetes mellitus	9	3
Glucocorticoid therapy	7	1
Liver disease	1	7
Iron overload (ferritin > 1000 µg/litre	6	15
Splenectomy	1	4
Acidosis ($HCO_3 \leq 17$ mmol/litre)	2	3
Immunosuppressive medication	2	0
Neutropenia	0	1

*Nine patients had one risk factor; eight had two; one had three or more.
[†]16 patients had one risk factor; six had two; two had three or more.

Risk factors for the occurrence of mucormycosis, other than renal failure or desferrioxamine therapy, were commonly present among the afflicted dialysis patients. These are listed in Table 9.2, with the patients separated into those treated with desferrioxamine and those without. Among the desferrioxamine-treated patients, 52% had no risk factor other than receiving desferrioxamine. Among the dialysis patients not given desferrioxamine, only 10% lacked any known risk factor. Of interest, about 30% of both groups had evidence of iron overload, as indicated by a serum ferritin level above 1000 µg/litre; thus, iron overload may be a predisposing factor in these patients. Diabetes was relatively common among the dialysis patients who had not been treated with desferrioxamine. Among the 71 dialysis patients reviewed, only 3% had no risk factor other than renal failure and treatment with dialysis. These data suggest that end-stage renal failure that is managed with dialysis is not an important factor predisposing to the development of mucormycosis. It should be emphasized, however, that such a collection of patients from literature citations or reported to a registry may not provide an accurate estimate of the true prevalence of mucormycosis among dialysis patients.

Diagnosis

Early diagnosis and aggressive treatment are very important if a dialysis patient with mucormycosis is to survive. The threshold for suspicion of mucormycosis should be low when an infection at any site does not respond to antibiotic therapy. Infection of a progressive nature that exhibits areas of apparent vasculitis, with thrombosis, haemorrhage, and infarction, are important clues to suggest the presence of mucormycosis. Another highly suspicious sign of mucormycosis is the lack of bleeding of an affected tissue during a biopsy or surgical debridement. A definitive diagnosis of mucormycosis is made most readily by visualization of the unique and characteristic hyphae in sections of a biopsy specimen; less commonly, a specific diagnosis can be made by culturing the fungus with appropriate culture media; however, a negative culture does not exclude this disorder. Serology has no role in the diagnosis of mucormycosis. The methods for the recognition and diagnosis of the different syndromes of mucormycosis are described below.

A definitive diagnosis of **rhinocerebral mucormycosis** can be difficult. A diagnosis can be proven from a biopsy sample of tissue from a nasal turbinate or sinus. Computed tomography (CT) of the sinus can demonstrate thickening of the sinus mucosa and/or osseous destruction; an air–fluid level in the sinus is usually lacking. In the orbit, there may be swelling of the orbital muscle or a space-occupying lesion. The typical findings of cavernous sinus thrombosis on contrast-enhanced CT include multiple irregular filling defects or complete non-opacification of one or both sides of the cavernous sinus. Gadolinium-enhanced MRI is helpful for the early detection of intraparenchymal lesions that involve the cerebral cortex, meninges, or the orbit and for the identification of intracranial vascular occlusion; such abnormalities may be detected even before clinical signs appear. From a retrospective review of patients with rhinocerebral mucormycosis, frequent and serial follow-up MRI was recommended in patients with rhinocerebral mucormycosis for the early recognition of intracranial extension and to provide a guide for necessary debridement.

For **pulmonary mucormycosis**, the diagnosis can be established by direct visualization of the lesion at flexible fiberoptic bronchoscopy, with transbronchial biopsy, brush biopsy, or bronchoalveolar lavage. Open lung biopsy, transthoracic needle aspiration of a lesion, or thoracocentesis may be needed to obtain samples or tissue for the specific diagnosis of mucormycosis. The radiographic features are generally non-specific; chest radiographs are generally abnormal, with findings of infiltrates, effusion, consolidation, nodules, a fungal ball, a mass, or cavitation. Some so-called 'specific' features on chest radiographs include an 'air crescent' sign, which is air between a radiodense parenchymal lesion and normal lung tissue, or a 'halo' sign, which is an area of low attenuation surrounding an infiltrate. In one case, the diagnosis of pulmonary mucormycosis was suggested by the findings of multiple segmental ventilation–perfusion defects on a ventilation–perfusion lung scan; such features were consistent with pulmonary emboli.

The abnormalities probably occurred due to the vaso–occlusive pathological process of mucormycosis.

Mucormycosis involving the **central nervous system** can be diagnosed by the demonstration of a low-density mass with variable peripheral enhancement and/or the finding of ischaemic infarction of various regions of the brain by CT or MRI. Lumbar puncture is usually not helpful for the diagnosis of cerebral mucormycosis. Involvement of the spinal cord with mucormycosis can be detected with CT or by myelography.

The endoscopic appearance of giant gastric ulcer may suggest a diagnosis of gastric mucormycosis; this should be confirmed by a gastric biopsy which often demonstrates the characteristic appearance of Mucorales. Culture of peritoneal fluid, the peritoneal membrane, or the peritoneal dialysis catheter can be the means to detect peritoneal mucormycosis. It may be necessary to obtain a large volume of seffluent peritoneal dialysate and submit this to sterile filtration through a pump, with the filter cultured to demonstrate the specific fungus.

The biopsy of a suspicious skin lesion with histological examination and culture can be used to diagnose cutaneous mucormycosis.

The diagnosis of disseminated mucormycosis during life is difficult, and most cases are only recognized at postmortem examination. Blood cultures are usually negative; in a susceptible patient who is worsening, there should be an attempt to identify an affected organ or tissue in order to obtain a tissue sample for the diagnosis.

Therapy of mucormycosis

The successful treatment of mucormycosis must involve aggressive and coordinated actions that include both medical and surgical approaches (Lee *et al.* 1999)[8]. It is imperative that aggressive surgical debridement be considered as an important option early in the evaluation of a patient in whom this disorder is suspected. Indeed, a surgical procedure that is being done to obtain tissue for diagnostic purposes can often be extended to include the excision of necrotic and devitalized tissue. A goal should be the surgical excision of all devitalized tissue. In many cases of rhinocerebral mucormycosis, surgical debridement may be required two or more times (Gupta *et al.* 1999)[13]. The reported data on successful treatment of mucormycosis have included all patients, some with renal failure and some treated with dialysis. These data on therapy of mucormycosis are reviewed, since the principles apply to patients undergoing dialysis.

With pulmonary mucormycosis, which has a poor prognosis when managed with antifungal therapy alone, fatal pulmonary haemorrhage can occur suddenly in a patient who has been showing evidence of clinical improvement. Patients with pulmonary mucormycosis who have received amphotericin B in combination with surgery, e.g. lobectomy or even pneumonectomy, have shown a more favourable outcome than patients treated with amphotericin B therapy alone. There is evidence from a review of the outcome of rhinocerebral mucormycosis in patients lacking renal failure that the survival is worse in patients treated with amphotericin B alone compared with those who had combination therapy that includes surgical debridement and amphotericin B.

Medical therapy should include the early consideration of starting antifungal therapy with amphotericin B. The initiation of treatment with amphotericin B should not be delayed in a susceptible dialysis patient who presents with clinical features suggestive of rhinocerebral mucormycosis until a tissue or biopsy sample is available or until a tissue sample has been processed to document the diagnosis of mucormycosis. This would be the case in particular for a dialysis patient who has received desferrioxamine, glucocorticoids, or other immunosuppressive treatment, or a dialysis patient with concomitant diabetes mellitus, evidence of iron overload, or liver disease. Therapy with conventional intravenous amphotericin B should be initiated utilizing relatively high doses. It has been recommended that the starting dose is 1.0 mg/kg/day, with daily doses increased as high as 1.5 mg/kg in patients with a rapidly progressive infection. When the status of such a patient improves or stabilizes, the dose of amphotericin B can be reduced to 0.8 to 1.0 mg/kg/day. The duration of therapy must depend on the condition of the patient, the location of the disease, and the apparent toxicity with amphotericin B. With a patient who is undergoing haemodialysis, concern about the nephrotoxicity of amphotericin B may not be relevant, and potential toxicity to other tissues must receive attention. It has been suggested that he mortality of mucormycosis in a general patient population lacking renal failure can be reduced to 20 to 25%, a rate much lower than the 70 to 90% mortality noted in patients undergoing dialysis.

Rhinocerebral mucormycosis has been treated successfully using lipid formulations of amphotericin B (Gonzalez *et al.* 1997)[11]. However, the patients reported did not have renal failure; it is not certain that there is an advantage of the lipid formulations of amphotericin B in dialysis patients. In general, the doses of the various lipid formulations used have been two to four times higher than the conventional dose of amphotericin B. It is uncertain whether the higher doses may make one or more of the lipid formulations more effective than the conventional amphotericin B. It is apparent, however, that the nephrotoxicity of lipid formulations is considerably less than that of conventional amphotericin B (Hiemenz *et al.* 1996)[12]. Further experience with the lipid formulations is clearly needed in patients with mucormycosis.

Adjunctive treatment modalities noted in case reports to 'aid' in the management of mucormycosis include hyperbaric oxygen (Ferguson *et al.* 1988)[15] for patients with rhinocerebral mucormycosis and the use of combined rifampin and amphotericin B for pulmonary mucormycosis (Christenson *et al.* 1987)[14]. Currently, there are no data to prove that these treatment modalities have altered the prognosis of this infection, and there are no data about their use in dialysis patients. There are a few reports of 'successful treatment' of mucormycosis using fluconazole; however, all patients eventually died, albeit most of causes other than mucormycosis. At this time, treatment of mucormycosis with drugs in this azole class of antifungal agents is not warranted. Since mucormycosis is quite rare, controlled trials will never be undertaken to evaluate the efficacy of any specific form or combination of therapy, particularly in dialysis patients.

It has become common to administer intravenous iron dextran or ferrous gluconate to dialysis patients receiving erythropoietin to maintain the transferrin saturation above 25 to 30%; it would seem prudent that intravenous iron should be discontinued in a patient suspected of having mucormycosis.

Prevention

Desferrioxamine therapy is a major risk factor for the development of progressive and fatal mucormycosis in dialysis patients, and it would be best to avoid both aluminium toxicity and iron overload that would necessitate the use of desferrioxamine in such patients. However, the high mortality among patients with acute aluminium neurotoxicity may make it necessary to treat dialysis patients with desferrioxamine when high aluminium levels in the dialysate lead to severe aluminium toxicity in a dialysis unit. Also, one encounters patients with both severe secondary hyperparathyroidism requiring parathyroidectomy and evidence of significant aluminium accumulation; ideally, such patients would need the removal of aluminium with desferrioxamine before undergoing parathyroid surgery. The recommended procedures for desferrioxamine treatment, shown in Table 9.3, are designed to minimize the exposure of a dialysis patient both to ferrioxamine, which markedly enhances the risk for mucormycosis, and to aluminoxamine, which can precipitate acute aluminium neurotoxicity. In comparison to the methods used before 1993 for both diagnosis and treatment using desferrioxamine, the current procedures are designed to reduce the length of time for which a dialysis patient is exposed to significant levels of ferrioxamine and/or to high concentrations of aluminoxamine. The doses of desferrioxamine, both for the desferrioxamine infusion test and for continued treatment, are low (5 mg/kg or 10 mg/kg), and the time between the infusion of desferrioxamine and the next dialysis is shortened (Barata *et al.* 1996)[17]. Also, a high-flux dialyser, with or without charcoal haemoperfusion, should be employed to maximize the removal of both ferrioxamine and aluminoxamine (Vasilakakis *et al.* 1992)[16]. The next treatment with desferrioxamine should not be given until after two or three dialysis procedures without desferrioxamine to ensure that the serum levels of both ferrioxamine and aluminoxamine are maximally reduced.

Ideally, aluminium-containing phosphate binders should be abandoned altogether and only calcium-containing phosphate binders and/or newer phosphate binders, such as sevelamer or lanthanum, that contain no aluminium, should be used. This practice would eliminate or greatly reduce any risk of sporadic aluminium loading arising from the oral intake of aluminium gels.

The availability and use of recombinant human erythropoietin should obviate the need for multiple blood transfusions; hence, desferrioxamine treatment should not be needed for iron overload in dialysis patients.

Table 9.3   Changes in the practice of desferrioxamine therapy to reduce the risk of mucormycosis

	Before 1993: mucormycosis encountered	After 1993: mucormycosis absent*
Dose of desferrioxamine (test does and treatment)	40 mg/kg	15 mg/kg 5 mg/kg
Frequency of dosing	One dose per dialysis	One dose per three to four dialysis sessions
Schedule of dosing in relation to dialysis	Last 1–2 h of dialysis (44 h before next dialysis)	1 to 5 h before dialysis
Dialyser used during desferrioxamine treatment	Standard low flux	High flux (with/without charcoal haemoperfusion)

* These changes also result in lower aluminoxamine levels and thereby minimize the risk of acute aluminium neurotoxicity.

Greater and greater numbers of diabetic patients are encountered with renal failure and therefore require treatment with dialysis; attention to careful control of blood glucose and the avoidance of significant metabolic acidosis would minimize the risks for mucormycosis in dialysis patients with concomitant diabetes mellitus. With these manoeuvres, it would be hoped that mucormycosis may become even rarer in patients managed with dialysis.

References

1. Sugar AM. Mucormycosis. *Clin Infect Dis* 1992; **14** (suppl. 1):S126–S129.
2. Boelaert JR. Mucormycosis (zygomycosis): Is there news for the clinician? *J Infect* 1994; **28** (suppl. 1):1–6.
3. Artis WM, Fountain JA, Delcher HK, Jones HE. A mechanism of susceptibility to mucormycosis in diabetic ketoacidosis: transferrin and iron availability. *Diabetes* 1982; **31**:1109–1114.
4. Jorens PG, Boelaert JR, Halloy V, Zamora R, Schneider Y-J, Herman AG. Human and rat macrophages mediate fungistatic activity against *Rhizopus* species differently: *in vitro* and *ex vivo* studies. *Infect Immun* 1995; **63**:4489–4494.
5. Van Cutsem J, Boelaert JR. Effects of deferoxamine, feroxamine and iron on experimental mucormycosis (zygomycosis). *Kidney Int* 1989; **36**:1061–1068.
6. Yokei RA, Bullock JD, Aziz AA, Markert RJ. Survival factors in rhino-orbital-cerebral mucormycosis. *Surv Ophthalmol* 1994; **39**:3–22.
7. Tedder M, Spratt JA, Anstadt MP, Hegde SS, Tedder SD, Lowe JE. Pulmonary mucormycosis: results of medical and surgical therapy. *Ann Thorac Surg* 1994; **57**:1044–1050.
8. Lee FYW, Mossad SB, Adal KA. Pulmonary mucormycosis. *Arch Intern Med* 1999; **159**:1301–1309.
9. Boelaert JR, Fenves AZ, Coburn JW. Deferoxamine therapy and mucormycosis in dialysis patients: report of an international registry. *Am J Kidney Dis* 1991; **18**:660–667.
10. Polo JR, Luno J, Menarguez C, Gallego E, Robles R, Hernandez P. Peritoneal mucormycosis in a patient receiving continuous ambulatory peritoneal dialysis. *Am J Kidney Dis* 1989; **13**:237–239.
11. Gonzalez CE, Couriel DR, Walsh TJ. Disseminated zygomycosis in a neutropenic patient: successful treatment with amphotericin B lipid complex and granulocyte colony-stimulating factor. *Clin Infect Dis* 1997; **24**:192–196.
12. Hiemenz JW, Walsh TJ. Lipid formulations of amphotericin B: recent progress and future directions. *Clin Infect Dis* 1996; **22** (suppl. 2):S133–S144.
13. Gupta AK, Mann SBS, Khosla VK, Sastry KVSSRK, Hundal JS. Non-randomized comparison of surgical modalities for paranasal sinus mycoses with intracranial extension. *Mycoses* 1999; **42**:225–230.
14. Christenson JC, Shalit I, Welch DF, Guruswamy A, Marks MI. Synergistic action of Amphotericin B and Rifampin against rhizopus species. *Antimicrob Agents Chemother* 1987; **31**:1775–1778.
15. Ferguson BJ, Mitchell TG, Moon R, Camporesi EM, Farmer J. Adjunctive hyperbaric oxygen for treatment of rhinocerebral mucormycosis. *Rev Infect Dis* 1988; **10**:551–559.
16. Vasilakakis DM, D'Haese PC, Lamberts LV, Lemoniatou E, Digenis PN, De Broe ME. Removal of aluminoxamine and ferrioxamine by charcoal hemoperfusion and hemodialysis. *Kidney Int* 1992; **41**:1400–1407.
17. Barata JD, D'Haese PC, Pires C, Lamberts LV, Simoes J, De Broe ME. Low dose (5 mg/kg) desferrioxamine treatment in acutely aluminium-intoxicated haemodialysis patients using two drug administration schedules. *Nephrol Dial Transplant* 1996; **11**:125–132.

10

Hepatitis C in end-stage renal disease

Svetlozar N. Natov and Brian J.G. Pereira

Biology of the hepatitis C virus and tests for the detection of hepatitis C infection

Structure of the hepatitis C virus genome

Hepatitis C virus (HCV) is a small spherical virus, 40–60 nm in size, with a lipid envelope and a single-stranded RNA. The virus exhibits structural and sequence homology with the Flavivirideae family—human flaviviruses and animal pestiviruses—and therefore is considered to be a member of this family.[1] The viral genome containing approximately 9400 nucleotides is organized in a long reading frame coding for a 3000-amino-acid polyprotein bracketed at the ends by two non-coding regions (NCR) in 5′ and 3′ terminus (5′ NCR and 3′ NCR respectively).[1,2] The 5′ end of the genome encodes the major structural proteins and is described as the structural region of the viral genome. It includes the basic nucleocapsid (C) followed by two envelope glycoprotein domains (E1 and E2/NS1 regions).[1] Downstream to the envelope protein genes and towards the 3′ end of the genome is the non-structural region with the non-structural genes *NS2*, *NS3*, *NS4*, and *NS5* respectively. Variable degrees of genetic heterogeneity have been observed over the entire viral genome.[3–5] The 5′ non-coding region (5′NCR) represents the most conserved sequence.[6–9] The nucleocapsid is likewise highly conserved. The E2/NS1 region followed by the E1 are the most variable sequences of the viral genome.[10,11] Among the non-structural regions, the NS3 region, and parts of the NS4 and NS5 regions display significant genetic heterogeneity.[12,13] However, the c33 protein encoded by the NS3 region appears to contain well-conserved immunogenic epitopes.[12]

A number of distinct HCV variants have been isolated by nucleotide sequence analysis of the viral genome and a variety of classification systems have been introduced.[1,4,5,7,14–18] Based on the data from an international collaborative study, which compared the nucleotide sequences in the NS5 region of a worldwide panel of HCV variants and other published isolates, an universal system for the nomenclature of hepatitis C viral isolates has been proposed, and recommended for future use in studies related to HCV genotypes.[5,14] This consensus classification defines six HCV phenotypes with mean sequence homology of 65% (range from 55% to 72%). These are designated as HCV types and numbered in Arabic numerals 1 to 6. Each type consists of two or more clusters of variants, subtypes, which are named with lower case letters a, b, c, etc., in order of discovery and have mean sequence homology of 80% (range from 75% to 86%).

Finally, each subtype includes individual isolates sharing sequence homology of 88%. Virus genotypes have been assigned in order of discovery, so that the prototype strain is 1a and the distinct variant first described in Japan is 1b.[14]

Tests for antibodies to HCV

The clinical diagnosis of HCV infection is routinely based on tests detecting the presence of antibodies to HCV (anti-HCV), rather than the viral RNA (HCV RNA) itself, as the latter is subjected to significant technical difficulties.[19] Both enzyme-linked immunosorbent assays (ELISA) and recombinant immunoblot assays (RIBA) have been used to detect non-neutralizing antibodies. ELISA detects antibody to a specific HCV antigen (first-generation tests) or a combination of antigens (second- and third-generation tests) in a standard ELISA plate. In contrast, RIBA detects antibodies to one or more HCV antigens on a strip that is read visually. While ELISA have been used as screening tests, RIBA have been considered confirmatory tests by virtue of their increased specificity.

The first-generation anti-HCV tests (ELISA1, RIBA1) detect non-neutralizing antibodies to the C100-3 (and 5-1-1) protein(s) encoded by the NS3/NS4 region of the HCV prototype isolate (i.e. HCV genotype 1a). Since there is a substantial heterogeneity in C100-3 sequences of different genotypes, the first-generation tests would most readily detect antibodies induced by infection with HCV genotype 1 and would lack sensitivity due to their genotype dependence.[12] The performance of the first-generation anti-HCV tests is further compromised by the delay in antibody production to C100-3 antigen in response to HCV infection, resulting in a longer 'window' period (i.e. the early stage of the infection, when viraemia is present, but antibody response is not yet manifest).[20] In fact, the mean interval from transfusion with HCV-infected blood products to seroconversion detected by first-generation tests is 16 weeks, but could be as long as 1 year. Overall, with the use of these assays, anti-HCV was ultimately detected in 46–89% of the patients with HCV infection.[21,22]

The second-generation tests have overcome some of these limitations. ELISA2 includes c22 antigen from the nucleocapsid region and c200, which is a composite of c33 and c100-3 antigens from the NS3 and NS4 region. RIBA2 uses four recombinant HCV antigens (c22, c33, c100, and 5-1-1). There are at least two good reasons for the better sensitivity of these second-generation tests. First, the increased number of incorporated antigens with highly conserved protein sequences negates any dependence on genotype in the performance of these tests. Second, the 'window period' is shortened as the production of antibodies to c22 or c33 proteins precedes by at least 1 month the production of antibodies to c100-3.[23] Indeed, seroconversion can be detected with the use of second-generation tests as early as 4 weeks after exposure.[21] In addition, the antibodies to the c22 or c33 proteins remain detectable in the serum for a longer period of time.[24]

Recently, third-generation anti-HCV tests have become available. They incorporate an additional recombinant antigen from the NS5 region, and an improved c33 antigen corresponding to the NS3 region. In theory, the improvement of c33, as well as the inclusion of antigens from regions of the HCV genome not represented in the previous tests, could further improve the sensitivity.

A number of supplementary tests detecting specific antibodies have been developed to facilitate a more precise diagnosis of HCV infection. Thus, the presence of IgM antibody to the NS3 region has been used for early diagnosis of HCV infection after exposure to the virus.[25] Likewise, the duration of HCV infection could be estimated with the use of an IgG antibody avidity test.[26] Patients with recent infection (within 50 days of seroconversion) demonstrate a low avidity index as opposed to patients with long-term infection (at least 300 days after seroconversion) who have a high avidity index. Indeed, longitudinal follow-up of a cohort of patients with newly acquired HCV infection revealed that the avidity index increased significantly as time elapsed after primary infection. This antibody test was also shown to distinguish between primary antibody response and passively acquired antibody.[26]

Tests for HCV RNA

Polymerase chain reaction

The detection of HCV RNA by reverse transcriptase polymerase chain reaction (PCR) is considered to be the 'gold standard' in the diagnosis of current HCV infection.[27–29] In post-transfusion hepatitis C, HCV RNA can be detected in the circulation within a week after exposure, and precedes the production of antibodies.[20,27] The PCR uses 'universal' primers which are derived from the highly conserved 5' end shared by all known HCV variants. It is very sensitive and can detect HCV RNA levels as low as 2000 copies/ml.[30] However, this extreme sensitivity is a relative limitation of the test, as even minor contamination could result in false positives.[31] On the other hand, imperfect handling and/or storage of blood samples can result in up to 40% false negative results, thus substantially jeopardizing the reliability of the test.[32] Finally, PCR testing is available only in select institutions, its performance is labour intensive, and protocols vary from one laboratory to another.[33]

Quantitation of HCV RNA titers

The branched-chain DNA assay (bDNA assay) is a quantitative assay for HCV RNA in which, the signal/probe rather than the viral nucleic acid is amplified.[34,35] The assay is simple, automated, and reproducible.[35] It has a cut-off limited to 350 000 molecules/ml, and therefore appears to be less sensitive than PCR.[35] Yet, this decreased sensitivity could be regarded as an advantage as false positive results due to contamination are unlikely.[35] The sensitivity of the bDNA assay, based on a positive PCR, is 72%.[35] However, the bDNA-negative, PCR-positive patients could be those with very low circulating HCV RNA load. In addition to the bDNA assay, quantitative PCR has also been used to measure the level of HCV RNA in serum.[27]

Tests for HCV genotypes

Several different methods have been used to identify the specific HCV type and subtype. Some of them are commercially available. Sequence analysis of the viral genome is the most precise assay, but also the most expensive, time-consuming, and fraught with the problem of mutations.[4,36–41] Other techniques for HCV genotyping include PCR using type- and subtype-specific primers, PCR using universal primers, followed by digestion of the PCR product by restriction enzymes (restriction fragment length polymorphism, RFLP), PCR using universal primers, followed by hybridization with type- or subtype-specific probes, and enzyme-linked immunosorbent assay that detects antibodies to serotype-specific immunodominant epitopes from the NS4 region of the HCV genome.[4,12,41–43]

Epidemiology and clinical features of HCV infection

Prevalence

Hepatitis C is a ubiquitous infection whose prevalence varies widely between different countries and geographical areas. Using first-generation anti-HCV tests, the prevalence of anti-HCV among blood donors was found to be 0.47–1.4% in North America, 1.2% in South America, 0–1.3% in Europe, 0.28% to 1.3% in Asia, 2.2% in Africa, and 0.5% in New Zealand. The newer generation anti-HCV tests have revealed similar prevalence of anti-HCV in the general population: 0.03% to 1.03% in Europe, and 0.5% to 0.98% in Asia by second-generation tests, and 0.4% to 1% in Europe by third-generation tests.[44,45] However, comparative data with the new third-generation anti-HCV tests are insufficient at the present time.

Routes of transmission and clinical course

Hepatitis C, the principal cause for parentally transmitted non-A, non-B hepatitis (NANBH), is a bloodborne infection which accounts for more than 90% of cases of post-transfusion hepatitis, and for the majority of all cases of NANBH in the United States.[46] Although blood transfusion is by and large the most important route of transmission of HCV, other modes of parenteral exposure such as intravenous drug abuse and needle-stick injuries, and more rarely professional exposure to blood, as well as sexual and household contacts with a person who has hepatitis C have resulted in acquisition of HCV. The incubation period of HCV ranges from 15 to 150 days (mean 50 days). Clinical symptoms in patients with acute hepatitis C tend to be mild. In fact, most cases are asymptomatic, and fulminant and subacute liver failure is rare. In transfusion-associated hepatitis C, HCV RNA levels become detectable in the serum as early as 1 to 3 weeks after the exposure, and are commonly followed by increase in serum alanine aminotransferase (ALT) levels.[20] If a chronic HCV carrier state is established, HCV RNA levels are usually sustained in serum over the time.[47] Anti-HCV antibody production typically begins at 4 weeks, but can be delayed as long as 1 year.[21,22] Anti-HCV antibodies are directed towards multiple viral proteins, commonly persist indefinitely or at least over a long period of time, and their presence is unrelated to the course or outcome of the disease.[24,48–51] In about half of patients the disease will take a self-limited course and ALT activity will return to normal. In the other half of patients, ALT levels will remain persistently elevated and a relatively slow, sequential progression from acute hepatitis C to chronic HCV infection—chronic hepatitis, cirrhosis, and hepatocellular carcinoma—will take place over the years.[52] The mean interval from the time of trans-fusion to the diagnosis of liver disease was 10 to 13.7 years for patients with chronic hepatitis, 18.4 years for those with chronic active hepatitis, 20.6 to 21.2 years for those with cirrhosis, and 28.3 to 29 years for those with hepatocellular carcinoma.[53,54] Regardless of the relentless progression of HCV-induced liver disease, a recent long-term study with an average follow-up of 18 years has failed to show any increase in all-cause-mortality after transfusion-associated non-A, non-B hepatitis. However, the frequency of death from liver disease, although low (3.3%), was significantly higher than that in the control groups (1.1% and 2.0%). It is possible that with time, the difference between groups in all-cause mortality could reach statistical significance, as an increase in mortality among the subjects with transfusion-associated NANBH can be expected with the progression of liver disease.[55] Hence, longer follow-up might be required to reveal differences in mortality between groups.

Numerous studies have consistently found that ALT levels, in the general population as well as in patients with end-stage renal disease (ESRD), have limited value for the diagnosis of HCV infection. Indeed, increased ALT activity was detected in only 20% of anti-HCV-positive blood products and 33% of anti-HCV-positive blood donors.[56,57] Similarly, among patients on haemodialysis, serum ALT levels are elevated in only 4–67% of the anti-HCV-positive patients, 12–31% of the HCV RNA-positive ones, and one-third of those with biopsy-proven hepatitis.[51,58–64] Likewise, biochemical evidence of liver disease is present in only 42–52% of the HCV RNA-positive transplant recipients.[65,66] In addition, no association has been found between HCV genotype and liver enzyme activity.[67] The discrepancy between serum ALT levels and the presence of anti-HCV is due to several factors:

1. Chronic hepatitis C characteristically has a fluctuating course with multiple peaks and troughs in ALT levels, and therefore patients with normal ALT levels may have severe histological lesions.[20]
2. HCV infection is not always associated with chronic liver disease. In fact, only 69% of anti-HCV-positive symptom-free blood donors who underwent liver biopsy had histological evidence of chronic hepatitis, all of whom had HCV RNA in the serum.[68] Therefore, it is likely that a carrier state can exist with viral replication occurring at extrahepatic sites and no apparent liver damage; this can be explained by the inability of some patients to mount a strong immune response to HCV and thus allowing the virus to cause hepatic injury.[69]
3. Some anti-HCV-positive patients may have cleared the infection and anti-HCV may be the remnant of past infection.
4. Baseline ALT levels are depressed in patients on dialysis.[70] Interestingly, elevated ALT levels have also been observed in 4–23% of anti-HCV-negative dialysis patients.[58,63,64,71,72] These patients could be carriers of HCV infection in whom anti-HCV production is absent, or the liver disease might be due to a non-A, non-B virus other than HCV, or to non-viral causes.

Consequently, in patients with HCV infection, liver biopsy remains the only reliable method of confirming the presence of liver disease and assessing its severity. Indeed, liver histology at the time of initial presentation has been shown to be a good predictor of intermediate and long-term outcome in transplant recipients with liver disease.[73]

Immunity

The immune mechanisms triggered by HCV infection involve humoral and cellular responses targeted at multiple determinants of the viral genome. Yet in the majority of cases these responses are insufficient to provide protective immunity and fail to control the HCV infection, allowing the development of a chronic carrier state. A number of studies in humans and animals have documented the development of reinfection (new infection after the previous infection has cleared) with the same or a different HCV strain as well as superinfection (infection with a new HCV strain in the presence of current infection).[40,74,75] Indeed, Farci and colleagues confirmed the occurrence of reinfection in chimpanzees with convalescent HCV infection by demonstrating that rechallenge with the same or a different HCV genotype consistently resulted in the recurrence of viraemia and biochemical and histological evidence of hepatitis.[40] Superinfection has been also well documented, both in animals and in humans.[74-76]

The lack of protective immunity, although incompletely elucidated, can possibly be attributed to the following:

1. The majority of the anti-HCV antibodies are non-neutralizing and hence they do not provide immunity despite their presence. Even though neutralizing antibodies to the envelope regions of HCV have been recently identified, they seem to circulate at a titre which is too low to neutralize the infecting virus and therefore have no role in providing protective immunity.[77]
2. Compelling evidence is now available that the cellular responses of the host are inadequate and directly contribute to the pathogenicity associated with the viral infection.
3. The existence of extrahepatic replication sites, now generally accepted, is likely to promote the chronicity of the infection.
4. The emergence of mutant forms able to resist neutralization has been suggested by the existence of two groups of viral particles—low-density particles (1.08–1.11 g/ml), representing the intact virions and high-density particles (1.22–1.25 g/ml) corresponding to virions complexed with immunoglobulins. The presence of low-density particles (unbound forms) has been associated with a stronger infectious potency and the highest heterogenicity of the hypervariable region of the viral genome. While providing additional evidence for the existence of neutralizing antibodies capable of complexing with the virus, this observation suggests that mutations in the hypervariable region of the viral genome may be creating mutants capable of escaping effective neutralization.

HCV genotypes—epidemiology and clinical significance

The clinical significance of the genomic diversity of HCV has yet to be elucidated. The existing biological differences between viral genotypes may play an important role in the epidemiology and natural history of HCV infection. Indeed, HCV genotype-related differences in the severity of disease, clinical outcomes, and response to interferon therapy have been observed in patients with HCV infection.[78-81]

HCV genotypes have distinct geographical distribution.[2,17,79,81-86] HCV genotype 1a is the most common genotype in the United States and Western Europe.[2,79,81,86] For the most part, HCV genotype 1b shares the geographical distribution of 1a in the United States and Europe, but is also frequently seen in Japan. In fact, this is the predominant HCV genotype in Japan and the second most common genotype in the United

States.[79,81,82] The other HCV genotypes, less frequent in the United States, are typically found in certain parts of the world. In particular, HCV genotypes 2a and 2b are commonly seen in Western Europe, Japan, China, and Taiwan, 3a in Western Europe, Thailand, Singapore, India, and Bangladesh, 4a in the Middle East, Egypt, and Central Africa, 5a in South Africa, and 6a in Hong Kong.[2,17,79,81–85]

Some investigators have hypothesized that each HCV genotype has a preferential route of transmission and thus the mode of acquisition of HCV infection could predict the distribution of HCV genotype in high-risk populations. Indeed, a significant difference has been reported between intravenous drug abusers and patients who have acquired HCV by other means. In particular, among patients who were infected with HCV via blood transfusions, 1b is the predominant HCV genotype in contrast to intravenous drug abusers among whom coexistence of different HCV genotypes (1b, 2b, 3, and 4) can be frequently seen.[81,87–89]

Demographic differences between HCV genotypes have been noted in some but not all studies. Indeed, it has been reported that HCV genotype 1b is highly predominant in patients older than 40 years and in those with a long duration of HCV infection, while HCV genotype 3 is usually seen in younger patients, frequently with history of drug abuse.[88,90,91] A progressively decreasing relative prevalence of HCV genotype 1b has been observed in large reference centres in France and Italy.[88] In contrast, Mahaney and colleagues failed to detect any genotype-related differences in patients with HCV infection.[81] Also, Dusheiko *et al.* could not find any significant differences in age, serum albumin, and ALT levels in patients infected with different HCV genotypes.[85] Furthermore, no significant differences in the geographical distribution of HCV genotypes across the United States, and no substantial changes in the spectrum of the infecting HCV genotypes have been detected over a period of 2 to 20 years.[90] Genotype 1 has been consistently the most common HCV genotype in patients with chronic hepatitis C in the United States across different time periods.[81]

Several studies have attempted to correlate the severity of HCV disease to the genotype of the virus. HCV genotype 1b has been associated with a higher prevalence of severe liver disease (i.e. cirrhosis and hepatocellular carcinoma), a greater cytopathic effect in liver transplant recipients, and a lower rate of initial and long-term sustained response to interferon-α treatment, while patients infected with HCV genotypes other than 1 have shown approximately equal distribution of severe and mild liver disease. [78,80,81,85,88,92] In contrast, other investigators have reported that genotype 2 usually causes more serious liver disease (chronic active hepatitis or cirrhosis), despite significantly lower levels of circulating HCV RNA, and paradoxically better long-term response to treatment with interferon-α when compared with other genotypes. [81] In addition, ALT levels were found to be higher in asymptomatic Scottish blood donors infected with HCV genotype 3 than in those infected with HCV genotype 1.[79] Obviously, clinical evaluation of the virulence of HCV genotypes is difficult and complex, as it is conceivable that not the HCV genotype *per se*, but other confounding variables such as duration of infection, viral load, mode of acquisition, reinfections, host immunity, genetic factors, age, coexisting viral, bacterial, or parasitic infections, alcohol consumption, etc. may ultimately determine the outcomes of HCV infection.

As discussed earlier, HCV infection does not provide protective immunity and therefore both reinfection and superinfection can occur.[40,74,76] In fact, in thalassaemic children and haemophiliacs, reinfection and superinfection have been reported after multiple blood transfusions.[74] Yet detailed epidemiological analysis has demonstrated that the observed prevalence of mixed infections among HCV-infected individuals is lower than the estimated one, suggesting that some particular genotype(s) may suppress infection with other genotypes, a clinical phenomenon with conceivably significant therapeutic implications in the future.[93] Importantly, some investigators have suggested that the presence of multiple genotypes, rather than of a specific genotype, determines the outcomes of treatment.[94] However, in the absence of enough data at the present time, the clinical significance of mixed infections remains to be clarified.

Finally, the genetic variations of HCV have important implications for the development of vaccines. Due to the lack of cross-immunity between the different HCV genotypes, it is likely that a vaccine against one HCV genotype would not protect against infection with the others. Therefore, to provide effective protection against the full range of HCV genotypes, it might be necessary to develop multivalent vaccines.

HCV infection in dialysis

Prevalence in dialysis patients

It has been consistently found that the prevalence of anti-HCV in patients on dialysis is higher than that in the healthy population, thus suggesting that dialysis patients have an increased risk of acquiring HCV infection.[19] Using first-generation ELISA, the prevalence of anti-HCV in dialysis patients in North America was found to be 8–36%, in South America 39%, in Europe 1–54%, in Asia 17–51%, and in New Zealand/Australia 1.2–10%.[19] In most studies, the use of second-generation anti-HCV tests has detected even higher seroprevalence of HCV in patients on maintenance dialysis: 25–36 % in the United States, 2–63% in Europe, and 22–55.5% in Asia.[19,95–102] In a recent study from France using third-generation tests, a 42% prevalence of anti-HCV was reported.[48] Using third-generation ELISA, we have found a 19% prevalence of anti-HCV among dialysis patients in the northeastern region of the United States between 1986 and 1990.[103]

Remarkable geographical variations in the prevalence of HCV infection have been observed in the above-mentioned studies (Fig. 10.1).[104] The European Dialysis and Transplantation Association (EDTA) data have revealed that the prevalence of anti-HCV by second-generation anti-HCV tests varied widely in the different European and Mediterranean countries—between 2 and 63% in 1992, and between 2 and 44% in 1993.[102,105] Wide differences in the prevalence of HCV infection have been also observed between dialysis units within a single country. For example, the Centers for Disease Control and Prevention (CDC) reported that the prevalence of anti-HCV by ELISA2 in dialysis centres with 40 or more patients in the United States ranged from 0% to 64% (mean 10%) in 1995.[106] In Portugal, the prevalence of HCV infection in haemodialysis units ranged from 0 to 75.5%, being lowest in the northern regions of the country and particularly high in the southern and central regions.[107] Likewise, the prevalence of anti-HCV in haemodialysis units in Saudi Arabia ranged from 15.4–94.7%.[108]

The incidence and prevalence of HCV infection in patients on dialysis is steadily declining. Among member nations in the EDTA, the prevalence of anti-HCV in

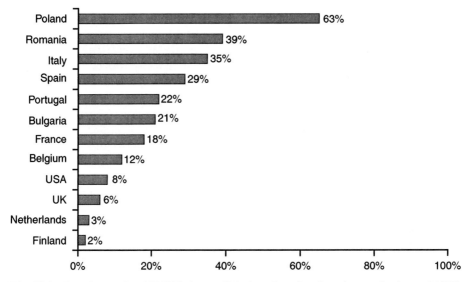

Fig. 10.1 Prevalence of anti-HCV in haemodialysis patients in selected countries (around 1992). (Reprinted from Pereira[104] with permission.)

haemodialysis patients declined from 21% in 1992 to 17.7% in 1993.[102,105] Similarly, in haemodialysis units in Portugal, the incidence of HCV infection decreased from 11.2% in 1991 to 7.2% in 1992 and 6.5% in 1993.[107] In haemodialysis patients in the United States, the incidence of NANBH, the major cause of which is HCV, declined from 1.7% in 1982 to 0.3% in 1995.[106] This decline in the incidence of HCV infection was initially due to the reduction in post-transfusion HCV infection; however, subsequently it reflected the implementation of infection control measures for the prevention of nosocomial transmission within dialysis units. Nonetheless, the 0.4–15% incidence of anti-HCV in some haemodialysis units continues to be a cause for concern.[109–116]

Prevalence in dialysis unit staff

The prevalence of anti-HCV in dialysis staff ranges from 0% to 4.1% and is comparable to that in blood donors.[19,117,118] According to the National Surveillance of Dialysis Associated Diseases conducted by the CDC, the incidence of NANBH in dialysis staff members has declined from 0.5% in 1983 to 0.05% in 1995, while the prevalence of anti-HCV has remained low and relatively stable: 1.6% with a range of 0 to 6% in centres with more than 20 staff members in 1992, and 2.0% in 1995.[106,119,120] The declining incidence and the low prevalence reflect the adequacy of general infection control strategies and precautions in preventing transmission of HCV infection from dialysis patients to staff members.

Accidental transmission of HCV infection from infected patients to healthcare workers by needlestick injuries has been reported and more recently confirmed with the help of genotypic analysis, which has shown that the acquired viral strain was identical to that in the index patient.[4,121,122] The risk of transmission of HCV by needlestick injuries appears to be between 2.7% and 10%, which is extremely low compared with a 67% risk in needlestick accidents involving HBe antigen-positive individuals.[122–124] The infective risk of 2.7% was computed based on first-generation anti-HCV testing over an observation period which might not have been long enough to detect all cases of seroconversion. Indeed, using both HCV core antibodies and HCV RNA as markers of HCV infection and a longer observation period, Mitsui and colleagues have reported a much higher risk (10%) of HCV transmission to medical staff after needlestick exposure.[123] In summary, although the risk of transmission of HCV by needlestick injury to medical staff is important, it is much lower than that for HBV. This is probably due to the low circulating titre of HCV in humans which reduces the likelihood of HCV transmission by accidental small-volume inoculation.[125] Chimpanzee transmission studies have shown that the viral titre of human non-A, non-B hepatitis sera is generally less than 10^2 chimpanzee-infective units compared with 10^8 chimpanzee-infective units for Hbe antigen-positive sera and 10^{11} chimpanzee-infective units for hepatitis D virus-infected sera.[126–128] Nonetheless, the need for strict adherence to the general infection control strategies and precautions in order to protect healthcare workers cannot be overemphasized (see Chapter 17).

HCV genotypes in ESRD patients—epidemiology and clinical significance

Although it is inaccurate to extrapolate the characteristics of HCV infection observed in non-renal patients to patients with renal failure, in whom the natural course of this infection is likely to be different, some common features related to the HCV genotype have been reported.[86,129] Typically, the geographical distribution of HCV genotypes in patients on renal replacement therapy closely follows that in non–dialysis patients.[129,130] Indeed, we have found that genotypes 1a and 1b were the two predominant genotypes in renal transplant candidates which corresponds to the distribution of HCV genotypes in the general population across the United States.[103] This observation probably reflects the fact that prior to implementation of screening of blood and blood products for anti-HCV, hepatitis C in dialysis patients was mainly a post-transfusion infection.[19] In contrast, the distribution of HCV genotypes in a group of haemodialysis patients from northern Italy was found to be markedly different from that in the background population with community-acquired HCV infection, which was attributed to possible transmission of rare genotypes by imported blood products or to migration of patients who had already acquired HCV infection.[131]

Demographic differences between HCV genotypes have been observed in ESRD patients. In haemodialysis patients in Morocco, HCV genotype 1b was most prevalent in older patients, whereas 2a/2c was mainly seen in the younger ones.[132] In accordance with this observation, a temporally related pattern of HCV genotype prevalence has been documented in haemodialysis patients and kidney transplant recipients in France. Genotype 1b, which initially accounted for more than two-thirds of HCV infection in patients who started dialysis prior to 1977, was found in less than one-third of those who began haemodialysis after 1985, whereas genotype 2a demonstrated increasing prevalence in this group. Furthermore, while genotype 1b persisted throughout the study period, genotypes 1a and 2a emerged in the 1970s and genotypes 3a, 4a, and 5a in the 1980s.[86]

The same phenomenon has been observed in haemodialysis patients in northern Italy: genotype 1b accounted for 75% of cases before 1985, yet there was an equal prevalence of genotype 1 and genotype 2 after 1985, and in Belgium, where genotype 4 has shown an increasing prevalence in more recent years.[129,133] However, the clinical significance of these findings is currently unclear. In contrast to these reports, a study of renal transplant candidates from the New England region of the United States found a relatively constant distribution of HCV genotypes over the years, with no temporal relationship to the year of initiation of renal replacement therapy.[103]

There are only limited data on the impact of HCV genotype on the clinical course and outcomes of HCV infection in dialysis patients and renal transplant recipients. HCV genotype-related differences in the severity of disease have been observed in some but not all studies. Colleoni and colleagues reported that HCV genotype 1 was associated with higher ALT levels both in the acute phase and after more than 10 years of HCV infection.[129] However, since liver histology was not available, no precise assessment of the severity of liver disease could be made. More recently, in renal transplant recipients with HCV infection, Rostaing and colleagues were unable to find any correlation between severity of liver disease and HCV genotype over a period of more than 10 years.[134] However, these studies were limited to liver disease and did not address survival. Although patient survival in anti-HCV-positive ESRD patients is subjected to a number of confounding variables, it is conceivable that HCV genotype-related differences in the severity of liver disease and in the response to therapy could ultimately influence the outcomes of HCV infection in this population. A study from the New England Organ Bank in the United States failed to detect any significant HCV genotype-related differences in the relative risk of death in renal transplant candidates.[135] Consequently, HCV genotyping of HCV RNA-positive dialysis patients does not appear to have any direct implication for the overall management of these patients, and might be unnecessary for practical purposes. As in patients without renal failure, because of the lack of protective immunity, reinfection and superinfection can occur in HCV-infected ESRD patients. Indeed, infection with two or three different HCV genotypes was present in 10% of HCV RNA-positive renal transplant candidates.[135] However, mixed infection was not associated with a significantly increased relative risk of death, but the small number of patients with mixed HCV infection, as well as the wide confidence intervals, preclude a definitive conclusion.[135] This observation may have important implications for the development of dialysis unit and transplant policies.

Risk factors

The high incidence and prevalence of anti-HCV in patients on dialysis can be attributed to several risk factors (Table 10.1) which are discussed below.

Number of blood transfusions

Numerous studies have shown that anti-HCV-positive haemodialysis patients have received significantly more units of blood products than anti-HCV-negative patients.[59,60,71,111,136–142] The advent of erythropoietin therapy and the implementation of screening of blood products for anti-HCV have resulted in a decline in the incidence of

Table 10.1   Risk factors for HCV infection in dialysis patients

---

Number of blood transfusions

Duration of hemodialysis

Mode of dialysis
  Haemodialysis versus peritoneal dialysis
  In-centre haemodialysis versus home haemodialysis

Prevalence of HCV infection in the dialysis unit

Previous organ transplantation

Intravenous drug abuse

Gender

---

post-transfusion hepatitis. Currently, the risk of acquiring post-transfusion hepatitis C infection is estimated at less than one per 3000 units of blood products transfused.[143]

Duration of haemodialysis

Anti-HCV-positive patients have spent a significantly longer time on dialysis than seronegative patients.[59,71,137–142,144–150] With an estimated risk of acquiring HCV infection of 10% per year, the likelihood of HCV seroconversion increases considerably after a decade of haemodialysis treatment.[151,152] Although a longer time on dialysis could potentially increase the risk of acquiring HCV infection due to a higher number of blood transfusions, stepwise regression analysis has shown that the prevalence of anti-HCV was independently associated with both factors, but had a stronger correlation with increasing years on haemodialysis than with the number of blood transfusions (Fig. 10.2).[57,137,153] Further, in patients without a history of blood transfusion, intravenous drug abuse, or any other obvious parenteral exposure to HCV infection, the interval since beginning dialysis correlated directly with the prevalence of HCV infection.[144,151,154] These data suggest that time on haemodialysis is an independent risk factor for acquiring HCV infection.

Mode of dialysis

Haemodialysis versus CAPD.   Data from centres that studied the prevalence of anti-HCV in both their haemodialysis and peritoneal dialysis patients revealed that peritoneal dialysis patients had consistently lower HCV seroprevalence than haemodialysis patients (Fig. 10.3).[111,114,149,150,153–162] Indeed, in a group of 129 anti-HCV-negative patients on chronic dialysis, the rate of seroconversion was 0.15 per patient year on haemodialysis compared with 0.03 per patient-year on CAPD and a hazard ratio for HCV infection of 5.7 in haemodialysis patients.[114] Some investigators have reported that the prevalence of anti-HCV in peritoneal dialysis patients drops further if patients with prior haemodialysis are excluded.[161] Further, in one study, none of the anti-HCV-positive peritoneal dialysis patients had received peritoneal dialysis as the sole form of replacement therapy, suggesting that the majority of anti-HCV-positive CAPD patients might have acquired HCV infection while on haemodialysis.[136] Further, the duration of dialysis does not

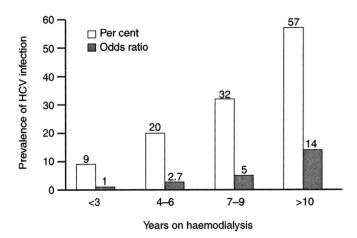

Fig. 10.2 Duration of haemodialysis as a risk factor for HCV infection. Based on data from Dussol *et al.*[153]

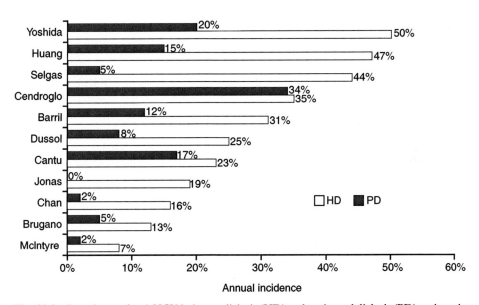

Fig. 10.3 Prevalence of anti-HCV in haemodialysis (HD) and peritoneal dialysis (PD) patients in the same dialysis programmes. Data from references 114, 149, 150, 153–156, 158, 160–162. (Reprinted from Pereira and Levey[249] with permission.)

appear to be a risk factor for acquiring HCV infection.[19,153,160] The lower risk for acquiring HCV infection in peritoneal dialysis patients can be explained by the following. First, peritoneal dialysis patients have a lower requirement for blood transfusion than haemodialysis patients do.[158] Second, the absence of an access site and extracorporeal blood circuit reduces the risk for parenteral exposure to the virus. Third, because CAPD is primarily a home procedure, it offers a more isolated environment.[19]

Home dialysis versus in-centre dialysis. The prevalence of anti-HCV in patients on home-haemodialysis is significantly lower than that in patients receiving in-centre haemodialysis. It appears that, similar to CAPD, home haemodialysis provides an isolated environment, and thus protects against patient-to-patient transmission of HCV infection.[19]

Prevalence of HCV infection in the dialysis unit

A recent survey by the Portuguese Society of Nephrology found that the incidence of HCV correlated directly with the prevalence of the infection in the haemodialysis unit.[163] These findings suggest that patients treated in haemodialysis units with a high prevalence of HCV infection appear to be at an increased risk of acquiring infection, and therefore favour the possibility of patient-to-patient transmission of HCV infection.[163] In contrast, in a multicentre study from Belgium, HCV seroconversion occurred in only three out of the 15 participating haemodialysis units, with no significant differences being present in the initial prevalence of anti-HCV by ELISA2 between haemodialysis units with and without seroconversions.[110]

Other factors

A history of previous organ transplantation is a risk factor for HCV infection in dialysis patients, possibly reflecting transmission of HCV with infected donor organs.[160,164] Intravenous drug abuse has been identified as an important risk factor for HCV infection in haemodialysis patients. A history of intravenous drug abuse was present in 30% of anti-HCV-positive patients receiving haemodialysis at the Northwest Kidney Center, Seattle, and 73% in two urban haemodialysis units in Miami.[60,69] Gender differences in HCV infection have been reported, with male haemodialysis patients being more frequently affected than females.[24,46] Further, male haemodialysis patients infected with HCV have a significantly higher concentration of serum HCV RNA than females.[69] However, there is currently no other data available regarding gender-related differences in the natural history of HCV.

Nosocomial transmission of HCV in haemodialysis units

The screening of blood and blood products for anti-HCV has significantly decreased the risk of post-transfusion HCV infection. Nonetheless, the prevalence of anti-HCV in dialysis patients in general, and particularly in those who have never been transfused, has remained considerably higher than in the general population.[19,72,137,149,152,159,165–167] In addition, the seroprevalence of HCV in the dialysis population varies widely between countries and even between dialysis units within the same country, and does not correlate with the prevalence of anti-HCV in the general population of the area. Therefore, these variations do not simply reflect differences in the thoroughness of screening blood products and transfusion practices across countries and dialysis units, but suggest that some aspects of the dialysis process are involved in the transmission of HCV infection. Proof of the nosocomial mode of transmission of HCV in dialysis units has been provided by numerous epidemiological and genetic studies and case observations in dialysis patients:

1. Some investigators have failed to show any correlation between anti-HCV and a history of previous blood transfusions.

2. Home dialysis and peritoneal dialysis, both limiting patient-to-patient contact by creating an isolated environment, have been associated with a lower prevalence of anti-HCV compared with in-centre haemodialysis.[72,112,114,153,154,158]

3. The incidence of HCV has been directly correlated with the prevalence of the infection in haemodialysis units.[107]

4. Outbreaks of HCV infection in haemodialysis units have occurred as a result of multiple breaks in infection control policies.[72,111,168]

5. The use of dedicated machines and isolated rooms has been associated with a lower incidence of anti-HCV.[169,170]

6. Studies using genotypic analysis of HCV strains have shown relative homogeneity of HCV variants in patients receiving treatment in the same haemodialysis unit.[171–173]

Although the exact vectors of nosocomial transmission in haemodialysis units have not yet been clarified, a variety of potential modes of transmission have been implicated (Table 10.2) which are discussed below.

Breakdown in standard infection control practices

Implementation of universal precautions has led to a decline in the incidence of NANBH in dialysis units, and therefore appears to play a crucial role in preventing transmission of HCV.[174] Indeed, breakdowns in standard infection control practices, such as sharing of a multidose heparin vial between patients with and without HCV infection and failure to change gloves between patients while performing haemodialysis treatments, have resulted in outbreaks of hepatitis C in haemodialysis units.[72,168] In each case, adherence to rigorous infection- control measures, cleaning and disinfection of all instruments and environmental surfaces that are routinely touched, and a ban on sharing of articles between patients decreased the incidence of HCV infection in dialysis units.[111,169] More recently, a multicentre prospective study from Belgium unequivocally demonstrated that enforcement of universal precautions alone could fully prevent transmission of HCV in haemodialysis units.[175]

Physical proximity to an infected patient

In a multicentre study in Belgium, HCV seroconversion in haemodialysis patients occurred only in dialysis units treating anti-HCV-positive patients. More importantly, 38% of the seroconverters had been never transfused and had no other apparent risk factor for HCV infection. Patients who had been dialysed at a station adjacent to that of an

Table 10.2 Risk factors for nosocomial transmission in haemodialysis units

---

Breakdown in standard infection control policies

Physical proximity to an infected patient

Dialysis machines and equipment

Dialyser membranes, haemodialysis ultrafiltrate, and peritoneal fluid

Reprocessing of dialysers

---

anti-HCV-positive patient had a higher incidence of seroconversion than the other patients in the unit.[110] Epidemiological studies have found that the lowest incidence of HCV infection occurred in haemodialysis units using isolated rooms to treat anti-HCV-positive patients.[163] These data demonstrate that the nosocomial transmission of HCV is possible, and that the close physical proximity, probably by allowing direct patient-to-patient contact, has facilitated nosocomial viral transmission through environmental contamination (blood spillage, etc.) and/or failure to comply strictly with universal precautions.

Dialysis machines and equipment

Sharing of dialysis machines and equipment appears to play a role in the transmission of HCV.[149,157,176] Haemodialysis units that routinely use dedicated machines for anti-HCV-positive patients have a significantly lower incidence of HCV infection than those that do not practice such a policy. Further, implementing the use of dedicated machines and isolated areas for anti-HCV-positive patients, along with strict enforcement of universal precautions, has led to a drop in the incidence of seroconversion from 20–25% to 0% at some centres.[169,170,177] However, the need for isolation has recently been challenged. In a multicentre study from Belgium, over the 54-month study period, none of the participating haemodialysis centres used dedicated machines for anti-HCV-positive patients, and over 70% of the patients were dialysed in units whose monitors were not disinfected after each session.[175] Despite this practice, no new cases of HCV transmission were observed. These data argue against any significant role of haemodialysis machines in the nosocomial transmission of HCV infection.

Dialyser membranes, haemodialysis ultrafiltrate, and peritoneal fluid

Theoretically, the passage of HCV through intact dialyser membranes seems improbable as the viral particles have an estimated size of 35 nm which is much higher than the pores of even the most porous dialysis membrane (polysulfone 3 nm, PAN 1.8–2.2 nm, AN69 2.9 nm, polyamide 3 nm, polymethyl methacrylate 1.7–7 nm).[178] However, any alteration in pore size or disruption of the integrity of the membrane associated with the process of filter assembly, the dialysis session itself, or with dialyser reuse, could presumably permit the passage of the virus into the dialysate compartment. Two recent studies have reported that neither low-flux (cellulose) nor high-flux (cellulose-diacetate, polysulfone, and polyacrilonitrile) dialysers permit contamination of the dialysis ultrafiltrate with HCV.[179,180] In contrast, others have detected HCV RNA by PCR in the dialysate of apparently intact polyacrilonitrile membranes, but not cellulose membranes.[181] It is important to emphasize that detection of HCV RNA in the dialysate by PCR may only imply the presence of fragments of viral RNA, and not necessarily the infective virus itself, a situation which is unlikely to result in transmission of the infection. On the other hand, a negative PCR test does not absolutely rule out the presence of viral RNA in the dialysis ultrafiltrate as minimal amounts of HCV RNA, below the detection threshold of the PCR assay, may have crossed through the dialysis membrane. However, such a low viral load in the dialysis ultrafiltrate may represent only a negligible risk of transmission of HCV infection. To date, there has been no association between any particular dialysis membrane and a higher prevalence of anti-HCV in haemodialysis patients.[59,72,107,110,113]

HCV has been found in several organic fluids, including ascites, and therefore, the peritoneal fluid of HCV-infected peritoneal dialysis patients could possibly represent a potential infectious risk in the dialysis environment.[182] Most studies suggest that HCV RNA is present in the CAPD effluent of some patients and hence the effluent should be considered as infectious material.[183]

Reprocessing of dialysers

In a multicentre prospective study from Belgium, dialyser reuse was not a risk factor for seroconversion.[110,175] Likewise, a survey by the Portuguese Society of Nephrology found that the incidence of HCV infection in patients in haemodialysis units which reprocessed dialysers was not significantly different from that in haemodialysis units which did not reprocess dialysers.[163] However, in units that did reprocess dialysers, the lowest incidence was observed in patients in units that used separate rooms to reprocess dialysers from anti-HCV-positive and anti-HCV-negative patients or had a ban on reprocessing dialysers from anti-HCV-positive patients. These data suggest that contamination in the reprocessing room may be a vector for the transmission of HCV in haemodialysis units.

Strategies to control the transmission of HCV infection in haemodialysis units

The shortcomings in our knowledge about the modes of transmission of HCV infection within dialysis units, and the limitations of the current tests for the timely identification of HCV-infected patients, have created significant difficulties in the formulation of policies for the prevention and control of HCV infection in haemodialysis units. The debate on the efficacy of patient isolation, use of dedicated machines, and ban on reuse of dialysers in controlling HCV infection in haemodialysis units has not been resolved. Arguments in favour of such measures are based on prior experience and excellent results achieved with the use of similar strategies in decreasing the incidence of HBV infection in haemodialysis units.[184] However, there are strong arguments against a policy of isolating anti-HCV-positive patients and use of dedicated machines for three major reasons:

1. HCV is not as infective as HBV, it circulates in low titres in infected serum, and is rapidly degraded at room temperature.[125,185]
2. Currently licensed anti-HCV tests detect only non-neutralizing antibodies, do not distinguish between current and past infection, and lack sufficient sensitivity to unequivocally exclude HCV infection. Consequently, isolation of anti-HCV-positive patients will not eliminate the risk of transmission. Although this problem could potentially be avoided by testing for HCV RNA by PCR, this test is not licensed for clinical use, is expensive, requires a specialized laboratory, and technical limitations can lead to false positive and false negative results.
3. Although isolation may protect uninfected patients, it might also increase the risk of superinfection in patients originally infected with a single strain.[40] Although, the clinical impact of such polygenotype infections are currently incompletely defined, we have recently shown that this may not be clinically important.

In view of the above debate, the CDC do not recommend dedicated machines, patient isolation, or a ban on dialyser reuse in haemodialysis patients with HCV infection.[174] Meanwhile, strict adherence to 'universal precautions', careful attention to hygiene, and strict sterilization of dialysis machines are mandatory.[58,72,110] Conventional cleansing and sterilization appear to be adequate to inactivate the virus.[72,110] However, eliminating the spread of HCV infection in haemodialysis units may ultimately require the development of treatments to eradicate the virus or vaccines to prevent infection.

HCV infection in kidney transplantation

Transmission of HCV infection by organ transplantation

Shortly after the introduction of the first-generation anti-HCV tests, the New England Organ Bank initiated studies to evaluate the risk of transmission of HCV infection by anti-HCV-positive cadaver organ donors. Stored sera from 716 consecutive cadaver organ donors between 1986 and 1990 (prior to the availability of anti-HCV tests) were screened for anti-HCV using ELISA1, and 13 (1.8%) anti-HCV-positive donors were identified.[66,186] Of the 29 recipients of organs from these anti-HCV-positive donors, 14 (48%) developed post-transplantation non-A, non-B hepatitis within a mean follow-up interval of 20 months, a prevalence that was seven- to eight-fold higher than that among recipients of untested donors in previous studies.[187,188] Further, of the 14 recipients who developed NANBH, two (14%) died from subfulminant liver failure and 12 (86%) developed chronic liver disease. Liver pathology was available in eight patients and revealed chronic active hepatitis in six patients and cirrhosis in two patients. Among the 24 recipients in whom post-transplantation sera were available, 16 (67%) tested positive for anti-HCV, and 23 (96%) tested positive for HCV RNA by PCR. All 13 HCV RNA-negative recipients of organs from HCV RNA-positive donors tested positive for HCV RNA after transplantation. These observations unequivocally demonstrated the transmission of HCV by organ transplantation. Similar studies have been undertaken by other organ procurement organizations and transplant centres. Overall, among recipients of organs from anti-HCV-positive donors, 35% (range 0–55%) developed post-transplant liver disease, 50% (range 14–100%) tested positive for anti-HCV after transplantation, and 74% (range 57–96%) tested positive for HCV RNA by PCR.[65,66,186,189–200]

The differences in the rate of transmission of HCV infection by anti-HCV-positive donors reported by different centres could be due to several factors. First, clinical or laboratory evidence of liver disease, and testing for anti-HCV in organ transplant recipients significantly underestimates the prevalence and transmission of HCV infection.[66] Hence, failure to test recipients for HCV RNA at some centres could erroneously suggest a low rate of transmission of HCV infection. Second, the risk of transmission of HCV infection by anti-HCV-positive cadaver organ donors could be related to the prevalence of HCV RNA in these donors.[201] A lower prevalence of HCV RNA in anti-HCV-positive cadaver organ donors at some centres could explain the lower rate of transmission of HCV by anti-HCV-positive donors reported by these centers.[190,202,203] Finally, some authors have suggested that reduction of the viral inoculum by pulsatile perfusion of the organs as opposed to cold storage could reduce the transmission of HCV by infected organs.[190] This possibility, however, remains to be proven.

Clinical impact of transmission of HCV infection

Long-term studies from the New England Organ Bank have compared post-transplantation clinical outcomes in the 29 recipients of organs from the 13 anti-HCV-positive cadaver organ donors with 74 recipients from 37 randomly selected anti-HCV-negative donors.[66,189] After a median follow-up of 42 and 49 months respectively, the relative risk of liver disease was increased four-fold in recipients from anti-HCV-positive donors and four (14%) of the 29 patients died due to or with liver failure. However, there was no increase in graft loss (relative risk 0.93, 95% confidence intervals of 0.51 to 1.70) or death (relative risk 0.89, 95% confidence intervals of 0.41 to 1.93) among recipients from anti-HCV-positive donors. Mendez and colleagues prospectively studied 42 anti-HCV-negative recipients of kidneys from anti-HCV-positive donors.[204] After 4 years of follow-up, the prevalence of liver disease was higher than in controls, but patient survival was not significantly different. Pirsch and colleagues prospectively transplanted 69 kidneys from anti-HCV-positive donors into anti-HCV-negative recipients who were considered to have a limited life expectancy.[199] After a short follow-up, one patient died of fulminant hepatitis and two patients developed cirrhosis.[199] Survival in recipients from anti-HCV-positive donors was significantly lower than in recipients from anti-HCV-negative donors.[199] Overall, these data indicate a higher risk of liver disease, but no significant adverse effect on patient or graft survival. However, it is noteworthy that subfulminant hepatitis was reported only in patients who received organs from anti-HCV-positive donors.

Transplantation of kidneys from anti-HCV-positive donors into recipients with pretransplantation HCV infection

In chimpanzees, previous infection with HCV does not protect from reinfection with a different strain or even the same strain of the virus.[40] Likewise, dialysis and transplant patients with pre-existing HCV infection are not protected from superinfection with a new HCV genotype.[205,206] Indeed, two recent reports have demonstrated that among HCV RNA-positive recipients of kidneys from HCV RNA-positive donors, the viral genotype present post-transplantation was either the same genotype present pretransplantation, the genotype from the donor, or both.[205,206] The clinical implications of superinfection in transplant recipients are not well defined. In a prospective study from Spain, there were no differences in the post-transplantation prevalence of liver disease, graft, or patient survival between 24 anti-HCV-positive recipients who received kidneys from anti-HCV-positive donors and 40 anti-HCV-positive recipients of kidneys from anti-HCV-negative donors.[207] However, four (80%) of five anti-HCV-positive but PCR-negative recipients from PCR-positive donors acquired HCV RNA.[207] These data suggest that superinfections do occur, but they may not have any serious clinical consequences, at least in the short-term.

HCV infection in renal transplant recipients

Effect of pretransplantation anti-HCV status on post-transplantation clinical outcomes

In renal transplant recipients, the prevalence of pretransplantation anti-HCV is 11–49%.[147,208–214] Pretransplantation anti-HCV is associated with an increased risk of post-transplant liver disease and is reported in 19–64% of recipients compared with 2–19% of recipients without anti-HCV.[208,209,211,213,214] Indeed, studies from the New England Organ Bank have shown that for recipients with anti-HCV prior to transplantation, the relative risk of post-transplantation liver disease was 5.0 (95% confidence intervals of 2.4–10.5).[208] In patients with pretransplantation HCV RNA in the serum, kidney transplantation was associated with a 1.8- to 30.3-fold increase in viral titre, suggesting that kidney transplantation is associated with proliferation of the hepatitis C virus. However, among patients with HCV RNA detected in the serum, the titre of HCV RNA did not differ between patients with and without post-transplantation liver disease. These data suggest that factors other than the viral load determine the risk of liver disease in transplant recipients with HCV infection.

Although pretransplantation anti-HCV is consistently associated with an increased risk of post-transplantation liver disease, post-transplantation patient survival was adversely affected in only some studies. Studies from Roth and colleagues at the University of Miami, Ynares and colleagues at Vanderbilt University, and Stempel and colleagues at the University of California, San Francisco, failed to detect significant differences in patient survival between recipients with and without anti-HCV prior to renal transplantation.[209,211,213] In contrast, studies from Fritsche and colleagues at the Medical College of Wisconsin reported a lower 8-year patient survival for the anti-HCV-positive recipients compared with anti-HCV-negative controls.[214] Likewise, our results from the New England Organ Bank study revealed that recipients with pretransplantation anti-HCV had a 3.3-fold higher risk of death (95% confidence intervals of 1.4 to 7.9) and a 9.9-fold higher risk of death due to sepsis (95% confidence intervals of 2.6 to 38.3).[208] Interestingly, infection rather than liver failure was the leading cause of death in anti-HCV-positive recipients. The differences between studies in patient survival could be due to several factors: differences in study design such as selection of patients, and length and completeness of follow-up; virus and test factors such as sensitivity and specificity of the anti-HCV test, prevalence of serum HCV RNA, genotype of the infecting virus, and single or mixed infection; and the presence and severity of pretransplant liver disease, HLA matching, and immunosuppression protocols. Indeed, the severity of pretransplant liver disease has been shown to be an important predictor of adverse post-transplant outcomes.[73]

Effect of renal transplantation on the course of HCV infection in dialysis patients

Port and colleagues have observed that in the general ESRD population, compared with patients on the waiting list for dialysis, those who underwent renal transplantation had a higher relative risk of death in the first month post-transplantation (relative risk of 2.43), but a lower relative risk thereafter (relative risk 0.96 between 1 to 12 months and 0.36 after 12 months). These results clearly demonstrated the long-term benefit of kidney transplantation on patient survival.[215] On the other hand, there exists evidence that transplantation, by virtue of the necessity for continuous immunosuppressive therapy, can worsen the course of some viral infections, including infection with HCV. Indeed, as discussed earlier, in some studies HCV infection at the time of renal transplantation has been associated with an increased risk of liver disease and death in the post-transplantation period. However, a number of studies have found that the prevalence of liver disease in anti-HCV-positive transplant recipients (19–66%) does not exceed the prevalence in anti-HCV-positive dialysis patients (18–80%).[60,145,147,156,216–223] Consequently, transplant physicians are faced with the dilemma of whether or not to offer renal transplantation to anti-HCV-positive ESRD patients. With 34766 patients on the waiting list for renal transplant in the United States alone, it is important to clarify the merits of allocation kidneys to anti-HCV-positive patients.[224] To evaluate the relative effect of dialysis versus transplantation on patient survival, we studied a cohort of 496 ESRD patients referred for renal transplantation between 1986 and 1990 to the transplant centres served by the New England Organ Bank. We found that the presence of anti-HCV was associated with a 1.41-fold (1.01- to 1.97-fold) increased risk of death, irrespective of whether the patients remained on dialysis or underwent renal transplantation (Fig. 10.4).[225] The HCV genotype and the type of HCV infection had no significant impact on patient survival.[135] Further, the analysis of the effect of treatment modality (dialysis versus transplantation) on patient survival revealed that, in the anti-HCV-positive renal transplant candidates, those who received a transplant had an initially higher risk of death (4.75 between 0 to 3 months and 1.76 between 4 to 6 months), but a lower risk thereafter (0.31 between 7 months and 4 years, and 0.84 after

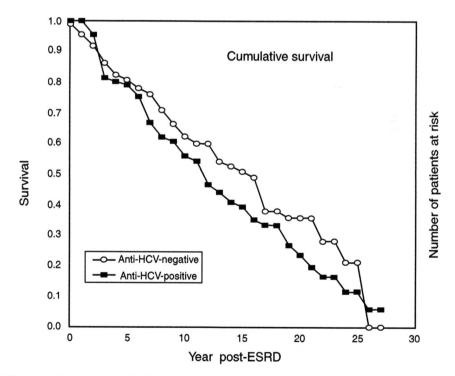

Fig. 10.4 Survival in anti-HCV-negative and -positive patients referred for renal transplantation (ESRD = end-stage renal disease). The unadjusted actuarial survival from the time of first initiation of renal replacement therapy (dialysis or transplantation) until death, loss to follow-up, or 31 December 1995, whichever occurred earlier. (Reprinted from Pereira *et al.*[225] with permission.)

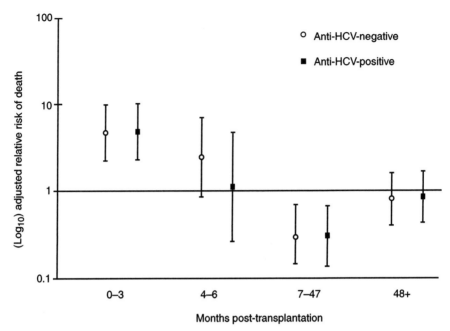

Fig. 10.5 Relative risk of death for transplantation versus dialysis in anti–HCV-negative and-positive patients referred for renal transplantation. The relative risk of death (and 95% confidence intervals) for different time intervals after transplantation are adjusted for age and the presence of diabetes. The relative risk of death for transplantation versus dialysis was similar for anti-HCV-positive and -negative patients at all intervals after transplantation. (Reprinted from Pereira *et al.*[225] with permission.)

4 years).[225] This pattern was not affected by the HCV genotype or type of HCV infection (mixed versus single).[135] Our results demonstrate that the association between transplantation and survival was no different between anti-HCV-positive and anti-HCV-negative patients and was not influenced by the genotype or the number of infecting HCV strains (Fig. 10.5). These findings suggest that the possible detrimental effect of transplantation on the course of HCV infection does not appear to outweigh its long-term beneficial effect on survival in ESRD. Hence, in the absence of definite studies demonstrating worse outcomes after renal transplantation, anti-HCV-positive status alone should not be considered a contraindication for renal transplantation, and anti-HCV-positive ESRD patients should be allowed to make an informed choice between dialysis or transplantation. However, because the histological severity of liver damage is a strong predictor of liver failure and death after transplantation and dialysis patients and transplant recipients can have histological evidence of liver disease in the absence of increased ALT levels, there may be merit in a policy of performing liver biopsies on anti-HCV-positive patients awaiting renal transplantation. In patients with histological evidence of liver disease, the decision to proceed with renal transplantation should be made cautiously, after taking into consideration the influence of immunosuppression on viral replication and consequent exacerbation of liver disease.

Role of interferon-α in the treatment of chronic hepatitis C infection in patients with ESRD

The efficacy of interferon-α (IFN-α) therapy in chronic hepatitis C has been demonstrated in a number of randomized controlled trials, and its use is currently recommended in anti-HCV-positive patients with abnormal serum aminotransferase and well-compensated chronic hepatitis on biopsy.[226,227] Four forms of IFN-α have been evaluated for clinical use in large trials: α-2b (most commonly used), α-2a, α-nl, and consensus interferon (CIFN).[226] They appear to be similarly effective. A number of other α and β interferons are under evaluation. [226]

Response to treatment is defined on the basis of ALT and HCV RNA testing as biochemical (normalization of serum ALT) and virological (lack of detectable serum HCV RNA by PCR) and on the basis of the timing of testing in relation to the treatment course as end-of-treatment response (ETR) (at the end of the treatment) and sustained response (SR) (6 or 12 months after stopping therapy).[227] Two therapeutic regimens using identical dosing (3 MU of IFN- α administered subcutaneously three times weekly) but a different duration of treatment (either 6 or 12 months) have been studied. [226,227] Six-month treatment courses have resulted in biochemical and virological ETR rates of 40–50% and 30–40% respectively, and biochemical and virological SR of 15–20% and 10–20% respectively.[227] The biochemical and virological responses have been accompanied by histological improvement. The 12-month treatment regimen has not produced higher biochemical or virological ETR, but has increased SR rates to 20–30%.[227] The benefit of treatments of longer duration and with higher doses are currently being evaluated.[228] Although IFN-α treatment has demonstrated favourable biochemical and virological results, its effects on paramount clinical outcomes such as quality of life and disease progression have not been ascertained. [227]

In patients with chronic hepatitis C, the pretreatment clinical, biochemical, histological, and viral characteristics that predict the success of interferon treatment have been the subject of intense investigation. Patients with lower levels of viral RNA in the serum and a lower concentration of HCV antigens in the liver are more likely to respond to interferon treatment.[229] Preliminary results of a large European multicentre study suggest that age under 40 years, absence of cirrhosis, pretreatment ALT levels less than three times the upper limit of normal, post-transfusion rather than sporadic infection, and infection with the genotypes 1, 5, and 6, are predictors of response to interferon treatment.[92] However, others have shown that patients infected with genotypes 2 and 3 have a better response to interferon than those infected with genotype 1.[230] Some of the differences in the relationship between HCV subtypes and response to interferon treatment could be related to the lack of uniformity in the viral nomenclature followed by different groups, and the different types of interferon used. Nevertheless, tailoring interferon treatment based on viral type promises to be an exciting possibility.

IFN-α has pleiotropic effects including antiproliferative and immunomodulatory properties as well as antiviral activity. [231] Indeed, IFN-α induces cytokine gene expression, increases cell surface expression of HLA antigens, and enhances the functions of natural killer cells, cytotoxic T cells, and monocytes. Further, the use of IFN-α as prophylaxis against cytomegaloviral disease in renal transplant recipients has been associated with a high incidence of steroid-resistant allograft rejection resulting in graft loss.[232,233] Since IFN-α treatment carries a risk of inducing or facilitating rejection in allograft recipients, questions have been raised regarding the efficacy, tolerance, safety, and timing of IFN-α therapy in dialysis and transplant patients.

As shown in Table 10.3, the initial response of dialysis and transplant patients to IFN-α treatment has been encouraging, with a majority of patients demonstrating a decrease in serum ALT levels and an improvement in liver histology.[234-245] However, as in the case with non-renal patients, relapses are common after stopping treatment and long-term outcomes are not yet adequately defined.[235,236,243] Further, although disappearance of HCV RNA from the serum is common, recurrence of viraemia from extravascular sites remains a distinct possibility.[236,246]

A major stumbling block to IFN-α treatment in transplant recipients has been the occurrence of acute rejection. A majority of studies have observed an increased risk of acute rejection (40% to 100%) in transplant recipients treated with IFN-α for chronic liver disease due to hepatitis C.[236,240,242,247] In contrast, Rao and colleagues did not encounter allograft rejection in six renal transplant recipients treated with IFN-α 2 to 15 years after transplantation.[234] The absence of rejection in the study by Rao and colleagues could be attributed to the fact that the patients had stable renal function for several years prior to the start of IFN-α therapy and were hence at low risk of rejection. However, others have demonstrated irreversible rejection and return to dialysis in patients

Table 10.3   Initial response to interferon-α treatment in dialysis and transplant patients with chronic hepatitis C

Study	Study population	N	Decrease in serum ALT*	Improvement in liver histology*	Clearing of serum HCV RNA*
Rao and Anderson[234]	HD + Tx	10	100%	80%	NA
Pol et al.[235]	HD	19	85%	NA	53%
Rostaing et al.[236]	Tx	16	100%	NA	0%
Casanovas et al.[237]	HD	10	90%	NA	10%
Koenig et al.[238]	HD	37	71%	NA	65%
Duarte et al.[239]	HD	5	100%	NA	NA
Harihara et al.[240]	Tx	3	67%	NA	NA
Raptopoulou-Gigi et al.[241]	HD	19	100%	NA	77%
Ozgur et al.[242]	Tx	5	100%	100%	NA
Umlauft et al.[243]	HD	33	NA	NA	73%
Rostaing et al.[244]	HD	10	NA	NA	90%
Hanafusa et al.[245]	Tx	10	80%	NA	20%

*Among patients who had an abnormal test prior to treatment and who completed the course of treatment.
Abbreviations: HD, haemodialysis patients; Tx, transplant recipients; ALT, alanine aminotransferase; NA, not applicable.

treated with IFN-α as late as 8 years after transplantation.[240,242] Similarly, patients treated with IFN-α to prevent post-transplantation infection with cytomegalovirus or Epstein–Barr virus also experienced an increased incidence of acute rejection.

Treatment with IFN-α is also associated with a 'flu-like' syndrome with aesthenia, myalgia, headache, neutropenia, thrombocytopenia, and depression, and is partly related to the dose administered.[248] Despite these side-effects, the dropout rate among non-renal patients treated with IFN-α has been surprisingly low.[248] In contrast, treatment was stopped for reasons other than transplant rejection in 0–54% of dialysis and transplant recipients treated with IFN-α.[234–238] The reasons for this difference between non-renal and renal patients are currently unclear.

Overall, the limited efficacy of IFN-α, together with its high cost, risk of acute rejection, and side-effects have diminished enthusiasm for its use in transplant recipients with chronic HCV infection. In fact, the NIH Consensus Statement on management of hepatitis C currently lists renal transplant as a contraindication to treatment with interferon.[227] A safer, but probably less cost-effective strategy, might be to treat dialysis patients with chronic hepatitis C prior to transplantation. Indeed, two recent studies in patients with chronic hepatitis C who were treated with IFN- α while on dialysis did not observe recurrence of liver disease or an increased risk of rejection after subsequent transplantation.[237,239] Controlled studies will be required to evaluate the long-term effects of this strategy on the course of liver disease, rates of transplantation, and graft and patient survival.

Other treatment approaches to chronic hepatitis C including steroids, ursodiol, thymosin, iron reduction therapy, and the new oral antiviral drug ribavirin alone have led to either disappointing or inconclusive results.[227] However, recent studies using ribavirin as an adjunctive drug to IFN- α have reported promising preliminary data showing that the combination of IFN-α and ribavirin leads to virological SR rates of 40–50% which are higher than those observed with 6-month treatment courses with IFN-α alone. Large-scale trials of this combination in hepatitis C are now under way.

References

1. Houghton M, Weiner A, Han J, Kuo G, Choo QL. Molecular biology of the hepatitis C viruses: implications for diagnosis, development and control of viral disease. *Hepatology* 1991; 14:381–388.
2. Choo Q, Kuo G, Weiner AJ, Overby LR, Bradley DW, Houghton M. Isolation of a cDNA clone derived from a blood-borne non-A, non-B viral hepatitis genome. *Science* 1989; 244:358–362.
3. Okamoto H, Okada S, Sugiyama Y, *et al.* Nucleotide sequence of the genomic RNA of hepatitis C virus isolated from a human carrier: comparison with reported isolates for conserved and divergent regions. *J Gen Virol* 1991; 72:2697–2704.
4. Okamoto H, Sugiyama Y, Okada S, *et al.* Typing hepatitis C virus by polymerase chain reaction with type-specific primers: application to clinical surveys and tracing infectious sources. *J Gen Virol* 1992; 73:673–679.
5. Simmonds P, Holmes EC, Cha TA, *et al.* Classification of hepatitis C virus into six major region genotypes and a series of subtypes by phylogenetic analysis of the NS5 region. *J Gen Virol* 1993; 74:2391–2399.

6. Okamoto H, Okada S, Sugiyama Y, *et al.* The 5'-terminal sequence of the hepatitis C virus genome. *Japan J Exp Med* 1990; **60**:167–177.

7. Cha TA, Kolberg J, Irvine B, *et al.* Use of a signature nucleotide sequence of hepatitis C virus for detection of viral RNA in human serum and plasma. *J Clin Microbiol* 1991; **29**:2528–2534.

8. Han JH, Shyamala V, Richman KH, *et al.* Characterization of the terminal regions of hepatitis C viral RNA: identification of conserved sequences in the 5' untranslated region and poly(A) tails at the 3' end. *Proc Natl Acad Sci USA* 1991; **88**:1711–1715.

9. Bukh J, Purcell RH, Miller RH. Importance of a primer selection for the detection of hepatitis C virus RNA with the polymerase chain reaction assay. *Proc Natl Acad Sci USA* 1992; **89**:187–191.

10. Hijikata M, Kato N, Ootsuyama Y, *et al.* Hypervariable regions in the putative glycoprotein of hepatitis C virus. *Biochem Biophys Res Commun* 1991; **175**:220–228.

11. Weiner AJ, Brauer MJ, Rosenblatt J, *et al.* Variable and hypervariable domains are found in the regions of HCV corresponding to the flavivirus envelope and NS1 proteins and the pestivirus envelope glycoproteins. *Virology* 1991; **180**:842–848.

12. Nagayama R, Tsuda F, Okamoto H, *et al.* Genotype dependence of hepatitis C virus antibodies detectable by the first generation enzyme-linked immunosorbent assay with C100–3 protein. *J Clin Invest* 1993; **92**:1529–1533.

13. Simmonds P, Rose KA, Graham S, *et al.* Mapping of serotype-specific, immunodominant epitopes in the NS-4 region of hepatitis C virus (HCV)—use of type-specific peptides to serologically differentiate infections with HCV type 1, type 2, and type 3. *J Clin Microbiol* 1993; **31**:1493–1503.

14. Simmonds P, Alberti A, Alter HJ, *et al.* A proposed system for the nomenclature of hepatitis C virus genotypes. *Hepatology* 1994; **19**:1321–1324.

15. Chan SW, McOmish F, Holmes EC, *et al.* Analysis of a new hepatitis C virus type and its phylogenetic relationship to existing variants. *J Gen Virol* 1992; **73**:1131–1141.

16. Mori A, Yamada K, Kimura J, *et al.* Enzymatic characterization of purified NS3 serine proteinase of hepatitis C virus expressed in *Escherichia coli. FEBS Letters* 1996; **378**:37–42.

17. Enomoto N, Takada A, Nakao T. There are two major types of hepatitis C virus in Japan. *Biochem Biophy Res Commun* 1990; **170**:1021–1025.

18. Kohara KT, Kohara M, Yamaguchi K, *et al.* A second group of hepatitis C viruses. *Virus Genes* 1991; **5**:243–254.

19. Natov SN, Pereira BJG. Hepatitis C infection in patients on dialysis. *Semin Dial* 1994; **7**:360–368.

20. Farci P, Alter HJ, Wong D, *et al.* A long-term study of hepatitis C virus replication in non-A, non-B hepatitis. *New Engl J Med* 1991; **325**:98–104.

21. Aach RD, Stevens CE, Hollinger FB, *et al.* Hepatitis C virus infection in post-transfusion hepatitis. *New Engl J Med* 1991; **325**:1325–1329.

22. Esteban JI, Gonzales A, Hernandez JM, *et al.* Evaluation of antibodies to hepatitis C virus in a study of transfusion-associated hepatitis. *New Engl J Med* 1990; **323**:1107–12.

23. Nasoff MS, Zebedee SL, Inchauspé G, *et al.* Identification of an immunodominant epitope within the capsid protein of hepatitis C virus. *Proc Natl Acad Sci USA* 1991; **88**:5462–5466.

24. Alter MJ, Margolis HS, Krawczynski K, *et al.* The natural history of community-acquired hepatitis C in the United States. The Sentinel Countries Chronic non-A, non-B Hepatitis Study Team. *New Engl J Med* 1992; **327**:1899–1905.

25. Oliva JA, Ercilla G, Mallafre JM, Bruguera M, Carrió J, Pereirs BJG. Markers of hepatitis C infection among hemodialysis patients with acute and chronic infection: Implications for infection control strategies in hemodialysis units. *Int J Artif Org* 1995; **18**:73–77.

26. Ward KN, Dhaliwal W, Ashworth KL, *et al.* Measurment of antibody avidity for hepatitis C virus distinguishes primary antibody responses from passively acquired antibody. *J Med Virol* 1994; 43:367–72.

27. Weiner AJ, Kuo G, Bradley DW, *et al.* Detection of hepatitis C viral sequences in non-A, non-B hepatitis. *Lancet* 1990; 335:1–3.

28. Simmonds P, Zhang LQ, Watson HG, *et al.* Hepatitis C quantification and sequencing in blood products, hemophiliacs, and drug users. *Lancet* 1990; 336:1469–1471.

29. Ulrich PP, Romeo JM, Lane PK, Kelly I, Danial LJ, Vyas GN. Detection, semiquantitation, and genetic variation in hepatitis C virus sequences amplified from the plasma of blood donors with elevated alanine aminotransferase. *J Clin Invest* 1990; 86:1609–1614.

30. Lau JYN, Davis GL, Orito E, Qian KP, Mizokami M. Significance of antibody to the host cellular gene derived epitope GOR in chronic hepatitis C virus infection. *J Hepatol* 1993; 17:253–257.

31. Kwok S, Higuchi R. Avoiding false positives with PCR. *Nature* 1989; 339:237–238.

32. Busch MP, Wilber JC, Johnson PJ, Tobler L, Evans CS. Impact of specimen handling and storage on detection of hepatitis C virus RNA. *Transfusion* 1992; 32:420–425.

33. Wright TL. Hepatitis C virus infection and organ transplantation. *Prog Liver Dis* 1993; 11:215–230.

34. Urdea MS, Horn T, Fultz TJ, *et al.* Branched DNA amplication multimers for the sensitive, direct detection of human hepatitis viruses. *Nucleic Acids Research Symposium Series* 1991; 24:197–200.

35. Lau JYN, Davis GL, Kniffen J, *et al.* Significance of serum hepatitis C virus RNA levels in chronic hepatitis C. *Lancet* 1993; 341:1501–1504.

36. Feray C, Samuel D, Thiers V, *et al.* Reinfection of liver graft by hepatitis C virus after liver transplantation. *J Clin Invest* 1992; 89:1361–1365.

37. Inoue Y, Miyamura T, Unayama T, Takahashi K. Maternal transmission of HCV. *Nature* 1991; 353:609.

38. Widell A, Shev S, Mansson S, *et al.* Genotyping of hepatitis C virus isolates by a modified polymerase chain reaction assay using type specific primers: epidemiological applications. *J Med Virol* 1994; 44:272–279.

39. Weiner AJ, Geysen HM, Christopherson C, *et al.* Evidence for immune selection of hepatitis C virus (HCV) putative envelope glycoprotein variants: Potential role in chronic HCV infections. *Proc Natl Acad Sci USA* 1992; 89:3468–3472.

40. Farci P, Alter HJ, Govindarajan S, *et al.* Lack of protective immunity against reinfection with hepatitis C virus. *Science* 1992; 258:135–140.

41. Kurosaki M, Enomoto N, Marumo F, Sato C. Rapid sequence variation of the hypervariable region of hepatitis C virus during the course of chronic infection. *Hepatology* 1993; 18:1293–1299.

42. Nakao T, Enomoto N, Takada N, *et al.* Typing of hepatitis C virus genomes by restriction fragment length polymorphism. *J Gen Virol* 1991; 72:2105–2112.

43. Stuyver L, Rossau R, Wyseur A, *et al.* Typing of hepatitis C virus isolates and characterization of new. *J Gen Virol* 1993; 74:1093–1102.

44. Salleras L, Bruguera M, Vidal J, *et al.* [Seroepidemilogy of hepatitis C infection in pregnant women in Catalonia]. *Medicina Clinica* 1994; 103:721–724. (In Spanish.)

45. Uyttendaele S, Claeys H, Mertens W, *et al.* Evaluation of third-generation screening and confirmatory assays for HCV antibodies. *Vox Sang* 1994; 66:122–129.

46. Alter M, Hadler SC, Judson FN, *et al.* Risk factors for acute non-A, non-B hepatitis in the United States and association with hepatitis C virus infection. *J Am Med Assoc* 1990; 264:2231–2235.

47. Yoshimura E, Hayashi J, Ueno K, *et al.* No significant changes in levels of hepatitis C virus (HCV) RNA by competitive polymerase chain reaction in blood samples from patients with chronic HCV infection. *Digest Dis Sci* 1997; **42**:772–7.

48. Courouce A-M, Bouchardeau F, Chauveau P, *et al.* Hepatitis C (HCV) infection in haemodialysed patients: HCV-RNA and anti-HCV antibodies (third-generation assays). *Nephrol Dial Transplant* 1995; **10**:234–239.

49. Courouce AM, Barin F, Botte C, *et al.* A comparative evaluation of the sensitivity of seven anti-hepatitis C virus screening tests. *Vox Sang* 1995; **69**:213–6.

50. Carrera F, Silva JG, Oliveira C, Frazao JM, Pires C. Persistence of antibodies to hepatitis C virus in a chronic hemodialysis population. *Nephron* 1994; **68**:38–40.

51. Simon N, Couroucé AM, Lemarrec N, *et al.* A twelve year natural history of hepatitis C virus infection in hemodialyzed patients. *Kidney Int* 1994; **46**:504–511.

52. Alter HJ. Chronic consequences of non-A, non-B hepatitis. In: LB S, JH L (eds) *Current perspectives in hepatology*, 1989:83–97. Plenum Medical Books, New York.

53. Kiyosawa K, Sodeyama T, Tanaka E, *et al.* Interrelationship of blood transfusion, non-A, non-B hepatitis and hepatocellular carcinoma: analysis by detection of antibody to hepatitis C virus. *Hepatology* 1990; **12**:671–675.

54. Tong MJ, el-Farra NS, Reikes AR, Co RL. Clinical outcomes after transfusion-associated hepatitis C. *New Engl J Med* 1995; **332**:1463–6.

55. Seeff LB, Buskell-Bales Z, Wright EC, *et al.* Long-term mortality after transfusion-associated non-A, non-B hepatitis. *New Engl J Med* 1992; **327**:1906–1911.

56. van der Poel CL, Reesink HW, Schaasberg W, *et al.* Infectivity of blood seropositive for hepatitis C virus antibodies. *Lancet* 1990; **335**:558–560.

57. Alter MJ, Favero MS, Maynard JE. Impact of infection control strategies on the incidence of dialysis-associated hepatitis in the United States. *J Infect Dis* 1986; **153**:1149–1151.

58. Pol S, Romeo R, Zins B, *et al.* Hepatitis C virus RNA in anti-HCV positive hemodialyzed patients: Significance and therapeutic implications. *Kidney Int* 1993; **44**:1097–1100.

59. Muller GY, Zabaleta ME, Arminio A, *et al.* Risk factors for dialysis-associated hepatitis C in Venezuela. *Kidney Int* 1992; **41**:1055–1058.

60. Jeffers LJ, Perez GO, de Medina MD, *et al.* Hepatitis C infection in two urban hemo-dialysis units. *Kidney Int* 1990; **38**:320–322.

61. Ayoola EA, Huraib S, Arif M, *et al.* Prevalence and significance of antibodies to hepatitis C virus among Saudi haemodialysis patients. *J Med Virol* 1991; **35**:155–159.

62. Roger SD, Cunningham A, Crewe E, Harris DC. Hepatitis C virus infection in haemo-dialysis patients. *Aust NZ J Med* 1991; **21**:22–24.

63. Vasile A, Allegra V, Canciani D, Forchi G, Mengozzi G. Prospective and retrospective assessment of clinical and laboratory parameters in maintenance hemodialysis patients with and without HCV antibodies. *Nephron* 1992; **61**:318–319.

64. Colombo P, Filiberti O, Porcu M, *et al.* Prevalence of hepatitis C infection in a hemo-dialysis unit. *Nephron* 1992; **61**:326–327.

65. Aeder MI, Shield CF, Tegtmeier GE, *et al.* The incidence and clinical impact of hepatitis C virus (HCV) positive donors in cadaveric transplantation. *Transplant Proc* 1993; **25**:1469–1471.

66. Pereira BJG, Milford EL, Kirkman RL, *et al.* Prevalence of HCV RNA in hepatitis C antibody positive cadaver organ donors and their recipients. *New Eng J Med* 1992; **327**:910–915.

67. Fabrizi F, Lunghi G, Andrulli S, *et al.* Influence of hepatitis C virus (HCV) viraemia upon serum aminotransferase activity in chronic dialysis patients. *Nephrol Dial Transplant* 1997; **12**:1394–1398.

68. Alberti A, Morsica G, Chemello L, *et al.* Hepatitis C viraemia and liver disease in symptom-free individuals with anti-HCV. *Lancet* 1992; **340**:697–698.

69. DuBois DB, Gretch D, dela Rosa C, *et al.* Quantitation of hepatitis C viral RNA in sera of hemodialysis patients: gender-related differences in viral load. *Am J Kidney Dis* 1994; **24**:795–801.

70. Wolf PL, William D, Coplon N, *et al.* Low aspartate transaminase activity in serum of patients undergoing chronic hemodialysis. *Clin Chem* 1972; **18**:567–573.

71. Mondelli MU, Smedile V, Piazza V, *et al.* Abnormal alanine aminotransferase activity reflects exposure to hepatitis C virus in haemodialysis patients. *Nephrol Dial Transplant* 1991; **6**:480–483.

72. Gilli P, Moretti M, Soffritti S, *et al.* Non-A, non-B hepatitis and anti-HCV antibodies in dialysis patients. *Int J Artif Organs* 1990; **13**:737–741.

73. Rao KV, Anderson RW, Kasiske BL, Dahl DC. Value of liver biopsy in the evaluation and management of chronic liver disease in renal transplant recipients. *Am J Med* 1993; **94**:241–250.

74. Lai ME, Mazzoleni AP, Argiolu F, *et al.* Hepatitis C virus in multiple episodes of acute hepatitis in polytransfused thalassaemic children. *Lancet* 1994; **343**:388–390.

75. Kao JH, Chen PJ, Lai MY, Chen DS. Superinfection of heterologous hepatitis C virus in a patient with chronic type C hepatitis. *Gastroenterology* 1993; **105**:583–587.

76. Okamoto H, Mishiro S, Tokita H, *et al.* Superinfection of chimpanzees carrying hepatitis C virus of genotype II/1b with that of genotype III/2a or I/1a. *Hepatology* 1994; **20**:1131–1136.

77. Zibert A, Schreier E, Roggendorf M. Antibodies in human sera to hypervariable region 1 of hepatitis C virus can block viral attachment. *Virology* 1995; **208**:653–661.

78. Yoshioka K, Kakumu S, Wakita T, *et al.* Detection of hepatitis C virus by polymerase chain reaction and response to interferon-alpha therapy: relationship to genotypes of hepatitis C virus. *Hepatology* 1992; **16**:293–299.

79. McOmish F, Chan SW, Dow BC, *et al.* Detection of three types of hepatitis C virus in blood donors: investigation of type-specific differences in serologic reactivity and rate of alanine aminotransferase abnormalities. *Transfusion* 1993; **33**:7–13.

80. Feray C, Grigou M, Samuel D, *et al.* HCV type II has a more pathogenic course after liver transplantation (abstract). *Hepatology* 1993; **18**:59.

81. Mahaney K, Tedeschi V, Maertens G, *et al.* Genotypic analysis of hepatitis C virus in American patients. *Hepatology* 1994; **20**:1405–1411.

82. Li J, Tong S, Vitvitski L, *et al.* Two French genotypes of hepatitis C virus: homology of the predominant genotype with the prototype American strain. *Gene* 1991; **105**:167–172.

83. Tsukiyama Kohara K, Kohara M, Yamaguchi K, *et al.* A second group of hepatitis C viruses. *Virus Genes* 1991; **5**:243–254.

84. Takada N, Takase S, Enomoto N, *et al.* Clinical backgrounds of the patients having different types of hepatitis C virus genomes. *J Hepatol* 1992; **14**:35–40.

85. Dusheiko G, Schmilovitz-Weiss H, Brown D, *et al.* Hepatitis C virus genotypes: an investigation of type-specific differences in geographic origin and disease. *Hepatology* 1994; **19**:13–18.

86. Pol S, Thiers V, Nousbaum JB, *et al.* The changing relative prevalence of hepatitis C virus genotypes: evidence in hemodialyzed patients and kidney recipients. *Gastroenterology* 1995; **108**:581–583.

87. Sallie R. Hepatitis C: IIb (IV) or not IIb (IV) that is the question. *Hepatology* 1995; **22**:671–4.

88. Nousbaum J, Pol S, Nalpas B, *et al.* Hepatitis C virus type 1b (II) infection in France and Italy: Collaborative Study Group (see commments). *Ann Intern Med* 1995; **122**:161–168.

89. Pawlowska M, Halota W, Bulik F, Topczewska-Staubach E. Hepatitis C virus (HCV) serotype in the asymptomatic HCV-infected patients from selected groups. *Arch Immunol Ther Exp* 1997; **45**:455–457.

90. Zein NN, Rakela J, Krawitt EL, *et al.* Hepatitis C virus genotypes in the United States: epidemiology, pathogenicity, and response to interferon therapy. *Ann Intern Med* 1996; **125**:634–639.

91. Pontisso P, Ruvoletto MG, Nicoletti M, *et al.* Distribution of three major hepatitis C virus genotypes in Italy: a multicentre study of 495 patients with chronic hepatitis. *J Vir Hepatitis* 1995; **2**:33–38.

92. Brouwer JT, Nevens F, Kleter GEM, Elewaut A, Adler M, Brenard Rea. Treatment of chronic hepatitis C: efficacy of interferon dose and analysis of factors predictive of response. Interim report of 350 patients treated in a Benelux multicenter study. *44th Annual Meeting of the American Association for the Study of Liver Diseases, Chicago, Nov. 4–7 1993.*

93. Liaw YF. Role of hepatitis C virus in dual and triple hepatitis virus infection (review). *Hepatology* 1995; **22**:1101–8.

94. Okada S, Akahane Y, Suzuki H, Okamoto H, Mishiro S. The degree of variability in the amino terminal region of the E2/NS1 protein of hepatitis C virus correlates with responsiveness to interferon therapy in viremic patients. *Hepatology* 1992; **16**:619–624.

95. Mazzotta L, Landucci G, Pfanner L, *et al.* Comparison between first and second generation tests to determine the frequency of anti-HCV antibodies in uremic patients in replacement dialytic therapy. *Nephron* 1992; **3**:354–355.

96. Chauveau P, Couroucé AM, Lemarec N, *et al.* Antibodies to hepatitis C virus by second generation test in hemodialyzed patients. *Kidney Int* 1993; **43** (suppl. 41):S149–S152.

97. Schneeberger PM, Vos J, van Dijk WC. Prevalence of antibodies to hepatitis C virus in a Dutch group of haemodialysis patients related to risk factors. *J Hosp Infect* 1993; **25**:265–270.

98. Kolho E, Oksanen K, Honkanen E ea. Hepatitis C antibodies in dialysis patients and patients with leukemia. *J Med Virol* 1993; **40**:318–321.

99. Hruby Z, Sliwinski J, Molin I, *et al.* High prevalence of antibodies to hepatitis C virus in three haemodialysis centres in south western Poland. *Nephrol Dial Transpl* 1993:740–743.

100. Spanish MSG. Prevalence of hepatitis C virus in dialysis patients in Spain. *Nephrol Dial Transplant* 1995; **10** (suppl 6):78–80.

101. Hayashi J, Nakashima K, Yoshimura E, Kishihara Y, Ohmiya M, Hirata M. Prevalence and role of hepatitis C viraemia in haemodialysis patients in Japan. *J Infect* 1994; **28**:271–277.

102. Geerlings W, Tufveson G, Ehrich JHH, *et al.* Report on the management of renal failure in Europe, XXIII. *Nephrol Dial Transpl* 1994; **9**:6–25.

103. Natov SN, Lau J, Bouthot BA, *et al.* Serological and virological profiles of hepatitis C infection in renal transplant candidates. *Am J Kidney Dis* 1998; **31**:920–927.

104. Pereira B. Hepatitis C virus infection in dialysis: a continuing problem. *Artif Organs* 1999; **23**:1–10.

105. Valderrábano F, Jones EHP, Mallick NP. Report on management of renal failure in Europe, XXIV, 1993. *Nephrol Dial Transplant* 1995; **10** (suppl. 5):1–25.

106. Tokars JI, Miller ER, Alter MJ, Arduino MJ. National surveillance of dialysis associated diseases in the United States, 1995. *ASAIO J* 1998; **44**:98–107.

107. Loureiro A, Pinto dos Santos J, Schmid CS, *et al.* Trends in incidence of hepatitis C (HCV) infection in hemodialysis (HD) units (abstract). *J Am Soc Nephrol* 1995; **6**:547.

108. Huraib S, al-Rashed R, Aldrees A, Aljefry M, Arif M, al-Faleh FA. High prevalence of and risk factors for hepatitis C in haemodialysis patients in Saudi Arabia: a need for new dialysis strategies. *Nephrol Dial Transplant* 1995; 10:470–4.

109. Fabrizi F, Lunghi G, Guarnori I, et al. Incidence of seroconversion for hepatitis C virus in chronic haemodialysis patients: a prospective study. *Nephrol Dial Transplant* 1994; 9:1611–1615.

110. Jadoul M, Cornu C, Van Ypersele de Strihou C, the UCL Collaborative Group. Incidence and risk factors for hepatitis C seroconversion in hemodialysis: A prospective study. *Kidney Int* 1993; 44:1322–1326.

111. Niu MT, Alter MJ, Kristensen C, Margolis HS. Outbreak of hemodialysis-associated non-A, non-B hepatitis and correlation with antibody for hepatitis C virus. *Am J Kidney Dis* 1992; 19:345–352.

112. Pascual J, Teruel JL, Mateos M, et al. Nosocomial transmission of hepatitis C virus (HCV) infection in a hemodialysis (HD) unit during two years of prospective follow-up (abstr). *J Am Soc Nephrol* 1992; 3:386.

113. Lin DY, Lin HH, Huang CC, Liaw YF. High incidence of hepatitis C virus infection in hemodialysis patients in Taiwan. *Am J Kidney Dis* 1993; 21:288–291.

114. Cendoroglo-Neto M, Draibe SA, Silva AE, et al. Incidence of and risk factors for hepatitis B virus and hepatitis C virus infection among haemodialysis and CAPD patients: evidence for environmental transmission. *Nephrol Dial Transplant* 1995; 10:240–6.

115. Vandelli L, Medici G, Savazzi AM, et al. Behavior of antibody profile against hepatitis C virus in patients on maintenance hemodialysis. *Nephron* 1992; 61:260–262.

116. Fabrizi F, Martin P, Dixit V, et al. Acquisition of hepatitis C virus in hemodialysis patients: a prospective study by branched DNA signal amplification assay. *J Am Soc Nephrol* 1997; 8:234A.

117. Incandela L, Giomi S, Nencioni C, et al. [Incidence and prevalence of anti-HCV antibodies and HBV markers in patients undergoing extracorporeal hemodialysis]. *Minerva Med* 1994; 85:505–509. (In Italian.)

118. Schlipkoter U, Gladziwa U, Cholmakov K, et al. Prevalence of hepatitis C infections in dialysis patients and their contacts using a second generation enzyme-linked immunosorbent assay. *Med Microbiol Immunol* 1992; 181:173–180.

119. Tokars J, Alter M, Favero M, Moyer L, Miller E, Bland L. National Surveillance of Dialysis Associated Diseases in the United States, 1993. *ASAIO J* 1996:219–229.

120. Tokars JI, Alter MJ, Miller E, Moyer LA, Favero MS. National surveillance of dialysis associated diseases in the United States, 1994. *ASAIO J* 1997; 43:108–119.

121. Schlipköter U, Roggendorf M, Cholmakow K, Weise A, Dienhardt. Transmission of hepatitis C virus (HCV) from a haemodialysis patient to a medical staff member. *Scand J Infect Dis* 1990; 22:757–758.

122. Kiyosawa K, Sodeyama T, Tanaka E, et al. Hepatitis C in hospital employees with needle-stick injuries. *Ann Intern Med* 1991; 115:367–369.

123. Mitsui T, Iwano K, Masuko K, et al. Hepatitis C virus infection in medical personnel after needlestick accident. *Hepatology* 1992; 16:1109–1114.

124. Masuko K, Mitsui T, Iwano K, et al. Factors influencing postexposure immunoprophylaxis of hepatitis B virus infection with hepatitis B immune globulin. High deoxyribonucleic acid polymerase activity in the inocula of unsuccessful cases. *Gastroenterology* 1985; 88:151–155.

125. Bradley DW. Hepatitis non-A, non-B viruses become identified as hepatitis C and E viruses. *Prog Med Virol* 1990; 37:101–135.

126. Yoshizawa H, Otoh Y, Iwakiri K, Tanaka A, Tachibana T. Non-A, non-B (type 1) hepatitis agent capable of inducing tubular structures in the hepatocyte cytoplasm of chimpanzees: inactivation by formalin and heat. *Gastroenterology* 1982; **82**:502–506.

127. Shikata T, Karasawa T, Abe K, *et al.* Hepatitis B e antigen and infectivity of hepatitis B virus. *J Infect Dis* 1977; **136**:571–576.

128. Ponzetto A, Hoyer BH, Popper H, Engle R, Purcell RH, Gerin JL. Titration of the infectivity of hepatitis D virus in chimpanzees. *J Infect Dis* 1987; **155**:122–128.

129. Colleoni N, Bucci R, Ribero M, Zhou J, D'Amico G, Tagger A. Hepatitis C virus genotype in anti-HCV-positive haemodialysis patients. *Nephrol Dial Transplant* 1996; **11**:2258–2264.

130. Bouchardeau F, Chauveau P, Couroucé AM, Poignet J-L. Genotype distribution and transmission of hepatitis C virus (HCV) in French haemodialysis patients. *Nephrol Dial Transplant* 1995; **10**:2250–2252.

131. Fabrizi F, Lunghi G, Guarnori I, *et al.* Hepatitis C virus genotypes in chronic dialysis patients. *Nephrol Dial Transplant* 1996; **11**:679–683.

132. Benani A, El-Turk J, Benjelloun S, *et al.* HCV genotypes in Marocco. *J Med Virol* 1997; **52**:396–398.

133. Bosmans J, Nouwen E, Behets G, *et al.* Prevalence and clinical expression of HCV-genotypes in hemodialysis-patients of two geographically remote countries: Belgium and Saudi-Arabia. *Clin Nephrol* 1997; **47**:256–262.

134. Rostaing L, Izopet J, Cisterne J-M, *et al.* Impact of hepatitis C virus duration and hepatitis C virus genotypes on renal transplant patients: correlation with clinicopathological features. *Transplantation* 1998; **65**:930–936.

135. Natov SN, Bouthot BA, Lau JYN, *et al.* Effect of HCV genotype on patient survival among renal transplant candidates. in press 1998.

136. Conway M, Catterall AP, Brown EA, *et al.* Prevalence of antibodies to hepatitis C in dialysis patients and transplant recipients with possible routes of transmission. *Nephrol Dial Transplant* 1992; **7**:1226–1229.

137. Oguchi H, Miyasaka M, Tokunaga S, *et al.* Hepatitis virus infection (HBV and HCV) in eleven Japanese hemodialysis units. *Clin Nephrol* 1992; **38**:36–43.

138. Knudsen F, Wantzin P, Rasmussen K, *et al.* Hepatitis C in dialysis patients: Relationship to blood transfusions, dialysis and liver disease. *Kidney Int* 1993; **43**:1353–1356.

139. Dussol B, Chicheportiche C, Cantaloube JF, *et al.* Detection of hepatitis C infection by polymerase chain reaction among hemodialysis patients. *Am J Kidney Dis* 1993; **22**:574–580.

140. Dentico P, Buongiorno R, Volpe A, *et al.* Prevalence and incidence of hepatitis C virus (HCV) in hemodialysis patients: study of risk factors. *Clin Nephrol* 1992; **61**:49–52.

141. Mosconi G, Campieri C, Miniero R, *et al.* Epidemiology of hepatitis C in a population of hemodialysis patients. *Nephron* 1992; **61**:298–299.

142. Scotto G, Savastano AM, Forcella M, *et al.* HCV infections in dialysis patients. *Nephron* 1992; **61**:320–321.

143. Donahue JG, Muñoz A, Ness PM, *et al.* The declining risk of post-transfusion hepatitis C virus infection. *New Engl J Med* 1992; **327**:369–373.

144. Niu MT, Coleman PJ, Alter MJ. Multicenter study of hepatitis C virus infection in chronic hemodialysis patients and hemodialysis center staff members. *Am J Kidney Dis* 1993; **22**:568–573.

145. Schlipkoter U, Roggendorf M, Ernst G, *et al.* Hepatitis C virus antibodies in haemodialysis patients. *Lancet* 1990; **335**:1409.

146. Elisaf M, Tsianos E, Mavridis M, Dardamanis M, Pappas M, Siamopoulos KC. Antibodies against hepatitis C virus (anti-HCV) in haemodialysis patients: association with hepatitis B serological markers. *Nephrol Dial Transplant* 1991; **6**:476–479.

147. Ponz E, Campistol JM, Barrera JM, *et al.* Hepatitis C virus antibodies in patients on hemodialysis and after transplantation. *Transplant Proc* 1991; 23:1371–1372.

148. Yamaguchi K, Nishimura Y, Fukuoka N, *et al.* Hepatitis C virus antibodies in haemodialysis patients. *Lancet* 1990; 335:1409–1410.

149. Brugnano R, Francisci D, Quintaliani G, *et al.* Antibodies against hepatitis C virus in hemodialysis patients in the central Italian region of Umbria: evaluation of some risk factors. *Nephron* 1992; 61:263–265.

150. Cantu P, Mangano S, Masini M, Limido A, Crovetti G, DeFilippo C. Prevalence of antibodies against hepatitis C virus in a dialysis unit. *Nephron* 1992; 61:337–338.

151. Hardy NM, Sandroni S, Danielson S, Wilson WJ. Antibody to hepatitis C virus increases with time on dialysis. *Clin Nephrol* 1992; 38:44–48.

152. Medici G, Depetri GC, Mileti M. Anti-hepatitis C virus positivity and clinical correlations in hemodialyzed patients. *Nephron* 1992; 61:363–364.

153. Dussol B, Berthezène P, Brunet P, *et al.* Hepatitis C virus infection among chronic dialysis patients in the south-east of France. *Nephrol Dial Transplant* 1995; 10:477–478.

154. Selgas R, Martinez-Zapico R, Bajo MA, *et al.* Prevalence of hepatitis C antibodies (HCV) in a dialysis population at one center. *Peritoneal Dial Int* 1992; 12:28–30.

155. Yoshida CFT, Takahashi C, Gaspar AMC, Schatzmayr HG, Ruzany F. Hepatitis C virus in chronic hemodialysis patients with non-A, non-B hepatitis. *Nephron* 1992; 60:150–153.

156. Jonas MM, Zilleruelo GE, LaRue SI, Abitbol C, Strauss J, Lu Y. Hepatiis C infection in pediatric dialysis population. *Pediatrics* 1992; 89:707–709.

157. Mitwalli A, Al-Mohaya S, Al Wakeel J, *et al.* Hepatitis C in chronic renal failure patients. *Am J Nephrol* 1992; 12:288–291.

158. Chan TM, Lok ASF, Cheng IKP. Hepatitis C infection among dialysis patients: A comparison between patients on maintenance haemodialysis and continuous ambulatory peritoneal dialysis. *Nephrol Dial Transplant* 1991; 6:944–947.

159. Besso L, Rovere A, Peano G, *et al.* Prevalence of HCV antibodies in a uraemic population undergoing maintenance dialysis therapy and in staff members of the dialysis unit. *Nephron* 1992; 61:304–306.

160. McIntyre PG, McCruden EA, Dow BC, *et al.* Hepatitis C virus infection in renal dialysis patients in Glasgow. *Nephrol Dial Transplant* 1994; 9:291–295.

161. Huang CC, Wu MS, Lin DY, Liaw YF. The prevalence of hepatitis C virus antibodies in patients treated with continuous ambulatory peritoneal dialysis. *Peritoneal Dial Int* 1992; 12:31–33.

162. Barril G, Traver JA. Prevalence of hepatitis C virus in dialysis patients in Spain. *Nephrol Dial Transplant* 1995; 10 (suppl. 6):78–80.

163. Pinto dos Santos J, Loureiro A, Cendoroglo M, Pereira BJG. Impact of dialysis room and reuse strategies on the incidence of HCV infection in haemodialysis units. *Nephrol Dial Transplant* 1996; 11:2017–2022.

164. Cendoroglo Neto M, Manzano SI, Canziani ME, *et al.* Environmental transmission of hepatitis B and hepatitis C viruses within the hemodialysis unit. *Artif Organs* 1995; 19:251–5.

165. Mondelli MU, Cristina G, Pazza V, Cerino A, Villa G, Salvadeo A. High prevalence of antibodies to hepatitis C virus in hemodialysis units using a second generation assay. *Nephron* 1992; 61:350–351.

166. Machida J, Yamaguchi K, Uerda S, *et al.* High incidence of hepatitis C virus antibodies in hemodialysis patients. *Nephron* 1992; 60:117–118.

167. Ruffatti A, Bortolotti F, Bianco A, *et al.* Hepatitis C virus infection in hemodialyzed patients detected by first and second generation assays. *Nephron* 1992; 61:344–345.

168. Okuda K, Hayashi H, Yokozeki K, *et al.* Mode of nosocomial HCV infection among chronic hemodialysis patients and its prevention. *Hepatology* 1994; **19**:293.

169. Garcia-Valdescasas J, Bernal MC, Cerezo S, Garcia F, Pereira BJG. Strategies to reduce the transmission of HCV infection in hemodialysis (HD) units (abstract). *J Am Soc Nephrol* 1993; **4**:347.

170. Vagelli G, Calabrese G, Guaschino R, Gonella M. Effect of HCV+ patients isolation on HCV infection incidence in a dialysis unit (letter). *Nephrol Dial Transplant* 1992; **7**:1070.

171. Corcoran GD, Brink NS, Millar CG, *et al.* Hepatitis C virus infection in hemodialysis patients: a clinical and virological study. *J Infect Dis* 1994; **28**:279–285.

172. Sampietro M, Badalamenti S, Salvadori S, *et al.* High prevalence of a rare hepatitis C virus in patients treated in the same hemodialysis unit: Evidence for nosocomial transmission of HCV. *Kidney Int* 1995; **47**:911–917.

173. de Lamballerie X, Olmer M, Bouchouareb D, Zandotti C, De Micco P. Nosocomial transmission of hepatitis C virus in hemodialysis patients. *J Med Virol* 1996; **49**:296–302.

174. Alter MJ, Favero MS, Moyer LA, Bland LA. National surveillance of dialysis-associated diseases in the United States, 1989. *ASAIO Trans* 1991; **37**:97–109.

175. Jadoul M, Cornu C, Van Ypersele de Strihou C, Group. atUCUC. Universal precautions prevent hepatitis C virus transmission: a 54 month follow-up of the Belgian multicenter study. *Kidney Int* 1998; **53**:1022–1025.

176. Chiaramonte S, Tagger A, Ribero ML, Grossi A, Milan M, La Greca G. Prevention of viral hepatitis in dialysis unit: isolation and technical management of dialysis. *Nephron* 1992; **61**:287–289.

177. Calabrese G, Vagelli G, Guaschino R, Gonella M. Transmission of anti-HCV within the household of hemodialysis patients. *Lancet* 1991; **338**:1466.

178. Yuasa T, Ishikawa G, Manabe S, Sekiguchi S, Takeuchi K, Miyamura T. The particle size of hepatitis C virus estimated by filtration through microporous regenerated cellulose fibre. *J Gen Virol* 1991; **72**:2021–2024.

179. Hubmann R, Zazgornik J, Gabriel C, *et al.* Hepatitis C virus-does it penetrate the haemodialysis membrane? PCR analysis of haemodialysis ultrafiltrate and whole blood. *Nephrol Dial Transplant* 1995; **10**:541–542.

180. Caramelo C, Navas S, Alberola ML, *et al.* Evidence against transmission of hepatitis C virus through hemodialysis ultrafiltrate and peritoneal fluid. *Nephron* 1994; **66**:470–473.

181. Lombardi M, Cerrai T, Dattolo P, *et al.* Is the dialysis membrane a safe barrier against HCV infection? *Nephrol Dial Transplant* 1995; **10**:578–579.

182. Liou T, Chang T, Young T, Lin X, Lin C, Wu H. Detection of HCV RNA in saliva, urine, seminal fluid and ascites. *J Med Virol* 1992; **37**:197–202.

183. Castelnovo C, Sampietro M, De Vecchi A, *et al.* Diffusion of HCV through peritoneal membrane in HCV positive patients treated with continuous ambulatory peritoneal dialysis. *Nephrol Dial Transplant* 1997; **12**:978–980.

184. Tokars J, Alter MJ, Favero MS, Moyer LA, Bland LE. National surveillance of hemodialysis associated diseases in the United States, 1990. *ASAIO J* 1993; **39**:71–80.

185. Cuypers HTM, Bresters D, Winkel INea. Storage conditions of blood samples and primer selection affect the yield of cDNA polymerase chain reaction products of hepatitis C virus. *J Clin Microbiol* 1992; **30**:3220–3224.

186. Pereira BJG, Milford EL, Kirkman RL, Levey AS. Transmission of hepatitis C virus by organ transplantation. *New Eng J Med* 1991; **325**:454–460.

187. LaQuaglia MP, Tolkoff-Rubin NE, Dienstag JL, *et al.* Impact of hepatitis on renal transplantation. *Transplantation* 1981; **32**:504–507.

188. Weir MR, Kirkman RL, Strom TB, Tilney NL. Liver disease in recipients of long-surviving renal allografts. *Kidney Int* 1985; **28**:839–844.

189. Pereira BJG, Wright TL, Schmid CH, Levey AS, for The New England Organ Bank Hepatitis C Study Group. A controlled study of hepatitis C transmission by organ transplantation. *Lancet* 1995; 345:484–87.

190. Roth D, Fernandez JA, Babischkin S, *et al.* Detection of hepatitis C infection among cadaver organ donors: evidence for low transmission of disease. *Ann Intern Med* 1992; 117:470–475.

191. Huang CC, Lai MK, Lin MW, Pao CC, Fang JT, Yao DS. Transmission of hepatitis C virus by renal transplantation. *Transplant Proc* 1993; 25:1474–1475.

192. Vincenti F, Lake J, Wright T, Kuo G, Weber P, Stempel C. Nontransmission of hepatitis C from cadaver kidney donors to transplant recipients. *Transplantation* 1993; 55:674–675.

193. Gomez E, Aguado S, Gago E, *et al.* A study of renal transplants obtained from anti-HCV positive donors. *Transplant Proc* 1991; 23:2654–2655.

194. Triolo G, Squiccimarro G, Baldi M, *et al.* Antobodies to hepatitis C virus in kidney transplantation. *Nephron* 1992; 61:276–277.

195. LeFor W, Wright C, Shires D, Kahana L, Spoto E, Ackermann J. A preliminary outcome evaluation of the impact of HCV-AB studied in 521 cadaver vascular organ donors over a 6 year period. *American Society of Transplant Physicians, 10th Annual Meeting, Chicago, May 28–29 1991.*

196. Tesi R, Waller K, Morgan C, *et al.* Transmission of hepatitis C by kidney transplantation— the risks. *Transplantation* 1994; 57:826–831.

197. Wreghitt TG, Gray JJ, Allain J-P, *et al.* Transmission of hepatitis C virus by organ transplantation in the United Kingdom. *J Hepatology* 1994; 20:768–772.

198. Prados MC, Franco A, Perdiguero M, Munoz C, De la Sen ML, Olivares J. Transmission of hepatitis C virus by kidney transplantation. *Transplant Proc* 1992; 24:2650–2651.

199. Pirsch JD, Heisey D, D'Allesandro AM, Knechtle SJ, Sollinger HW, Belzer FO. Transplantation of hepatitis C (HCV) kidneys: defining the risks. *14th Annual Meeting of the American Society of Transplant Physicians, Chicago, May 14–17, 1995.*

200. Otero J, Roderiguez M, Escudero D, Gomez E, Aguado S, Ona MD. Kidney transplants with positive anti-hepatitis C virus donors. *Transplantation* 1990; 50:1086–1087.

201. Pereira BJG, Wright TL, Schmid CH, *et al.* Screening and confirmatory testing of cadaver organ donors for hepatitis C virus infection: A U.S. National Collaborative Study. *Kidney Int* 1994; 46:886–892.

202. Mendez R, Aswad S, Bogaard T, *et al.* Donor hepatitis C antibody virus testing in renal transplantation. *Transplant Proc* 1993; 25:1487–1490.

203. Tesi RJ, Waller MK, Morgan CJ, *et al.* Use of low-risk HCV-positive donors for kidney transplantation. *Transplant Proc* 1993; 25:1472–1473.

204. Mendez R, El-Shahawy M, Obispo E, Aswad S, Mendex RG. Four years follow up of hepatitis C positive kidneys into hepatitis C negative recipients-prospective study. *J Am Soc Nephrol* 1995; 6:1105.

205. Widell A, Mansson S, Persson NH, Thysell H, Hermodsson S, Blohme I. Hepatitis C superinfection in hepatitis C virus (HCV)-infected patients transplanted with an HCV-infected kidney. *Transplantation* 1995; 60:642–647.

206. Oldach D, Constantine N, Schweitzer E, *et al.* Clinical and virological outcomes in hepatitis C virus (HCV)-infected renal transplant recipients. *14th Annual Meeting of the American Society of Transplant Physicians, Chicago, May 14–17, 1995.*

207. Morales JM, Campistol JM, Castellano G, *et al.* Transplantation of kidneys from donors with hepatitis C antibody into recipients with pre-transplantation anti-HCV. *Kidney Int* 1995; 47:236–240.

208. Pereira BJG, Wright TL, Schmid CH, Levey AS, for the New England Organ Bank Hepatitis C Study Group. The impact of pretransplantation hepatitis C infection on the outcome of renal transplantation. *Transplantation* 1995; 60:799–805.

209. Stempel CA, Lake J, Kuo G, Vincenti F. Hepatitis C—its prevalence in end-stage renal failure patients and clinical course after kidney transplantation. *Transplantation* 1993; 55:273–276.

210. Huang C-C, Liaw Y-F, Lai M-K, Chu S-H, Chuang C-K, Huang J-Y. The clinical outcome of hepatitis C virus antibody-positive renal allograft recipients. *Transplantation* 1992; 53:763–765.

211. Roth D, Zucker K, Cirocco R, *et al*. The impact of hepatitis C virus infection on renal allograft recipients. *Kidney Int* 1994; 45:238–244.

212. Roth D. Hepatitis C virus: the nephrologist's view. *Am J Kidney Dis* 1995; 25:3–16.

213. Ynares C, Johnson HK, Kerlin T, Crowe D, MacDonell R, Richie R. Impact of pretransplant hepatitis C antibody status upon long-term patient and renal allograft survival–a 5- and 10-year follow-up. *Transplant Proc* 1993; 25:1466–1468.

214. Fritsche C, Brandes JC, Delaney SR, *et al*. Hepatitis C is a poor prognostic indicator in black kidney transplant recipients. *Transplantation* 1993; 55:1283–1287.

215. Port F, Wolfe R, Mauger E, Berling D, Jiang K. Comparison of survival probabilities for dialysis patients vs cadaveric renal transplant recipients. *J Am Med Assoc* 1993; 270:1339–1343.

216. Mondelli MU, Cristana G, Filice G, Rondanelli EG, Piazza V, Barbieri C. Anti-HCV positive patients in dialysis units? *Lancet* 1990; 336:244.

217. Zeldis JB, Depner TA, Kuramoto IK, Gish RG, Holland PV. The prevalence of hepatitis C virus antibodies among hemodialysis patients. *Ann Intern Med* 1990; 112:958–960.

218. Alivanis P, Derveniotis V, Dioudis Cea. Hepatitis C virus in antibodies in hemodialyzed and renal transplant patients: correlation with chronic liver disease. *Transplant Proc* 1991; 23:2662–2663.

219. Medici G, Vandelli L, Savazzi AM, Lusvarghi E. Hepatitis C virus (HCV) infection on maintenance hemodialysis: biological results and clinical remarks (abstract). *J Am Soc Nephrol* 1990; 1:368.

220. Lilis D, Hadjiconstantinou V, Kravaritis A, *et al*. Prevalence of anti-HCV antibodies in four hemodialysis units in Athens (abstract). *Kidney Int* 1991; 39:192.

221. Pouteil-Noble C, Tardy JC, Chossegros P, Trepo C, Aymard M, Touraine JL. Hepatitis C virus infection in renal transplantation (abstract). *Kidney Int* 1991; 39:1318.

222. Lozano L, Nieto J, Sanchez M, Martin JE, Granizo V, Jarillo MD. Evaluation of incidence of hepatitis C in dialysis (abstract). *Kidney Int* 1991; 40:379.

223. Cordero Sanchez M, Bondia Roman A, Lopez Ochoa J, Martin Sanchez AM, Nunez Garcia J. Anti-hepatitis C antibodies in hemodialysis (abstract). *Kidney Int* 1991; 40:361.

224. Bulletin TU. 1997; 2.

225. Pereira BJG, Natov SN, Bouthot BA, *et al*. Effect of hepatitis C infection and renal transplantation on survival in end-stage renal disease. *Kidney Int* 1998; 53:1374–1381.

226. Lindsay KL. Therapy of hepatitis C: overview. *Hepatology* 1997; 26 (suppl. 1):71S–77S.

227. Anonymous. Management of hepatitis C. *NIH Consensus Statement* 1997; 15:1–41.

228. Di Bisceglie AM. Interferon therapy for chronic viral hepatitis. *New Engl J Med* 1994; 330:137–138.

229. Di Bisceglie AM, Hoofnagle JH, Krawczynski K. Changes in hepatitis C virus antigen in liver with antiviral therapy. *Gastroenterology* 1993; 105:858–862.

230. Chemello L, Alberti A, Rose K, Simmonds P. Hepatitis C serotype and response to interferon therapy. *New Engl J Med* 1994; 330:143.

231. Black M, Peters M. Alpha-interferon treatment of chronic hepatitis C: need for accurate diagnosis in selecting patients. *Ann Intern Med* 1992; 116:86–88.

232. Kramer P, ten Kate FJW, Bijnen AB, Jeekel J, Weimar W. The pathology of interferon-induced renal allograft lesions. *Transplant Proc* 1985; **17**:58.
233. Kovarik J, Mayer G, Pohanka E, *et al.* Adverse effect of low-dose prophylactic human recombinant leukocyte interferon-alpha treatment in renal transplant recipients. Cytomegalovirus infection prophylaxis leading to an increased incidence of irreversible rejections. *Transplantation* 1988; **45**:402–405.
234. Rao VK, Anderson WR. Clinical and histological outcome following interferon treatment of chronic viral hepatitis, in uremic patients, before and after renal transplantation (abstract). *14th Annual Meeting of the American Society of Transplant Physicians, Chicago, May 15–17, 1995.*
235. Pol S, Thiers V, Carnot F, *et al.* Efficacy and tolerance of alpha-2b interferon therapy on HCV infection of hemodialyzed patients. *Kidney Int* 1995; **47**:1412–1418.
236. Rostaing L, Izopet J, Baron E, *et al.* Preliminary results of treatment of chronic hepatitis C with recombinant interferon alpha in renal transplant patients. *Nephrol Dial Transplant* 1995; **10**:93–96.
237. Casanovas TT, Baliellas C, Sese E, *et al.* Interferon may be useful in hemodialysis patients with hepatitis C virus chronic infection who are candidates for kidney transplant. *Transplant Proc* 1995; **27**:2229–2230.
238. Koenig P, Vogel W, Umlauft F, Weyrer K, Prommegger R, Lhotta K. Interferon treatment for chronic hepatitis C virus infection in uremic patients. *Kidney Int* 1994; **45**:1507–1509.
239. Duarte R, Huraib S, Said R, *et al.* Interferon-alpha facilitates renal transplantation in hemodialysis patients with chronic viral hepatitis. *Am J Kidney Dis* 1995; **25**:40–45.
240. Harihara Y, Kurooka Y, Yanagisawa T, Kuzuhara K, Otsubo O, Kumada H. Interferon therapy in renal allograft recipients with chronic hepatitis C. *Transplant Proc* 1994; **26**:2075.
241. Raptopoulou-Gigi M, Spaia S, Garifallos A, *et al.* Interferon-alpha2b treatment of chronic hepatitis C in haemodialysis patients. *Nephrol Dial Transplant* 1995; **10**:1834–1837.
242. Ozgur O, Boyacioglu S, Telatar H, Haberal M. Recombinant alpha-interferon in renal allograft recipients with chronic hepatitis C. *Nephrol Dial Transplant* 1995; **10**:2104–2106.
243. Umlauft F, Gruenewald K, Weiss G, *et al.* Patterns of hepatitis C viremia in patients receiving hemodialysis. *Am J Gastroenterol* 1997; **92**:73–78.
244. Rostaing L, Chatelut E, Payen J, *et al.* Pharmacokinetics of alfa-interferon-2b in chronic hepatitis C virus patients undergoing chronic hemodialysis or with normal renal function: clinical implications. *J Am Soc Nephrol* 1998; **9**:2344–2348.
245. Hanafusa T, Ichikawa Y, Kishikawa H, *et al.* Retrospective study on the impact of hepatitis C virus infection on kidney transplant patients over 20 years. *Transplantation* 1998; **66**.
246. Oesterreicher C, Hammer J, Koch U, *et al.* HBV and HCV genome in peripheral blood mononuclear cells in patients undergoing hemodialysis. *Kidney Int* 1995; **48**:1967–1971.
247. Chan TM, Lok ASF, Cheng IKP, Ng IOL. Chronic hepatitis C after renal transplantation. Treatment with alpha-interferon. *Transplantation* 1993; **56**:1095–1098.
248. Poynard T, Bedrossa P, Chevallier M, *et al.* A comparison of three interferon alpha-2b regimens for the long-term treatment of chronic non-A, non-B hepatitis. *New Engl J Med* 1995; **332**:1457–1462.
249. Pereira BJG, Levey AS. Hepatitis C infection in dialysis and renal transplantation. *Kidney Int* 1997; **51**:981–999.

11

Hepatitis B in end-stage renal disease

Svetlozar N. Natov and Brian J.G. Pereira

Biology of the hepatitis B virus and tests for the detection of hepatitis B infection

Structure of the hepatitis B viral genome

Hepatitis B virus (HBV) is a spherical, small, enveloped DNA virus, which belongs to the family Hepadnaviridae (hepatotropic DNA viruses). The complete virion or Dane particle is 42 nm in diameter and consists of a surface and a core. The surface incorporates the envelope protein, referred to as hepatitis B surface antigen (HBsAg). It is antigenically complex and has different antigenic determinants—a common antigenic determinant, named *a*, and four other subdeterminants, designated *d*, *y*, *w*, and *r*. The possible combinations of these determinants have led to the recognition of four subtypes of HBsAg, i.e. *adw*, *adr*, *ayw*, and *ayr*. These subtypes have epidemiological significance as additional markers in evaluating the transmission of HBV, but no clinical relevance. Antibodies to the *a* determinant confer protection to all HBsAg subtypes.

The core contains the polymerase protein (a DNA polymerase), the viral genome (a double-stranded DNA) and the nucleocapsid protein, which embodies a core antigen (HBcAg) and another antigen called 'e' (HBeAg), which is a protein subunit of the core.

Although the viral genomic structure is relatively stable, mutations in various regions of the viral genome can still occur and give origin to variants of HBV. These mutations can potentially alter the level of HBV replication or the expression of immunogenic epitopes and thus modulate the severity of liver disease. Indeed, some viral mutants have been incriminated in causing severe forms of liver injury.[1,2] In contrast, other mutants have been found in asymptomatic HBsAg carriers, suggesting that not all mutations necessarily lead to increased pathogenicity.[3]

Tests for detection of HBV infection

Three antigen–antibody systems characterize serologically the different stages of HBV infection.[4]

The presence of HBsAg in the serum indicates current HBV infection and implies potential infectivity of the blood. Antibody to HBsAg (HBsAb) reveals past infection with HBV or immune response to HBV vaccine, or may result from passive antibody transfer with hepatitis B immune globulin (HBIG).

HBeAg can be detected exclusively in HBsAg-positive individuals, usually in association with HBV DNA present in the serum. Therefore, it is generally regarded as a marker of HBV replication and a state of high infectivity. The appearance of antibody to HBeAg (anti-HBe) in the serum of an HBsAg carrier is usually indicative of decreasing titres or eventual disappearance of HBV DNA, thus suggesting a lower degree of infectivity.

Hepatitis B core antigen (HBcAg) is an intracellular antigen, expressed in infected hepatocytes, and is not detectable in serum. Antibody to HBcAg (anti-HBc) can be detected throughout the course of HBV infection. Acute or recent infection with HBV is associated with the presence of anti-HBc of IgM class. IgM anti-HBc is the sole marker of HBV infection during the 'window' period between the disappearance of HBsAg and the appearance of anti-HBs. However, the titre of IgM anti-HBc may increase to detectable levels during exacerbations of chronic hepatitis B, which can incorrectly be interpreted as acute hepatitis B and thus may create a diagnostic problem.[5] Anti-HBc of IgG class is a marker of past infection with HBV at some undefined time. Usually, it is present along with anti-HBs in patients who recover from acute hepatitis B, but can also be found in association with HBsAg in those who progress to chronic HBV infection. In some instances, anti-HBc can be present in the absence of HBsAg and anti-HBs. This can occur in three settings:

(1) during the window period of acute hepatitis B when the anti-HBc is predominantly IgM class;
(2) many years after recovery from acute hepatitis B when anti-HBs has fallen to undetectable levels; and
(3) after many years of chronic HBV infection when the HBsAg titre has decreased below the cut-off level for detection.

The isolated presence of anti-HBc has been observed in 0.4% to 1.7% of blood donors in low-prevalence areas and in 10% to 20% of the population in endemic countries.[6–8] The clinical significance of isolated anti-HBc is uncertain.

Epidemiology and clinical features of HBV infection

Routes of transmission

HBV is a bloodborne infection with ubiquitous distribution. The modes of HBV transmission vary between different populations and geographical areas in relation to risk factors, cultural habits, and endemic regions. In general, HBV is mainly parenterally transmitted. Blood transfusion was a major route of HBV transmission in the past. However, in the United States, as a result of routine screening of blood donors for HBV infection, it is currently associated with only a very small risk (1 in 63 000) of post-transfusion hepatitis B.[9] Consequently, the role of blood transfusion in the spread of HBV, particularly in developed countries, seems to be negligible. Percutaneous inoculation of blood and body fluid as a result of needlestick injury, needle sharing between intravenous drug users, or the use of contaminated needles for tattoos, acupuncture, and ear piercing has become an increasingly important mode of HBV transmission. The risk of acquiring HBV after accidental needlestick exposure to contaminated blood is as high as 78%.[10] At present, sexual contact is the most important mode of HBV transmission in developed countries.[11,12] Horizontal transmission between household contacts of HBV carriers has been reported.[13,14] HBV can be transmitted by organ transplantation.[15] Transmission via casual contact or food has never been documented.

Natural course of HBV infection

HBV causes acute and chronic infections. Acute infection is associated with acute hepatitis defined as a self-limiting disease characterized by acute inflammation and hepatocellular necrosis. The diagnosis rests upon detecting HBsAg and anti-HBc of IgM class in the serum of a patient with clinical and laboratory evidence of acute hepatitis. More than half (50% to 70%) of the patients with acute HBV infection respond with production of protective antibodies (HBsAb and anti-HBc) and are ultimately able to clear the virus. Consequently, they develop only a silent and self-limiting infection, which does not result in clinically apparent acute hepatitis. In another 0.1% to 0.5% of patients with acute hepatitis, the disease will take a fulminant course with a high mortality rate, most likely arising from massive immune-mediated lysis of infected hepatocytes. Viral mutants, particularly those resulting from mutation in the precore region of the HBV DNA, have been implicated in these cases.[1,2]

Fewer than 5% of adults (but 80% to 90% of infants) fail to mount an adequate immunological response to HBV infection and develop persistent or chronic infection. This causes hepatocellular injury and inflammation resulting in chronic hepatitis. The diagnosis is based on detecting persistently elevated serum transaminases and the presence of HBsAg in the serum for a period of 6 months or more. The interaction between viral replication and the immune response of the host determines two phases in the natural course of chronic HBV infection. The initial 'replicative' phase is characterized by active viral replication that may continue for a number of months or years. This is manifested by the presence of HBeAg and high levels of circulating HBV DNA, which makes patients in this phase highly infectious to others. Necroinflammatory changes in the liver and elevated serum aminotransferase levels are often present. Eventually, viral replication diminishes and the chronic HBV infection enters a 'non-proliferative' phase. During this second phase in the course of the chronic HBV infection, HBeAg is cleared in most cases, usually at a rate of 10 to 15% per year, and transient increase in disease activity with a rise in serum transaminase levels becomes often apparent. The clearance of HBeAg, which may be accompanied by the appearance of anti-HBe in the serum, is associated with a significant drop in HBV DNA levels, resulting in reduced infectivity. Liver disease activity usually subsides and some patients will ultimately enter a phase of remission despite persistence of HBsAg. These individuals are commonly referred to as 'healthy' chronic HBsAg carriers. However, this term is in a way misleading because they are still at risk of reactivating their infection, and if cirrhosis has already developed, they are also at risk of developing hepatocellular carcinoma (HCC). Chronic HBsAg carriers can still loose detectable HBsAg at some later point in time; however, the annual rate of HBsAg loss is very low—approximately 0.5%.[16] Although, the degree and the evolution of hepatocellular injury in patients with chronic HBV infection are variable, about 15 to

20% of those who acquire the infection in adulthood and up to 40% of those who become infected in childhood will ultimately progress to liver cirrhosis. In addition, the annual probability of HCC in patients with HBV-related chronic hepatitis is 0.5% and that in patients with cirrhosis is 2.4%.[17] In some geographical regions endemic for HBV infection, HCC in HBV-infected individuals develops at a rate as high as 5.7% per year.[18] Finally, mortality rates from HBV-related disease vary largely between studies, but they are consistently remarkably high. Indeed, HBsAg carriers, as compared with normal individuals, have relative risks of death due to cirrhosis of between 12 and 79 and of death due to HCC of between 30 and 148.[19]

HBV infection in dialysis

Prevalence of HBV infection in dialysis patients and dialysis unit staff

Viral hepatitis was recognized as a major health problem in dialysis patients and staff, both in the United States and elsewhere soon after the establishment of dialysis centres as healthcare settings providing maintenance haemodialysis (HD) treatment for patients with end-stage renal disease (ESRD). Indeed, a United States national survey conducted in 1967 and 1968, i.e. before the implementation of serological testing for HBsAg, found that cases of hepatitis in dialysis patients or staff members were observed in 41% and 19% respectively of the participating HD centres.[20] Another survey of HD-associated hepatitis in the United States, conducted by the Centers for Disease Control (CDC) after the advent of serological testing for HBV infection, reported that the attack rates of HBV infection in 1972, ascertained by the incidence of HBsAg seropositivity, were 2.8% in dialysis patients and 1.9% in dialysis staff.[21] Alarmingly, between 1972 and 1974, the incidence of HBs antigenaemia in the United States increased by more than 100%, among both patients and staff, and reached 6.2% and 5.8% respectively.[22] In keeping with these observations, a point-prevalence study of 15 dialysis centres in the United States, which included 583 patients and 451 staff members screened for serological markers of HBV infection between 1972 and 1973, reported that HBsAg was present in 16.8% of the patients and in 2.4% of the dialysis staff.[23] Similarly, for the period 1967–1971, the European Dialysis and Transplant Association (EDTA) reported a 5–10% annual incidence of HBV infection in patients on maintenance HD.[24] In addition, in 1971, HBV infection was endemic in 43% of 367 dialysis centres in 24 European countries.[25,26] The HBsAg carrier state at these centres was 20 to 40%, and the infection rate in staff members was close to 30%. In 1976, the CDC annual survey of dialysis-associated hepatitis in the United States reported that, for the 750 participating dialysis centres, HBs antigenaemia had a 7.8% prevalence and a 3.0% annual incidence in HD patients, and a 2.6% incidence in HD staff.[27] It is obvious that in these studies dialysis staff members had an almost equal risk of acquiring HBV infection as dialysis patients.[21,22] Further, the risk of hepatitis B for dialysis staff was clearly correlated to job category and the function of the dialysis unit.[22] Dialysis technicians and nurses, i.e. the personnel who were potentially coming in to close contact with HBV while attending HBsAg-positive patients during dialysis or while manipulating HBsAg contaminated dialysis machines or other equipment, had indeed the greatest risk of acquiring HBV infection. In addition, staff employed in HD units with several functions (i.e. HD units which combined chronic inpatient, home training, and acute dialysis) had significantly higher rates than staff in other units, particularly in those providing only acute or transplant-support dialysis.

A significant drop in the incidence and the prevalence of HBV infection in both dialysis patients and staff occurred following the implementation of control measures for hepatitis B in dialysis centres as recommended by CDC in 1977. By 1980, the incidence and prevalence of HBsAg positivity had impressively decreased to 1% and 3.8% respectively in dialysis patients and to 0.7% each in dialysis staff members.[27] This decline in the incidence and the prevalence of HBV infection in HD centres in the United States has continued uninterrupted over the last two decades as a result of a large number of policies and practices implemented in HD centres with the aim of preventing the spread of bloodborne infections. Thus, by 1997, the incidence and the prevalence of HBsAg positivity had further decreased to 0.05% and 0.9% respectively in patients, and 0.4% and 0.05% respectively in staff.[28]

Clinical course of HBV infection in dialysis patients

Because of an impaired immune system and consequent inability to produce antibodies, patients on maintenance dialysis who contract infection with HBV typically develop a disease with attenuated clinical presentation but demonstrate a high rate of chronicity. Indeed, the majority of these patients either manifest very mild illness and only occasionally become jaundiced or remain asymptomatic with normal or slightly elevated serum transaminase levels.[29] However, it has been well documented that a remarkably high percentage (80% to 90%) of HD patients who become infected with HBV do not respond with protective antibody production, fail to clear the virus within 3 to 6 months from the onset of HBV infection, and, consequently, become persistent HBsAg carriers.[21,22,29,30] Very few of these chronic HBsAg carriers will subsequently clear the virus. In one study, only 7% (3 out of 42) of the patients who remained HBsAg-positive for more than 6 months were able to clear the virus 21, 52, and 55 months respectively after becoming HBsAg-positive, while none of the patients who developed chronic enzyme elevations were able to do so.[29] In fact, it appears that the longer the duration of HBsAg positivity, the higher the risk of an HBsAg-positive HD patient remaining an HBsAg carrier indefinitely.[29]

Commonly, HBsAg-positive HD patients experience persistent viral replication and, as a result, test positive for HBeAg. In general, patients with chronic HBV infection (i.e. chronic HBsAg carriers), who are also HBeAg-positive, have extremely high titres of HBV circulating in their blood (approximately 10^8 virions/ml), and consequently, considerable HBV levels in body fluids containing their serum or blood.[31]

The existence of chronic HBsAg carriers in the HD population has substantial epidemiological implications. These patients, who are usually highly infectious, particularly if they are also HBeAg-positive, serve as a reservoir of HBV infection within the HD centre, from where the virus can be transmitted to other patients and staff members. Therefore, recognition of every chronic HBsAg carrier in the HD population is of major importance for the prevention of nosocomial transmission of HBV.

Effect of HBV infection on clinical outcomes in dialysis patients

The impact of chronic HBs antigenaemia on clinical outcomes of patients on maintenance dialysis has been a matter of debate. Despite the fact that HD patients with HBV
infection have a high rate of chronicity, several studies have demonstrated that a chronic
HBsAg carrier state in this population is not associated with increased morbidity and
mortality.[29,32,33] Indeed, over a study period of 8 years, Josselson and colleagues could not
detect any significant differences between HD patients who were HBsAg-positive,
persistently or transiently (mean duration of HBsAg positivity 31 months, range 2 to 120
months), and those who were persistently HBsAg-negative in terms of mortality, causes
of death, hospitalizations, or hospitalized days.[32] However, among HBsAg-positive
patients, death rates for those who were persistently positive were higher than for those
who were only transiently positive. Although transient elevations in serum alanine aminotransferase (ALT) levels were observed in 76% of the HBsAg-positive HD patients, none
of them developed persistently elevated serum ALT levels or died of liver-related causes
during the follow-up period. Similarly, in a study conducted by Harnett and colleagues,
only a minority of HBsAg-positive HD patients (29%) developed chronic elevations of
liver enzymes during a mean follow-up of 52 months after acquisition of the virus. Thirty-
seven per cent of chronic HBsAg carriers for 2 years or more developed chronic hepatitis, but only one died from liver failure secondary to liver cirrhosis. Thus, the risk of death
from liver disease among these patients was low (3%).[29] Likewise, Parfrey and colleagues
reported that of the 3.4% (out of 295) of dialysis patients who developed chronic
hepatitis, only half were HBsAg-positive. No patient died from chronic liver disease.[33]

Because serum ALT levels in HD patients tend to underestimate the prevalence and
severity of liver disease (due to suppressed transaminase activity at baseline), the lack of
serum ALT elevations in HBsAg-positive HD patients cannot reliably exclude the presence of liver disease or the progression of already existing liver pathology. Indeed, serial
liver biopsies in HBsAg-positive HD patients have provided histological evidence of slow
but relentless progression of liver disease.[29] Nonetheless, the observed low mortality rate
from liver disease in this study argues against the existence of aggressive liver disease.
Yet, due to the slow progression of HBV-induced liver disease, a potential adverse effect
of HBV infection on patient morbidity and mortality that extends beyond the observation period or the mean life duration of HD patients could remain undetected.
Therefore, with longer follow-up periods and, even more importantly, with the
improved survival of HD patients due to the constantly improving quality of dialysis
treatment, the burden of HBV infection is likely to become more apparent.

Risk factors for acquiring HBV infection

Significant success has been achieved in identifying the risk factors implicated in the
spread of HBV between dialysis patients. This has made possible the development of
preventive measures and infections control strategies that have proved to be very
successful in controlling HBV infection in this population. However, the relative importance of the different risk factors has changed over the years. Today, while some of the
risk factors are only of historical interest, others are gaining increasing importance, which
mandates constant updates of the current infections control policies and practices.

Number of blood transfusions

In the early surveys of dialysis-associated hepatitis serological evidence of HBV infection was strongly correlated with the number of units of blood transfused. However, the implementation of mandatory blood donor screening for HBsAg and ALT and the exclusion of those who are HBsAg-positive or have elevated serum ALT activity from the blood donor pool almost eliminated the risk of HBV transmission with blood transfusions. Indeed, as we already noted, the risk of acquiring post-transfusion HBV infection in the United States is currently estimated at 1 in 63 000.[9] In addition, more recently the significant decrease in blood transfusion requirements of ESRD patients associated with the advent of erythropoietin for treatment of chronic anaemia in these patients has further reduced the importance of blood transfusions for the spread of HBV infection in dialysis patients. Today, blood transfusions play a negligible role in HBV transmission in the dialysis population.

Duration of HD

Several studies have found that HBsAg-positive patients have spent a significantly longer time on dialysis than HBsAg-negative ones.[23,32,34] Hence, the duration of HD treatment appears to be an important risk factor for contracting HBV infection. It is plausible that a longer time on dialysis apparently increases the hazard of exposure to HBV within the dialysis unit. This is of particular relevance for HBV-susceptible patients.

Mode of dialysis

Patients receiving in-centre chronic dialysis treatment have been found to have a higher risk of contracting HBV infection than patients on home dialysis.[21] Similarly, a number of studies have shown that HD patients, compared with those on PD, are at an increased risk of contracting HBV and have, indeed, a higher incidence and prevalence of HBV infection.[35-38] Since the CDC do not report currently on the incidence and prevalence of HBs antigenaemia in PD patients, no national data are available to compare the risk of acquiring HBV infection with respect to the mode of dialysis. Yet it seems likely that PD patients have an overall reduced risk for parenteral or nosocomial transmission of the virus because of their lower requirement for blood transfusions, absence of an access site and extracorporeal blood circuit, and the more isolated environment in which they receive their renal replacement therapy.[39]

Other factors

Other known risk factors refer mostly to acquiring HBV from community sources. These include the incidence and prevalence of HBV infection in the background population and high-risk behaviour, such as intravenous drug use, body piercing and tattoos, promiscuity, homosexuality, etc. Their relative role in the transmission of HBV in dialysis patients varies between dialysis centres depending on the location of the dialysis centre and the population served.

Nosocomial transmission of HBV in HD units

HBV is the most efficiently transmitted bloodborne infection in the dialysis setting. Consequently, nosocomial transmission within the dialysis unit continues to be an important mode of HBV transmission. It usually occurs through several mechanisms involving the following risk factors.

Breakdown in standard infection control practices

Outbreaks of HBV infection in dialysis units can occur as a result of non-compliance of dialysis staff with preventive measures and infection control strategies. For example, in one study, an outbreak of hepatitis B caused by one specific HBV subtype was observed in a group of patients who were clustered geographically in one dialysis unit and were attended by the same dialysis staff during the dialysis session. After excluding other risk factors for nosocomial transmission of HBV, dialysis staff seemed to be the most probable vector of HBV transmission in this instance.[40]

Outbreaks of HBV infection in HD centres have typically occurred among patients receiving dialysis treatment on the same shift, in the same room, or using a specific chair location in the room.[40–42] HBV transmission in these cases is likely to have occurred via contaminated environmental surfaces and equipment as a result of unintentional breaks in technique. Similarly, sharing articles between patients, sometimes facilitated by physical proximity in the unit, has been incriminated in the transmission of HBV. Indeed, HBsAg can be recovered from a wide variety of surfaces and equipment routinely handled in the dialysis centre even though no visible blood can be observed.[43] This is well in accordance with the observation that HbsAg-infected blood diluted to the point of becoming invisible and chemically undetectable still contains $10^2–10^3$ HBV virions/ml. In addition, the virus is very durable in the environment and can survive for at least 7 days on environmental surfaces at room temperature.[44]

Obviously, in the dialysis centre, where there is typically a high degree of exposure to blood, an overlooked route of HBV transmission may be inadvertently created starting from HBsAg-positive patients, going to dialysis machine, system, equipment and external surfaces, then to staff members' hands, and from there extending to a HBV-susceptible patient. Thus, contaminated environmental surfaces, equipment, or articles may serve as an important source of infection in the dialysis unit. This environmental mode of HBV transmission is much more important than the internal contamination of dialysis machines and equipment. Its significance is further amplified if disinfection of environmental surfaces is not routinely performed after each use and if equipment is shared between patients.

At least three outbreaks of HBV infection in HD centres have resulted from the use of contaminated multiple-dose injectable vials of local anaesthetic or heparin.[40–42] In each outbreak, the HBV isolates from all infected patients had identical or very closely related DNA sequences, favouring an infection from a common source.

Size of the dialysis centre

The size of the dialysis centre (as measured by the number of patients receiving dialysis) was initially found to correlate directly with the incidence and prevalence of HBsAg in dialysis patients and staff.[27] However, in subsequent surveillance studies this correlation was no longer present.[27] More recently, the size of the dialysis centre has not been reported as an independent risk factor for acquiring HBV infection.[45–48]

Dialysis machines and equipment

In the national survey of dialysis-associated hepatitis in the United States conducted by CDC the type of machine used, i.e. single-pass versus recirculating, was not correlated with the incidence or prevalence of HBV infection in the dialysis centres.[27] However, malfunctioning of dialysis machines with occurrence of blood leaks has resulted in nosocomial spread of HBV infection within dialysis centres. Blood leaks, which occur due to breaks or ruptures of the dialysis membrane, are likely to result in contamination of staff and the environment, from where the virus is subsequently passed to susceptible patients. As proof, the investigation of an outbreak of hepatitis B in a dialysis unit in Philadelphia found a temporal relationship of blood leaks with onset of HBs antigenaemia, consistent with the length of the incubation period of hepatitis B. Furthermore, there was a correlation between the increasing rates of blood leaks and the occurrence of new cases of hepatitis. These observations have provided evidence in support of the importance of blood leaks for the dissemination of HBV within the dialysis unit.[49]

Dialyser membranes, HD ultrafiltrate, and peritoneal fluid

In the 1976 annual survey of dialysis-associated hepatitis in the United States conducted by CDC parallel-plate dialysers were associated with a higher incidence and prevalence of HBs antigenaemia in patients and a higher incidence in staff.[27] This association remained unexplained. However, in 1980 these differences were no longer observed.[27]

There has never been an association of a specific dialyser membrane with a higher incidence or prevalence of HBV infection in HD patients. Indeed, all dialysis membranes should be considered impermeable to HBV since the viral particle has a diameter of 42 nm, exceeding several times the size of the pores of even the most porous dialysis membrane (polysulfone 3 nm, PAN 1.8–2.2 nm, AN69 2.9 nm, polyamide 3 nm, polymethyl methacrylate 1.7–7 nm). Nonetheless, tiny alterations in membrane integrity, which can occur during dialyser manufacture, shipping, storage, utilization, or reprocessing, may result in pore defects that are small enough to be detected but large enough to allow the passage of the virus across the membrane.

Reprocessing of dialysers

Data from the 1976 CDC survey of dialysis-associated hepatitis and a Renal Physicians Association survey on dialyser reuse in the United States demonstrated that the practice of reusing disposable dialysers was not associated with an increased risk of HBV infection in HD patients or staff.[50] Similarly, the national survey on dialysis-associated hepatitis and other diseases in 1980, conducted jointly by CDC and the Health Care Financing Administration, failed to reveal any association of dialyser reuse with increased incidence and prevalence of HBs antigenaemia or prevalence of HBsAb in patients or staff.[27] More recent reports confirm the lack of association of dialyser reuse with an increased risk of HBV infection in both patients and staff.[46–48]

Hepatitis B vaccination

The incidence of HBV infection in dialysis patients has been correlated to the rate of hepatitis B vaccination in the dialysis unit. Centres where 50% or fewer of patients were vaccinated against HBV have higher incidence of HBV than centres with vaccination rates above 50%.[47,48] Furthermore, a logistic regression model of data that were pooled from 1992 to 1994 demonstrated that having fewer than 50% of HD patients vaccinated for HBV was an independent risk factor for acute HBV infection.[47] Vaccination is dealt with in Chapter 21.

Treatment of HBV infection in HD patients

Antiviral therapy is the mainstay in the treatment of chronic HBV infection. The goal of this therapy is to eradicate HBV and thus on the one hand to eliminate infectivity, which will consequently limit the spread of HBV, and on the other hand to induce remission of the liver disease and prevent progression to cirrhosis and HCC. Ultimately, this will improve survival in patients with chronic HBV infection.

Interferon-α (IFN-α) is the first antiviral therapy of proven benefit in the treatment of chronic HBV infection. IFN-α is usually administered as subcutaneous injections in doses of 5 million units (MU) daily or 10 MU three times a week for 16 weeks. Prolonging treatment beyond 24 weeks has not been shown to increase the response rate. In the general population, IFN-α is recommended early in the course of HBV infection and is indicated in patients with chronic HBV infection (HBsAg-positive for more than 6 months), who have evidence of active virus replication (HBeAg-positive and HBV DNA-positive), and active liver disease (elevated serum ALT concentration and chronic hepatitis on liver biopsy). In patients who have cirrhosis on liver biopsy but no clinical evidence of decompensation this treatment is considered to be safe. In other clinical settings (HBeAg-positive and HBV DNA-positive patients with normal serum ALT; HBeAg-negative, but HBV DNA-positive patients, with elevated serum ALT, and HBV DNA-positive patients wth decompensated cirrhosis), the efficacy of IFN-α therapy is variable.

In the general population, IFN-α therapy has been associated with an overall response rate of 30 to 40%. A positive response is commonly defined as the loss of viral replication markers (HBeAg and serum HBV DNA) within 12 months of the initiation of treatment.[51] Sustained response has been associated with improved overall survival.[51,52] About 30 to 50% of patients receiving IFN-α therapy may demonstrate at least two-fold increase in serum ALT levels, which probably reflects immune-mediated lysis of infected hepatocytes.[53] If this increase in serum ALT concentration becomes severe and is accompanied by symptoms or a substantial hyperbilirubinaemia, IFN-α may need to be discontinued or the dose reduced. In cases that respond successfully to IFN-α therapy, there is subsequent normalization of serum ALT and decreased necroinflammatory activity.

IFN-α is an expensive treatment. In addition, it may be frequently accompanied by side-effects. As new therapies emerge, the role of IFN-α in the treatment of chronic HBV infection should be revisited.

New therapeutic approaches include lamivudine and famciclovir and have shown promising preliminary results.[54] Lamivudine is a nucleoside analogue, which inhibits viral DNA synthesis. Long-term trials have demonstrated the safety and effectiveness of this drug in the treatment of chronic hepatitis B.[55,56] Lamivudine was recently approved by the United States Food and Drug Administration for the treatment of chronic hepatitis B. Famciclovir, another nucleoside analogue with antiviral properties, is currently in phase III clinical trials and has shown promise in the treatment of chronic HBV infection.

Although the same principles of therapy apply to HBV-infected dialysis patients, data on the use of lamivudine in patients on renal replacement therapy are limited. It is note-worthy that decreasing renal function has been found to be associated with a proportional reduction in lamivudine clearance in an apparently linear relationship. In addition, it has been demonstrated that lamivudine is well dialysable, but because of its large volume of distribution (approximately 100 litres), a 4-h hemodialysis session cannot significantly affect lamivudine blood concentrations in most subjects. Therefore, in patients with renal dysfunction the lamivudine dose should be adjusted to the degree of renal impair-ment. However, no further dose modification is needed for patients undergoing chronic HD treatment.[57] An important problem with lamivudine treatment is the emergence of lamivudine-resistant HBV strains. A recent study has reported that this phenomenon occurs frequently in HD patients.[58] Because of the high risk of HBV genotypic resistance to lamivudine in this population, the authors of this study have suggested that lamivu-dine therapy should be restricted to only those patients who have severe liver disease.

Currently, no information is available on the safety and effectiveness of the use of famciclovir in patients of maintenance dialysis.

HBV infection in kidney transplantation

Prevalence of HBV infection

The prevalence of HBs antigenaemia in renal transplant recipients is in the range of 1.8% to 18%.[33,59–63] This wide variation reflects differences between studies with respect to transplant policies, study populations, and geographical areas.

Transmission of HBV by organ transplantation

Hepatitis B is transmitted by solid organ transplantation. The risk of transmission is a function of the serological status of both donor and recipient. As an example, in one study, five HBsAg-negative/HBsAb-negative ESRD patients were transplanted with kidneys from three HBsAg-positive cadaver donors, two of whom were also HBeAg-positive.[64] The single recipient from the first HBsAg-positive/HBeAg-positive donor had anti-HBc antibody prior to transplantation and remained HBsAg-negative in the post-transplant period. Both recipients of kidneys from the second HBsAg-positive/HBeAg-positive donor became positive for HBsAg after transplantation. Furthermore, the HBV subtypes in these recipients were identical to the subtype of the donor. The third donor was HBsAg-positive/HBeAg-negative, and neither of his two recipients became HBsAg-positive following transplantation. However, one of the patients developed HBsAb. The antibody production in this case was presumably triggered by exposure to the donor's HBsAg. This observation clearly demonstrates that transmission of HBV infection does occur and is more likely to happen with the use of allografts from HBsAg-positive donors who are also HBeAg-positive as HBe antigenaemia is a marker of active viral replication and consequently associated with high degree of infectivity.[65,66]

The kidney tissue itself is unlikely to carry HBV. Presumably, the vehicle of transmission is the residual blood retained in the transplant. If this is true, certain techniques for handling and preservation of the kidney allografts after harvesting may have impact on the risk of allograft infectivity by modulating the infectious burden transmitted to the recipients. In support of this possibility, is a case report by Lutwick and colleagues wherein two kidneys were harvested from an HBsAg-positive/HBeAg-positive donor in whom serological results were not available at the time of organ procurement.[67] Both kidneys were transplanted into HBsAg-negative/HBsAb-negative recipients. One of the kidneys was packed in ice and transplanted 6 h later. Post-transplantation, the recipient developed asymptomatic HBs-antigenaemia. HBsAg subtyping revealed that both recipient and donor had the same subtype. The other kidney was mechanically perfused for 40 h prior to transplantation. The recipient of this kidney subsequently became positive for HBsAb but never developed HBs-antigenaemia. Importantly, HBsAg was present in the perfusate from that kidney. As a certain amount of infectious load is probably needed to ensure viral transmission, the continuous mechanical perfusion may have cleared some of the virus, thus reducing the infectious burden to an extent insufficient to establish infection in the recipient. Nevertheless, the production of HBsAb in the post-transplant period indicates that the recipient was exposed to HBsAg, most probably from the donor, as no other source of infection could be identified.

Transplantation policies

Although the majority of organ procurement organizations do not accept kidneys from HBsAg-positive donors, such a moratorium has been recently questioned. Based on published data, it seems that only chronic HBsAg carriers who are HBeAg-positive can transmit hepatitis B infection to their recipients.[64,67] On the other hand, in areas endemic for hepatitis B, such as Hong Kong and Saudi Arabia, the chronic HBsAg carrier rate is so high that it is difficult to reject all HBsAg-positive donors (10% of all potential donors are HBsAg-positive), especially when they are HLA-matched living relatives.[68–70] At the same time, the prevalence of naturally occurring immunity to hepatitis B virus infection in the adult population in these areas is as high as 40 to 50%, which makes it easy to find immune patients who could potentially receive allografts from HBsAg-positive donors with no or a low risk of acquiring new infection with the donor strain.[70,71] Therefore, the potential exists for the use of kidneys from HBsAg-positive/HBeAg-negative donors in HBsAg-negative patients who are immune to hepatitis B virus. Chan and Chang reported four HBsAg-negative recipients of kidneys from living related HBsAg-positive/HBeAg-negative donors.[69] All but one of the recipients had serological evidence of exposure to HBV prior to transplantation. Hyperimmune gammaglobulin was given to all patients at the time of transplantation. None of the recipients became HBsAg-positive or manifested any evidence of hepatic dysfunction after transplantation. In a similar study, Al-Khader and colleagues reported post-transplantation outcomes in three HBsAg-negative recipients of kidneys from HBsAg-positive/HBeAg-negative donors (two cadaver and one living-related).[68] Post-transplantation, all three patients remained negative for HBsAg and had normal liver function. Hyperimmune gammaglobulin and a booster dose of recombinant hepatitis B vaccine (to boost the pre-existing immunity) were simultaneously administered to all patients at the time of transplantation. In another study 10 out of 11 recipients of kidneys from HBsAg-positive donors were HBsAg-negative with pre-existing immunity from a previous contact with the virus or active immunization with subsequent adequate antibody response.[72] Only one recipient was HBsAg-positive at the time of transplantation. All 10 HBsAg-negative recipients remained HBsAg-negative after transplantation and no case of active HBV disease was observed, including in the HBsAg-positive patient. The allograft apparently did not transmit HBV to any of the recipients. Obviously, none of the recipients acquired HBV infection transmitted with the kidney allograft.

In conclusion, HBV can be transmitted via organs donated from HBsAg-positive donors who are simultaneously positive for HBeAg. However, kidneys from HBsAg donors who are negative for HBeAg may be considered for transplantation in HBsAg-negative recipients with pre-existing naturally acquired or postvaccination immunity to HBV. Perioperative hyperimmune globulin is recommended in both of these groups.

Since HBsAg carriage can be associated with delta agent (hepatitis D virus) super-infection, simultaneous transmission of delta agent with HBsAg can occur.[73] Lloveras and colleagues reported transmission of delta agent to two healthy HBsAg carriers by kidneys procured from a single HBsAg-positive donor with known heroin addiction.[74] One of the recipients developed severe hepatitis. Liver histology was consistent with severe acute hepatitis. Aminoperoxidase staining identified the presence of delta agent. Thirteen months later, antidelta antibodies were present in the blood. The other recipient developed fulminant hepatitis 14 weeks post-transplantation and died within 48 h. Liver histology was not reported. The authors recommend that routine serological screening for delta infection should be performed whenever organs from HBsAg-positive donors are to be used for transplantation into HBsAg-positive recipients, particularly if risk factors such as a history of drug addiction are present in the donors.

Clinical course of HBV infection in renal transplant recipients

The clinical presentation of hepatitis B in renal transplant recipients is commonly insidious because of the state of immunosuppression. In general, clinically recognizable acute hepatitis is almost never observed. Jaundice is rarely manifested and clinical symptoms tend to be mild, usually consisting only of vague complaints of general fatigue, malaise, or anorexia. Not uncommonly, the disease is asymptomatic and remains undiagnosed until its chronic phase.[70] In fact, frank liver disease becomes clinically apparent only when it reaches its advanced stages, late after transplantation.[75] Laboratory tests typically show only mild elevations in the serum ALT activity, sometimes associated with increased serum bilirubin concentrations. Occasionally, serum ALTs do not return to normal values, but demonstrate fluctuating levels at different times.[76] Liver dysfunction usually presents within the first 12 months. The presence of abnormal liver function tests (LFT) for more than 6 months defines the liver disease as chronic.

Among HBV-infected renal transplant recipients, HBs antigenaemia commonly persists, indicating uninterrupted viral replication, most likely secondary to iatrogenic immunosuppression.[77,78] In some studies, enhanced HBV replication has been associated both with increased prevalence and accelerated progression of liver disease and therefore, was found to be a predictor of poor prognosis.[59,79–81]

Compared with an HBsAg-negative patient, a patient who is HBsAg-positive on the day of renal transplantation has a 30-fold increased relative risk of developing post-transplant chronic hepatitis.[82] The mechanisms of liver injury are not well understood, but it is believed that liver destruction is immune-mediated and occurs at the peak of intrahepatic viral reproduction. On the other hand, it is also possible that the enhanced viral replication somehow arises from the increased immunological reaction to HBV-infected hepatocytes.[80] Since the degree of viral replication can be precisely estimated by HBV DNA concentration, serial determinations of HBV DNA levels might be useful for non-invasive monitoring of the activity of liver disease. Peaks in HBV DNA concentrations may correctly identify transition from a relatively quiescent liver disease to an active phase and alert the clinician to the need for liver biopsy or adjustment of the immuno-suppressive regimen.[79] However, a marked decline in the serum HBV DNA concentration in those with previously diagnosed chronic active hepatitis may signify progression to cirrhosis and probably reflects loss of hepatic mass harbouring the virus.[79]

The time of acquisition of HBV infection, as evidenced by the appearance of HBsAg, emerges as an important prognostic factor. Renal transplant recipients who became HBsAg-positive in the post-transplantation period as compared with those who acquired HBs antigenaemia prior to transplantation have demonstrated higher mortality rates.[81,83] Most probably this reflects substantial differences in virus–host interaction with respect to whether HBV is acquired in the early post-transplant period when large doses of immunosuppressive drugs are administered or HBV infection has existed for a long period of time prior to renal transplantation.[78]

Overall, the clinical presentation and LFT have shown poor correlation with liver morphology and are poor predictors of the activity of liver disease. Often, the histo-pathological findings on liver biopsy can unexpectedly demonstrate advanced disease. In fact, silent (i.e. in the absence of any overt clinical symptoms or LFT abnormalities) morphological progression of liver disease to cirrhosis is not infrequently seen among HBsAg-positive renal transplant recipients.[75,77] On the contrary, in a few patients with biochemical evidence of hepatic dysfunction, liver biopsy failed to document any patho-logical changes.[75,77] Evidently, liver biopsy is the only means for precise diagnosis and monitoring the degree of liver injury in HBsAg-positive renal transplant recipients.[75,76,79]

Occasionally, hepatitis B in renal transplant recipients may take a fulminant course with fatal outcome.[62,80,84–87] In these rare cases, liver histology at postmortem examina-tion has shown massive hepatic necrosis.[80,85] The pathogenesis of the fulminant liver failure in HBsAg-positive renal transplant recipients is not quite clear. Some cases with fulminant hepatitis have been related to coinfection or superinfection with delta agent.[86] In addition, it has been speculated that massive hepatic necrosis could possibly result from rapid cessation of immunosuppressive therapy with subsequent restoration of cell-mediated immunity and massive destruction of HBV-infected hepatocytes.[85]

HBsAg-positive renal transplant recipients have also demonstrated variable, but mostly, relatively high frequency (1 to 23%) of HCC, which can be attributed to the unique combination of rapid histological deterioration to liver cirrhosis (the most important risk factor for HCC) and increased hepatocarcinogenesis (secondary to persistent or enhanced HBV replication).[30,76,77,88–91] Moreover, transplantation by itself carries an increased risk of malignancy.[88] Despite discontinuation of immunosuppressive drugs and institution of chemotherapy, HCC in this population has demonstrated an accelerated course with fatal outcome.[30,77]

Factors affecting the course of hepatitis B in renal transplant recipients

Several factors can affect the course of HBV infection in renal transplant recipients. The most important among these are duration of HBV infection, type of immunosuppressive regimen, and type of HBV infection (reactivation vs. *de novo* infection).

Duration of HBV infection

Because of the insidious course of hepatitis B in renal transplant recipients, HBV-induced liver disease in this population becomes manifest only after advanced stages have been reached, usually as a result of a long-lasting HBV infection and in the late post-transplant period. Therefore, a sufficiently long follow-up period is crucial for the precise assessment of the relative risk of post-transplant liver disease in HBsAg-positive renal transplant recipients. Indeed, only studies with follow-up extending beyond 3 years have been able to demonstrate an increased incidence of liver disease in general, and of more severe forms of liver disease in particular.[75]

Type of immunosuppressive regimen

A number of studies have examined the association between the type of immunosuppressive regimen and the incidence and progression of liver disease. Early series, in which patients were receiving the combination of azathioprine and prednisone, have reported a high incidence of chronic liver disease in HBsAg-positive patients which could have been, at least in part, related to the hepatotoxic effect of azathioprine and the enhanced viral replication induced by high-dose prednisone treatment.[77,92,93] Furthermore, immunosuppressive regimens using antilymphocyte preparations in HBsAg-positive renal transplant recipients in addition to azathioprine and prednisone have been associated with a high frequency of progression to liver cirrhosis and a high mortality from liver disease.[76,94] The use of cyclosporine A (CsA) in the triple-therapy regimen (CsA, azathioprine, and prednisone) has allowed a decrease in both azathioprine and prednisone doses. Therefore, CsA-based triple therapy is believed to be less hepatotoxic and to have less of an enhancing effect on viral replication, and consequently to be associated with a lower incidence of post-transplant liver disease in HBsAg-positive renal transplant recipients.[94] Indeed, there has been a trend towards a lower incidence of liver disease in HBsAg-positive patients in more recent studies, in which most of the patients are on triple therapy, as compared with the older ones that have traditionally used a regimen of azathioprine and prednisone.[94] In addition, a regimen only of CsA and prednisone has been associated with a low (27%) incidence of chronic liver dysfunction in HBsAg-positive renal transplant recipients.[94] Therefore, the combination CsA and prednisone might be the optimal immunosuppressive regimen for HBsAg-positive patients undergoing renal transplantation. However, other investigators have observed no correlation between the type of immunosuppressive regimen and the occurrence of hepatitis in HBsAg-positive renal transplant recipients. Further, they have been unable to demonstrate any statistically significant difference in the risk of developing chronic hepatitis and cirrhosis in those treated with azathioprine as compared with those treated with CsA.[70,78]

Type of HBV infection—reactivation and de novo infection

Reactivation of HBV in the post-transplant period occurs frequently in chronic HBsAg carriers and is commonly attributed to the ability of immunosuppressive drugs, azathioprine, CsA, and prednisone, to cause enhanced and sustained viral replication.[78,95] Serologically, HBV reactivation manifests with reappearance of HBeAg and/or HBV DNA in the serum.[30,59,61,70,79,80] Both persistence and reactivation of viral replication post-transplantation are implicated in the overwhelming majority of cases of chronic hepatitis B among renal transplant recipients.[30,59,61,70,80,85,86] In contrast, *de novo* HBV infection in renal transplant recipients is relatively rare, which suggests that despite the state of iatrogenic immunosuppression, HBsAb can confer protection against hepatitis B.[70,80] Importantly, as previously stated, *de novo* HBV infection in the post-transplant period seems to be associated with a more aggressive clinical course and a worse prognosis.[81,83]

Liver histology

HBs antigenaemia in renal transplant recipients has been associated with more advanced histological forms of liver disease and marked tendency to morphological progression.[30,76,77] Indeed, in renal transplant recipients with clinical evidence of post-transplant chronic liver disease, benign histological lesions (fat metamorphosis and chronic portal triaditis) were predominant on liver biopsies of HBsAg-negative patients, while more severe histological forms of liver disease (chronic persistent hepatitis, chronic active hepatitis, and cirrhosis) were commonly associated with the presence of HBs antigenaemia. In addition, HBsAg-positive recipients, as compared with those who were HBsAg-negative, demonstrated not only a higher incidence of liver cirrhosis (42% versus 19%) on initial liver biopsy, but also a trend towards more frequent progression to cirrhosis during histological follow-up.[76] Indeed, serial liver biopsies have shown that 82% of the HBsAg-positive renal transplant recipients who initially presented with only benign histological lesions (virus only, reactive hepatitis, or chronic persistent hepatitis) progressed to aggressive liver disease (chronic active hepatitis or cirrhosis) after a mean follow-up period of 83 months.[77] Likewise, Fornairon and colleagues have reported an 85% rate of histological deterioration.[30] Hence, HBsAg-positive renal transplant recipients appear to be at an increased risk of developing advanced stages of liver disease and in particular liver cirrhosis.[77] Increased HBV replication, concomitant chronic HCV infection, and chronic alcohol consumption have been recognized as precipitating factors for rapid histological deterioration in HBsAg-positive renal transplant recipients.[30]

In contrast, Dhar and colleagues did not observe any significant tendency to histological progression on serial liver biopsies performed in a group of 16 HBsAg-positive renal transplant recipients with a mean follow-up of 2.1 years.[97] Even in those who were

HBeAg-positive, reactive changes were predominant (in 85% of the cases) and in only one out of seven patients (15%) were histological lesions consistent with chronic active hepatitis. In the few cases where histological progression did, however, occur, it was generally not silent.[97] In fact, patients with chronic active hepatitis had persistently abnormal LFT, cirrhotic patients demonstrated only marginal elevations in liver biochemistry, and patients with normal liver histology had normal liver biochemical tests. A major criticism of this study is the short follow-up period, which might not have allowed enough time for morphological progression to become apparent.

In an attempt to correlate liver histopathology in HBsAg-positive renal transplant recipients with the type of immunosuppressive regimen, Stempel and colleagues reported that in a small group of HBsAg-positive renal transplant recipients receiving CsA-based immunosuppressive therapy, liver biopsy revealed milder histological lesions than those reported in previous studies.[98] Because these earlier studies had included mostly patients treated with azathioprine (known to be hepatotoxic) and prednisone (known to increase HBV replication), the authors postulated that the decrease in the doses of both medications, allowed by the introduction of CsA to the immunosuppressive regimen, might have accounted for the lesser degree of liver impairment. Thus, it appears that HBsAg-positive renal transplant recipients who are treated with CsA might have a lower risk of liver damage than those whose immunosuppressive regimen has included azathioprine and prednisone alone. However, conclusions should be guarded because of the small size and the relatively short follow-up period of this study.[98]

Effect of HBV infection on post-transplantation clinical outcomes in renal transplantation

Patient survival and causes of death

The impact of HBV infection on graft and patient survival following renal transplantation has been a matter of debate for almost three decades. In a number of studies, HBs antigenaemia in renal transplant recipients has not been found to affect adversely graft and patient survival up to 2 years post-transplantation.[59,75,99] However, studies with an extended follow-up period (from 3 years upward) have indeed associated HBs antigenaemia with decreased patient survival in the late post-transplant period.[75] In some other studies, the decrease in patient survival in HBsAg-positive renal transplant recipients, as compared with those who were HBsAg-negative, could in fact be appreciated only after the follow-up period was extended beyond 5 to 15 years.[100,101] Thus, it appears that the adverse effect of HBs antigenaemia in renal transplant recipients mostly affects the long-term survival (beyond 3 years post-transplantation).

In contrast, other investigators have reported significantly higher mortality rates for HBsAg-positive renal transplant recipients, as compared with those who were HBsAg-negative, regardless of the duration of follow-up.[59,79,102] In one study, the accelerated mortality observed in renal transplant recipients who were HBsAg-positive at the time of transplantation, as compared with those who were HBsAg-negative, began shortly after transplantation and was attributed to the combination of pre-existing HBs antigenaemia and the onset of immunosuppression induced by the institution of immunosuppressive therapy.[92] Consequently, the presence of HBs antigenaemia at the time of transplantation appears to be a predictor of poor survival.[92] Likewise, for renal transplant recipients with clinical evidence of post-transplant chronic liver disease, HBsAg-positive patients have shown a higher overall mortality rate than those who were HBsAg-negative.[76] The highest mortality rate (60%) has been reported in HBsAg-positive renal transplant recipients who acquired their disease in the early post-transplant period.[81] It is noteworthy that the association of HBs antigenaemia with a higher mortality in renal transplant recipients has not been uniformly observed. Several studies have failed to detect any significant difference in patient survival between HBsAg-positive and HBsAg-negative renal transplant recipients.[30,70,78,103–105]

In some studies, but not all, mortality due to liver failure was significantly higher for HBsAg-positive renal transplant recipients as compared with HBsAg-negative ones, not infrequently with more than half of all deaths in the HBsAg-positive group attributable to liver disease.[30,75–77,100,105] However, the death rates from causes other than hepatitis were found to be virtually the same in HBsAg-positive and HBsAg-negative renal transplant recipients.[75] In contrast, other studies have demonstrated that the increased mortality in HBsAg-positive renal transplant recipients was not related to hepatic dysfunction, but to other non–hepatic causes, such as sepsis, infections, and vascular pathological events.[92,100,102,106,107] Interestingly, in one report, no deaths due to liver disease occurred in a group of renal transplant recipients who were HBsAg-positive at the time of transplantation.[106]

These controversial data can only be reconciled if the increased risk of developing fatal liver disease were exclusively present in a particular subgroup of renal transplant candidates, namely those with active viral replication as assessed by the presence of HBeAg and/or HBV DNA.[93] Consequently, the wide variation in the incidence of fatal liver disease observed across studies is likely to be related to differences uniquely in the prevalence of HBeAg and/or HBV DNA. These speculations are supported by the observations that survival in HBsAg-positive renal transplant recipients with markers of active viral replication was lower (although not significantly so) than in recipients without these markers. Because an excellent correlation between HBe antigenaemia and serum HBV DNA concentrations has been documented, HBeAg testing, which is relatively easy to perform, widely available, and cheaper, has been recommended as a good and reliable marker of viral replication. It appears that among chronic HBsAg carriers who undergo renal transplantation, increased mortality from liver disease may be confined to patients who are HbeAg- and/or HBV DNA-positive before transplantation. Therefore, a policy not to transplant these patients but to treat and follow them until they become negative for these markers seems reasonable. Once this occurs, the relative risk of fatal post-transplantation liver disease could be significantly decreased.[93]

Effect of renal transplantation on the course of HBV infection in dialysis patients

Although not unanimously supported, some studies have suggested that HBV infection may take an accelerated course after renal transplantation.[77,79,106] Indeed, Harnett and colleagues observed that the mortality rate in HBsAg-positive renal transplant recipients, as compared with that in HBsAg-positive HD patients was significantly higher (64% versus 19%).[79] This difference was attributed to deaths from liver disease (57% versus 17%), which implied that HBV infection in HD patients had a less aggressive course than in renal transplant recipients. These observations raised the question of whether HBsAg-positive ESRD patients should be offered renal transplantation or maintained on chronic dialysis. To date, there is no easy answer to this dilemma. Based on currently available data, several suggestions regarding the management of HBsAg-positive ESRD patients have been made. Overall, the prevailing feeling is that transplantation should not be denied categorically to all HBsAg-positive ESRD patients. The following categories deserve specific consideration. Patients who clinically present with cirrhosis, portal hypertension, or liver failure should be advised to continue on dialysis or should be offered combined liver–kidney transplantation. Patients, who are older, of female sex, or have chronic active hepatitis on liver histology, appear to be at an increased risk of developing cirrhosis in the post-transplant period.[108] The decision whether to transplant them should be made very cautiously. Patients with serological markers of viral replication should first be treated with antiviral agents or IFN-α and offered transplantation once

Table 11.1 Incidence and prevalence of HBsAg in haemodialysis patients and staff, 1976–1997, United States. (Data from Tokars *et al.*[28])

Year	Patients		Staff	
	Incidence	Prevalence	Incidence	Prevalence
1976	3.0	7.8	2.6	ND
1980	1.0	3.8	0.8	0.9
1982	0.5	2.7	0.6	0.5
1983	0.5	2.4	0.5	0.6
1984	0.3	2.3	0.3	0.5
1985	0.3	2.1	0.2	0.3
1986	0.3	1.9	0.1	0.4
1987	0.2	1.7	0.1	0.4
1988	0.2	1.5	0.1	0.3
1989	0.1	1.4	0.1	0.3
1990	0.2	1.2	0.04	0.3
1991	0.2	1.3	0.04	0.3
1992	0.1	1.2	0.03	0.3
1993	0.1	1.2	0.02	0.3
1994	0.1	1.1	0.02	0.3
1995	0.06	1.1	0.02	0.4
1996	0.08	1.1	0.05	0.3
1997	0.05	0.9	0.05	0.4

Table 11.2 Recommendations for serological surveillance for hepatitis B in chronic haemo-dialysis centres. (Reprinted from Moyer LA, Alter MJ, Favero MS. Hemodialysis-associated hepatitis B: revised recommendations for serological screening. *Semin Dial* 1990; 3:201–204, with permission)

Vaccination and serological status	Frequency of screening			
	HBsAg		Anti-HBs	
	Patients	Staff	Patients	Staff
Unvaccinated				
Susceptible	Monthly	Semiannually	Semiannually	Semiannually
HBsAg carrier	Annually	Annually	None	None
Anti-HBs-positive*	None	None	Annually	None
Vaccinees				
Anti-HBs-positive*	None	None	Annually	None
Low level or no anti-HBs	Monthly	Semiannually	Semiannually	Semiannually

*At least 10 SRUs by RIA or positive by EIA.

Table 11.3 Recommended doses and schedules for adults of currently licensed hepatitis B vaccines. (Reprinted from Moyer LA, Alter MJ, Favero MS. Hemodialysis-associated hepatitis B: revised recommendations for serological screening. *Semin Dial* 1990; 3:201–204, with permission)

Group	Heptavax-B[a,b]	Recombivax HB[a]	Energix-B[a,c]
Dialysis patients	40 mg (2 ml)[d,e]	40 mg (1 ml)[d]	40 mg (2 ml)[f]
Healthy adults	20 mg (1 ml)	10 mg (1 ml)	20 mg (1 ml)

[a]Usual schedule: three doses at 0, 1, 6 months.
[b]Available only for haemodialysis and other immunocompromised patients and for persons with known allergy to yeast.
[c]Alternative schedule: four doses at 0, 1, 2, 12 months.
[d]Two 1.0 ml doses given at different sites.
[e]Special formulation for dialysis patients.
[f]Four-dose schedule recommended at 0, 1, 2, 6 months.

these markers become negative. Patients with advanced histological forms of liver disease will probably fit in one of the above categories, and although they are expected to do poorly after transplantation, this may not necessarily happen. Therefore, the decision whether to transplant them should be individualized and made in harmony with the patient's desires.

In conclusion, since no general principles can apply to the selection of HBsAg-positive patients for renal transplantation, each case should be decided individually with the participation of a well informed patient capable of understanding and weighing the risks and benefits of transplantation and comparing the expected quality of life with renal transplant to the current and projected quality of life on dialysis.

Prevention and treatment of HBV infection in ESRD patients

Hepatitis B is a preventable disease. Large-scale vaccination of all susceptible predialysis and dialysis patients can increase the percentage of immune individuals, and thus prevent the spread of HBV infection in the ESRD population. This practice is particularly important because, due to the existing immunosuppression, hepatitis B vaccination of renal transplant recipients is associated with a poor antibody response (18 to 36%).[109,110] On the other hand, it has been shown that since secondary immune responses are relatively well maintained under immunosuppression, renal transplant recipients successfully vaccinated before transplantation, who had subsequently lost their protective immunity, could benefit from a booster dose. In this scenario, a booster injection of 40 µg given intramuscularly resulted in a rise in the HBsAb titre above the protective level in 86% of the patients.[110] In addition, strict enforcement of and adherence to HD unit precautions is crucial in preventing the spread of HBV infection in dialysis units and consequently in renal transplant candidates.

As already discussed, IFN-α is an antiviral therapy of proven benefit in the treatment of chronic hepatitis B. However, this therapy has been associated with risk of inducing acute transplant rejection. Consequently, IFN-α should be avoided in renal transplant recipients.

Among the newer therapies, the effectiveness of lamivudine has been studied in a small group of six HBV DNA-positive cadaver renal transplant recipients. Lamivudine therapy led to rapid disappearance of HBV DNA from the serum in all patients and normalization of ALT in four of five patients with initial elevation of ALT levels. Importantly, there were no changes in renal function and no adverse effects associated with this treatment. Discontinuation of lamivudine after a 6-month course resulted in biochemical and virological relapse within weeks, which required reinstitution of lamivudine therapy.[111] As in HD patients, because of frequent emergence of lamivudine-resistant HBV strains in renal transplant recipients, treatment with lamivudine should be restricted to patients with severe liver disease.[58]

References

1. Sato S, Suzuki K, Akahane Y, *et al.* Hepatitis B virus strains with mutations in the core promoter in patients with fulminant hepatitis. *Ann Intern Med* 1995; **122**:241–248.
2. Baumert TF, Rogers SA, Hasegawa K, Liang TJ. Two core promoter mutations identified in a hepatitis B virus strain associated with fulminant hepatitis result in enhanced viral replication. *J Clin Invest* 1996; **98**:2268–2276.
3. Akarca US, Greene S, Lok AS. Detection of pre-core hepatitis B virus mutants in asymptomatic HBsAg-positive family members. *Hepatology* 1994; **19**:1366–1370.
4. Locarnini SA, Gust ID. Hepadnaviridae: hepatitis B virus and delta virus. In: Balow A, Hausler WJJ, Lennette EH (eds) *Laboratory diagnosis of infectious diseases. Principles and practice*, vol. 2, 1988:750–796. Springer, New York.
5. Maruyama T, Schodel F, Iino S, *et al.* Distinguishing between acute and symptomatic chronic hepatitis B virus infection. *Gastroenterology* 1995; **106**:1006–1015.
6. Hadler SC, Murphy BL, Schable CA, Heyward WL, Francis DP, Kane MA. Epidemiological analysis of the significance of low positive test results for antibody to hepatitis B surface and core antigens. *J Clin Microbiol* 1984; **19**:521–525.

7. Joller-Jemelka HI, A.N. W, Grob PJ. Detection of HBs antigen in 'anti-HBc alone' positive sera. *J Hepatol* 1994; 21:269–272.

8. Lok ASF, Lai CL, Wu PC. Prevalence of isolated antibody to hepatitis B core antigen in an area endemic for hepatitis B virus infection: Implication in hepatitis B vaccination programs. *Hepatology* 1988; 8:766–770.

9. Schreiber GB, Busch MP, Kleinman SH, Korelitz JJ. The risk of transfusion-transmitted viral infections. The Retrovirus Epidemiology Donor Study (see comments). *New Engl J Med* 1996; 334:1685–1690.

10. Alter HJ, Seef LB, Kaplan PM, *et al*. Type B hepatitis: the infectivity of blood positive for e antigen and DNA polymerase after accidental needlestick exposure. *New Engl J Med* 1976; 295:909–913.

11. Kingsley LA, Rinaldo CR, Lyter DW, Valdiserri RO, Belle SH, Ho M. Sexual transmission efficiency of hepatitis B virus and HIV among homosexual men. *J Am Med Assoc* 1990; 264:230–234.

12. Rosenblum L, Darrow W, Witte J, *et al*. Sexual practices in the transmission of hepatitis B virus and prevalence of hepatitis Delta virus infection in female prostitutes in the United States. *J Am Med Assoc* 1992; 267:2477–2481.

13. Botha JF, Ritchie MJJ, Dusheiko GM, Mouton HWK, Kew MC. Hepatitis B virus carrier state in black children in Ovamboland: Role of perinatal and horizontal infection. *Lancet* 1984; i:1210–1212.

14. Tabor E, Bayley AC, Cairns L, Gerety RJ. Horizontal transmission of hepatitis B virus among children and adults in five villages in Zambia. *J Med Virol* 1985; 15:113–120.

15. Natov SN, Pereira BJG. Transmission of disease by organ transplantation. In: Chapman JR, Deierhoi M, Wight C (eds) *Organ and tissue donation for transplantation*, 1997:120–151. Edward Arnold, London.

16. Liaw YF, Sheen IS, Chen TJ, Chu CM, Pao CC. Incidence, determinants and significance of delayed clearance of serum HBsAg in chronic hepatitis B virus infection: A prospective study. *Hepatology* 1991; 13:627–631.

17. Di Bisceglie AM, Rustgi VK, Hoofnagle JH, Dusheiko GM, Lotze MT. NIH conference: hepatocellular carcinoma. *Ann Intern Med* 1988; 108:390–401.

18. Dusheiko G. Hepatitis B. In: Bircher J, Benhamou J-P, McIntyre N, Rizzetto M, Rodes J (eds) *Oxford textbook of clinical hepatology*, vol. 1, 1999:876–903. Oxford University Press, Oxford.

19. Lee WM. Hepatitis B virus infection. *New Engl J Med* 1997; 337:1733–1745.

20. CDC. *Hepatitis Surveillance Report*, No. 30, 1969:15–20. US Department of Health, Education and Welfare, Atlanta.

21. Snydman DR, Bryan JA, Hanson B. Hemodialysis-associated hepatitis in the United States—1972. *J Infect Dis* 1975; 132:109–113.

22. Snydman DR, Bregman D, Bryan JA. Hemodialysis-associated hepatitis in the United States, 1974. *J Infect Dis* 1977; 135:687–691.

23. Szmuness W, Prince AM, Grady GF, *et al*. Hepatitis B infection: A point-prevalence study in 15 US hemodialysis centers. *J Am Med Assoc* 1974; 227:901–906.

24. Marmion BP, Tonkin RE. Control of hepatitis in dialysis units. *Br Med Bull* 1972; 28:169–179.

25. Soulier JP, Jungers P, Zingraff J. Virus B hepatitis in hemodialysis centers. *Adv Nephrol* 1976; 6:383–405.

26. Kleinknecht D, Courouce AM, Delons S, *et al*. Prevention of hepatitis B in hemodialysis patients using hepatitis B immunoglobulin: A controlled study. *Clin Nephrol* 1977; 8:373–376.

27. Alter MJ, Favero MS, Petersen NJ, Doto IL, Leger RT, Maynard JE. National surveillance of dialysis-associated hepatitis and other diseases, 1976 and 1980. *Dial Transplant* 1983; 12:860–866.
28. Tokars JI, Miller ER, Alter MJ, Arduino MJ. National surveillance of dialysis associated diseases in the United States, 1997. *Semin Dial* 2000; 13:75–85.
29. Harnett JD, Parfrey PS, Kennedy M, Zeldis JB, Steinman TI, Guttmann RD. The long-term outcome of hepatitis B infection in hemodialysis patients. *Am J Kidney Dis* 1988; 11:210–213.
30. Fornairon S, Pol C, Legendre C, *et al.* The long-term virologic and pathologic impact of renal transplantation on chronic hepatitis B virus infection. *Transplantation* 1996; 62:297–299.
31. Favero MS, Maynard JE, Leger RT, Graham DR, Dixon RE. Guidelines for patients hospitalized with viral hepatitis. *Ann Intern Med* 1979; 91:872–876.
32. Josselson J, Kyser BA, Weir MR, Sadler JH. Hepatitis B antigenemia in a chronic hemodialysis program: lack of influence on morbidity and mortality. *Am J Kidney Dis* 1987; 9:456–461.
33. Parfrey PS, Farge D, Forbes C, Dandavino R, Kenick S, Guttman RD. Chronic hepatitis in end-stage renal disease: comparison of HBsAg-negative and HBsAg-positive patients. *Kidney Int* 1985; 28:959–967.
34. Garibaldi RA, Forrest NJ, Bryan AJ, *et al.* Hemodialysis-associated hepatitis. *J Am Med Assoc* 1973; 225:384–389.
35. Mioli VA, Balestra E, Bibiano L, *et al.* Epidemiology of viral hepatitis in dialysis centers: a national survey. *Nephron* 1992; 61:278–283.
36. Cendoroglo Neto M, Manzano SI, Canziani ME, *et al.* Environmental transmission of hepatitis B and hepatitis C viruses within the hemodialysis unit. *Artif Organs* 1995; 19:251–255.
37. Cendoroglo-Neto M, Draibe SA, Silva AE, *et al.* Incidence of and risk factors for hepatitis B virus and hepatitis C virus infection among haemodialysis and CAPD patients: evidence for environmental transmission. *Nephrol Dial Transplant* 1995; 10:240–246.
38. Ambuhl PM, Binswanger U, Renner EL. Epidemiology of chronic hepatitis B and C among dialysis patients in Switzerland. *Schweiz Med Wochenschr* 2000; 130:341–348.
39. Chan TM, Lok ASF, Cheng IKP. Hepatitis C infection among dialysis patients: A comparison between patients on maintenance haemodialysis and continuous ambulatory peritoneal dialysis. *Nephrol Dial Transplant* 1991; 6:944–947.
40. Rosenberg J, Gilliss DL, Moyer L, Vugia D. A double outbreak of hepatitis B in a dialysis center. *SHEA J* 1995; 16:19.
41. Alter MJ, Ahtone J, Maynard JE. Hepatitis B virus transmission associated with a multiple-dose vial in a hemodialysis unit. *Ann Int Med* 1983; 99:330–333.
42. Danzig LE, Tormey MP, Sinha SD, *et al.* Common source transmission of HBV infection in a hemodialysis unit. *SHEA J* 1995; 16:19.
43. Favero MS, Maynard JE, Peterson NJ, *et al.* Hepatitis B antigen on environmental surfaces. *Lancet* 1973; 2:1455.
44. Bond WW, Favero MS, Peterson NJ, Gravelle CRR, Ebert JW, Maynard JE. Survival of hepatitis B after drying and storage for one week. *Lancet* 1981; 1:550–551.
45. Tokars J, Alter MJ, Favero MS, Moyer LA, Miller E, Bland L. National surveillance of hemodialysis associated diseases in the United States, 1992. *ASAIO J* 1994; 40:1020–1031.
46. Tokars J, Alter M, Favero M, Moyer L, Miller E, Bland L. National Surveillance of Dialysis Associated Diseases in the United States, 1993. *ASAIO J* 1996:219–229.
47. Tokars JI, Alter MJ, Miller E, Moyer LA, Favero MS. National surveillance of dialysis associated diseases in the United States—1994. *ASAIO J* 1997; 43:108–119.

48. Tokars JI, Miller ER, Alter MJ, Arduino MJ. National surveillance of dialysis associated diseases in the United States, 1995. *ASAIO J* 1998; **44**:98–107.

49. Snydman DR, Bryan JA, London WT, *et al.* Transmission of hepatitis B associated with hemodialysis: role of malfunctioning (blood leaks) in dialysis machines. *J Infect Dis* 1976; **134**:562–570.

50. Favero MS, Deane N, Leger RT, Sosin AE. Effect of multiple use of dialyzers on hepatitis B incidence in patients and staff. *J Am Med Assoc* 1981; **245**:166–167.

51. Niederau C, Heintges T, Lange S, *et al.* Long-term follow-up of HBeAg-positive patients treated with interferon alfa for chronic hepatitis B. *New Engl J Med* 1996; **334**:1422–1427.

52. Fattovich G, Realdi G, Corrocher R, Schalm SW. Long-term outcome of hepatitis B e antigen-positive patients with compensated cirrhosis treated with interferon alfa. European Concerted Action on Viral Hepatitis (EUROHEP). *Hepatology* 1997; **26**:1338–1342.

53. Perrillo RP. The management of chronic hepatitis. *Am J Med* 1994; **96**:34S–40S.

54. Hoofnagle JH. The treatment of chronic viral hepatitis. *New Engl J Med* 1997; **336**:347–356.

55. Lai CL, Chien RN, Leung NWY, *et al.* A one-year trial of lamivudine for chronic hepatitis B. *New Engl J Med* 1998; **339**:61–68.

56. Dienstag JL, Schiff ER, Wright TL, *et al.* Lamivudine as initial treatment for chronic hepatitis B in the United States. *New Engl J Med* 1999; **341**:1256–1263.

57. Johnson MA, Verpooten GA, Daniel MJ, *et al.* Single dose pharmcokinetics of lamivudine in subjects with impaired renal function and the effect of haemodialysis. *Br J Clin Pharmacol* 1998; **46**:21–27.

58. Fontaine H, Thiers V, Chretien Y, *et al.* HBV genotypic resistance to lamivudine in kidney recipients and hemodialysis patients. *Transplantation* 2000; **69**:2090–2094.

59. Degos F, Lugassy C, Degott C, *et al.* Hepatitis B virus and hepatitis B-related viral infection in renal transplant recipients. *Gastroenterology* 1988; **94**:151–156.

60. Pol S, Debure A, Degott C, *et al.* Chronic hepatitis in kidney allograft recipients. *Lancet* 1990; **335**:878–880.

61. Durlik M, Gaciong Z, Soluch L, *et al.* Risk of chronic liver disease in HBsAg and/or anti-HCV-positive renal allograft recipients. *Transplant Proc* 1996; **28**:50–51.

62. Yagisawa T, Toma H, Tanabe K, *et al.* Long-term outcome of renal transplantation in hepatitis B surface antigen-positive patients in the cyclosporin era. *Am J Nephrol* 1997; **17**:440–444.

63. Mathurin P, Mouquet C, Poynard T, *et al.* Impact of hepatitis B and C virus on kidney transplantation outcome. *Hepatology* 1999; **29**:257–263.

64. Wolf JL, Perkins HA, Schreeder MT, Vincenti F. The transplanted kidney as a source of hepatitis B infection. *Ann Intern Med* 1979; **91**:412–413.

65. Shikata T, Karasawa T, Abe K, *et al.* Hepatitis B e antigen and infectivity of hepatitis B virus. *J Infect Dis* 1977; **136**:571–576.

66. Fairley CK, Mijch A, Gust ID, Nichilson S, Dimitrakakis M, Lucas CR. The increased risk of fatal liver disease in renal transplant patients who are hepatitis B e antigen and/or HBV DNA positive. *Transplantation* 1991; **52**:497–500.

67. Lutwick LI, Sywassink JM, Corry RJ, Shorey JW. The transmission of hepatitis B by renal transplantation. *Clin Nephrol* 1983; **19**:317–319.

68. Al-Khader AA, Dhar JM, Al-Sulaiman M, Al-Hasani MK. Renal transplantation from HBsAg positive donors to HBsAg negative recipients. *Br Med J* 1988; **297**:854.

69. Chan MK, Chang WK. Renal transplantation from HBsAg positive donors to HBsAg negative recipients. *Br Med J* 1988; **297**:522–523.

70. Chan PC, Lok AS, Cheng IK, Chan MK. The impact of donor and recipient hepatitis B surface antigen status on liver disease and survival in renal transplant recipients. *Transplantation* 1992; **53**:128–131.

71. Talukder MA, Gilmore R, Bacchus RA. Prevalence of hepatitis B surface antigen among male Saudi Arabians. *J Infect Dis* 1982; 146:446.

72. Bedrossian J, Akposso K, Metivier F, Moal MC, Pruna A, Idatte JM. Kidney transplantation with HBsAg positive donors. *Transplant Proc* 1993; 25:1481–1482.

73. Rizzetto M, Canese MG, Arico S, et al. Immunofluorescence detection of new antigen-antibody system (gamma/anti-gamma) associated to hepatitis B virus in liver and in serum of HBsAg carriers. *Gut* 1977; 18:997–1003.

74. Lloveras J, Momteis J, Sanchez-Tapias JM, et al. Delta agent transmission through renal transplantation with severe hepatitis induction in two HBsAg healthy carriers. *Transplant Proc* 1986; 18:467–468.

75. Pirson Y, Alexandre GP, van Ypersele de Striou C. Long-term effect of HBs antigenemia on patient survival after renal transplantation. *New Engl J Med* 1977; 296:194–196.

76. Rao KV, Kasiske BL, Andreson WR. Variability in the morphological spectrum and clinical outcome of chronic liver disease in hepatitis B-positive and B-negative renal transplant recipients. *Transplantation* 1991; 51:391–396.

77. Parfrey PS, Forbes RDC, Hutchinson TA, et al. The impact of renal transplantation on the course of hepatitis B liver disease. *Transplantation* 1985; 39:610–615.

78. Huang C, Lai M, Fong M. Hepatitis-B liver disease in cyclosporine-treated renal allograft recipients. *Transplantation* 1990; 49:540–544.

79. Harnett JD, Zeldis JB, Parfrey PS, et al. Hepatitis B in dialysis and transplant patients. *Transplantation* 1987; 44:369–376.

80. Dusheiko G, Song E, Bowiers S, et al. Natural history of hepatitis B virus infection in renal transplant recipients—a fifteen-year follow-up. *Hepatology* 1983; 3:330–336.

81. Scott D, Mijch A, Lucas CR, Marshall V, Thomson N, Atkins R. Hepatitis B and renal transplantation. *Transplant Proc* 1987; 19:2159–2160.

82. Degos F, Degott C, Bedrossian J, et al. Is renal transplantation involved in post-transplantation liver disease? A prospective study. *Transplantation* 1980; 29:100–102.

83. Anuras S, Piros J, Bonney WW, Forker L, Colville DS, Corry RJ. Liver disease in renal transplant recipients. *Arch Intern Med* 1977; 137:42–48.

84. Ware AJ, Luby JP, Hollinger B, et al. Etiology of liver disease in renal transplant patients. *Ann Intern Med* 1979; 91:364–371.

85. Hanson CA, Sutherland DE, Snover DC. Fulminant hepatic failure in an HBsAg carrier renal transplant patient following cessation of immunosuppressive therapy. *Transplantation* 1985; 39:311–312.

86. Kharsa G, Degott C, Degos F, Carnot F, Potent F, Kreis H. Fulminant hepatitis in renal transplant recipients. The role of the Delta agent. *Transplantation* 1987; 44:221–223.

87. Hung YB, Liang JT, Chu JS, Chen KM, Lee CS. Fulminant hepatic failure in a renal transplant recipient with positive hepatitis B surface antigens: a case report of fibrosing cholestatic hepatitis. *Hepato-Gastroenterology* 1995; 42:913–918.

88. Penn I. The occurrence of cancer in immune deficiencies. *Curr Probl Cancer* 1982; 6:1–64.

89. Schroter GPJ, Weil RI, Penn I, Speers WC, Waddell WR. Hepatocellular carcinoma associated with chronic hepatitis B virus infection after kidney transplantation. *Lancet* 1982; 2:381–382.

90. Colombo M. Hepatocellular carcinoma. *J Hepatol* 1992; 15:225–236.

91. Brechot C. Hepatitis B virus (HBV) and hepatocellular carcinoma: HBV DNA status and its implications. *J Hepatol* 1987; 4:269–279.

92. Hillis W, Hillis A, Walker G. Hepatitis B surface antigenemia in renal transplant recipients. Increased mortality risk. *J Am Med Assoc* 1979; 242:329–332.

93. Fairley C, Mijch A, Gust ID, Nichilson S, Dimitrakakis M, Lucas CR. The increased risk of fatal liver disease in renal transplant patients who are hepatitis Be antigen and/or HBV DNA positive. *Transplantation* 1991; 52:497–500.

94. Hsieh H, Chen CH, Huang HF, Tseng YJ. Optimal immunosuppression regimen for hepatitis B-positive kidney transplant recipients. *Transplant Proc* 1996; 28:1495–1497.
95. Sagnelli E, Mauzillo G, Maio G, *et al.* Serum levels of hepatitis B surface and core antigens during immunosuppressive treatment of HBsAg positive chronic active hepatitis. *Lancet* 1980; 2:395–397.
96. Marcellin P, Giostra E, Martinot-Peignoux M, *et al.* Redevelopment of hepatitis B surface antigen after renal transplantation. *Gastroenterology* 1991; 100:1332–1434.
97. Dhar JM, Al-Khader AA, Al-Sulaiman MH, Al-Hasani MK. The significance and implications of hepatitis B infection in renal transplant recipients. *Transplant Proc* 1991; 23:1785–1786.
98. Stempel C, Lake J, Ferrell L, *et al.* Effect of cyclosporin on the clinical course of HBsAg-positive renal transplant patients. *Transplant Proc* 1991; 23:1251–1252.
99. Chatterjee SN, Payne JE, Bischel MD, *et al.* Succesful renal transplantation in patients positive for hepatitis B antigen. *New Engl J Med* 1974; 291:62–65.
100. Sengar DPS, Couture RA, Lazarovitz AI, Jindal SL. Long-term patient and renal allograft survival in HBsAg infection: a recent update. *Transplant Proc* 1989; 21:3358–3359.
101. Gagnadoux MF, Guest G, Ronsse-Nussenzveig P, Mitsioni A, Broyer M. Long-term outcome of hepatitis B after renal transplantation during childhood. *Transplant Proc* 1993; 25:1454–1455.
102. White AG, Kumar MSA, Stranneegard O, Abouna GM. Renal transplantation in hepatitis B surface antigen-positive patients. *Transplant Proc* 1987; 19:2150–2152.
103. Flagg GL, Silberman H, Takamoto SK, Berne TV. The influence of hepatitis B infection on the outcome of renal allotransplantation. *Transplant Proc* 1987; 19:2155–2158.
104. Ranjan D, Burke G, Esquenazi V, *et al.* Factors affecting the ten-year outcome of human renal allografts. The effect of viral infections. *Transplantation* 1991; 51:113–117.
105. Rivolta E, De Vecchi A, Tarantino A, Castelnovo C, Berardinelli L, Ponticelli C. Prognostic significance of hepatitis B surface antigenemia in cadaveric renal transplant patients. *Transplant Proc* 1987; 19:2153–2154.
106. Friedlaender MM, Kaspa RT, Rubinger D, Silver J, Popovtzer MM. Renal transplantation is not contraindicated in asymptomatic carriers of hepatitis B surface antigen. *Am J Kidney Dis* 1989; 14:204–210.
107. Nelson SR, Snowden SA, Sutherland S, Smith HM, Parsons V, Bewick M. Outcome of renal transplantation in hepatitis BsAg-positive patients. *Nephrol Dial Transplant* 1994; 9:1320–1323.
108. Rao KV, Anderson RW, Kasiske BL, Dahl DC. Value of liver biopsy in the evaluation and management of chronic liver disease in renal transplant recipients. *Am J Med* 1993; 94:241–250.
109. Jacobson IM, Jaffers G, Dienstag JL, *et al.* Immunogenicity of hepatitis B vaccine in renal transplant recipients. *Transplantation* 1985; 39:393–395.
110. Lefebure AF, Verpooten GA, Couttenye MM, De Broe ME. Immunogenicity of a recombinant DNA hepatitis B vaccine in renal transplant recipients. *Vaccine* 1993; 11:397–399.
111. Rostaing L, Henry S, Cisterne JM, Duffaut M, Icart J, Durand D. Efficacy and safety of lamivudine on replication of recurrent hepatitis B after cadaveric renal transplantation. *Transplantation* 1997; 64:1624–1627.

12

Management of renal disease in patients with human immunodeficiency virus infection

T.K. Sreepada Rao

Introduction

The expansion of human immunodeficiency virus (HIV) infection worldwide has led to an increase in the recognition of both the spectrum and the number of patients developing renal diseases. In HIV-infected patients, renal damage can result both as a direct consequence of viral-mediated glomerular/tubular/interstitial injury, and indirectly from the wide systemic derangements induced in the host by the virus, as well as from the therapeutic agents employed in their treatment. Furthermore, well-defined intrinsic primary renal diseases can also occur in patients with prior HIV infection. In addition, patients receiving renal replacement therapy may acquire HIV infection through various routes.

Renal impairment in HIV patients can vary from a mild asymptomatic azotaemia or fluid-electrolyte acid–base disturbances, to severe uraemia necessitating temporary dialysis in those with acute reversible renal failure, or to permanent maintenance dialysis in those who develop end-stage renal disease (ESRD). Renal disorders in patients with HIV infection can be categorized into two broad groups (Table 12.1):

(1) HIV (specific) associated glomerulopathies;
(2) coincidental renal disorders.

Table 12.1 Renal disorders in HIV infection

HIV-specific glomerulopathy	I. HIV-associated nephropathy
	    Focal and segmental glomerulosclerosis
	II. Immune complex glomerulonephritis
	    a. IgA nephropathy
	    b. Other glomerular lesions

Coincidental renal diseases	Infections/Infiltrations in the kidney Fluid-electrolyte, acid–base disturbances Acute renal failure syndromes Intrinsic renal diseases in patients with prior HIV infection HIV infection in patients undergoing maintenance dialysis therapy HIV infection in patients receiving renal transplantation

This chapter will primarily deal with the management of patients with HIV (specific) associated glomerulopathies but will give brief comments on the coincidental renal disorders.

HIV-associated glomerulopathies

Although a variety of glomerular diseases have been reported in HIV patients, one lesion that has been most extensively studied and investigated is focal and segmental glomerulosclerosis (FSGS). We strongly believe that the term HIV-associated nephropathy (HIVAN) should be confined to the description of renal disease manifesting FSGS. HIVAN refers to a syndrome of massive proteinuria, microscopic or gross haematuria, normotension, and an unusually rapid deterioration in renal functional leading to the development of ESRD.[1-6] The disease occurs predominantly in black patients with HIV infection, and is distinctively rare among Caucasians. In one-third of patients, nephropathy may be the initial manifestation prompting clinicians to investigate for the presence of HIV infection. HIVAN is seen in patients irrespective of the route of HIV infection, namely sexual contacts (homo- and heterosexual), needle sharing by intravenous drug abusers, recipients of contaminated blood/blood products, and children born to HIV-infected mothers. Intravenous drug abusers are also at an increased risk of developing another distinct form of FSGS, namely heroin-associated nephropathy. A recent longitudinal study revealed that intravenous drug abusers were three times more likely to develop renal disease if they were infected with HIV as compared to those who were persistently seronegative.[7]

Common clinical feature of HIVAN is nephrotic syndrome, consisting of massive proteinuria, hypoalbuminaemia, and generalized oedema, with or without microscopic or gross haematuria. Occasionally, mild proteinuria (<2 g/day) may be discovered during the evaluation of a non-renal medical problem. Proteinuria is accompanied by either normal creatinine clearance, or varying degrees of azotaemia. Most subjects with HIVAN are young black men (mean age 33 years, male:female ratio of 10:1), and approximately 50% are intravenous drug abusers, while the remaining are either homosexual or bisexual men, heterosexual contacts of infected persons, or children with AIDS. In centres both in the United States and elsewhere, where a majority of patients with HIV are white, nephropathy is distinctly rare. An analysis of published work from within and outside the United States reveals that more than 95% of patients with HIVAN are black, which has prompted some to suggest that genetic factors may be a cofactor in the pathogenesis of renal disease.[8] In the United States, HIVAN is now the third leading cause of renal failure in blacks between the ages of 20 and 64.[9] In HIVAN, investigations fail to find other known causes of renal disease. The serum complement levels are normal, and concentrations of circulating immunoglobulins (IgA, IgG, and IgM) are increased. There is a diminution in the absolute number of CD4+ lymphocytes, with reversal of the CD4/CD8 cell ratio in the blood. Although HIVAN is seen in asymptomatic HIV-seropositive individuals, studies indicate that renal disease is a late manifestation as evidenced by low levels of CD4 cells.[9] No correlation exists between the severity of renal disease and the levels of viraemia. Patients are usually normotensive, and even in the presence of severe azotaemia, hypertension is rare. Ultrasonography shows enlarged and highly echogenic kidneys despite severe uraemia, a non-specific finding.

From the onset of proteinuria, HIVAN follows a malignant course of rapid decline in glomerular filtration rate (GFR) leading to ESRD in 3 to 4 months (median of 11 weeks), although wide variations in the time course are seen. In children the mean duration from onset of proteinuria to ESRD is 8–9 months. One prominent clinical feature is the absence of high blood pressure despite advanced uraemia in a majority of patients with HIVAN, while moderate to severe hypertension is present in more than 85% of subjects with renal failure from other causes.

Renal pathology in HIVAN is a constellation of unusual glomerular and tubulointerstitial changes and electron microscopic features. The commonest lesion is a collapsing form of FSGS (> 90% of renal histology reported). There is a varying degree of focal and global collapse of glomerular capillary tufts accompanied by global glomerulosclerosis, dilated Bowman spaces filled with eosinophilic proteinaceous material. Visceral epithelial cells are markedly hypertrophied, focally hyperplastic, and contain abundant protein resorption droplets. The most striking feature is the presence of enormously dilated tubules reaching microcystic proportions filled with large hyaline casts, and lined by flattened or swollen reactive epithelium. Interstitial infiltrate consists mostly of CD8+ T lymphocytes mixed with few plasma cells, and B cells. The monocyte infiltration varies from moderately dense in early lesions to scant as the disease approaches end-stage. Severe interstitial fibrosis, renal tubular atrophy, and vascular changes of arteriolosclerosis are minimally present, or strikingly absent.

The most frequent immunofluorescent finding is the immunostaining for albumin, IgG, and IgA in hypertrophic and hyperplastic visceral epithelial cells, and segmental coarse granular deposition of IgM and C3 in the mesangium and sclerotic areas. The nature of these immune deposits is unknown. They may represent deposited immune complexes or non-specific trapping of immunoglobulins in the mesangium or sclerotic areas. In HIV-associated IgA nephropathy, immunecomplexes circulating in the blood are composed of IgA idiotypic antibodies, and glomerular mesangial IgA deposits contain HIV antigens.

Ultrastructurally, there is wrinkling and collapse of the glomerular basement membrane (GBM) with excessive accumulation of mesangial matrix in the sclerosed glomeruli, along with effacement and focal detachment of epithelial foot processes. Visceral epithelial cells are markedly swollen, hypertrophic with frequent villous transformation, and contain protein absorption droplets. But the most striking feature is the presence of abundant tubuloreticular inclusions (TRI) in endothelial cells, occasionally in peritubular capillaries, and in the infiltrating leucocytes. The demonstration of abundant TRI is of high predictive value in suspecting HIV infection in otherwise asymptomatic individuals. A variety of unusual (distinctive?) ultrastructural changes best described as viral footprints noted in HIVAN include presence of complex nuclear bodies, a peculiar granulofibrillary transformation of nuclear chromatin in the tubular and interstitial cells, and intanuclear crystalline and fibrillary inclusions in the interstitial fibroblasts. Based on these findings, a viral aetiology for HIVAN has been strongly suggested. Some *in situ* hybridization studies showing replication of HIV in the glomerular and renal tubular cells offer strong support to the viral theory of the causation of HIVAN.[10,11]

The pathogenesis of HIVAN is poorly understood. Although nephropathy may be an initial manifestation, marked depletion of CD4 cells (generally fewer than 200) suggests that renal disease occurs late. Lack of immune glomerular deposits speaks against an antigen–antibody-mediated mechanism. Since viral genomes have been demonstrated in renal biopsies from patients with HIVAN by *in situ* hybridization, or by techniques involving microdissection and polymerase chain reaction, a direct role for virus has been advanced.[10,11] HIV genomes are, however, also seen in renal tissues of patients without nephropathy, which indicates that in addition to viral infection, individual host responses or other triggering mechanisms are also necessary to induce glomerulopathy. The nature of HIV infection of various renal cells which lack CD4 receptors is also poorly understood. *In vitro* studies have suggested that HIV can infect and replicate in glomerular endothelial cells and to a lesser extent in mesangial cells, but not in epithelial cells. Paradoxically, in HIVAN there is extensive epithelial cell injury. Since mesangial cells and monocytes share many common features, HIV-infected monocytes may serve as reservoirs in the glomeruli and facilitate infection of mesangial cells. Genetic and environmental factors may play a major role, as the disease is very rare among Caucasians.[8] It is likely that the critical factor which determines who develops nephropathy may be the nature of host response to HIV infection.

Transgenic mice produced with a non-infectious HIV-1 construct (lacking certain structural proteins, but preserving the envelope and regulatory genes), develop FSGS with mesangial hypercellularity and epithelial cell hypertrophy, along with microcystic dilatation of renal tubules. Proteinuria detectable within a month progresses to nephrotic syndrome with the development of ESRD, all features resembling HIVAN in humans.[12,13] Viral genomes are expressed in renal tissues, and there is up-regulation of basic fibroblast growth factor (bFGF), and TGF-β. From this model, it can be inferred that the whole virus may not be necessary to evoke nephropathy, rather one or more viral proteins can trigger renal disease by acting either directly on renal cells, or indirectly through the release of soluble mediators that affect the kidney. Subsequently, other workers have demonstrated increased levels of cytokines (TGF-β, IL-8), as well as over-expression of TGF-β in renal cells in humans with HIVAN. HIV proteins have multiple nephropathogenic effects *in vitro*. The HIV transactivator protein that stimulates cell proliferation and production of TGF-β by macrophages, and GP120 can modulate immune cell functions, promote apoptosis, and decrease extracellular matrix degradation. TGF-β is one of the major cytokines implicated in matrix protein synthesis and glomerulosclerosis in experimental renal disease. Increased renal cellular expression of TGF-β as a result of either direct viral infection or exposure to circulating HIV peptides may be one of the mechanisms responsible for glomerulosclerosis seen in HIVAN.

One of the major unresolved issues in the pathogenesis of HIVAN is whether the kidney disease is due to direct viral infection of renal tissues or is a secondary phenomenon mediated by dysregulated cytokines. From the recent work by Bruggerman *et al.* in the transgenic mice model, the evidence seem to favour a direct viral effect.[14] Normal kidneys transplanted into HIV transgenic mice remain disease free, while HIVAN develops in transgenic kidneys transplanted into non-transgenic litter mates.[26] In brief, the pathogenesis of HIVAN is complex and may involve an interplay of direct viral infection, modulation by various HIV proteins, dysregulated cytokines, and environmental and genetic factors.

Treatment of HIVAN

From the above discussion of the pathogenesis of HIVAN, the goals of treatment should be:

1. Eradication of virus (replication), to prevent further viral-mediated renal injury.
2. Stop or minimize the effects of cytokine-mediated glomerular injury.
3. Eliminate or prevent interstitial injury by infiltrating cells.
4. Stop or minimize proteinuria.

Unfortunately, in addition to symptomatic treatment of oedema and hypoalbuminaemia, (low-salt diet, diuretics), specific treatment options for HIVAN are limited because of a lack of prospective controlled studies. Therefore our management strategies are primarily derived from anecdotal and retrospective observations. We can speculate that the beneficial results reported in a limited number of studies (patients) may be due to achievement of one or more the goals cited above.

Role of antiretroviral agents in HIVAN

Three early reports indicated some beneficial effects of prolonged zidovudine (AZT), the only antiretroviral drug available then) in HIVAN.[15–17] In one patient with biopsy-proven HIVAN and a serum creatinine (Scr) of 8.1 mg/dl, AZT in a dose of 200 mg every 4 h resulted in stabilization of the slope of decline of 1/cr. In a second report from France, one patient with HIVAN had remission of nephrotic syndrome and maintainance of normal renal function for 11 months with AZT (800 mg/day). But when AZT was stopped because of severe anaemia, there was a rapid decline in renal function leading to ESRD within a month. These authors also commented on another patient in whom AZT therapy for 5 months led to a temporary discontinuation of chronic haemodialysis therapy. In the third study, of the six patients treated with AZT, two did not respond, and in four others the disease progressed slowly. These workers stressed the importance of treating HIVAN early. We also reported 15 HIV-infected patients treated for over 2 years with AZT, who did not progress to ESRD despite continued proteinuria in some of them.[18] From these anecdotal observations, we suggested that AZT may offer hope in some patients with HIVAN. These not so encouraging results may be explained by our current understanding that AZT monotherapy is ineffective in reducing the viral load. Some of the beneficial effects reported may be due to the *in vitro* demonstration of AZT reducing mesangial cell proliferation and matrix synthesis.

While the deployment of highly active antiretroviral therapy (HAART) has clearly improved survival in HIV patients, its impact on the natural history of HIVAN is less clear. Isolated case reports have shown the efficacy of HAART in reducing proteinuria and dramatically improving renal function, including discontinuation of dialysis support in some patients with ESRD.[19–21] Currently, many prospective studies evaluating the efficacy of HAART in HIVAN are in progress, which should lead to meaningful recommendations.

Two pertinent issues are whether antiretroviral therapy can prevent the development of nephropathy if it is administered prior to the onset of renal markers (proteinuria, azotaemia, haematuria), and whether these drugs alter the course in established HIVAN. Some recent observations provide partial answers to these questions. At our institution, the incidence of HIVAN as a cause of ESRD remained fairly constant at 22% per year for a decade (1986 to 1995, an average of 75 new patients per year). During the past 4 years (1996 to 1999), the incidence has declined to 12% per year. Similar observations have also been made at other centres which treat large numbers of HIV patients. The incidence of severe acute renal failure (described later) has also declined by 50% over the same period at our centre. One other indirect evidence in favour of effective antiretroviral therapy is the fact that HIVAN in children has almost disappeared over the past several years at our hospital and at other institutions. The speculation is that in children HIV infection is diagnosed at birth, and treatment is initiated very early before the development of renal lesions. In patients with established nephropathy, data from current studies may be able to answer the question of efficacy of HAART.

Role of corticosteroids in HIVAN

In addition to several isolated case reports, two important studies have addressed the role of corticosteroids in HIVAN. In one study, 20 consecutive HIVAN patients (one with normal Scr and 19 with varying degrees of azotaemia) were treated with prednisone 60 mg/day for a median of 4 weeks, with a follow-up of 44 weeks (range 8–107). The response to prednisone therapy in this study is very impressive when contrasted with historical controls in a disease noted for fulminant loss of renal function. Only two patients with severe azotaemia progressed to ESRD in 4–5 weeks, while in the other 17 Scr declined from 8.1 mg/dl to 3.0 mg/dl. In five patients who relapsed after stopping initial therapy, with a second course of prednisone treatment, Scr decreased from 8.2 mg/dl to 3.9 mg/dl. In 12 patients, 24-h urinary protein excretion diminished from 9.1 g/day to 3.2 g/day along with an increase in serum albumin concentration. Six patients developed serious infectious complications related to prednisone therapy. A total of seven patients were alive free of ESRD 8–81 weeks from the initiation of prednisone therapy.[22] In the other retrospective study of 102 patients with HIVAN from France, the main independent factors associated with better renal outcome were steroid therapy and a lower magnitude of proteinuria.[23] The author is aware of another study from Baltimore which also showed favourable effects of steroids in HIVAN. Our own personal experience indicates that steroid therapy is associated with dramatic results including discontinuation of dialysis support in several of our patients with advanced renal failure.

It is important to note that corticosteroids can be effectively utilized with caution in patients with immunodeficiency. Steroids have been used in HIV patients in the management of thrombocytopenia, lymphomas, *pneumocystis carinii* pneumonia and others. In selected patients with HIVAN, and no evidence of active infection, corticosteroid therapy is beneficial. The benefits of steroids may be due to their effects on the interstitial infiltrating cells (mostly CD8+ T lymphocytes mixed with plasma cells, B cells, and monocytes), and their antiinflammatory properties.

Another non-specific therapy which has shown promise in reducing proteinuria and preserving renal function is the use of angiotensin-converting enzyme (ACE) inhibitors. Both experimental and clinical studies have shown that ACE inhibitors are effective agents in HIVAN.[24-26] The efficacy of ACE inhibitors is attributable to their haemo-dynamic effects of lowering of intraglomerular pressure and reducing proteinuria, and possibly in modulating cytokine-mediated renal injury.

Our current approach is to document HIVAN by renal biopsy, assess the patient's immune status (viral load, CD4 count), and administer prednisone 60 mg/day for 4–8 weeks in patients who have massive proteinuria and show evidence of renal deterioration. All patients receive HAART in consultation with our infectious disease consultants, along with appropriate antimicrobial prophylaxis. Prednisone therapy is gradually tapered over the next several weeks. In those who relapse, a second course of prednisone therapy is offered if no contraindications are present. Patients are carefully monitored so that any infectious complications can be identified and treated early and steroid therapy discontinued. Obviously, a compliant patient who can follow this complicated polyphar-macy regimen and keep clinic appointments is a prerequisite for success. ACE inhibitors in varying doses are also employed to reduce further the proteinuria.

Many glomerular diseases including postinfectious immune-complex glomerulo-nephritis, membranoproliferative glomerulonephritis, membranous glomerulonephritis, mesangial proliferative glomerulonephritis, minimal change disease, systemic lupus erythematosus and, IgA nephropathy, have been described in patients with HIV disease manifesting proteinuria and an acute onset of azotemia.[27-30] Membranoproliferative glomerulonephritis and membranous glomerulonephritis in association with either hepatitis C or hepatitis B infection in patients with HIV have also been reported. In all the reports, there is a preponderance of Caucasians in whom these miscellaneous glomerular lesions are seen, suggesting a different immunological renal response (more proliferative than sclerosing glomerulonephritis) to HIV. These observations once again add confirmation to the fact that HIV-associated FSGS is very rare in whites. Other than some well-studied cases of IgA nephropathy in HIV patients, it is difficult to say whether or not these primary glomerular diseases are incidental, or whether there is a direct relationship to viral infection. In published reports, the striking feature about HIV-associated IgA nephropathy is that the disease has been observed in whites and Hispanics but not in blacks or intravenous drug abusers. In some patients both circulating IgA immune complexes and those eluted from the glomeruli are directed against HIV anti-gens. The renal histology in HIV-associated IgA nephropathy reveals the presence of TRI in glomerular cells, a feature not generally seen in idiopathic IgA nephropathy. In addi-tion, progression to ESRD has not been observed in HIV patients with IgA nephropathy.

Coincidental renal disorders

A review of published work reveal a heterogenous collection of renal abnormalities which can be coincidental in patients with HIV disease (Table 12.2). Renal lesions included under the category of infections/infiltrations are reflections of systemic processes (infection or malignancy) in the host, a consequence of the HIV-induced severe immuno-suppressive state. Some are evident and symptomatic during life, but others may be identified only during autopsy examinations. A variety of fluid-electrolyte and acid–base disturbances observed in patients with the acquired immunodeficiency syndrome (AIDS) are of practical relevance to clinicians because these abnormalities predispose

Table 12.2   Coincidental renal diseases

Infections in the kidney	Renal microabcesses from bacterial infections
	Tuberculosis of the kidney (both typical and atypical *Mycobacterium*)
	Cytomegalovirus, other viruses
	Candida, cryptococci, aspergillosis, mucormycosis, Nocardia, other fungi
	Mycoplasma
	Microsporidia
Infiltrative lesions of the kidney	Calcifications
	Amyloidosis
	Light chains
	Lymphoma
	Kaposi's sarcoma
	Hypernephroma
	Other malignancies
Fluid-electrolyte and acid–base derangements	Hypo- and hypernatraemia
	Inappropriate secretion of antidiuretic hormone (ADH)
	Hypo- and hyperkalaemia
	Type IV renal tubular acidosis (hyporeninaemic hypoaldosteronism)
	Metabolic acidosis and alkalosis
	Hypo- and hypercalcaemia
	Hypomagnesaemia
	Hypo- and hyperuricaemia
	Lactic acidosis

patients to renal injury and contribute to the pathogenesis of acute renal failure. An understanding of virtually every type of fluid-electrolyte, simple, and mixed acid–base disorders in AIDS patients is essential because they reflect not only the gravity of underlying primary illnesses but also are major risk factors (directly or indirectly) to subsequent development of acute tubular necrosis. These derangements are almost always found in patients with advanced clinical AIDS, suffering from hypovolaemia/hypotension secondary to gastrointestinal losses (vomiting, diarrhoea, malnutrition, malabsorption), poor fluid intake from central nervous system involvement with mental obtundation, haemodynamic compromise from multiple infections/septicaemia and respiratory failure. It is also important to recognize that fluid and electrolyte abnormalities can be iatrogenically induced in stable outpatients receiving various drugs. A classification of these abnormalities is listed in Table 12.3. An expanded discussion of management of these coincidental renal disorders is beyond the scope of this chapter. More details are found in the paper by Rao.[31]

Acute renal failure syndromes

The spectrum of acute renal failure encountered in HIV patients in most cases is similar to that in general nephrology practice, except for certain unique associations. As listed in

Table 12.3 Drug-induced electrolyte disorders

Disorder	Drug
Hyponatraemia	DDI TMP-SMX Itraconazole
Hypernatraemia	Foscarnet Rifampin Amphotericin B
Hypokalaemia	Amphotericin B DDI Foscarnet, itraconazole
Hyperkalaemia	TMP-SMX Pentamidine
Hypocalcaemia	Amphotericin B Pentamidine Foscarnet
Hypercalcaemia	Foscarnet
Hypo/hyperphosphataemia	Foscarnet
Hypomagnesaemia	Amphotericin B Pentamidine Foscarnet
Hyperuricaemia	DDI

DDI, didanosine; TMP-SMX, trimethoprim-sulphamethoxazole.

Table 12.4, the aetiology of acute renal failure in HIV disease can be categorized into prerenal, postrenal (both intra- and extrarenal obstruction), and intrinsic renal causes. Prerenal azotaemia is due to volume depletion from gastrointestinal bleeding, vomiting, diarrhoea, high fever, and poor intake (mental obtundation secondary to CNS lesions). Occasionally, azotaemia may result from sequestration of fluids into the third space in patients with massive proteinuria, hypoalbuminaemia, and cachexia. Prerenal azotaemia is a harbinger of acute tubular necrosis, especially if nephrotoxic agents are also administered prior to the correction of hypovolaemia. Causes of postrenal failure include extrinsic compression of ureters (retroperitoneal fibrosis, lymph nodes/tumours), or intrinsic ureteral blockage (fungus balls/blood clots), or bladder outlet and urethral obstruction. Most pertinent to patients with HIV disease is the syndrome of intrarenal obstruction from crystal deposits in the tubules, an iatrogenic complication of drug therapy. These include acute uric acid deposition in renal tubules from hyperuricosuria secondary to chemotherapy-induced tumour lysis in AIDS-associated lymphoma, and renal insufficiency secondary to foscarnet crystals deposits in the tubules. More often, crystal-induced acute renal failure in HIV disease is attributable to sulfadiazine, parenteral acyclovir, and protease inhibitors. Predisposing factors include pre-existing renal insufficiency, dehydration, and hypoalbuminaemia. It is essential for clinicians to be aware of this complication, because not only is it preventable, but it is also effectively treatable by

Table 12.4   Acute renal failure syndromes

Prerenal	Hypovolaemia (diarrhoea, vomitting, infections)
	Hypotension (sepsis, bleeding, fluid loss)
	Hypoalbuminaemia (cachexia, third space fluid loss)
Renal	Acute tubular necrosis from hypovolaemic, anoxic, and toxic injuries
	Rhabdomyolysis and myoglobinuric renal failure
	Allergic interstitial nephritis from drugs: rifampicin, trimethoprim
	sulphamethaxazole, phenytoin, and others
	Acute azotaemia from non-steroidal anti-inflammatory drugs
	Plasmacytic interstitial nephritis
	Haemolytic uraemic syndrome
	Thrombotic thrombocytopenic purpura
	Postinfectious immune complex glomerulonephritis
	Renal oedema from massive proteinuria and severe hypoalbuminaemia
	Multiple myeloma
	Leptospirosis
Postrenal	Crystal-induced renal failure (foscarnet, sulphadiazine, acyclovir,
	protease inhibitors)
	Tumour lysis syndrome (urate deposit-induced renal failure)
	Retroperitoneal fibrosis
	Obstructive nephropathy
	Extrinsic ureteral compression (lymph nodes, tumours)
	Intrinsic obstruction (fungus balls, blood clots)
	Bladder and ureteral obstruction

adequate hydration. Renal failure from crystalluria is rarely severe enough to warrant dialysis intervention. When the offending agent is discontinued and fluids are administered, renal function is rapidly reversible. A detailed description can be found in Rao.[31]

The leading cause of acute renal failure in HIV disease is acute tubular necrosis secondary to the use of nephrotoxic agents (antibiotics, radiocontrast agents) in patients prone to renal injury from anoxic insults such as obvious or unrecognized prerenal azotemia (volume depletion), and hypotension from sepsis and respiratory failure.

Acute tubular necrosis

Among the intrinsic renal causes, acute tubular necrosis is the commonest acute renal failure syndrome, and is a problem often avoidable in clinical practice.[32] In asymptomatic HIV-seropositive individuals, acute tubular necrosis is generally not seen. But patients with advanced AIDS are acutely ill from multiple infections and neoplasms. Their clinical course is often complicated by hypovolaemia, severe metabolic/respiratory acidosis, and multiorgan failure with compromised cerdiorespiratory status. Moreover, these patients may be subjected to invasive diagnostic procedures resulting in blood loss, thus sustaining additional anoxic/ischaemic insult to the kidneys. Furthermore, administration of multiple nephrotoxic agents such as pentamidine, aminoglycoside antibiotics, and radiocontrast agents contributes to toxic renal injury. It is not surprising, therefore, that severe and life-threatening acute tubular necrosis is not an uncommon event in such patients. In one of the earlier studies, Valeri and Neusy found a 20% (88 of 449) incidence of acute renal failure (defined as a 2 mg/dl or greater rise in baseline Scr concentration) in hospitalized AIDS patients. The causes of acute renal failure were hypovolaemia (38%), toxicity from pentamidine (17%), amphotericin B (11%), radio-contrast agents (4%), shock and/or sepsis (8%), and allergic interstitial nephritis from trimethoprim-sulfamethaxazole (TMP-SMX) in 9%.[33] Other observations reveal a 6 to 20% incidence of acure renal failure in hospitalized AIDS patients from ischaemic/toxic renal injuries. In recent years, the incidence of severe acute tubular necrosis has been decreasing, attributable to overall improvements in the care of AIDS patients.[32]

Both oliguric and non-oliguric forms of acute tubular necrosis are common, with a variable clinical course ranging from mild, self-limited, asymptomatic azotaemia manifested by elevated Scr, to one of life-threatening uraemia, requiring dialysis and other life support in an intensive care unit. The majority of patients with mild acute tubular necrosis regain kidney function with or without the need for dialysis interven-tion. Severe acute tubular necrosis can be a terminal event in AIDS patients who are confined to intensive care units with numerous complications and multiorgan failure. Death in such patients is primarily from the primary illnesses compounded by renal failure, and intensive management by dialysis and all other means fails to alter their prog-nosis. Despite high mortality, some gravely ill patients treated by dialysis and general supportive care recover sufficient renal function to survive the acute event. While in the early 1980s many studies reported a high mortality in acute tubular necrosis, wide deployment of chemoprophylaxis and newer antiretroviral agents, has vastly improved the prognosis of patients with HIV disease.[31] In our recent comparative study of 146 HIV and 340 non-HIV patients with severe acute renal failure (those with an Scr of 6 mg/dl or higher), major findings were:

1. Aggressive management by dialysis and other supportive care results in similar rates of recovery of renal function (56% and 46%), and mortality (38% and 47%) in AIDS and non-AIDS patients respectively.
2. Renal recovery and patient mortality in acute tubular necrosis are influenced by the patient's underlying illness and haemodynamic stability, and not by the presence or absence of infection.
3. In AIDS patients hospitalized for all causes, the incidence of severe acute renal failure has declined by 50% (from 2% in the years 1986–1989 to 1% during 1990–1993), presumably to an improvement in the overall comprehensive approach to the management of HIV infection.

In clinical practice, physicians caring for AIDS patients should be cognizant of the fact that acute tubular necrosis is avoidable when precautionary measures such as hydration prior to use of radiocontrast agents, exercising caution in the choice of antibiotics while treating serious infections, and following dosage guidelines of aminoglycoside and other nephrotoxic drugs (based on renal function and serum drug concentrations) are followed. While acute tubular necrosis is a major contributor to morbidity and mortality, aggres-sive measures such as correction of fluid-electrolyte and acid–base derangements, early dialysis intervention, and nutritional supplementation are associated with favourable outcome in many. The choice between peritoneal or haemodialysis depends on the patient's clinical status and the availability of institutional resources. An aggressive approach facilitates renal recovery from the acute insult, and surviving patients will have subsequent opportunities to receive the benefits of highly active antiretroviral therapy. At times, haemodialysis may be unsuitable because of a patient's haemodynamic instability and terminal illness. A decision to withhold dialysis and supportive therapy should be individualized based upon clinical circumstances, while respecting the wishes of the patient and their family.

Since nephrotoxic agents contribute greatly to the occurrence of acute renal failure, one should be familiar with their use while treating AIDS patients suffering from multiple infections. The drugs widely employed in HIV disease which can cause renal impairment include aminoglycoside antibiotics, amphotericin B, pentamidine, TMP-SMX, foscarnet, parenteral acyclovir, sulfadiazine, and protease inhibitors. Many excellent reviews provide recommendations about several aspects of their use in clinical practice.[34-36] Tables 12.5 and 12.6 lists the currently approved antiretroviral drugs and broad guidelines for their use in patients with renal failure. In general, it is better to avoid adeofir and hydroxyurea in patients with renal failure, while the other agents have no nephrotoxic potential.

Haemolytic uraemic syndrome (HUS) and thrombotic thrombocytopenic purpura (TTP)

The clinical distinction between HUS and TTP is imprecise, as both may represent a different spectrum of the same clinical entity. HUS and TTP leading to acute renal failure are being recognized with increasing frequency in HIV disease, and the topic has been reviewed in great detail recently.[37] Several authors have raised questions about a possible direct aetiological role of HIV in causing these disorders. In about 25% of cases, HUS/TTP may be the initial presenting illness subsequently leading to a diagnosis of HIV infection. The prevalence of HIV positivity has varied from 3 to 36% in all HUS/TTP patients seen at different centres. The disease has been seen in HIV-infected children. Thrombotic microangiopathy leading to ESRD has also been reported in renal allografts in two transplant recipients who were HIV-positive.

HIV-associated HUS/TTP is similar to the idiopathic variety in clinical presentation, laboratory findings, and pathological features. Salient points differentiating between the two include a striking preponderance of young men (male to female ratio of 9:1, mean age of 35 years), and a higher prevalence in whites than in black and Hispanic patients. In addition, TRI are present in the renal endothelial cell cytoplasm in HIV-associated HUS/TTP, which are not generally seen in the idiopathic variety. TRI are considered to represent alterations induced by interferon-α, indirect evidence for viral infection.

In most patients renal impairment has been mild to moderate with Scr between 2 and 5 mg/dl. Occasionally, oliguria and azotaemia are severe needing dialysis intervention. In reported studies, the management of HIV patients has included various combinations of plasmapheresis with fresh frozen plasma replacement, aspirin, dipyridamole, and corticosteroids. Additionally, in some patients vincristine, prostacyclin, and intravenous gamma globulin have also been administered. Such a regimen has resulted in serious complications such as PCP, cytomegalovirus, fungal (*Candida*, *Aspergillus*), *Listeria monocytogenes* and bacterial infections. Several patients have also required dialysis with

Table 12.5(a) Currently approved (in the United States) antiretroviral drugs

Nucleoside analogue RTI (NRTI)	Zidovudine (AZT) (Retrovir*)
	Didanosine (DDI) (Videx*)
	Dideoxycytidine (ddC, Zalcitabine) (Hivid*)
	Stravudine (d4T) (Zerit*)
	Lamivudine (3TC) (Epivir*)
	Abacavir(Ziagen*)
Non-nucleoside analogue RTI (NNRTI)	Nevirapine (Viramune*)
	Delaviridine (Rescriptor*)
	Efavirenz (sustiva*)
Protease inhibitors (PI)	Indinavir (Crixivan*)
	Ritonavir (Norvir*)
	Saquinavir (Invirase* hard gel)
	Saquinavir (Fotovase* soft gel)
	Nelfinavir (Viracept*)
	Ampenavir (Agenerase*)
Nucleotide RTI (Nu RTI)	Adeofir (Preveon*)
Ribonucleotide reductase inhibitors (RRI)	Hydroxuurea (Hydrea*)

*Brand names. RTI=reverse transcriptase inhibitor.

Table 12.5(b) Dosage modification in patients with Ccr < 50 ml/min

Reduced dosage	Probably++	No reduction in dose	Avoid
Zidovudine	Nevirapine++	Indinavir	Adeofir
Didanosine	Delaviridine++	Ritonavir	Hydroxuurea
Dideoxycytidine		Saquinavir	
Stravudine		Nelfinavir	
Lamivudine		Ampenavir	
		Efavirenz	
		Abacavir	

Renal calculi is a risk with protease inhibitors in all patients including those with impaired renal function. It is not a consideration in dialysis patients.
In general the dialyser clearance of most drugs (limited information) is not clinically significant, additional dosage is not necessary in maintenance dialysis patients. Generally, it is advisable to administer the drug following dialysis.
++ In view of high urinary excretion, dosage should probably be reduced.

recovery of renal function in some and development of ESRD in others. In some, renal failure was a terminal event.

The prognosis in HIV-related HUS/TTP is much worse than in the idiopathic variety. Sudden death within hours of admission has been stressed in some reports. Despite aggressive management, more than a third of patients have died during the acute phase because of septicaemia, shock/cardiac arrest, and bleeding. In most studies, the

Table 12.6   Currently approved antiretroviral drugs (United States)

Drug	Class	Half-life		Urinary excretion	Dialyser clearance	
		Normal	Renal failure		Haemo	PD
Zidovudine	NRTI	1 h	6–8 h	63%	102 ml/min	< 5 ml/min
Didanosine	NRTI	1.4 h	4–5 h	61%	107 ml/min	Negligible
Dideoxycytidine	NRTI	1–3 h	8 h	80%	NA	NA
Stravudine	NRTI	1.4 h	8 h	40%	NA	NA
Lamivudine	NRTI	5–7 h	22 h	71%	NA	NA
Abacavir	NRTI	1.5 h	NA	2%	NA	NA
Nevirapine	NNRTI	25 h	NA	82%	NA	NA
Delaviridine	NNRTI	2–11 h	NA	51%	NA	NA
Efavirenz	NNRTI	40–55 h	NA	2%	NA	NA
Indinavir	PI	1.8 h	NC	9%	NA*	NA*
Ritonavir	PI	3–5 h	NC	11%	NA*	NA*
Saquinavir	PI	2–3 h	NC	3%	NA*	NA*
Nelfinavir	PI	2–11 h	NC	2%	NA*	NA*
Ampenavir	PI	7–10 h	NC	3%	NA*	NA*
Adeofir	Nu RTI	NA	NA	98%	NA	NA
Hydroxuurea	RRI	NA	NA	82%	NA	NA

Abbreviations: NC, no change; NA, not available; NA*, not available but heavy protein binding indicate that it is not dialysable; NRTI, nucleoside analogue RTI; NNRTI, non-nucleoside analogue RTI; Nu RTI, nucleotide RTI; RRI, ribonucleotide reductase inhibitor.

mortality rate has been 67 to 100% in HIV patients in contrast to long-term survival of over 75% seen in non-HIV-associated HUS/TTP.

Other coincidental renal diseases

Many intrinsic renal diseases such as polycystic kidney disease, essential hypertension, amyloidosis, idiopathic glomerulonephritis, and others, all leading to ESRD in patients with prior HIV infection have been noted. In addition, patients undergoing maintenance dialysis therapy and renal transplantation have acquired HIV infection from contaminated blood transfusion, intravenous drug abuse, sexual contacts, or through the allograft. At present, these modes of HIV transmission are most unlikely in view of routine screening of all transfused blood and transplanted organs. Maintenance dialysis therapy, once considered futile in many, is now a viable choice in a large number of such patients. From the USRDS registry, we note that the number of ESRD patients with AIDS receiving maintenance dialysis in the United States has increased steadily from 0.1% during the years 1987–1991, to 0.9% between 1991 and 1995 (2646 patients), and to 1.06% (3629 patients) between 1993 and 1997.[38] From the data available, both maintenance haemodialysis and peritoneal dialysis are effective modalities in HIV patients with ESRD. The choice of therapy should depend on the individual patient's lifestyle, preference, and availability of family and other support, and should not be based on HIV seropositivity. Also noteworthy is the fact that the survival of HIV-infected ESRD patients undergoing maintenance dialysis has improved significantly over the years. It is not unusual to find HIV patients with ESRD surviving beyond 6–7 years at many centres. ESRD patients with HIV who are undergoing maintenance dialysis should be treated with HAART (dose modification), chemoprophylaxis, and other supportive care similar to those without renal failure.

Therapeutic strategies in ESRD patients with HIV

HIV patients with ESRD offer many challenges to nephrologists which are manageable with a comprehensive approach to patient care. Some general issues which are relevant in HIV patients include: early creation of autogenous arteriovenous access, avoidance of in-dwelling catheters and PTFE grafts whenever possible, improvement of the nutritional status during maintenance dialysis, and preference of MH over CAPD in patients with severe malnutrition. In addition to delivering adequate dialysis, HIV patients require a higher dose of erythropoietin to maintain haematocrit. HIV-infected ESRD patients, those with lower serum erythropoietin levels respond better to exogenous erythropoietin than those with higher baseline levels.

The specific overall aim in ESRD patients infected with HIV should be to reduce the viral load to undetectable levels in the blood, and prevent associated infections. These complicated regimens involving multiple combinations of antiretroviral drugs and chemoprophylactic agents are best achieved by a comprehensive approach involving collaboration with infectious disease consultants, nutritionists, and primary physicians. The reluctance on the part of nephrologists to employ antiretroviral therapy due to a lack of pharmacokinetic information in ESRD patients is also changing. Currently, even with the limited available data, these agents are being more widely employed. Table 12.6 lists the approved antiretroviral drugs in the United States, and summarizes broad criteria for their use in renal failure. Guidelines for the deployment of other agents commonly used in HIV patients with renal impairment/ESRD are discussed in greater detail in recent excellent reviews.[34–36]

All the published studies of renal transplantation in patients with HIV are retrospective observations in asymptomatic patients in whom infection was neither obvious nor suspected. In some instances, HIV infection was present prior to transplantation, and in others, infection developed at the time of or following transplantation. From the two excellent reviews summarizing the results of solid organ transplantation, 1-year patient survival of 90% in 61 recipients who became infected was similar to that reported in non-HIV patients by the UNOS network.[39,40] Currently, United States centres routinely screen all potential recipients, and are reluctant to transplant even asymptomatic HIV patients. Over the past 8 years there has been a glaring absence of information in the literature about HIV and renal transplantation. Recently, 144 out of all 248 United States renal transplant centres (58%) responded to a mailed a questionnaire asking for their views and practices regarding transplantation in HIV patients. All responding centres required HIV testing of prospective recipients, but 11% would consider transplanting those who refused screening. Only 10 centres (7%) would consider a cadaver donor renal transplant in HIV patients and even fewer centres (six), a live donor transplant. But in actual practice, not a single centre had performed a renal transplant in an HIV-positive patient in the prior year.[41] This survey sums up the sentiments of United States transplant centres' reluctance to transplanted HIV patients with ESRD. But in view of advances in the management of HIV patients, especially HAART, this approach must be reconsidered.

In summary, renal manifestations of HIV disease are diverse. Great progress has been made in identifying specific glomerular lesions and their pathogenesis. Newer antiretroviral agents offer great promise both in preventing renal disease and possibly in patients with established HIVAN. Prognosis in HIV patients with ESRD irrespective of cause has improved remarkably over the years. Acute reversible renal failure, a preventable complication, is also declining in hospitalized HIV patients. More and more physicians who were reluctant in the past, are now employing antiretroviral and other agents widely in complicated patients with renal failure because of better understanding of drug pharmacokinetics in uraemia.

References

1. Rao TKS, Filippone EJ, Nicastri AD, Landesman SH, Frank E, Chen CK, Friedman EA (1984). Associated focal and segmental glomerulosclerosis in the acquired immunodeficiency syndrome. *New Engl J Med* 310:669–73.
2. Rao TKS, Friedman EA, Nicastri AD (1987). The types of renal disease in the acquired immunodeficiency syndrome. *New Engl J Med* 316:1062–73.
3. Rao TKS (1996). Renal complications in HIV disease. *Med Clin N Am* 80:1437–51.
4. D'Agati V, Appel GB (1997). HIV infection and the kidney. *J Am Soc Nephrol* 8:138–52.
5. Klotman PE (1999). HIV associated nephropathy. *Kidney Int* 56:1161–76.
6. D'Agati V, Appel GB (1998). Renal pathology of human immunodeficiency virus infection. *Semin Nephrol* 18:406–21.
7. Coresh J, Caiaffa WT, Vlahov D, Astemborski J, Schaeffer M, Jarr B (1997). HIV infection and the risk of renal disease among injection drug users: a prospective study in the alive cohort. *J Am Soc Nephrol* 8:135A.
8. Bourgoignie JJ, Ortiz C, Green DF, Roth D (1989). Race a cofactor in HIV-1 associated nephropathy. *Transplant Proc* 21:3899–901.
9. Winston JA, Bums GC, Klotman PE (1998). The human immunodeficiency virus (HIV) epidemic and HIV-associated nephropathy. *Semin Nephrol* 18:373–77.
10. Cohen AH, Sun NCJ, Shapshak P, Imagawa DT (1989). Demonstration of human immunodeficiency virus in renal epithelium in HIV-associated nephropathy. *Mod Pathol* 2:125–28.
11. Kimmel PL, Ferreira-Centeno A, Farkas-Szallasi T, Abraham AA, Garreh CT (1993). Viral DNA in microdissected renal biopsy tissue from HIV infected patients with nephrotic syndrome. *Kidney Int* 43:1347–52.
12. Dickie P, Felser J, Eckhaus M, Bryant J, Silver J, Marinos N, Notkins AL (1991). HIV-associated nephropathy in transgenic mice expressing HIV-1 genes. *Virology* 185:109–19.
13. Kopp JB, Ray PE, Adler SH, Bruggeman LA, Mangurian CV, Owens JW, et al. (1994). Nephropathy in HIV-transgenic mice. *Contrib Nephrol* 107:194–204.
14. Bruggeman LA, Dickman S, Meng C, Quaggin SE, Coffman TM, Klotman PE (1997). Nephropathy in human immunodeficiency virus-1 transgenic mice is due to transgene expression. *J Clin Invest* 100:84–92.

15. Lam M, Park MC (1990). HIV associated nephropathy—beneficial effect of zidovudine therapy. *New Engl J Med* 323:1775–76.

16. Babut-Gay ML, Echard M, Kleinknechl D, Meyrier A (1989). Zidovudine and nephropathy with human immunodeficiency virus (HIV) infection. *Ann Intern Med* 111:856–57.

17. Michel C, Dosquet P, Ronco P, Mougenolt B, Viron B, Mignon F (1992). Nephropathy associated with infection by human immunodeficiency virus: a report on 11 cases including 6 treated with zidovudine. *Nephron* 62:434–40.

18. Ifudu O, Rao TKS, Tan CC, Fleischman H, Chirgwin K, Friedman EA (1995). Zidovudine is beneficial in human immunodeficiency virus associated nephropathy. *Am J Nephrol* 15:217–21.

19. Wali RK, Drachenberg CI, Papadimitriou JC, Keay S, Ramos E (1998). HIV-1-associated nephropathy and response to highly-active antiretrovital therapy. *Lancet* 352:783–84.

20. Dellow E, Unwin R, Miller R, Williams I, Griffiths M (1999). Protease inhibitor therapy for HIV infection: the effect on HIV-associated nephrotic syndrome. *Nephrol Dial Transplant* 14:744–47.

21. Viani RM, Dankner WM, Muelenaer PA, Spector SA (1999). Resolution of HIV-1-associated nephrotic syndrome with highly active antiretroviral therapy delivered by gastrostomy tube. *Pediatrics* 104:1394–96.

22. Smith MC, Austen JL, Corey JT, Emancipator SN, Herbener T, Gripshover B, et al. (1996). Prednisone improves renal function and proteinuria in human immunodeficiency virus-associated nephropathy. *Am J Med* 101:41–48.

23. Laradi A, Mallet A, Beaufis H, Allouache M, Martinez F (1998). HIV-associated nephro-pathy: outcome and prognosis factors. *J Am Soc Nephrol* 9:2327–35.

24. Kimmel PL, Mishkin GJ, Umana WO (1996). Captopril and renal survival in patients with human immunodeficiency virus nephropathy. *Am J Kidney Dis* 28:202–08.

25. Bums GC, Paul SK, Toth IR, Sivak SL (1997). Effect of angiotensin-converting enzyme inhibition in HIV-associated nephropathy. *J Am Soc Nephrol* 8:1140–46.

26. Kopp JB, Ray PE, Adler SH, Bruggeman LA, Mangurian CV, Owens JW, et al. (1994). Nephropathy in HIV-transgenic mice. *Contrib Nephrol* 107:194–204.

27. Kimmel PL, Phillips TM (1995). Immune complex glomerulonephritis associated with HIV infection. In: Kimmel PL and Berns JS (eds) *Renal and urologic aspects of HIV infection*, pp. 77–110. Churchill Livingstone, New York.

28. Stokes MB, Chawla H, Brody RI, Kumar A, Genner R, Goldfarb DS, Gallo G (1997). Immune complex glomerulonephritis in patients coinfected with human immunodeficiency virus and hepatitis C virus. *Am J Kidney Dis* 29:514–25.

29. Morales E, Alegre R, Herrero JC, Morales JM, Ortuno T, Praga M (1997). Hepatitis C virus associated cryoglobulinemic membranoproliferative glomerulonephrits in patients infected with HIV. *Nephrol Dial Transplant* 12:1980–84.

30. Kimmel PL, Phillips TM, Centeno AF, Szallasi TF, Abraham AA, Garrett CT (1992). Brief report: Idiotypic IgA nephropathy in patients with Human immunodeficiency virus infection. *New Engl J Med* 327: 702–06.

31. Rao TKS (1998). Acute renal failure syndromes in human immunodeficiency virus infection. *Semi Nephrol* 18:378–95.

32. Rao TKS, Friedman EA (1995). Outcome of severe acute renal failure in patients with the acquired immunodeficiency syndrome. *Am J Kidney Dis* 25:390–98.

33. Valeri A, Neusy AJ (1991). Acute and chronic renal disease in hospitalized AIDS patients. *Clin Nephrol* 35:110–18.

34. Berns JS, Cohen RM, Rudnick MR, Bennett WM (1995). Renal aspects of antimicrobial therapy for HIV infection. In: Kimmel PL and Berns JS (eds) *Renal and urologic aspects of HIV infection*, pp. 195–235. Churchill Livingstone, New York.

35. Gurtman A, Borrego F, Klomtan ME (1998). Management of antiretroviral therapy. *Semin Nephrol* 18:459–80.
36. Jayasekara D, Aweeka FT, Rodriguez R, Kalayjian RC, Humphreys MH, Gambertoglio JG (1999). Antiviral therapy for HIV patients with renal insufficiency. *J Acquired Immune Defic Synd* 21:384–95.
37. Berns JS (1995). Hemolytic–uremic syndrome and thrombotic thrombocytopenic purpura associated with HIV infection. In: Kimmel PL and Berns JS (eds) *Renal and urologic aspects of HIV infection*, pp. 111–33. Churchill Livingstone, New York.
38. US Renal Data System (1999). *USRDS 1999 Annual Data Report.*
39. Erice A, Rhame FS, Heussner, Dunn DL, Balfour HH Jr (1991). Human immunodeficiency virus infection in patients with solid-organ transplants: report of five cases and review. *Rev Infect Dis* 13:537–47.
40. Simonds RJ (1993). HIV transmission by organ and tissue transplantation. *AIDS* 7 (suppl. 2):S35–S38.
41. Vijayvargiya R, Bosch JP (1995). Dialysis and transplantation in patients with HIV infection. In: Kimmel PL and Berns JS (eds) *Renal and urologic aspects of HIV infection*, pp. 253–77. Churchill Livingstone, New York.
42. Spital A (1998). Should all human immunodeficiency virus-infected patients with end-stage renal disease be excluded from transplantation? The views of US Transplant centers. *Transplantation* 15:65:1187–91.

13

Cytomegalovirus in the renal allograft recipient

Paul D. Griffiths and Vincent C. Emery

Cytomegalovirus (CMV) is often detected in renal transplant patients but it can be difficult to determine if this is clinically significant for an individual patient because of their complex medical history and multiple potential explanations for morbidity. In this chapter we will review the evidence that CMV is important because in some patients it both causes specific end-organ disease and triggers graft rejection, and in others possibly initiates accelerated atherosclerosis.

The virus

The strain Ad169 of CMV has been completely sequenced. It has the largest genome of any human virus, and only a few of its genes are used to produce the virus particle. Most of the remaining genes are probably important for interaction with the host, and so are potential pathogenicity genes, but the function of approximately only one-third has been identified to date. In addition, wild strains of CMV contain an additional 22 genes, which are also presumed pathogenicity factors, lost when the virus is passaged in the laboratory.[1] Some of the pathogenicity genes are known to help the virus evade immune responses (Table 13.1); in particular, CMV contains a series of genes which coordinate the down-regulation of class I human leucocyte antigen (HLA) molecules so that the infected cell cannot be recognized efficiently by cytotoxic T lymphocytes. To avoid lysis by natural killer (NK) cells, which recognize major histocompatibility complex (MHC) molecules in a non-antigen-specific way, the virus encodes at least two other genes which provide a negative signal to the NK cell. Thus, CMV has evolved to avoid the responses

Table 13.1 Human CMV immune evasion strategies

Defence	Response	Effect
Antibody	Fc receptor	Interfere with antibody function
Complement	CD55/CD46/CD59	Degrade complement bound to CMV
T-cytotoxic	UL83/US3/US6/US2/US11	Down-regulate class I HLA molecules
NK cells	UL18	Provide negative signal to NK cells
CC chemokines	US28	Act as chemokine sink

of individuals with normal immunity and so is well adapted to the normal human. However, when infection occurs in a host with iatrogenic immunosuppression, the stage is set for the full virulence of the virus to be expressed.

Epidemiology

Seroepidemiological studies show that CMV infection is common, with approximately 60% of adults in developed countries showing evidence of past infection, with virtually 100% in people brought up in developing countries.[2] In almost all cases this virus is acquired asymptomatically, so that only testing for IgG-specific antibodies can indicate who has been infected in the past.

CMV acquisition is more common in lower socioeconomic groups.[3] Natural routes of transmission include intrauterine (presumably through maternal viraemia in 0.3–1% of cases); perinatal (through contact with infected maternal genital secretions and/or breast milk in 10–20% of cases); horizontal in childhood (through saliva); horizontal in the sexually active (through saliva and/or genital secretions). In addition, iatrogenic sources of CMV include donated solid organs and blood transfusions.

In all cases, seropositive individuals should be regarded as possessing latent CMV capable of reactivation. Thus, if they become immunocompromised, CMV may reactivate from latency and may cause disease (reactivation infection). In addition, if their organs are harvested for transplantation, they may transmit virus, irrespective of whether the recipient is seronegative (primary infection) or seropositive (reinfection).[4]

Pathogenesis

Viraemia and viral load

Most CMV disease in the immunocompromised is attributable to viraemic spread to multiple organs (Table 13.2). In all populations, the risk of disease correlates strongly with high CMV viral loads. This was first described in 1975 by Stagno and colleagues, who compared serial viruria titrations in neonates with symptomatic congenital, asymptomatic congenital, or perinatal infection.[5] The group with CMV disease had, on average, one log higher viruria than those with asymptomatic congenital infection, who in turn had an average one log higher viruria than those with perinatal infection. This observation suggested that there might be a threshold viral load above which CMV disease became common, and this possibility has been investigated using quantitative-competitive polymerase chain reaction (QCPCR). After renal transplantation, there is a significant correlation between the median values of maximum viruria post-transplant and the presence of CMV disease (see Fig. 13.1) and the same is true for viral loads in the blood.[6,7] Similar results are found in liver transplant and bone marrow transplant patients, with CMV viral loads in the blood significantly greater in patients with CMV disease in each case.[8,9]

It is well known that donor/recipient serostatus at the time of transplant identifies patients at risk of CMV disease.[10] For recipients of solid organs, the group with highest risk are D+R− (i.e. donor seropositive, recipient seronegative), followed by D+R+, then D−R+. These groups correspond to those at risk of primary infection, reinfection plus reactivation, and reactivation infections respectively. In addition, multiple studies

Table 13.2   CMV diseases in the immunocompromised

Symptoms	Solid organ transplant	Bone marrow transplant	AIDS
Fever/hepatitis	++	+	+
Gastrointestinal	+	+	+
Retinitis	+	+	++
Pneumonitis	+	++	
Myelosuppression		++	
Encephalopathy			+
Polyradiculopathy			+
Addisonian			+
Immunosuppression	+		
Rejection/GvHD	+	?	
Atherosclerosis	+		
Death		+	+

GvHD = graft versus host disease.

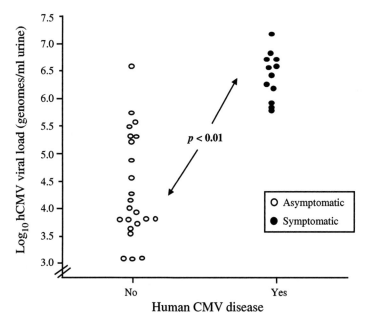

Fig. 13.1   Peak viral load in urine and human CMV disease in renal transplant patients.

in all transplant patient groups find that the detection of viraemia is a risk factor for CMV disease.[11] To determine if donor/recipient serostatus, viraemia, and high viral load were independent markers of high-risk patients or were different ways of measuring the same pathogenetic factor, multivariate statistical analyses were performed.

For all three patient populations, high viral load remained a risk factor for CMV disease after viraemia and donor/recipient serostatus had been controlled statistically. In contrast, donor/recipient serostatus and viraemia were no longer statistically significant once viral load had been controlled.[6,9] Thus, high viral load is the major determinant of CMV disease and the classically defined risk factors of donor/recipient serostatus and viraemia are markers of CMV disease because of their association with high viral load. Furthermore, the relationship between increasing viral load and disease is non-linear, showing that a threshold value exists above which CMV disease becomes more common.[8] This implies that marked prevention of disease could be obtained if drugs were deployed to prevent viral load reaching these critical values. Furthermore, serial measurements of viraemia in several groups of immunocompromised patients demonstrated that CMV replicates with rapid dynamics, approximating to a half-life of 1 day.[12] This means that its reputation as a 'slowly growing' virus is undeserved and that drugs of high potency are required to interfere with its replication. In addition, this high rate of replication explains how CMV variants resistant to ganciclovir (GCV) can evolve, and provides a basis for calculating their relative fitness compared with wild-type virus.[12] These mathematical modelling techniques can also be used to explain and predict the circumstances under which resistant strains become prominent.[13] In summary, short courses of GCV are unlikely to select resistant strains, but repeated courses, especially with oral GCV, provide ideal opportunities for resistant strains to flourish. They also demonstrate why resistant strains are cultured infrequently in practice; the process of incubating mixed populations of strains for 3–4 weeks in cell cultures lacking GCV allows the wild-type virus to out-compete the mutant strain, leading to the conclusion that resistance is not present. Thus, viral load measurements explain much of the pathogenesis of CMV disease, are important for understanding disease processes, for targeting the deployment of antiviral drugs, and for measuring the success of antiviral therapy and predicting the development of resistance.

Direct clinical effects

Much of the end-organ disease caused by CMV can be attributed to lysis, i.e. destruction of cells as a direct result of viral replication. This can be seen clearly in the special case of the retinal cells destroyed by CMV retinitis, but similar processes probably account for hepatitis, adrenalitis, gastrointestinal tract ulceration, encephalitis, and polyradiculopathy. In all of these cases, CMV can be seen histopathologically in biopsies (through the owl's eye inclusions formed when cells are producing CMV), can be cultured from biopsies (showing productive replication), and disease responds to antiviral therapy. In contrast, some other diseases (e.g. pneumonitis) associated with CMV may be triggered by the virus but be caused by immune responses.[14]

Indirect clinical effects

CMV is associated with an increased incidence of acute graft rejection. The presumed pathogenesis involves CMV infection of the transplanted organ acting like a transplantation antigen, marking the organ for immune attack. Evidence for CMV playing this pathogenic role includes statistical association, detection of CMV in organs undergoing rejection, apparent response of late rejection to ganciclovir therapy in an uncontrolled study, and a significant reduction in acute graft rejection in patients randomized to high-dose valaciclovir in a placebo-controlled trial of prophylaxis after renal transplant.[15–17]

CMV is also associated with accelerated atherosclerosis after heart transplantation.[15] Several potential pathogenic mechanisms could explain this association. CMV is found in monocytes/macrophages which could be attracted to sites of graft atheroma, either bringing CMV to that site or facilitating the formation of foam cells laden with oxidized lipids.[2] CMV major immediate-early protein binds p53 in arterial smooth muscle cells.[18] This suggests that CMV could reduce apoptosis leading to proliferation of such cells. The $U_S 28$ gene of CMV encodes a chemokine receptor, which once transferred experimentally to smooth muscle cells confers on them the ability to migrate towards a source of chemokines.[19] Thus, CMV infection might stimulate chemotactic mobility of these cells towards a site of inflammation. Finally, CMV stimulates the formation of reactive oxidized intermediates and could contribute further to the progression of atherosclerosis.[20] It should be noted that follow-up of heart allograft patients who took part in a placebo-controlled trial of GCV has recently reported reduced accelerated atherosclerosis in those allocated the drug.[21]

CMV is also associated with bacterial or fungal superinfection and follow-up of the heart allograft patients mentioned above has demonstrated reduced fungal infection in those randomized to GCV.[22] This implies that CMV is functionally immunosuppressive, although no immunological mechanism has ever been confirmed.

Clinical manifestations

The major clinical manifestations of CMV disease in different groups of immunocompromised patients are summarized in Table 13.2. These should be defined using criteria laid down at the International CMV Workshop which include: compatible clinical features plus signs of end-organ dysfunction plus demonstration of CMV in the affected organ (exception retina).[23] In particular, diseases should be described in terms of the body system affected and the term 'CMV syndrome' avoided.

Fever/leucopenia

CMV viraemia is often associated with prolonged spiking fever (e.g. > 38 °C on three consecutive days), with or without leucopenia. These constitutional symptoms may resolve spontaneously or may lead to end-organ disease. Other possible causes of fever (e.g. bacteraemia) and leucopenia (e.g. doses of immunosuppressive drugs) must be excluded.

Hepatitis

Typically, transaminases are raised by more than 2.5 times the upper limit of normal, with or without increased alkaline phosphatase. Hyperbilirubinaemia may be present but frank jaundice is uncommon. Hepatitis usually resolves spontaneously but may herald other end-organ disease.

Gastrointestinal disease

CMV may involve the gastrointestinal tract anywhere from the mouth to the anus. The presentation is usually with pain, often accompanied by fever. Oesophagitis, odynophagia, and abdominal pain mimicking perforation indicate involvement of the oesophagus/colon respectively. Endoscopy reveals mucosal ulcerations, with or without *Candida* superinfection. The ulcers respond slowly to treatment and may perforate and/or haemorrhage.

Pneumonitis

Most cases occur after bone marrow transplant with concurrent graft versus host disease, but can follow renal allografting. There is rapid onset of dyspnoea plus hypoxia. The chest radiograph may be relatively clear initially but progresses to show interstitial infiltrates. There is a high mortality, with poor response to treatment.[24]

Retinitis

This can occur in any immunocompromized patient but is most common in AIDS. Symptoms, if present, include 'floaters', flashing lights, and loss of central vision. Small peripheral lesions may be unnoticed by the patient; lesions involving the macula may be imminently sight-threatening and demand immediate treatment. Involvement of a large proportion of the retina interrupts retinal/scleral attachment and represents a risk factor for retinal detachment.

Diagnosis

Detection of viraemia

This can be performed by any published method shown to provide a good positive predictive value for CMV disease, e.g. 50–60% for the patient population to be followed. Thus, the rapid diagnostic techniques using cell culture amplification testing of virus (termed DEAFF testing in Europe and shell-vial in the United States) are no longer sufficiently sensitive and should be replaced with newer methods.[25,26] Examples include PCR in whole blood, PCR in plasma, and antigenaemia.[29,27–29] Note that a randomized trial in bone marrow transplant patients has shown PCR to be superior to conventional cell culture for deciding when to initiate pre-emptive therapy.[30] Laboratory protocols differ, and it is important that all aspects of each method are followed in detail including sample processing and virus detection. These have been optimized to avoid the detection of latent virus while providing good sensitivity for predicting disease but not necessarily the highest sensitivity for detecting asymptomatic infection. Thus, it is not possible to 'mix and match' different aspects of PCR protocols. Whichever method is chosen, the results must be audited at regular intervals to ensure that the anticipated positive predictive values are being attained, e.g. when any changes to immunosuppressive or antiviral protocols are being contemplated.

DEAFF/shell-vial

This method is still sufficiently sensitive and robust to diagnose CMV lung infection using bronchoalveolar lavage fluid. Cells from this fluid can also be cytocentrifuged and stained with monoclonal antibodies, but this approach, while more rapid, lacks sensitivity compared with DEAFF/shell–vial amplification.

Histopathology

This is performed on tissue biopsies to detect classic Cowdry type A intranuclear 'owl's eye' inclusion bodies. It is insensitive but has a high specificity for disease.[31]

Cell culture

This is performed on tissue biopsies after tissue is minced and inoculated directly on to cells. It is slow but sensitive.

Serology

Many enzyme immunoassays are commercially available for the detection of CMV IgG antibodies pretransplant in both donor and recipient. Serological testing has no role to play post-transplant.

Management

The principles of managing CMV infection and disease in the immunocompromised host are to anticipate their development, define policies for monitoring patients routinely for the presence of viraemia according to their baseline risk of CMV disease, and to enhance surveillance if patients develop a condition likely to increase their risk of CMV disease. Using the principles of evidence-based medicine, the patient will then be offered prophylaxis or pre-emptive therapy based upon an assessment of their individualized risk of disease, together with data from controlled clinical trials in the same patient group supporting the efficacy and safety of possible antiviral interventions.

Strategies for deploying antiviral agents

Different strategies have been devised for controlling CMV disease based on the efficacies and toxicities of the drugs available at present (summarized in Table 13.3).

True prophylaxis

This strategy may be used where an assessment at baseline shows that the risk of disease is high, the chance of severe disease is also high, and that at least one double-blind, randomized, placebo-controlled trial supports the efficacy and safety of prophylaxis in the target population. The patient will then be given the drug from the time of transplant until the time studied in the controlled clinical trial which provided evidence for its use. This is termed 'true prophylaxis' because, from a virological perspective, it administers the drug before there is active viral replication.

Delayed prophylaxis

At baseline, a decision was made that true prophylaxis was not indicated. However, the patient's situation has changed, e.g. because augmented immunosuppression is required to control an episode of graft rejection and so it is decided to start prophylaxis.[32] This is still termed 'prophylaxis' because the drug is given before there is active viral replication.

Table 13.3 Strategies for chemotherapy of CMV

Term used	When drug given	Risk of disease	Acceptable toxicity	Treatment decision prompted by
Prophylaxis	Before active infection	Low	None	Clinician
Delayed prophylaxis	Before active infection but after rejection	Medium	Low	Clinician
Suppression	After peripheral detection of virus	Medium	Low	Laboratory
Pre-emptive therapy	After systemic detection of virus	High	Medium	Laboratory
Treatment	Once disease is apparent	Established	High	Both

Suppression

The patient has been monitored by collecting weekly samples of urine and/or saliva and processing them by a laboratory method shown to provide a moderate positive predictive value for CMV disease, e.g. 30%.[11,27] It is decided to give an antiviral drug with the intention of suppressing virus replication below the level needed to cause viraemia. A drug more potent than that required for prophylaxis is needed because it will be deployed when the virus already has a 'head-start' in the race for control of replication.

Pre-emptive therapy

This term describes intervention when the results of laboratory tests indicate that a patient is at imminent risk of CMV disease.[33] It has been used in two circumstances: detection of viraemia in any immunocompromised patient and detection of asymptomatic lung infection after bone marrow transplant (an approach now superseded by testing for viraemia).[34] In either case, a highly potent drug is required, e.g. ganciclovir.

For detecting viraemia, patients should be monitored by collecting weekly samples of blood which are processed by laboratory methods known to provide a high positive predictive value for CMV disease, e.g. 50–60%.[11,27] If CMV is detected, an antiviral drug should be given with the intention of halting CMV viraemia before it reaches the high viral loads required to cause disease.

Decision points for starting pre-emptive therapy must be based upon the results of clinicopathological studies with the assay under evaluation. Examples include detection of viraemia by PCR or antigenaemia above a cut-off value associated with a high risk of disease or two consecutive samples PCR-positive (reviewed by Griffiths and Whitley).[35] More recently, the results of viral dynamic assessments have been applied to this problem; patients at risk of disease can be identified by the absolute value of viral load found in the first PCR-positive sample, coupled with an assessment of individual viral dynamics by calculating the rate of increase from the last PCR-negative sample.[36]

Treatment of established disease

A patient with compatible symptoms and signs, together with detection of CMV in the affected organ, meets the case definition of CMV disease. A highly potent drug is required which will penetrate the affected organ and resolve the disease, including any immunopathological components. As discussed below, no drug has been shown in a double-blind, placebo-controlled trial to be capable of meeting this objective.

Results of double-blind, randomized, placebo-controlled trials

Results of published trials defined according to these criteria are given in Tables 13.4–13.7. The most potent drug *in vitro*, GCV, has been subjected to several such clinical trials but the other licensed compounds, foscarnet and cidofovir, have not. Other agents such as interferon-α, acyclovir, valaciclovir, and immunoglobulin, have also been evaluated.

Table 13.4 shows that, in addition to ganciclovir, interferon-α, acyclovir, and valaciclovir have activity against CMV *in vivo*.[17,37–47] The only two studies not to show an effect were the two studies of immunoglobulin, which suggests that if immunoglobulin has a role in the prophylaxis of CMV disease it may not be working through inhibition of CMV replication.[48,49]

Table 13.5 shows that ganciclovir failed to demonstrate a significantly better resolution of established CMV disease than placebo.[37] Part of this disappointing outcome may be attributed to the low dose (2.5 mg/kg tid) and/or short duration used (14 days) to treat gastrointestinal disease in bone marrow transplant patients.[37] Nevertheless, it illustrates the difficulty of treating established CMV disease and so argues that the other strategies, which aim to prevent CMV disease, should always be pursued in preference to waiting for disease to establish itself. Ganciclovir did reduce CMV disease when used in the suppressive mode of bone marrow transplant patients.[38] It also had a significant benefit when

Table 13.4 Double-blind, placebo-controlled, randomized trials of CMV: infection end-point

Strategy	Drug	Bone marrow	Renal	Heart	Liver
Treatment	GCV	**Reed**[37]			
Suppressive	GCV	**Goodrich**[38]			
Prophylaxis	Interferon		**Cheeseman,**[43] **Hirsch,**[44] **Lui**[45]		
	ACV	**Prentice**[47]	**Balfour**[46]		
	VACV		**Lowance**[17]		
	Ig		Metselaar[49]		Snydman[48]
	GCV	**Winston,**[40] **Goodrich**[39]		**Merigan,**[41] **Macdonald**[50]	**Gane**[42]

Studies shown in bold reported a significant benefit.
Abbreviations: GCV, ganciclovir; ACV, acyclovir; VACV, valaciclovir, Ig, immunoglobulin.

Table 13.5 Double-blind, placebo-controlled, randomized trials of CMV: disease end-point

Strategy	Drug	Bone marrow	Renal	Heart	Liver
Treatment	GCV	Reed[37]			
Suppressive	GCV	**Goodrich**[38]			
Prophylaxis	Interferon		Cheeseman,[43] **Hirsch**,[44] Lui[45]		
	ACV	Prentice[47]	**Balfour**[46]		
	VACV		**Lowance**[17]		
	Ig		Metselaar[49]		**Snydman**[48]
	GCV	Winston,[40] Goodrich[39]		**Merigan**,[41] **Macdonald**[50]	**Gane**[42]

Studies shown in bold reported a significant benefit.
Abbreviations: GCV, ganciclovir; ACV, acyclovir; VACV, valaciclovir, Ig, immunoglobulin.

Table 13.6 Double-blind, placebo-controlled, randomized trials of CMV: survival end-point

Strategy	Drug	Bone marrow	Renal	Heart	Liver
Treatment	GCV	Reed[37]			
Suppressive	GCV	**Goodrich**[38]			
Prophylaxis	Interferon		Cheeseman,[43] Hirsch,[44] Lui[45]		
	ACV	**Prentice**[47]	Balfour[46]		
	VACV		Lowance[17]		
	Ig		Metselaar[49]		Snydman[48]
	GCV	Winston,[40] Goodrich[39]		Merigan,[41] Macdonald[50]	Gane[42]

Studies shown in bold reported a significant benefit.
Abbreviations: GCV, ganciclovir; ACV, acyclovir; VACV, valaciclovir, Ig, immunoglobulin.

used in one of two trials of prophylaxis after bone marrow transplant; the second study showed a strong trend in favour of ganciclovir which just failed to reach conventional statistical significance.[39,40] Ganciclovir also significantly reduced CMV disease following prophylaxis given orally to liver transplant patients and intravenously to heart transplant patients.[41,42,50] However, benefit after heart transplant was seen in the low-risk group only, with no effect in the D+R− group of one study, whereas the opposite outcome was seen in a second.[41,50] This difference might result from the longer treatment course in the later study, together with a design difference such that patients with rejection were given additional doses of GCV. Prophylactic acyclovir significantly reduced CMV disease after renal transplant, as did prophylactic

Table 13.7 Double-blind, placebo-controlled, randomized trials of CMV: indirect effects end-point

Strategy	Drug	Bone marrow	Renal	Heart	Liver
Treatment	GCV	Reed[37]			
Suppressive	GCV	Goodrich[38]			
Prophylaxis	Interferon		Cheeseman,[43] Hirsch,[44] Lui[45]		
	ACV	Prentice[47]	Balfour[46]		
	VACV		**Lowance**[17]		
	Ig		Metselaar[49]		**Snydman**[48]
	GCV	**Winston,**[40] Goodrich[39]		**Merigan,**[41] Macdonald[50]	Gane[42]

Studies shown in bold reported a significant benefit.
Abbreviations: GCV, ganciclovir; ACV, acyclovir; VACV, valaciclovir, Ig, immunoglobulin.

valaciclovir.[17,46] In a prophylaxis trial after bone marrow transplant, acyclovir significantly decreased CMV viraemia and showed a non-significant trend towards reduced CMV disease.[47] A trial of immunoglobulin prophylaxis showed reduced 'CMV syndrome', despite having no significant effect on CMV infection.[48] Subgroup analysis showed an effect on CMV-associated fungal superinfection (part of the predefined 'CMV syndrome'), so it remains possible that the immunoglobulin predominantly reduces fungal rather than CMV infection.

Table 13.6 examines whether these drugs demonstrated a survival benefit in the clinical trials. The number of deaths in the solid organ transplant populations is too low to provide the statistical power to address this issue. After bone marrow transplant, ganciclovir significantly improved survival when used suppressively but, when used prophylactically, no effect was seen.[38–40] This was not a problem of small sample size, and neither study demonstrated even a trend in favour of ganciclovir. The most likely explanations are that some patients with viraemia still received pre-emptive therapy so reducing CMV-induced mortality in both arms but that ganciclovir-induced neutropenia induced by prophylactic GCV predisposed patients to succumb to bacterial or fungal superinfections, so mitigating the potential benefits of this drug.[39] Overall, these studies indicate that ganciclovir is too toxic a compound to be used for prophylaxis after bone marrow transplant, although it is literally life-saving when used in suppressive mode.[38] This illustrates that, in prophylaxis, all patients are exposed to side-effects and that suppression, by limiting the number of patients exposed to the drug, can produce better therapeutic ratios. In contrast, acyclovir prophylaxis after bone marrow transplant produced a survival benefit, presumably because its more modest efficacy was not offset by serious toxicity.[47]

Table 13.7 summarizes the studies which have so far reported significantly reduced indirect effects of CMV. After renal transplant, valaciclovir produced a marked reduction in biopsy-proven acute graft rejection corresponding to a 50% decrease in incidence in seronegative recipients at risk of primary infection.[17] The effects in seropositive recipients were smaller, implying that CMV (rather than another herpesvirus susceptible to the drug) is responsible for this indirect effect and that most CMV-induced graft rejection occurs in the subset of patients with primary infection. Following heart transplantation, GCV significantly reduced fungal infections and accelerated atherosclerosis.[21,22]

Conclusions

Decisions about which drugs to recommend for particular treatment strategies must draw upon evidence-based medicine provided by the results of controlled clinical trials. Decisions must be based upon considerations of toxicity as well as on efficacy, and so may differ according to the therapeutic ratio of a compound in different populations.

The acyclovir and valaciclovir studies do show that potent inhibition of DNA polymerase by acyclovir triphosphate can have clinical utility under some circumstances. In the renal transplant study, the authors provide evidence that plasma levels of acyclovir were higher than expected because of poor renal clearance, but were still lower than would be required to inhibit CMV based on *in vitro* data, which demonstrate clearly that the IC50 levels produced by fibroblast cell cultures are misleadingly high.[51]

Antiviral prophylaxis can significantly reduce the incidence of biopsy-proven graft rejection in renal allograft patients. The same probably applies to pre-emptive therapy because the major effect was seen in the D+R− subgroup, whose need for therapy can be detected readily, but a controlled trial is needed to confirm this.

Overall, the clinical benefits of preventing CMV disease (including the indirect effects of CMV) are so clear that all patients at risk of CMV disease (e.g. those with seropositive donors) should either be given antiviral prophylaxis or be followed virologically and given pre-emptive therapy.

References

1. Cha TA, Tom E, Kemble GW, Duke GM, Mocarski ES, Spaete RR. Human cytomegalovirus clinical isolates carry at least 19 genes not found in laboratory strains. *Journal of Virology* 1996; **70**(1):78–83.
2. Guetta E, Guetta V, Shibutani T, Epstein SE. Monocytes harboring cytomegalovirus: interactions with endothelial cells, smooth muscle cells, and oxidized low-density lipoprotein. Possible mechanisms for activating virus delivered by monocytes to sites of vascular injury. *Circulation Research* 1997; **81**(1):8–16.
3. Stagno S, Cloud GA. Working parents: the impact of day care and breast-feeding on cytomegalovirus infections in offspring. *Proceedings of the National Academy of Sciences of the United States of America* 1994; **91**:2384–2389.
4. Grundy JE, Lui SF, Super M, Berry NJ, Sweny P, Fernando ON *et al.* Symptomatic cytomegalovirus infection in seropositive kidney recipients: reinfection with donor virus rather than reactivation of recipient virus. *Lancet* 1988; **2**:132–135.
5. Stagno S, Reynolds DW, Tsiantos A, Fuccillo DA, Long W, Alford CA. Comparative serial virologic and serologic studies of symptomatic and subclinical congenitally and

natally acquired cytomegalovirus infections. *Journal of Infectious Diseases* 1975; **132**(5):568–577.

6. Cope AV, Sweny P, Sabin C, Rees L, Griffiths PD, Emery VC. Quantity of cytomegalovirus viruria is a major risk factor for cytomegalovirus disease after renal transplantation. *Journal of Medical Virology* 1997; **52**:200–205.

7. Hassan-Walker AF, Kidd IM, Sabin C, Sweny P, Griffiths PD, Emery VC. Quantity of human cytomegalovirus (CMV) DNAemia as a risk factor for CMV disease in renal allograft recipients: relationship with donor/recipient CMV serostatus, receipt of augmented methyl-prednisolone and anti-thymocyte globulin (ATG). *Journal of Medical Virology* 1999; **58**:182–187.

8. Cope AV, Sabin C, Burroughs A, Rolles K, Griffiths PD, Emery VC. Interrelationships among quantity of human cytomegalovirus (HCMV) DNA in blood, donor-recipient sero-status, and administration of methylprednisolone as risk factors for HCMV disease following liver transplantation. *Journal of Infectious Diseases* 1997; **176**(6):1484–1490.

9. Gor D, Sabin C, Prentice HG, Vyas N, Man S, Griffiths PD *et al*. Longitudinal fluctuations between peak virus load, donor/recipient serostatus, acute GvHD and CMV disease. *Bone Marrow Transplantation* 1998; **21**:597–605.

10. Betts RF, Freeman RB, Douglas RG Jr, Talley TE. Clinical manifestations of renal allograft derived primary cytomegalovirus infection. *American Journal of Diseases of Children* 1977; **131**(7):759–763.

11. Meyers JD, Ljungman P, Fisher LD. Cytomegalovirus excretion as a predictor of cytomegalovirus disease after marrow transplantation: importance of cytomegalovirus viremia. *Journal of Infectious Diseases* 1990; **162**:373–380.

12. Emery VC, Cope AV, Bowen EF, Gor D, Griffiths PD. The dynamics of human cytomegalovirus replication *in vivo*. *Journal of Experimental Medicine* 1999; **190**(2):177–182.

13. Emery VC, Griffiths PD. Prediction of cytomegalovirus load and resistance patterns after antiviral chemotherapy. *Proceedings of the National Academy of Sciences of the United States of America* 2000; **97**(14):8039–8044.

14. Grundy JE, Shanley JD, Griffiths PD. Is cytomegalovirus interstitial pneumonitis in transplant recipients an immunopathological condition? *Lancet* 1987; **2**:996–999.

15. Grattan MT, Moreno-Cabral CE, Starnes VA, Oyer PE, Stinson EB. Cytomegalovirus infec-tion is associated with cardiac allograft rejection and atherosclerosis. *Journal of the American Medical Association* 1989; **261**:3561–3566.

16. Reinke P, Fietze E, Ode-Hakim S, Prosch S, Lippert J, Ewert R *et al*. Late acute renal allograft rejection and symptomless cytomegalovirus infection. *Lancet* 1994; **344**:1737–1738.

17. Lowance D, Neumayer H-H, Legendre C, Squifflet J-P, Kovarik J, Brennan PJ *et al*. Valaciclovir reduces the incidence of cytomegalovirus disease and acute rejection in renal allograft recipients. *New England Journal of Medicine* 1999; **340**:1462–1470.

18. Speir E, Modali R, Huang ES, Leon MB, Shawl F, Finkel T *et al*. Potential role of human cytomegalovirus and p53 interaction in coronary restenosis. *Science* 1994; **265**:391–394.

19. Streblow DN, Soderberg-Naucler C, Vieira J, Smith P, Wakabayashi E, Ruchti F *et al*. The human cytomegalovirus chemokine receptor US28 mediates vascular smooth muscle cell migration. *Cell* 1999; **99**:511–520.

20. Speir E, Shibutani T, Yu ZX, Ferrans V, Epstein SE. Role of reactive oxygen intermediates in cytomegalovirus gene expression and in the response of human smooth muscle cells to viral infection. *Circulation Research* 1996; **79**(6):1143–1152.

21. Valantine HA, Gao S-Z, Menon SG, Renlund DG, Hunt SA, Oyer P *et al*. Impact of prophylactic immediate posttransplant ganciclovir on development of transplant atherosclero-sis: A post-hoc analysis of a randomised, placebo-controlled study. *Circulation* 1999; **100**:61–66.

22. Wagner JA, Ross H, Hunt S, Gamberg P, Valantine H, Merigan TC *et al.* Prophylactic ganciclovir treatment reduces fungal as well as cytomegalovirus infections after heart transplantation. *Transplantation* 1995; **60**(12):1473–1477.

23. Ljungman P, Plotkin SA. Workshop of CMV disease: definitions, clinical severity scores, and new syndromes. *Scandinavian Journal of Infectious Diseases – Suppl.* 1995; **99** :87–89.

24. Ljungman P, Engelhard D, Link H, Biron P, Brandt L, Brunet S *et al.* Treatment of interstitial pneumonitis due to cytomegalovirus with ganciclovir and intravenous immune globulin: experience of European Bone Marrow Transplant Group. *Clinical Infectious Diseases* 1992; **14**:831–835.

25. Griffiths PD, Panjwani DD, Stirk PR, Ball MG, Ganczakowski M, Blacklock HA *et al.* Rapid diagnosis of cytomegalovirus infection in immunocompromised patients by detection of early antigen fluorescent foci. *Lancet* 1984; **2**:1242–1245.

26. Gleaves CA, Smith TF, Shuster EA, Pearson GR. Rapid detection of cytomegalovirus in MRC-5 cells inoculated with urine specimens by using low-speed centrifugation and monoclonal antibody to an early antigen. *Journal of Clinical Microbiology* 1984; **19**:917–919.

27. Kidd IM, Fox JC, Pillay D, Charman H, Griffiths PD, Emery VC. Provision of prognostic information in immunocompromised patients by routine application of the polymerase chain reaction for cytomegalovirus. *Transplantation* 1993; **56**(4):867–871.

28. Spector SA, Merrill R, Wolf D, Dankner WM. Detection of human cytomegalovirus in plasma of AIDS patients during acute visceral disease by DNA amplification. *Journal of Clinical Microbiology* 1992; **30**(9):2359–2365.

29. The TH, van der Bij W, van den Berg AP, van der Giessen M, Weits J, Sprenger HG *et al.* Cytomegalovirus antigenemia. *Reviews of Infectious Diseases* 1990; **12** Suppl 7:S734–S744.

30. Einsele H, Ehninger G, Hebart H, Wittkowski KM, Schuler U, Jahn G *et al.* Polymerase chain reaction monitoring reduces the incidence of cytomegalovirus disease and the duration and side effects of antiviral therapy after bone marrow transplantation. *Blood* 1995; **86**(7):2815–2820.

31. Mattes FM, McLaughlin JE, Emery VC, Clark DA, Griffiths PD. Histopathological detection of owl's eye inclusions is still specific for cytomegalovirus in the era of human herpesviruses 6 and 7. *Journal of Clinical Pathology* 2000; **53**:612–614.

32. Hibberd PL, Tolkoff-Rubin NE, Conti D, Stuart F, Thistlethwaite JR, Neylan JF *et al.* Preemptive ganciclovir therapy to prevent cytomegalovirus disease in cytomegalovirus antibody-positive renal transplant recipients. A randomized controlled trial. *Annals of Internal Medicine* 1995; **123**(1):18–26.

33. Rubin RH. Preemptive therapy in immunocompromised hosts [editorial]. *New England Journal of Medicine* 1991; **324**:1057–1059.

34. Schmidt GM, Horak DA, Niland JC, Duncan SR, Forman SJ, Zaia JA. A randomized, controlled trial of prophylactic ganciclovir for cytomegalovirus pulmonary infection in recipients of allogeneic bone marrow transplants; The City of Hope-Stanford-Syntex CMV Study Group. *New England Journal of Medicine* 1991; **324**:1005–1011.

35. Griffiths PD, Whitley RJ (ed.). *The challenge of CMV infection and disease in transplantation,* 2000. IHMF, Worthing, Sussex, UK

36. Emery VC, Sabin CA, Cope AV, Gor D, Hassan-Walker AF, Griffiths PD. Application of viral-load kinetics to identify patients who develop cytomegalovirus disease after transplantation. *Lancet* 2000; **355**(9220):2032–2036.

37. Reed EC, Wolford JL, Kopecky KJ, Lilleby KE, Dandliker PS, Todaro JL *et al.* Ganciclovir for the treatment of cytomegalovirus gastroenteritis in bone marrow transplant patients. A randomized, placebo-controlled trial. *Annals of Internal Medicine* 1990; **112**:505–510.

38. Goodrich JM, Mori M, Gleaves CA, Du-Mond C, Cays M, Ebeling DF *et al.* Early treatment with ganciclovir to prevent cytomegalovirus disease after allogeneic bone marrow transplantation. *New England Journal of Medicine* 1991; **325**:1601–1607.
39. Goodrich JM, Bowden RA, Fisher L, Keller C, Schoch G, Meyers JD. Ganciclovir prophylaxis to prevent cytomegalovirus disease after allogeneic marrow transplant. *Annals of Internal Medicine* 1993; **118**:173–178.
40. Winston DJ, Ho WG, Bartoni K, Du Mond C, Ebeling DF, Buhles WC. Ganciclovir prophylaxis of cytomegalovirus infection and disease in allogeneic bone marrow transplant recipients. Results of a placebo-controlled, double-blind trial. *Annals of Internal Medicine* 1993; **118**:179–184.
41. Merigan TC, Renlund DG, Keay S, Bristow MR, Starnes V, O'Connell JB *et al.* A controlled trial of ganciclovir to prevent cytomegalovirus disease after heart transplantation. *New England Journal of Medicine* 1992; **326**(18):1182–1186.
42. Gane E, Saliba F, Valdecasas GJ, O'Grady J, Pescovitz MD, Lyman S *et al.* Randomised trial of efficacy and safety of oral ganciclovir in the prevention of cytomegalovirus disease in liver-transplant recipients. The Oral Ganciclovir International Transplantation Study Group. *Lancet* 1997; **350**(9093):1729–1733.
43. Cheeseman SH, Rubin RH, Stewart JA, Tolkoff-Rubin NE, Cosimi AB, Cantell K *et al.* Controlled clinical trial of prophylactic human-leukocyte interferon in renal transplantation. Effects on cytomegalovirus and herpes simplex virus infections. *New England Journal of Medicine* 1979; **300**:1345–1349.
44. Hirsch MS, Schooley RT, Cosimi AB, Russell PS, Delmonico FL, Tolkoff-Rubin NE *et al.* Effects of interferon-alpha on cytomegalovirus reactivation syndromes in renal-transplant recipients. *New England Journal of Medicine* 1983; **308**:1489–1493.
45. Lui SF, Ali AA, Grundy JE, Fernando ON, Griffiths PD, Sweny P. Double-blind, placebo-controlled trial of human lymphoblastoid interferon prophylaxis of cytomegalovirus infection in renal transplant recipients. *Nephrology, Dialysis, Transplantation* 1992; **7**:1230–1237.
46. Balfour HHJ, Chace BA, Stapleton JT, Simmons RL, Fryd DS. A randomized, placebo-controlled trial of oral acyclovir for the prevention of cytomegalovirus disease in recipients of renal allografts. *New England Journal of Medicine* 1989; **320**:1381–1387.
47. Prentice HG, Gluckman E, Powles RL, Ljungman P, Milpied N, Fernandez Ranada JM *et al.* Impact of long-term acyclovir on cytomegalovirus infection and survival after allogeneic bone marrow transplantation. European Acyclovir for CMV Prophylaxis Study Group. *Lancet* 1994; **343**:749–753.
48. Snydman DR, Werner BG, Dougherty NN, Griffith J, Rubin RH, Dienstag JL *et al.* Cytomegalovirus immune globulin prophylaxis in liver transplantation. A randomized, double-blind, placebo-controlled trial. The Boston Center for Liver Transplantation CMVIG Study Group. *Annals of Internal Medicine* 1993; **119**:984–991.
49. Metselaar HJ, Rothbarth PH, Brouwer RM, Wenting GJ, Jeekel J, Weimar *et al.* Prevention of cytomegalovirus-related death by passive immunization. A double-blind placebo-controlled study in kidney transplant recipients treated for rejection. *Transplantation* 1989; **48**(2):264–266.
50. Macdonald PS, Keogh AM, Marshman D, Richens D, Harvison A, Kaan AM *et al.* A double-blind placebo-controlled trial of low-dose ganciclovir to prevent cytomegalovirus disease after heart transplantation. *Journal of Heart and Lung Transplantation* 1995; **14**(1):32–38.
51. Fletcher CV, Englund JA, Edelman CK, Gross CR, Dunn DL, Balfour HHJ. Pharmacologic basis for high-dose oral acyclovir prophylaxis of cytomegalovirus disease in renal allograft recipients. *Antimicrobial Agents and Chemotherapy* 1991; **35**:938–943.

14

Virus-related tumours

P. Sweny

Introduction

Most of the tumours that are encountered with a greatly increased frequency following renal transplantation have a viral aetiology (Table 14.1). In some cases these tumours behave more like infections in that they can regress completely on reduction or withdrawal of immunosuppression, particularly if this is embarked upon early in their natural history. Malignancy has been estimated to be about 100 times more frequent in the transplant population than in the non-immunosuppressed (Toukraine *et al.* 1996). No specific immunosuppressive agents appear to be responsible, but rather tumours develop in response to the total burden of immunosuppression however administered. In this respect azathioprine and prednisolone have a lower incidence and later presentation time than regimes based on calcineurin-blocking drugs. Increased TGF-β may contribute to this earlier presentation. Potent polyclonal antibodies such as antithymocyte globulin or antilymphocyte globulin and the monoclonal antibody OKT3 are associated with a further increase in virus-related tumours. It is too early to know whether newer agents such as mycophenolate mofetil, rapamycin, or the humanized/chimaeric antibodies to CD25 carry any increased risk.

Kaposi's sarcoma

Kaposi's sarcoma (KS) occurs as an endemic and sporadic tumour. It has been clearly related to immunosuppression both in organ transplant recipients (Francès 1998) and in HIV patients (Table 14.2).

Clinical features

KS presents on average some 20 months following transplantation (Gotti and Remuzzi 1997). In patients on prednisolone and azathioprine presentation is a little later, while those on the calcineurin blockers tend to present earlier. Clinical features are summarized in Table 14.3. In the transplant population 60% of patients have cutaneous limited disease and 40% have additional visceral involvement.

In the transplant population second malignancies are more common (6%) in KS patients, for example some 2% will have an associated lymphoma.

Table 14.1   Virus-related tumours

Tumour	Relative risk	Prevalence (%)	Relative proportion of post-transplant tumours (%)*	Virus	Other associated tumours related to virus
PTLD	300–400	1–2	40	EBV (HHV4)	Leiomyosarcoma in children, nasopharyngeal carcinoma, Burkitt's lymphoma, Hodgkin's lymphoma, T-cell lymphoma, NK lymphoproliferation
Kaposi's sarcoma	400–500			KSHV (HHV8)	Multicentric Castleman's disease, primary effusion lymphoma, ?POEMS syndrome
(i) Caucasian		0.4	3–5		
(ii) Arab, Jewish, Mediterranean		5.0	>65		
SCC of the cervix	14	10–50	10–20	HPV	Other anogenital sites (100×risk)
SCC of the skin	30	>15	Increase with time (~90%)	HPV	
Hepatoma	Unknown	Rare	Unknown	HBV, HCV	Plasmacytic lymphomas

*Excluding skin.
PTLD=post-transplant lymphoproliferative disorder; SCC=squamous cell carcinoma; EBV=Epsrtein–Barr virus; HPV=human papillomavirus; HBV=hepatitis B virus; HCV=hepatitis C virus.
POEMS syndrome: Peripheral neuropathy, Organomegaly, Endocrinopathy, Monoclonal plasmaproliferative disorder, Skin changes.

Aetiology of KS

Herpesvirus DNA sequences have been identified in the tissue of KS (Brooks *et al.* 1997; Ganem 1997). The virus is designated human herpesvirus 8 (HHV8) or Kaposi's sarcoma associated virus (KSHV). HHV8 belongs to the gamma herpesvirus group which all have oncogenic potential (e.g. Epstein–Barr virus (EBV) and herpesvirus saimian (HVS)). HHV8 sequences have also been detected in a variety of proliferative skin lesions in renal transplants (basal cell carcinoma, squamous cell carcinoma, actinic keratoses, verucca vulgaris, atypical squamous proliferations, and seborrhoeic keratosis). A number of these reports have, however, not been verified, e.g. squamous cell carcinoma. Transmission of the virus from donor to recipient has been demonstrated.

Table 14.2 Epidemiological classification of Kaposi's sarcoma

	Population affected	M:F	Survival
Classical	Elderly East European/ Meditteranean*	15:1	Years or decades
Endemic	Sub-Saharan African. Highly aggressive form in children	1:1	Months or years
Transplant	Solid organ transplant recipients. Marked ethnic susceptibility	3:1	Months or years
Epidemic	AIDS associated*	20:1	Weeks or months

*Both more prevalent in homosexual men.

Table 14.3 Clinical features of Kaposi's sarcoma

Site	Clinical features
Cutaneous (>90%)	Reddish blue macules or plaques. Nodules → ulcerating tumours. Deep infiltration. Multifocal. Local spread and expansion. Legs > trunk, face, arms. Associated oedema
Pulmonary (15–20%)	Dyspnoea. Haemoptysis. Chest pains. Stridor. Recurrent pleural effusions—subpleural nodules. Pulmonary oedema (lymphatic obstruction). Consolidation—collapse. Laryngeal involvement
Gastrointestinal (GI) (approximately 50%)	Asymptomatic. Non-specific upper GI symptoms. Bleeding. Perforation. Obstruction. Intussusception. Gum infiltration. Upper GI more common than lower GI
Lymph node (~30%)	
Other visceral: liver, spleen	

Geographical or racial factors are very important (Table 14.4) in determining exposure to HHV8.

A variety of growth factors and cytokines have been shown to promote the growth of KS tissue (IL-1b, oncostatin M, and GCSF). Additional angiogenic factors have also been shown to be important (TNF-α, EDGF, BFGF, vascular endothelial growth factor). It appears likely that many of these growth factors are produced locally in KS tissue from adjacent cells. KSHV itself encodes for proteins that play an important role in the proliferation and immortalization of KS tissue cells (Table 14.5) (Schultz 1998). HHV8-infected cells also express CD40 which promotes survival and proliferation as well as expressing integrins which bind to the extracellular matrix. A full understanding of these factors may open new therapeutic avenues (Bais *et al.* 1998).

Most workers consider that KS is not a true malignancy but rather a potentially reversible hyperplasia of the latently infected cells. Thus KS cells remain growth factor dependent, require anchorage, and do not result in stable tumours when injected into nude mice.

Table 14.4 Aetiological factors in post-transplant Kaposi's sarcoma

HHV8 viral load

Total burden of immunosuppression:
  Drugs
  Serotherapy

Geographical/racial:
  Jewish
  Mediterranean littoral
  African
  Arab (southern Arabian Peninsula)
  Eastern and Central Europe

HLA: A-2, A2 19, DR-5

Facilitating role of coinfection with EBV or CMV

Male > female (M:F 2:1)

Table 14.5 KSHV genes (modified from Schulz 1998)

Localization	Gene product	Expression	Function
ORF K4, K6	vMIP-1α	Lytic cycle	Angiogenic
ORF K4.1	vMIP-1β	Lytic cycle	Angiogenic
ORF K9	IRF	Lytic cycle	Prolongs survival of lytically infected cells
ORF K2	vII–6	PEL	B-cell stimulation
ORF 16	Vbcl-2	Lytic cycle	Antiapoptotic
ORF K1			Transforming/immortalizing gene?
ORF 72	vCyclin D	SC +ve	Continuous proliferation
ORF 74	vGCR		Chemokine receptor: secretion of VEGF
ORF K13	vFlip	SC +ve	Antiapoptotic
ORF 71	vFlip	SC +ve	Antiapoptotic
ORF K12	Kaposin-A	SC +ve	Unknown
ORF 73	LANA	SC +ve	
Numerous	Structural proteins	Lytic cycle	Viral replication

MIP=macrophage inflammatory protein; LANA=latency associated nuclear antigen; IRF=interferon regulatory protein; ORF=open reading frame; ORFK=open reading frame unique to KSHV; VEGF= vascular endothelial growth factor; GCR=G-protein coupled receptor; Flip=FLICE-inhibitor protein; SC=spindle cell; PEL=primary effusion lymphoma; v denotes viral homologue.

Diagnosis and investigation of KS

Diagnosis is usually by histology (Table 14.6). It is of note that KS tissue contains both lytically and latently infected cells which implies the likelihood of intense autocrine activity by a wide range of cytokines and growth factors encoded or induced by KSHV.

Table 14.6 Histological features of Kaposi's sarcoma

Thin-walled neovascular formations

Extravasated red blood cells

Inflammatory lymphocytic infiltration

Proliferating spindle cells (lymphatic endothelium)

Table 14.7 Investigation of Kaposi's sarcoma

Chest radiograph

Full blood count

PBL

   Immunophenotyping of peripheral blood mononuclear cells

   Activation markers

Endoscopy
   Upper GI tract
   Lower GI tract

CT of chest and abdomen

Whole body thallium scan

Biopsy

Serum Igs

PBL, peripheral blood lymphocytes; Igs, immunoglobulins; GI, gastrointestinal.

It is thought that at least in some patients the widespread nature of the tumour develops from the rapid early spread from a single monoclonal source. Circulating KS-like spindle cells can be isolated and cultured from the blood in some patients. HHV8 can be demonstrated in peripheral blood mononuclear cells particularly in HIV-associated KS but less commonly in transplant-associated cases. Serology for HHV8 is being more widely introduced and seroconversion in transplant recipients is associated with an increased risk of developing KS. More than one antibody test may be required, e.g. antibodies to capsid antigen (lytic cycle) and to latent antigens (e.g. latency-associated nuclear antigen (LANA)). PCR may be used to detect HHV8 in the tissues from KS lesions and also in normal adjacent skin. It is important to investigate patients fully (Table 14.7) so that accurate staging (Table 14.8) can be undertaken.

Epidemiology

Serology indicates a prevalence of KSHV infection in blood donors of 0 to 5% in the United Kingdom and the United States but higher elsewhere (Table 14.9). KSHV can be detected by PCR in semen in otherwise healthy subjects in areas where KS is endemic. The virus can therefore probably be transmitted sexually and more recently it has been shown to be transmissible by organ donation in addition to blood transfusion. In endemic areas horizontal transmission also occurs. The disease is endemic in Africa, particularly

Table 14.8   Staging of Kaposi's sarcoma

1. Limited cutaneous (one extremity only)
2. Disseminated cutaneous (involving more than one extremity)
3. Viscera and/or lymph nodes
4. Any of the above plus associated life-threatening infection or another neoplasm
5. Generalized Kaposi's sarcoma—skin plus viscera and/or nodes
   A. No associated life-threatening infection
   B. Associated life-threatening infection or malignancy

Table 14.9   Prevalence of KSHV infection

Country	Seropositivity for LANA (general population + blood donors) (%)	Post-renal transplant KS		KS in general population (% all tumours)
		Prevalence %	all tumours %	
USA (Caucasian). Northern Europe	0–3	<0.5	<1	0.02–0.06
Italy (south), Greece	5–35	1.5–5	3	
Saudi Arabia	3–7	~5	>80	0.2–0.38
Africa	20–50	Unknown	Unknown	3–9

LANA = latency-associated nuclear antigen.

in sub-Saharan regions. There is a much increased prevalence in the Mediterranean littoral and in the Arabic states (Al-Sulaiman and Al-Khader 1994).

Treatment

Immunosuppression should be reduced in a stepwise fashion or in more advanced life-threatening cases probably withdrawn fully. Regression can take several months to occur and is seen in less than half of cases. Peripheral blood monitoring of lymphocyte activation markers may help guide the rate of reduction of immunosuppression (see below). If lesions do not regress, chemotherapy can be tried but will further impair the immune responsiveness of the patient and is associated with a greatly increased risk of opportunistic infection and death. In anticipation of the possible need for cytotoxic chemotherapy, azathioprine and mycophenolate mofetil should be withdrawn early. Prophylaxis with cotrimoxazole should therefore be given and intravenous immunoglobulin may be of value in patients whose serum IgG is very low.

   Prior to starting cytotoxic chemotherapy it is appropriate to try immunostimulation with interferon-α2a (IFN-α2a). Retinoids may have a role to play (Nagpal *et al.* 1997)

Table 14.10   Treatment of Kaposi's sarcoma

Reduction or cessation of immunosuppression

Anti-viral agents: protease inhibitors, e.g. indinavir, foscarnet,
ganciclovir, cidovovir (NB: not aciclovir)

Stimulation of the immune system:
  Interferon-α
  IL-2

Local therapy
  Surgical excision of single lesions
  Radiotherapy
  Intralesional bleomycin
  Intralesional human chorionic gonadotrophin (hCG)
  Laser therapy (e.g. endobronchial)
  Cryotherapy

Inhibition of growth factors
  Retinoids
  ACE inhibitors
  IL-4
  PF-4

Antiangiogenic agents, e.g. thalidomide

Cytotoxic chemotherapy: adriamycin, bleomycin, vincristine
(ABV), or liposomal (doxorubicin or daunorubicin)

perhaps acting to block IL-6 dependent pathways. It is likely that such an approach will
be associated with an increased loss of grafts. A variety of chemotherapeutic regimes are
available (Table 14.10). On theoretical grounds it seems unlikely that antiviral agents will
be effective, as the HHV8 genome is present in an episomal form and will not be susceptible to antiviral agents. However, the presence of both lytic and latently infected cells
within the lesions may mean that some antiviral agents could be effective in reducing
viral load and may limit the spread of infection to new cells (e.g. ganciclovir, foscarnet,
cidofovir, and adefovir).

Prognosis

Prognosis can be related to staging. Stages IA and IIA usually regress with reduction of
immunosuppression. Stages IIIA and IVA may require cessation of immunosuppression.
Pulmonary involvement carries a particularly poor prognosis and immunosuppression
should probably be stopped at diagnosis. Stages IIIB and IVB also require immediate
cessation of immunosuppression. Regression on reduction or withdrawal of immunosuppression is seen in about 30–50% of cases but up to half may lose their grafts.
Mortality remains high at about 20% despite chemotherapy and full supportive
treatment. It remains to be seen if prognosis can be improved by a formalized stepwise
and monitored immunosuppression dose reduction as described for post-transplant
lymphoproliferative disorder (PTLD).

Retransplantation

Although there are only a few reports in the literature, most workers consider that KS will recur after subsequent retransplantation even if the tumour regressed completely following previous reduction or withdrawal of immunosuppression.

Prophylaxis

The widespread use of ganciclovir for the prevention of CMV disease post-transplant may reduce the viral load of certain viruses (e.g. EBV, KSHV) and in some studies has been reported to reduce the frequency of PTLD, but data on KS are not available (Kedes and Ganem 1997).

Post-transplant lymphoproliferative disorder (PTLD)

Introduction

The incidence of lymphomatous lesions is increased some 400-fold following renal transplantation. On analysis these 'lymphomas' are usually of B-cell origin (86%), but 13% are T cell and 1% null cell. Approximately 90% of all these 'lymphomas' are associated with the presence of EBV. Most do not possess the characteristics of a true malignancy (activation of oncogenes) and may regress spontaneously with reduction or cessation of immunosuppression, indicating that they behave more like an opportunistic infection. The term post-transplant lymphoproliferative disorder (PTLD) has been used in preference to lymphoma to describe these uninhibited proliferations of B cells.

Clinical features

The spectrum of lesions associated with EBV infection in allograft recipients is wide and encompasses asymptomatic seroconversion, classical glandular fever, and rapidly progressive lymphoproliferative lesions (PTLD) which can affect almost any tissue (Table 14.11). Within the syndrome of PTLD there are at least three subgroups based on histology which correlate moderately well with outcome (Table 14.12). PTLD has a marked predilection for the central nervous system, extranodal sites, and for the transplanted organ (Boubenider *et al.* 1997). In such circumstances, PTLD can mimic rejection. Because of the protean manifestations of PTLD, any suspicious lesion in an allograft recipient should be biopsied. It is important to send samples for immuno-fluorescence studies so that sections can be stained for expression of EBV-coded proteins. Onset is usually at about 24 months. Earlier onset and a more aggressive natural history is seen with the calcineurin-blocking drugs (15 months), and following potent serotherapy presentation can be earlier still (7 months).

EBV

EBV is a double-stranded DNA virus of the herpes family. Some 90–95% of the adult population carry the virus. EBV gains entry to the B lymphocyte via the C3d complement

Table 14.11 Spectrum of EBV infection

Asymptomatic seroconversion

Classical glandular fever

PTLD:
1. Lymphadenopathy: localized (any site) or generalized
2. Extranodal (70%): bone marrow infiltration, infiltration of other organs—gut, skin, eye, gums, lungs. Central nervous system (25%). Involvement of the transplanted organ (20%)
3. Systemic symptoms: PUO/malaise/weight loss

Endemic: African Burkitt's lymphoma (c-*myc* translocation)

Nasopharyngeal carcinoma

AIDS-related lymphoma

Hodgkin's disease (about 40% of cases)

Smooth muscle tumours (hepatic leiomyoma)

PUO = pyrexia of unknown origin; PTLD = post-transplant lymphoproliferative disorder.

Table 14.12 Post-transplant lymphoproliferative disorder (PTLD) (see Knowles *et al.* 1995)

1. Plasmacytic hyperplasia	Oropharynx, nodes (intact architecture)	Multiple EBV hits	OG no change TSG no change	Polyclonal
2. Polymorphic B-cell hyperplasia or polymorphic B-cell lymphoma	Nodes, extranodal	Single EBV hit	OG no change TSG no change	Monoclonal/ oligoclonal
3. Immunoblastic lymphoma (multiple myeloma)	Widely disseminated	Single EBV hit	OG altered TSG altered	Monoclonal

OG: oncogene, e.g. c-*myc*, N-*ras*.
TSG: tumour suppresser gene, e.g. p53.

receptor. Following infection, the virus remains latent for the life of the host. During the latency phase only a few viral antigens are expressed and the viral DNA persists in a circular or episomal form (Table 14.13). Prolonged latency may be related to the finding that the antigen-processing organelle, the proteosome, cannot process Epstein–Barr nuclear antigen 1 (EBNA 1) to antigenic particles and so the infected cell is poorly recognized by cytotoxic lymphocytes (CTL). The targets for CTL include EBNA 2–6 and latent membrane proteins (LMPs) and require expression of HLA and adhesion molecules on the infected cells. Of the two types of EBV most PTLD is associated with EBV type A (or 1) rather than type B (or 2). B-cell immortalization depends critically on EBNA 1. The *EBER* gene controls viral RNA processing during latency. LMP-1 plays a crucial role in the development of PTLD (Liebowitz 1998). LMP-1 is a member of the

Table 14.13   EBV genes: latent cycle viral proteins expressed in PTLD

EBV gene	Product/action
EBNA-1	Viral genome maintenance (episomal) required for replication of episome. Non-antigenic
EBNA-2 and *-3*	Transcriptional transactivator
EBNA-3, -4, and *-5*	Transcriptional transactivator. Main CTL targets
LMP-1	Constituitively active TNF-receptor homologue. Activation of NFκB, e.g. A20 inhibits p53 apoptosis
LMP-2A, LMP-2B	Blocks transactivation via Ig receptor, i.e. blocks B-cell activation
BHRF1	Sequence homology with *Bcl-2* (antiapoptotic)
BCRF1	IL-10 (B-cell growth factor, inhibition of T helper 1 and monocyte cytokine synthesis)
EBER-1 (mRNA), *EBER-2* (mRNA)	Controls viral RNA during latency

EBNA = Epstein–Barr nuclear antigen; LMP = latent membrane protein; CTL = cytotoxic lymphocytes.

TNF receptor family and binds to TNF receptor associated factors (TRAFs) which lead to the activation of broad spectrum transcriptional activators, NFκB and activator protein 1 (AP-1). One recent study suggests a direct effect of the calcineurin-blocking drugs on the growth of EBV-infected B-cell lymphoblastoid cell line. These drugs appear to protect against apoptosis (Beatty *et al.* 1998).

Aetiology

Most PTLD in solid organ transplantation is of host origin. EBV plays an important part in the immortalization and proliferation of infected B cells. In normal immunocompetent subjects infection with EBV causes B-cell proliferation, which is terminated by HLA-restricted specific CTL. EBV then remains as a latent infection for life. The sites of latency include the oropharyngeal epithelia, circulating B cells, and lymph nodes. Immunosuppressed recipients of organ transplants are unable to mount an effective antiviral CTL response and the B cells proliferate unchecked (Beatty *et al.* 1998). Following transplantation 25–30% of patients will show reactivation of EBV, but only a small proportion go on to develop PTLD.

It is thought that PTLD is a multistep process, which starts as an EBV-induced proliferation of immature B cells. Specific mutations may occasionally ensue at critical chromosomal loci. In late cases c-*myc*, *Bcl-2*, and N-*ras* may be involved (Knowles *et al.* 1995). It is thought that the c-*myc* oncogene is activated by juxtaposition to an immunoglobulin gene locus. Reduced B-cell expression of HLA antigens and adhesion molecules may play a role in promoting the development of PTLD and in resisting attack by CTL (Rickinson *et al.* 1992).

Clonality

Early studies suggest that not only does PTLD become increasingly monoclonal with the passage of time, but also the prognosis when immunosuppression is reduced is better with polyclonal rather than monoclonal tumours (Table 14.12). Clonality can be assessed by immunoglobulin gene rearrangement. Rearranged V, D, and J segments within a given B cell remain fixed for the lifespan of the cell and for its progeny. Clonality can also be assessed by looking for polymorphisms in the EBV genome. If all or most cells contain the same number of EVB genome terminal repeats, then the tumour is thought to be monoclonal (one hit). Recent studies suggest that most PTLD is monoclonal (Amlot *et al.* 2000).

Histology and immunophenotyping

Histology usually reveals a monomorphic mononuclear cell infiltrate replacing normal tissue architecture. In the renal allograft an expansile tumour-like interstitial mononuclear cell infiltrate displacing tubules with associated nuclear atypia and necrosis is typically seen. The absence of tubulitis should alert the clinician to the possibility of PTLD, although both tubulitis and intimal arteritis can occur in lesions with PTLD. In PTLD all nine latency-associated proteins may be expressed unlike in Burkitt's lymphoma and nasopharyngeal carcinoma (Table 14.14). The immunophenotype of EBV-infected lymphoblastoid cell lines is summarized in Table 14.15, but in PTLD major lineage antigens are often missing.

Diagnosis and investigation

Diagnosis is critically dependent on a tissue biopsy and the demonstration of viral proteins, DNA, or RNA in the appropriate tissue (Table 14.16). Serology is of little help. Biopsy specimens can be stained for EBV RNA (EBER-1 RNA) present in lymphocytes and this appears to predict the subsequent development of PTLD, particularly in liver transplants. This technique may also be of value for differentiating an atypical or resistant rejection episode from evolving PTLD. The quantitative analysis of EBER-1 in

Table 14.14 EBV latency

	Latency type		
	I	II	III
Expression	EBNA-1, EBER RNAs	EBNA-1, LMP-1, LMP-2, EBER RNAs	All latent genes, EBNA 1–6, LMP-1, -2, EBER RNAs
Clinical	Burkitt's lymphoma	Nasopharyngeal carcinoma, Hodgkin's disease, PTLD (some)	PTLD (most), *in vitro* B-cell line

Table 14.15   Immunophenotype of PTLD/EBV-infected B-cell lymphoblastoid cell line

CD19—Pan B

CD20—Pan B

CD21—C3d and EBV receptor

CD23—activation marker

CD54—ICAM-1 adhesion molecule

CD58—LFA-3 adhesion molecule

HLA class I reduced

HLA class II reduced

CD30—activation marker

CD39

CDW70

CD11a/CD18 (LFA-1) adhesion molecule

Surface immunoglobulin—variable sometimes monoclonal

Table 14.16   Investigation and monitoring of PTLD

Biopsy:
   Light microscopy
   Immunofluorescence: EBNA
   Molecular biology: Ig gene rearrangement, EBV terminal repeats
   In situ hybridization: EBER-1

Peripheral blood lymphocytes:
   CD4/CD8
   NK cells (CD16, CD57)
   Activation marker: CD 69, class II, CD 28

Saliva: EBV culture

PCR (EBV DNA): PBL, saliva

Staging
   CT chest and abdomen
   Gallium scanning

Serum Igs and plasma protein electrophoresis

β_2 microglobulin

Lactate dehydrogenase

PBL gives a measure of the EBV load and again may be of value diagnostically and for following response to therapy. Similarly quantitative PCR can be used to measure viral load in PBL. This approach can identify at-risk patients and be used to monitor response to treatment (Green *et al.* 1998). Immunophenotyping is required to demonstrate the B-cell lineage of PTLD. Surface staining of cells for IgG kappa or lambda light chains may reveal a monoclonal population. A monoclonal gammapathy may be detected in peripheral blood before PTLD is apparent. However, the presence of a monoclonal gammopathy is very common in transplant patients during the first year (approximately 40%).

Epidemiology

The incidence is critically dependent upon the total burden of immunosuppression, which may explain the varying incidence in different types of graft (Table 14.17). The incidence of PTLD is increased following a primary infection, which is more likely in paediatric practice as an EBV seropositive parent donating to an EBV-negative child is not uncommon (Ho *et al.* 1998).

The data from the European collaborative transplant study indicate that PTLD develops in about 0.2% of cadaver transplants in the first year and this reduces to 0.04% per year thereafter.

Retransplantation

Retransplantation has been attempted in a few patients and can be successful (Hickey *et al.* 1990). It is possible to harvest recipients' lymphocytes and grow EBV-specific CTLs from patients who have successfully eliminated PTLD with their first graft. Such cells may then be given should PTLD recur on subsequent grafting.

Prophylaxis

Restricting EBV seropositive donors to EBV seropositive recipients would reduce the risk of PTLD, but given the shortage of donors this not practical. In some studies of CMV prophylaxis with aciclovir or ganciclovir, authors have noticed a reduced incidence of PTLD perhaps due to reduced viral load (McDiarmid *et al.* 1998). Initial studies

Table 14.17   Incidence of PTLD

Renal allografts:
   Prednisolone/azathioprine: 1–2%
   Prednisolone/azathioprine/cyclosporine A: 2%
   Induction serotherapy: 5%
   Total dose of monoclonal antibody OKT3 > 7.5 mg: > 10%

Liver allograft: 2–3% (5–10% in children)

Heart: 2–3%

Heart–lung: 5–10%

Bone marrow:
   T-depleted donor: 12%
   Unmodified donor: 1%

Small bowel: 11%

suggest that a combination of mycophenolate mofetil (guanosine depletion) with antiviral drugs may act synergistically. No vaccine is available. Better HLA matching allowing reduced immunosuppression and more specific tailoring of potent immunosuppressive regimes to only the most high-risk patients may help reduce the incidence of PTLD.

Treatment

The initial step in treatment is the phased reduction of immunosuppression guided by careful monitoring of lymphocyte subsets and activation markers (Amlot *et al.* 2002, in press). Rapid reduction over 6 weeks or less appears more likely to lead to graft loss from acute rejection than a more gradual approach. Controlled trials are not available on which to base firm protocols. Careful lymphocyte monitoring can be a guide to immunosuppression dose reduction. An antiviral response is indicated by a reduction in CD69 expression on T cells and by an increase in cytotoxic T cells (CD8+) expressing HLA-DR and CD57 (an NK cell marker) (Rees *et al.* 1998). In the future specific anti-EBV response will be assessable by tetramer staining.

A variety of immunotherapies have been developed (Fischer *et al.* 1991). Anti-B-cell monoclonal antibodies may be successful when other treatments have failed (Table 14.18). Cytotoxic T-cell infusions have also been shown to be of benefit in several small studies. In some cases IL-2-stimulated autologous CTLs have been used and in others HLA-identical allogeneic cells have been given (Nalesnik *et al.* 1997). With this latter approach there is a risk of graft versus host disease.

Early recourse to chemotherapy or systemic radiotherapy is not recommended as this further immunosuppresses an already immunoincompetent patient. Outcomes are poor and death from overwhelming infection is common. Cytotoxic chemotherapy should be the approach of last resort.

Prognosis

Overall survival is 40% but may well be improved by a more structured approach to management. Adverse prognostic factors include presentation a long time after transplantation, monoclonality, chromosomal abnormalities, and multiple extranodal sites of

---

Table 14.18   The treatment of PTLD: sequential approach

1. Monitored and phased reduction of immunosuppression ± aciclovir. Local debulking: excision, local radiotherapy

2. Immunostimulation: interferon-α2a ± intravenous Ig ± IL-2

3. Immunotherapy:
   (a) Anti-B-cell antibodies: anti-CD21, 24, 37, 38, anti-CD20 (rituximab)
   (b) CTL (autologous or HLA matched heterologous)
   (c) Lymphokine-activated killer cells (LAK)

4. Chemotherapy: last resort, e.g. CHOP

---

disease. Localized polyclonal tumours occurring in renal transplant recipients should regress well with reduction of immunosuppression and are associated with a mortality of less than 25%.

Squamous cell carcinoma of the skin

Introduction

The incidence of squamous cell carcinoma (SCC) of the skin rises progressively with time after transplantation. In some countries with a potential for high sun exposure, the incidence may approach 100% at 20 years. Renal transplant recipients have a 100-fold increased risk of developing SCC. In the transplant population growth is more rapid and metastases to local nodes more prominent (6.4%).

Aetiology

Exposure to sunlight plays a crucial role. Ultraviolet light may induce chromosomal changes, increase AP-1, decrease retinoic acid receptor, deplete the skin's antigen-presenting cells (CD1+Langerhan's cells) and promote viral growth. The human papillomavirus (HPV) plays an important aetiological role (Euvrard *et al*. 1993). This has been most clearly delineated in the HPV-associated cervical and anogenital carcinomas but is also probably important in SCC of the skin.

Human papillomavirus

HPV is a large family of small DNA viruses. There are over 70 different types with different tissue specificities. They have been clearly linked with anogenital carcinoma including cervical intraepithelial neoplasia (CIN), condylomata acuminata, and non melanotic skin cancers. These associations are particularly strong in immunosuppressed individuals (Table 14.19). There are three main regions of the HPV genome:

1. Early region. This encodes for regulatory transforming and replicative proteins denoted E1–7 (see Table 14.20).
2. Late region. This area encodes for the capsid proteins denoted L1 and L2.
3. Upstream regulatory region. This region does not appear to encode for any proteins.

HPV infects the basal epithelial cells and causes epithelioid hyperplasia resulting in benign viral warts. Most of the HPV DNA is present as a free circular episomal form. The oncogenic potential for HPV can be shown for some types in that they can immortalize primary cell cultures of human keratinocytes. In malignant tissue the viral gene is no longer in an episomal form but becomes integrated in the host DNA. E1 and E2 are no longer expressed but E6 and E7 are. The E6 gene product targets and destroys p53 via the ubiquitin pathway. The E7 gene product on the other hand binds to pocket proteins including pRB (retinoblastoma tumour suppresser gene product). Binding of E7 gene products to pRB promotes increased DNA synthesis. HPV-immortalized cells are NK-cell resistant but remain sensitive to lymphokine activated killer cells (LAK).

Table 14.19 Lesions associated with human papillomavirus (HPV)

Hyperkeratotic common foot wart (HPV4)

Hyperkeratotic common hand wart (HPV1, 2, 3, 4, 5, 6, 27)

Flat planar wart (HPV3A, 10, 49)

Genital condylomata acuminata (HPV11)

Anogenital squamous cell carcinoma (HPV16, 18, 31, 33, 45, 54)

SCC in epidermodysplasia verruciformis (HPV5, 8, 14, 17, 20, 47)

SCC in transplant recipients (HPV5, 8, 14, 17, 20, 47 and others)

?SCC in normal individuals: uncertain

?Oral cavity and oesophagus: carcinoma of the epithelial cells (HPV16)

SCC = squamous cell carcinoma.

Table 14.20 HPV genes

Gene	Function
E1	ATPase and helicase activity—lost in malignancy
E2	Regulation of transcription and replication—lost in malignancy
E3	
E4	Maturation and release of viral particles—lost in malignancy
E5	Transforming potential—lost in malignancy
E6	Transforming protein (p53 degradation)—integrated in malignancy. Activation of telomerase
E7	Transforming protein (pRB inactivation)—integrated in malignancy. Increased AP-1 transcription

Clinical features

Transplant patients affected with SCC usually have a history of extensive viral warts. Other premalignant skin conditions may also be present, for example Bowen's disease or actinic keratoses (Table 14.19). A history of excessive sun exposure is common, so that squamous cell lesions have a predilection for sun exposed skin and the lips.

Management

Local surgical excision remains the mainstay of treatment. In patients where there are widespread or multifocal skin tumours or premalignant diffuse skin conditions a more systemic approach is needed. A careful reduction of immunosuppression can certainly allow regression of viral warts and may limit the spread of SCC. There is increasing use of retinoids both for the management of extensive viral warts and for the treatment of advanced or multifocal SCC (Table 14.21).

Table 14.21 Actions of retinoids

Bind to nuclear receptors (hormone response elements)

Inhibit the actions of AP-1 transcription factor

Upregulate retinoic binding protein mRNA

Synergistic inhibition of growth of cell lines with IFN-α, TGF-β, IL-1

Enhance natural killer cell activity (via IL-12)

Enhance cytotoxic lymphocyte activity (via IL-12)

Restore cutaneous Langerhan's cells (CD1+)

Increase Langerhan's cell IL-12 production

Blockade of IL-6 pathways

Increase collagen I synthesis

Retinoids bind to hormone response elements of DNA and initiate gene transcription. The process whereby these agents modify cellular proliferation and differentiation are not understood. 13-*cis*-retinoic acids (etidronate and acitretin) are of established value as preventive agents (Craven and Griffiths 1996). Retinoids are capable of promoting apoptosis and epidermal differentiation. Inhibition of the IL-6 signalling pathway appears important (Nagpal *et al.* 1997). They can also inhibit cellular proliferation by inhibiting the AP-1 transcription factor (a complex of c-*fos* and c-*jun* proteins). Retinoic acids can induce the synthesis of TGF-β, which may inhibit tumour cell growth. Treatment with retinoids is associated with repopulation of the skin with Langerhan's cells. The net effect of retinoids is to increase apoptosis and decrease proliferation.

High-dose systemic retinoids (etidronate 1 mg/kg/day) is associated with unpleasant side-effects (hyperlipidaemia and ligamentous calcification) so that a combination of low-dose oral therapy with topical therapy may be better (Rook *et al.* 1995). A suitable regime would be topical tretinoin at 0.25–0.05% plus oral etidronate 10 mg daily reduced to alternate days at 6 months if a satisfactory response has been obtained. Prolonged therapy is probably necessary, as relapse is common. For advanced disease with metastases reduction of immunosuppression combined with treatment using both retinoids and IFN-α2a may be of benefit (Lippman *et al.* 1992). It is likely that a significant number of patients will lose their grafts from rejection when IFN-α2a is used.

The prognosis for SCC in the immunosuppressed renal transplant recipient is not as good as in immunocompetent individuals. Widespread metastasis is not uncommon. Transplant patients need to be warned of the dangers of sun exposure, to wear appropriate clothing, and to use ultraviolet sun-block creams. It is important to examine transplant patients from head to toe at least once a year, particularly the long established transplants, to detect potentially malignant skin lesions at the earliest possible time.

Anogenital carcinoma

Twenty-nine per cent of renal transplant patients develop anogenital warts. There is a three-fold increased risk of developing cervical neoplasia with up to a half of the female final transplant recipients developing CIN. Characteristically CIN in transplant recipients is recurrent, persistent, and multifocal. It is closely related to infection with HPV of restricted types (Resnick *et al.* 1990) (Table 14.19). Studies have shown a direct correlation between HPV copy number and the severity of the cervical lesions. Part of the regular review of female renal transplant patients should include colposcopy and cervical smears. Early excision biopsies are important to prevent spread. The use of systemic and topical retinoids is currently being explored.

Hepatoma

Hepatitis C virus

Hepatitis C virus (HCV) is an RNA virus which is associated with the development of hepatoma usually in the context of cirrhosis (De Metri *et al.* 1995). It seems unlikely that the risk is greatly increased following renal transplantation in hepatitis C-positive recipients but there is a paucity of literature on the subject. It may also be that the duration of follow-up is insufficient to determine increased risk. HCV is also associated with plasmacytic lymphomas in transplant patients.

Hepatitis B virus

Hepatitis B virus (HBV) is the smallest DNA virus known. In the non-immunosuppressed HBV infection confers a 100-fold increased risk of hepatocellular carcinoma (HCC). The mechanism whereby HBV may induce HCC is unknown, but may include integration of HBV DNA adjacent to cellular oncogenes and lead to their activation (Hildt *et al.* 1996). The product of HBV x gene inhibits p53. In one long-term study eight of 151 HBV surface antigen-positive kidney transplant recipients developed HCC (Fornairon *et al.* 1996) which was felt to be higher and to occur earlier than would have been expected in a non-immunosuppressed population. Post-transplant monitoring for HBV DNA and α-fetoprotein may be appropriate. The efficacy of long-term antiviral treatment in the renal transplant population looks promising but awaits further studies.

References

Al-Sulaiman MH, Al-Khader AA. Kaposi's sarcoma in renal transplant recipients. *Transplantation Sciences* 1994 4(1): 46–60.

Amlot P.L, Rees L, Rawlings E, Tahami F, Thomas JA, Fernando ON *et al.* Management of renal transplant patients with EBV infection and post-transplant lymphoproliferative disease: superiority of gradual over rapid reduction in immunosuppression. 2002 In press.

Bais C, Santomasso B, Coso *et al.* G-protein-coupled receptor of Kaposi's sarcoma-associated herpes virus is a viral oncogene and angiogenesis activator. *Nature* 1998 391: 86–90.

Beatty PR, Krams SM, Esquivel CO, Martinez OL. Effect of cyclosporin and tacrolimus on the growth of Epstein–Barr virus-transfected B-cell lines. *Transplantation* 1998 65: 1248–1255.

Boubenider SA, Hiesse C, Goupy C, Kriaa F, Marchand S, Charpentier B. Incidence and consequence of post-transplant lymphoproliferative disorders. *Journal of Nephrology* 1997 10: 136–145.

Brooks LA, Wilson AJ, Crook T. Kaposi's sarcoma-associated herpes virus (KSHV)/human herpes virus (HHV8): a new human tumour virus. *Journal of Pathology* 1997 **182**: 262–265.

Craven NM, Griffiths CEM. The use of retinoids in the management of non-melanoma skin cancer and melanoma. *Cancer Surveys* 1996 **26**: 267–288.

De Metri M, Poussin K, Pontisso P. HCV associated liver cancer without cirrhosis. *Lancet* 1995 **345**: 413–415.

Euvrard S, Chardonnet Y, Poutil-Noble C. Associations of skin malignancies with various and multiple carcinogenic and non-carcinogenic human papilloma viruses in renal transplant recipients. *Cancer* 1993 **72**: 2198–2206.

Fischer A, Blanche S, Le Bidoix J. Anti B-cell monoclonal antibodies in the treatment of severe B-cell-lymphoproliferative syndrome following bone marrow and organ transplantation. *New England Journal of Medicine* 1991 **324**: 1451–1456.

Fornairon S, Pol S, Legendr C, Carnot F *et al.* The long-term virologic and pathologic impact of renal transplantation on chronic hepatitis B virus infection. *Transplantation* 1996 **62**(2): 297–299.

Francès C. Kaposi's sarcoma after renal transplantation. *Nephrolology Dialysis Transplantation* 1998 **13**: 2768–2773.

Ganem D. KSHV and Kaposi's sarcoma: the end of the beginning. *Cell* 1997 **91**: 157–160.

Gotti E, Remuzzi G. Post transplant Kaposi's sarcoma. *Journal of the American Society of Nephrology* 1997 **8**(1): 130–137.

Green M, Cacciarelli TV, Mazariegos GV *et al.* Serial measurement of Epstein–Barr viral load in peripheral blood in pediatric liver transplant recipients during treatment for post-transplant lymphoproliferative disease. *Transplantation* 1998 **66**: 1641–1644.

Hildt E, Hofschneider PH, Urban S. The role of hepatitis (HBV) in the development of hepatolcelluar carcinoma. *Seminars in Virology* 1996 **7**: 333–347.

Hickey DP, Nalensnik MA, Vivas CA *et al.* Renal re-transplantation in patients who lost their allografts during management of a previous post-transplant lymphoproliferative disease. *Clinical Transplantation* 1990 **4**: 187–190.

Ho M, Jaffe R, Miller G. The frequency of Epstein–Barr virus infection and associated lymphoproliferative syndrome after transplantation and its manifestation in children. *Transplantation* 1988 **45**: 719–727.

Kedes DH, Ganem D. Sensitivity of Kaposi's sarcoma associated herpes virus replication to antiviral drugs: implications for potential therapy. *Journal of Clinical Investigation* 1997 **99**: 2082.

Knowles DM, Cesarman E, Chadburn A *et al.* Correlative morphologic and molecular genetic analysis demonstrates three distinct categories of post-transplantation lymphoproliferative disorders. *Blood* 1995 **85**: 552–565.

Liebowitz D. Epstein–Barr virus and a cellular signaling pathway in lymphomas from immunosuppressed patients. *New England Journal of Medicine* 1998 **338**: 1413–1421.

Lippman SM, Parkinson DR, Itri LM *et al.* 13-*cis*-retinoic acid and interferon α-2a: Effective combination therapy for advanced squamous cell carcinoma of the skin. *Journal of the National Cancer Institute* 1992 **84**(4): 235–245.

McDiarmid SV, Jordan S, Lee GS *et al.* Prevention and pre-emptive therapy of post-transplant lymphoproliferative disease in paediatric liver recipients. *Transplantation* 1998 **66**: 1604–1611.

Nagpal S, Cai J, Zheng T *et al.* Retinoid antagonism of NF-IL-6: Insight into the mechanism of anti-proliferative effects of retinoids in Kaposi's sarcoma. *Molecular Cellular Biology* 1997 **17**: 159–168.

Nalesnik MA, Rao AS, Furukawa H *et al.* Autologous lymphokine-associated killer cell therapy of Epstein–Barr virus-positive and -negative lymphoproliferative disorders arising in organ transplant recipients. *Tranplantation* 1997 **63**: 1200–1205.

Rees L, Thomas JA, Amlot PL. Disappearance of an EBV+ post-transplant plasmacytoma with controlled reduction of immunosuppression. *Lancet* 1998; **352**(9130):789.

Resnick RM, Cornelissen MTE, Wright DK. Detection and typing of human papilloma virus in archival cervical cancer specimens by DNA amplification with consensus primers. *Journal of the National Cancer Institute* 1990 **82**: 1477–1484.

Rickinson AB, Murray RJ, Brooks J, Griffin H, Moss DJ, Maucci MG. T-cell recognition of Epstein–Barr virus-associated lymphomas. *Cancer Surveys* 1992 **13**: 53–80.

Rook AH, Jaworsky C, Nguyen T, Grossman RA, Wolfe JT, Witmer WK, Kligman AM. Beneficial effect of low dose systemic retinoid in combination with topica tretinoin for the treatment and prophylaxis of pre-malignant and malignant skin lesions in renal transplant recipients. *Transplantation* 1995 **59**: 179.

Schulz TF. Kaposi's sarcoma-associated herpes virus (human herpes virus 8). *Journal of General Virology* 1998 **79**: 1573–1591.

Toukraine JL *et al.* (eds). *Cancer in Transplantation; Prevention and Treatment*. Dordrecht, Kleuwer 1996.

15

Bacterial infections in renal allograft recipients

P. Sweny

Introduction

Timing

Bacterial infections may occur at any time following transplantation. In the early post-transplant period with the surgical breaches in natural defences (vascular access, surgical incisions, urethral catheters, and abdominal drains) the common bacterial organisms are seen as after any surgical procedure (Table 15.1). Similarly, a general anaesthetic exposes the patient to risks of postoperative chest infections. Common bacterial infections are more prevalent following transplantation than in other general surgical cases, reflecting the effects of uraemia and often malnutrition on the natural defence mechanisms. After the first few weeks the early intensive immunosuppression given both to prevent and to treat acute rejection crises significantly reduces the patient's resistance to infection. From this point more unusual opportunistic infections may occur, e.g. *Listeria*, reactivation of *Mycobacterium tuberculosis*, *Nocardia*, and non-typhoid salmonella. By 6-months post-transplant immunosuppression is approaching a lower baseline and opportunistic infections become increasingly uncommon but may still be seen.

Table 15.1 Classification of post-transplant bacterial infections

Perioperative and first month	Wound
	Lines—bacteraemia/septicaemia
	Urinary catheter
	Chest
	Perirenal haematoma
	Lymphocytes
1–6 months	'Malignant' urinary tract infection
	Bacteraemia/septicaemia
	Reactivation of mycobacterial infections
	Non-typhoid *Salmonella*
	Listeria
Late	'Benign' urinary tract infections
	Reactivation of mycobacterial infections
	Community acquired pneumonias

Predisposing factors

Predisposing factors have been dealt with elsewhere in this book. Suffice it to say here that pretransplant factors are important as well as the total burden of immunosuppression. It is important to remember that many of the herpes family of viruses are immunomodulating in their own right and increase the risk of bacterial infections (CMV, HHV8, EBV, and HBV). The hyperinfestation syndrome that may be seen with *Strongyloides stercoralis* may present with recurrent Gram-negative septicaemia as the larvae penetrate the gut wall. Table 15.2 summarizes the most important predisposing factors.

Infections transmitted by the donor organ

A wide variety of organisms can be transmitted by the donor organ. On occasions this can be bacterial contamination of the organ at harvesting (intestinal contents) or contamination of the perfusate and preservation fluid. Table 15.3 summarizes the most important bacterial organisms that may be transmitted by the donor organ. Organs can be used from donors with clearly defined bacterial infections provided that a specific microbiological diagnosis has been made and appropriate antimicrobial therapy has been given to the donor. The recipient must also receive prophylactic therapy for 1–2 weeks depending on the potential virulence of the identified organism. Urosepsis is particularly common, especially in a donor who has had prolonged urethral catheterization. Similarly, the risk of bacterial infection rises rapidly with the duration of ventilation and of in-dwelling venous lines. Highly resistant micro-organisms (vancomycin-resistant enterococci and methicillin-resistant *Staphylococcus aureus*) are present with increasing frequency in intensive care units and represent a serious potential threat to allograft recipients.

Table 15.2   Factors predisposing to infection

Pretransplantation	Protein–calorie malnutrition
	Uraemia (under dialysis)
	Previous immunosuppressive drugs for
	primary renal disease
Post-transplantation	Anaesthesia
	Venous access
	Abdominal wound
	Drains
	Urinary catheter
	Urinary stents
	Haematoma
	Total burden of immunosuppression: antilymphocyte
	preparations, numerous rejection episodes,
	combination therapy
	Coexisting infection: cytomegalovirus,
	Epstein–Barr virus, *Strongyloides stercoralis*

Table 15.3   Bacterial infections and organisms transmitted by the graft

Methicillin-resistant *Staphylococcus aureus*

Vancomycin-resistant enterococci

Brucella spp.

Listeria spp.

Bacterial meningitis

Mycobacterial species

Meliodosis

Typhoid and paratyphoid

Coxiella burnetti

Syphilis

Contamination at retrieval: faecal micro-organisms

Contamination of perfusate: pseudomonads

Donor urinary infection (upper tract)

Urinary tract infections

Urinary infections are an important and common complication of renal transplantation. They occur in 30–60% of patients and remain the commonest cause of bacteraemia.

Early

In the early post-transplant period, lower urinary tract infections are common and are clearly related to the length of time the urinary catheter is left *in situ*. Ureteric stenting may allow the earlier removal of urethral catheters. In some patients, such as diabetics, it may be preferable to consider using a suprapubic catheter rather than resort to prolonged urethral catheterization. In the early post-transplant period it is relatively unusual for a lower urinary tract infection to develop into severe sepsis or bacterial pyelonephritis, but this can occur. Prophylactic antibiotics should be considered for patients who have repeated urological intervention in the early post-transplant period. Treatment is to remove the catheter as soon as possible and to give a short course of treatment with an appropriate antibiotic for about 5 days.

Intermediate

During months 1–6 post-transplantation, immunosuppression is maximal. A lower urinary tract infection may ascend and can cause severe acute bacterial pyelonephritis. Clinical features include fever, impaired function, and in some cases a swollen, tender graft. Presentation may mimic acute rejection. Clearly an accurate diagnosis is vital. Graft biopsy should be considered to prove every acute rejection episode, if only to exclude other pathologies such as bacterial pyelonephritis or graft post-transplant lymphoproliferative disorder. It is important to be able to differentiate an upper tract urinary tract infection from graft rejection. In both cases there is an increase in IL-6 production and serum C-reactive protein rises. Measurement of urinary enzymes may be helpful, e.g. myeloperoxidase. This enzyme is predominantly derived from granulocytes and suggests the presence of graft pyelonephritis. During this intermediate post-transplant period, some 10% of urinary tract infections are complicated by bacteraemia. The inflammatory stimulus associated with a urinary tract infection may not only trigger acute rejection but can also play a role in the reactivation of latent herpesviruses. Serial ^{99m}Tc-DMSA scans can show progressive graft scarring and loss of renal tissue. Some surgical units implant the donor ureter with a long submucosal tunnel to try to reduce the risk of reflux up the transplant ureter, and thus reduce the risk of an ascending infection. Patients with recurring urinary tract infections present a special problem. Up to 60% of patients will experience a relapse. A micturating cystogram may show reflux to the transplanted kidney and also sometimes to the native kidneys. Reconstruction of the transplant ureter is seldom attempted, but gross reflux with infection to the native kidneys may prompt native nephroureterectomy. Gallium scintigraphy can sometimes help identify the native kidneys as a potential source of infection. A plain abdominal radiograph to include the bladder area should be performed to identify any calculi. Extensive pelvicalyceal or bladder encrustation/calcification indicates infection with urea splitting microorganisms e.g. Corynebacterium urealyticum. Patients with numerous infections justify cystoscopy. Occasionally a calcified bladder stitch may form a focus for multiple relapses.

Treatment of urinary tract infection in the intermediate period is usually prolonged for 2 weeks. If graft pyelonephritis has been demonstrated, then at least 6–8 weeks of antibiotic therapy is required. Multiple infections, for example more than three per year, call for 12 months of rotating antibiotics, after which resolution may occur. General measures are of course important, including a high fluid intake, scrupulous personal hygiene, and double micturition if reflux or poor bladder emptying is present. Treatment with an α-blocker or even prostatic resection in older male patients may be required. Prostatic-specific antigen should be checked in older males. Female patients with multiple infections should have a full pelvic examination so that local cervical pathology is not missed. Infections may become established in the patient's native kidney particularly in patients with polycystic kidneys or those with a history of stones and reflux. Even with a gallium scan (undertaken with the patient off antibiotics) it may be difficult to confirm infection in the native polycystic kidney. Immunosuppression clearly reduces the signs of inflammation and makes clinical diagnosis difficult. Bilateral native kidney nephrectomy for chronically infected polycystic kidneys can be helpful.

Late

A lower urinary tract infection which occurs months or years after a transplantation does not carry with it the same dire implications as infection occurring the second to sixth months. Males, of course, require a full investigation, but this seldom is necessary in females of child-bearing age who have isolated single infections. Recurrent infection requires a full urological investigation.

Prophylaxis

Most renal transplant centres advise cotrimoxazole 480 mg (trimethoprim 80 mg, sulfamethoxazole 400 mg) once daily for the first 3–6 months. Although originally intended for prophylaxis for Pneumocystis, clinical studies have shown that this reduces the incidence of urinary tract infection. Toxoplasmosis and wound infections are also significantly reduced by this prophylactic regime. Low-dose cotrimoxazole is rarely associated with nephrotoxicity even when given in combination with cyclosporine A or tacrolimus. Occasionally interstitial nephritis may occur.

Pulmonary infections

Chest infections are very common following renal transplantation. In the immediate post-transplant period the organisms responsible are likely to be the same as those after any general anaesthesic. Advice from the microbiologist is important in choosing first-line therapy for a hospital-acquired chest infection. Thereafter, as immunosuppression takes hold, a wide variety of opportunistic organisms may be involved (Table 15.4). Transplant patients are heir to community-acquired infections which occur with a greater frequency and severity than in the general population. During influenza outbreaks severe complicating bacterial pneumonia is not uncommon. *Streptococcus pneumoniae* remains the commonest cause of a bacterial pneumonia in renal transplant patients.

The differential diagnosis of pulmonary symptoms in the renal transplant patient is wide and important (Table 15.5). Most patients presenting to their unit with respiratory tract symptoms will have a self-limiting community-acquired infection which in most cases will

Table 15.4   Organisms causing pulmonary infections

Viral	Cytomegalovirus
	Respiratory syncytial virus
	Adenovirus
	Epstein–Barr virus (post-transplant lymphoproliferative disorder)
	Human herpesvirus 8
	Varicella zoster virus
	Herpes simplex virus
	Measles
	Influenza and parainfluenza
Bacterial	Mycobacteria: tuberculosis, atypicals
	Nocardia
	Nosocomial: *Klebsiella pneumiae*, *Legionella*, *Pseudomonas aeruginosa*
	Community acquired: *Haemophilus influenzae*, *Streptococcus pneumoniae* (commonest), *Chlamydia psittaci*
Fungal	*Aspergillus*
	Candida
	Mucormycosis
	Cryptococcus
	Pneumocystis carinii
Parasitic	*Toxoplasma gondii*
	Strongyloides stercoralis

Table 15.5 Non-infectious causes of pulmonary symptoms

Drug-induced pulmonary fibrosis

Non-cardiogenic pulmonary oedema:
  Cytokine release syndrome (OKT3)

Fluid overload:
  Iatrogenic
  Fluid retention with rejection
  Cardiac failure

Thromboembolic

Recurrence of original disease:
  Vasculitis
  Antiglomerular basement membrane antibody-mediated disease

Tumour:
  Kaposi's sarcoma
  Post-transplant lymphoproliferative disease

Prolonged drug activity (uraemia)
  Neuromuscular blockade
  Opiates (impaired respiratory effort)

---

be viral. Antibiotics will be of no value. Severe chest infections can develop rapidly and oxygen saturation (pulse oximetry) should be measured before and after exercise. Patients who desaturate after exercise are much more likely to be developing a severe interstitial pneumonitis than a simple community-acquired viral infection. Such patients warrant more detailed investigation with admission and possibly bronchoscopy and lavage. It is important that patients with these acute respiratory symptoms should have their treatment based on the microbiological isolate. Gallium scintigraphy can also detect an early *Pneumocystis carinii* infection and a fall in the diffusing capacity for carbon monoxide may also be helpful at identifying a potentially serious chest infection. A fine-cut CT scan of the chest can reveal lung pathology not evident on a standard chest radiograph.

Bacteraemia and septicaemia

Renal transplant patients are susceptible to bacteraemia/septicaemia from a variety of sources (Table 15.6). Presentation is dramatic, often with a minimal prodromal illness due to the masking effect of steroids on inflammation. Systemic symptoms, hypotension, and fever may herald imminent circulatory collapse. It is common clinical practice to undertake blood cultures with all pyrexial episodes in renal transplant patients. In the post-cyclosporine era of renal transplantation, acute rejection episodes are rarely associated with a high fever. Clinical experience suggests that bacteraemia/septicaemia is a more common complication of such intercurrent bacterial infections as pneumonia, wound infections, gastroenteritis, and diverticulosis than is usually seen in the general population. Following a bacteraemia, focal abscesses are more common in the immunocompromised particularly with non-typhoid salmonellae and *Listeria monocytogenes*.

Table 15.6 Causes of septicaemia and bacteraemia

Indwelling vascular access lines

Ascending urinary tract infection

Bacterial enteritis, e.g. non-typhoid *Salmonella*
Listeria

Associated with *Strongyloides stercoralis*

Steroid-induced bowel perforation

Associated overimmunosuppression

Associated cytomegalovirus leucopenia

Diverticulosis

Complicating bacterial pneumonia

Complicating wound and perirenal abscesses

Complicating cytomegalovirus colitis

Table 15.7 Initial treatment for suspected bacteraemia/septicaemia: related to likely primary source

Urinary tract	Cefotaxime or ciprofloxacin
Large bowel	Cefotaxime + metronidazole
Respiratory tract:	
Nosocomial	Penicillin V + doxycycline + clarithromycin
Community acquired	Penicillin V + cefotaxime
Unknown	Gentamicin + metronidazole + cefotaxime

Treatment needs to be initiated early and is usually chosen on the basis of the likely source of infection before an organism and sensitivities are available. Where possible, if graft function is poor, it is best to avoid aminoglycosides. Antimicrobial therapy is pruned or modified when the organism and sensitivities have been identified. Table 15.7 indicates possible choices of antimicrobial agents.

Central nervous system infections

Central nervous system infections (CNS) infections are common in renal transplants. A range of clinical syndromes from meningitis to encephalitis with focal neurological signs or subtle changes in behaviour can be encountered. Clinicians should have a low threshold for detailed investigation. A CT scan with contrast or an MRI scan are the investigations of choice. In the absence of evidence of raised intercranial pressure, a lumbar puncture is indicated. If an abscess is identified and the organism cannot be recovered from blood or cerebrospinal fluid then direct aspiration for a microbiological diagnosis should be undertaken. The range of organisms that may occur in the CNS is such that blind therapy is inappropriate (Table 15.8).

Table 15.8   Causes of central nervous system infections

Meningitis:	acute/subacute	*Listeria monocytogenes,* Cryptococcus
	subacute/chronic	Mycobacterial species Coccidioides immitis
Focal or space-occupying lesion		*Listeria monocytogenes* *Toxoplasma gondii* *Nocardia asteroides* Mycobacterium species *Aspergillus*
Progressive dementia		Polyomavirus (JC)
Encephalitis		Herpes simplex

Bacterial endocarditis

Bacterial endocarditis is surprisingly uncommon (Bishara *et al.* 1999). One might suspect that aortic valve sclerosis, immunosuppression, and a history of numerous central lines would predispose patients to bacterial endocarditis. When bacterial endocarditis does occur in renal transplant recipients, it usually involves an opportunistic infection (Prada *et al.* 1994, Niehues *et al.* 1996). Involvement of the transplant kidney by an associated glomerulonephritis has been reported (Ades *et al.* 1998).

Gastrointestinal infections

Acute diarrhoeal illnesses occur frequently. There is a wide range of micro-organisms that may be involved (Table 15.9). Ingestion of food contaminated with *Listeria monocytogenes* (soft cheeses), non-typhoid salmonellae (chicken), or *Cryptosporidium* (water) may lead to serious infection in the immunocompromised. The occurrence of hypovolaemia and hypotension are commonly associated with acute graft dysfunction. Prompt resuscitation with crystalloid and correction of electrolyte imbalance (acidosis, hypokalaemia, and hypomagnesaemia) is important. Both stool and blood should be cultured. Stools should be sent for microscopy for ova, cysts, and parasites. Renal patients receive many courses of antibiotics over their chronic illness and may become colonized with *Clostridium difficile*. In any diarrhoeal illness stool should be sent for identification of *Clostridium difficile* toxin. Diabetic patients with an autonomic neuropathy may develop a variety of bacterial overgrowth syndromes in the bowel. A hydrogen/urea breath test is helpful. There is a little anecdotal evidence to suggest that infections with *Helicobacter pylori* may be more common in renal patients than in the general population. A silent, ruptured diverticulum, presumably related to steroid therapy, can lead to rapidly deteriorating overwhelming sepsis, often with minimal symptoms and signs to point to the abdomen as the origin. A plain radiograph of the abdomen may reveal free gas. Most imaging techniques are unsatisfactory and early laparotomy is essential. Early peritoneal toilet and a defunctioning colostomy over the site of perforation can be lifesaving. Attempted

Table 15.9   Gastrointestinal infections in renal transplant patients

Food poisoning: staphylococcal toxin, pathogenic strains of
Escherichia coli, *Listeria monocytogenes*, non-typhoid *Salmonella*

Superinfection with *Clostridium difficile*

Giardia lamblia

Cytomegalovirus

Infiltration by post-transplant lymphoproliferative disorder

Rotavirus

Cryptosporidium

Small bowel bacterial overgrowth (diabetic autonomic neuropathy)

Reactivation of *Strongyloides stercoralis*

one-stage repairs with an intra-abdominal end-to-end anastomosis are liable to break down in a septic immunocompromised patient who may also be malnourished. In such situations early total parenteral nutrition may be needed if bowel function is slow to return. Mortality is high, so speed is of the essence. Included in the differential diagnosis of bowel syndromes is post-transplant lymphoproliferative disorder, which can present as obstruction, haemorrhage, or an abdominal mass.

Bone and joint infections

Inflammation of a single joint may be due to bacterial infection rather than gout in the renal transplant patient. Table 15.10 summarizes the range of organisms that has been identified. It is essential to aspirate an affected joint for culture. A bone scan or a gallium scan can be helpful at localizing potentially infected joints, particularly when signs and symptoms of inflammation are suppressed. The main differential diagnosis for a painful joint in the renal transplant patient is gout or avascular necrosis of the bone. Diabetic patients may develop progressive neuropathy resulting in a Charcot joint or foot. MRI is particularly helpful at assessing bony involvement in an arthritic joint.

Skin and soft tissue infections

Skin and subcutaneous infections are common. Table 15.11 indicates possible causes. Skin commensals frequently gain entry to the subcutaneous tissue through minor trauma, particulary in patients on long-term steroids. Skin staphylococci or streptococci can produce a spreading cellulitis as a complication of scabies. Mycobacterial species and *Nocardia* are also high on the differential diagnosis for both superficial and deep skin abscesses. Necrotizing fasciitis due to a combination of aerobic and non-aerobic organisms has been reported in transplant patients, particularly diabetics. Skin lesions can herald the development of severe infection of other organs, for example mycobacterial species, *Cryptococcus*, and *Nocardia*. Skin and subcutaneous infections may well require

Table 15.10   Causes of septic arthritis

Escherichia coli

Non-typhoid *Salmonella*

Serratia spp.

Haemophilus influenzae

Nocardia

Mycobacteria

Cryptococcus neoformans

Sporotrichosis schenckii

Table 15.11   Causes of skin and soft tissue infections

Mycobacterium spp.: tuberculosis and atypicals

Nocardia

Penetration by skin commensals

Gram-positive organisms: group A streptococcus, *Staphylococcus aureus*

Pseudomonas and other Gram-negative micro-organisms

Prototheca

Necrotizing fasciitis (combined anaerobe and aerobe)

Fungi: *Candida, Aspergillus, Rhizopus, Cryptococcus neoformans, Tinea, Paecilomyces*, mucormycosis

both culture and excision biopsy for a full diagnosis. Acid-fast bacilli and fungal elements may be identified with special stains.

Mycobacterial infections

Mycobacterium tuberculosis

Both reactivation and primary tuberculous infections are more common in dialysis and renal transplant patients (Table 15.12). The total burden of immunosuppression is probably more significant than any individual immunosuppressive agent. The estimated prevalence depends on the country in which the study has been performed. In Europe and the United States the ethnic origin of the patient is particularly important for first-generation immigrants, with reactivation of tuberculosis in Asians being particularly common. The excess risk of tuberculosis in allograft recipients appears to be about 20 times that of the general population.

Clinical features

Clinical features are essentially the same as in the non-immunosuppressed. A high index of suspicion in the at-risk population is essential. The commonest presentation will be pulmonary or pleural with dissemination common by the time of diagnosis (Table 15.13).

Table 15.12 Prevalence of tuberculosis in renal transplant recipients.* Adapted from Drobniewski and Ferguson (1996) and Aguado *et al.* (1997)

Origin	% of patients
Northern Europe	1–2.3
Spain	0.8–1.8
United States	0.2–0.5
Argentina	3.1
Saudi Arabia	3.5
Turkey	4.2
Pakistan	15
India	5–11.8
South Africa	4.3
Pakistan	14.5

*Approximately 20–50 times the prevalence of the general population.

Presentation is usually insidious and (initially) relatively asymptomatic. Once established progression is rapid and spread wide. Disseminated tuberculosis may be as frequent as 25–65%. Most commonly tuberculosis will represent reactivation, although transmission by the donor organ can occur and spread from patient to patient may occur in renal units. Tuberculosis, particularly in patients from endemic areas, can affect the transplanted kidney producing an interstitial nephritis that may mimic rejection. Strictures and obstructions may occur in the collecting system. Classical bilateral multifocal nodular lesions may develop on the chest radiograph, but single nodules, masses, or cavities may be present, often with an associated pleural effusion. Any delay in diagnosis may permit hospital spread from patient to patient (Jereb *et al.* 1993). Mild systemic features are common initially, with weight loss and a low-grade fever, although patients can remain relatively asymptomatic for quite prolonged periods. A bimodal time of onset is common, with early presentations being seen between 3 and 12 months after transplantation and then a further increase in incidence much later on. Coinfection is common, for example with CMV, *Nocardia*, or *Pneumocystis*. In the developing nations tuberculosis may be detected in the presence of other bacterial pneumonias.

Investigation of mycobacterial infections

In at-risk patients and those suspected of *Mycobacterium tuberculosis*, investigation may have to be exhaustive to prove infection (Table 15.14). Skin testing is usually of no value as immunosuppression blunts the response. An occasional patient has a vigorous response which can be suggestive of active infection. Gallium scanning can identify parenchymal involvement of various organs and tissues. CT examination of suspicious areas may indicate sites for biopsy or aspiration. It is increasingly important to culture the organism to define sensitivities and to identify atypical mycobacterial species. Table 15.14 summarizes the investigations which need to be considered. Smear-positive sputum correlates with the presence of pulmonary cavities. Cavities are, however, less

Table 15.13   Clinical features of mycobacterial infections

Pulmonary (40–60%):	Nodular infiltrates
	Consolidation
	Pleural effusion/pleurisy
	Laryngeal involvement
	Cavitation
Miliary/disseminated (25%):	Sepsis syndrome
	Adult respiratory distress syndrome
Extrapulmonary (10–15%):	
Glandular	Cervical/axillary
	Mediastinal
	Para-aortic
Central nervous system	Space-occupying lesion/abscess
	Meningitis
Cutaneous (10%)	Sinus
	Cold abscess
Musculoskeletal (3%)	Tenosynovitis, spinal abscess/cord compression
	Monoarthritis, deep fascial infiltration
	Osteomyelitis, myositis
Gastrointestinal tract	Hepatitis (increased ALP)
	Ileal lesions: mass or obstruction
	Peritoneum: diffuse infiltration/ascites
Genitourinary	Cystitis
	Epididymoorchitis
	Interstitial nephritis of graft
Non specific	PUO: malaise, weight loss, leucocytosis, night sweats
Asymptomatic (10%)	

ALP=alkaline liver phosphatase; PUO=pyrexia or unknown origin.

common in the transplant population as the concurrent immunosuppression reduces lung damage. The use of PCR has significantly speeded up investigation. In nearly two-thirds of patients, invasive investigation may be required. Diagnosis is often delayed unduly for want of a full investigation.

Prophylaxis

There is still controversy about prophylaxis (Higgins *et al.* 1991). Table 15.15 summarizes the main groups who may benefit from isoniazid prophylaxis. Isoniazid should probably be continued indefinitely in these high-risk groups. Up to 8.5% of patients receiving prophylaxis may develop a breakthrough infection (Edeltein *et al.* 1995). In one study, 11% of patients developed hepatic dysfunction (severe in 2.5%) on isoniazid prophylaxis (Thomas and Manko 1975). BCG cannot be used as it is a live vaccine and can cause spreading infection if given to the immunocompromised. One study from the Indian subcontinent, where there is an approximately 5.5% incidence of isoniazid

Table 15.14 Diagnosis of mycobacterial infections

Sputum if available

Chest radiograph (>80% show an abnormality)

Bronchoalveolar lavage

Pleural biopsy and culture of pleural effusion

Lymph node biopsy

Cutaneous biopsy

Bone marrow aspirate, trephine, and culture

Gastric lavage

Early morning urines for culture

Liver biopsy

Abdominal and chest CT scan (high resolution)

Gallium scan (may guide endoscopy, exploration, biopsy)

Aspiration, e.g. cerebral abscess, lumbar puncture

ADA: BAL fluid, ascitic fluid, CSF, pleural fluid, pericardial fluid

PCR: bronchoalveolar lavage fluid, sputum, urine, cerebrospinal fluid, bone marrow

ADA=adenine deaminase (ectoenzyme on the surface of macrophages and monocytes); BAL= bronchoalveolar lavage; CSF=cerebrospinal fluid; PCR=polymerase chain reaction.

Table 15.15 Indications for prophylaxis of tuberculosis

Past tuberculosis (even if treated): PPD positive

Recent PPD skin conversion (<2 years)

Residence in endemic area

History of inadequately treated tuberculosis

Family history of tuberculosis

Close contact with active tuberculosis

Abnormal chest radiograph compatible with past tuberculosis

Negative skin PPD recipient from a positive skin PPD donor

Parents born in endemic area

Strongly positive PPD test (>10 mm)

PPD=purified protein derivative.

resistance, showed a non-significant benefit of isoniazid prophylaxis in renal patients (John *et al.* 1994). Abnormal liver function tests are a common cause for having to suspend prophylaxis. Compliance is thought to be poor. Prophylaxis cannot be based on Mantoux testing alone, as up to 70% of renal transplant patients may be anergic.

Contact tracing

An outbreak of tuberculosis in a renal unit requires careful contact tracing but is expensive (Drobniewski *et al.* 1995).

Management of tuberculosis

Spread of tuberculosis from patient to patient and from patient to staff within renal units does occur, so that patients excreting bacteria should be isolated in a room ventilated to the outside. Treatment with standard triple therapy for 6–9 months is generally considered adequate, but many centres continue treatment for a full 12 months and some also use quadruple therapy, particularly if the chance of drug resistance is high (Table 15.16). The use of four drugs may double the incidence of hepatotoxicity (Aguado *et al.* 1997).

Rifampicin is a potent enzyme inducer and leads to rapid metabolic clearance of cyclosporine A, tacrolimus, Sirolimus, and prednisolone. Cyclosporine A and tacrolimus doses may need to be increased three- to five-fold, and in some patients the frequency of administration should be increased to three times daily. The dose of prednisolone is usually doubled. In some respects the goal may be to actually reduce the total burden of immunosuppression, for example stopping azathioprine or mycophenolate mofetil when given as part of a triple-dose regime, while at the same time trying to avoid the risk of acute allograft rejection by ensuring adequate blood levels of the calcineurin-blocking drugs and prednisolone. If tuberculosis is thought to involve the graft, serial renography should be performed to detect stricture formation and obstruction. A pelviureteric 'JJ' stent may be needed to ensure adequate drainage of urine.

Prognosis

Mortality is significant, and has been as high as 40% in some series (Aguado *et al.* 1997). There is a suggestion that shorter courses of therapy and the use of antilymphocyte preparations to treat acute rejection episodes prior to diagnosis is associated with increased mortality. With early diagnosis and optimum therapy mortality should be less than 1%. Mortality is significantly higher in disseminated disease. Graft loss is a real risk due to drug interactions between the calcineurin-blocking drugs and rifampicin. Mortality can occur from hepatotoxicity which may be present in up to one-third of patients in some studies, particularly those receiving quadruple therapy. Up to 15% of patients may need their therapy interrupting and alternative regimes devised. On a positive note, immunosuppression *per se* does not appear to affect the microbiological cure rate. It is important to remember that simultaneous infection can occur, for example, with CMV, HHV8, and CMV and that it is associated with an increased mortality.

Atypical mycobacterial infections

Nearly half the mycobacterial species isolated from renal transplant patients are atypical organisms, particularly *Mycobacterium kansasii* (Qunibi *et al.* 1990). Extrapulmonary presentations are particularly common, especially skin and joint. *Mycobacterium kansasii* can present as a disseminated infection. Skin infection alone may occur with *Mycobacterium marinum*, *Mycobacterium haemophilum*, and *Mycobacterium chelonae*. Criteria for diagnosis are summarized in Table 15.17. PCRs for atypical mycobacterial infections have not yet been developed. The onset of atypical mycobacterial infections can be from 3 months to many years postgrafting. Relapses are common, so prolonged treatment is usually recommended—often exceeding 2 years. Sensitivity testing will determine specific treatment.

Table 15.16(a)   Treatment of mycobacterial infections: *Mycobacterium tuberculosis*

First-line therapy:	
Standard triple therapy	Isoniazid, ?indefinite
	Rifamipicin, ≥ 12 months
	Ethambutol, 2 months
Quadruple therapy (if miliary)	Isoniazid, ?indefinite
	Rifampicin, ≥ 12 months
	Ethambutol, 2 months
	Pyrizinamide, 2 months
Rifampicin intolerance:	Isoniazid
	Pyrizinamide
	Ethambutol
	Streptomycin
	Ofloxacin
Resistance:	Quadruple therapy dictated by sensitivity testing

Table 15.16(b)   Treatment of mycobacterial infections: atypical mycobacteria*

Mycobacterium avium	Clarithromycin containing regimen
Mycobacterium intracellulare	Azithromycin + rifabutin, clofazimine, ciprofloxacin, amikacin
Mycobacterium xenopi	As for *Mycobacterium tuberculosis* (may be ethambutol resistant)
Mycobacterium kansasii	Ciprofloxacin + standard triple therapy
Mycobacterium chelonae	Doxycycline, clarithromycin, amikacin, cefoxitin
Mycobacterium fortuitum	Prothionamide containing regimen
Mycobacterium marinum	Triple therapy
Mycobacterium haemophilum	3 or 4 of isoniazid, ciprofloxacin, amikacin, doxycycline or clarithromycin

*Therapy should be dictated by the results of sensitivity testing.

Table 15.17   Criteria for the diagnosis of atypical mycobacterial infections (Yamamoto *et al.* 1967)

1. Clinical features compatible with atypical mycobacterial infection

2. Repeated isolation of atypical mycobacteria

3. Exclusion of other causes of the clinical syndrome

4. Biopsy evidence of acid-fast bacilli or compatible histology if conditions 1–3 have been fulfilled

Non-typhoid *Salmonella*

Non-typhoid *Salmonella* is usually a self-limiting disease in the non-immunocompromised. In the renal transplant population, however, severe septicaemia and metastatic abscesses may develop. Onset is usually within the first year, and more often than not within the first 6 months. Clinical presentations include fever, but diarrhoea is relatively uncommon. Other important features are summarized in Table 15.18. The organism may be recovered from urine, stool, blood, and from the fluid aspirated from joints or abscesses. Treatment needs to be prolonged (more than 6 weeks). Sensitivities will decide therapy and resistance is increasingly encountered. Ampicillin, cotrimoxazole, or ciprofloxacin is usually effective. Deep-seated infections or relapsing disease require treatment for at least 3 months. Relapses are common. Reservoirs include the gall-bladder, renal tract, and metastatic bone or joint infections. With effective antimicrobial therapy, a chronic carrier state is unusual. Persistence or relapse may be related to structural abnormalities in the renal or biliary tract. The organism can survive intracellularly for long periods of time. Effective cell-mediated immunity is required for eradication. Ciprofloxacin has been shown to kill organisms persisting within macrophages. The incidence of non-typhoid *Salmonella* varies between 0 and 4% in different units. It is clearly higher in tropical climates. In the United States it is estimated to be 20 times more common than in the general population. Investigation needs to be thorough, particularly in patients with a relapsing condition. Isotopic bone and gallium scanning may be quite helpful. A full urological work-up is needed for persistent infection. If a gall-bladder focus is suspected, CT, ultrasound, and duodenal aspirations may be helpful. A native kidney nephrectomy or cholecystectomy may be required to eradicate the infection. Even with effective antimicrobial therapy, mortality is reported at 5–10%.

Listeriosis

Listeria monocytogenes is a Gram-positive rod which in normals produces little in the way of symptoms. Infection is usually via the ingestion of contaminated foods, e.g. dairy products and precooked meats. In the immunocompromised state it is not uncommon

Table 15.18   Clinical features of non-typhoid *Salmonella*

Fever	
Septicaemia	Disseminated intravascular coagulation
Bacteraemia	Metastatic infections:
	Lung: pneumonia, abscess, septic pulmonary emboli
	Genitourinary tract: pyelonephritis, orchitis, prostatitis
	Blood vessels: mycotic aneurysms, phlebitis
	Gastrointestinal tract: cholecystis, peritonitis
	Multiple abscesses: soft tissues, sacrum, perianal, dental, perinephric
	Joints: septic arthritis

and may present with a bacteraemic/septicaemic-like illness and be complicated by spread to the central nervous system, causing meningitis or focal abscesses. Spread to bone and joints may occur. Listeria may also present as a febrile diarrhoeal syndrome, or with endocarditis. Central nervous system seeding is so common in the renal transplant population (about 30%) that a lumbar puncture should be performed in most, if not all, cases. The presence of cerebrospinal fluid infection will require longer and more intensive antimicrobial therapy. *Listeria* remains the commonest cause of post-transplant meningitis. Seeding of the brainstem can produce a pseudopolio-like syndrome (low-dose cotrimoxazole is very effect prophylaxis). Mortality is significant at 30–50% in the presence of central nervous system involvement. Persistent neurological sequelae are common. Treatment is usually with a combination of ampicillin and gentamicin and should continue for at least 6 weeks.

Nocardiosis

Prevalence

Prevalence varies in different series in different parts of the world with 0–20% of transplant patients being affected. Most units have an incidence of less than 4%.

Aetiology

Nocardia is a widely distributed free-living micro-organism. Infection is most likely by inhalation (e.g. aerosols of soil). Overimmunosuppression and exposure are clearly important factors in the generation of nocardiosis. Diabetic transplant recipients may be at a further increased risk. The presence of other immunomodulating cofactors, such as CMV or hepatitis, is important.

Clinical features

Nocardia is an important bacterial disease in the transplant population with a significant morbidity and mortality. Presentation can mimic tuberculosis or staphylococcal abscesses so that an accurate microbiological diagnosis is essential. *Nocardia* runs a chronic debilitating course and can sometimes be mistaken for underlying malignancy or fungal disease. A wide variety of different nocardial species may be present (Table 15.19). The commonest site of infection is the lung, with haematogenous spread to the central nervous system and soft tissues occurring (Table 15.20). Nosocomial spread is likely, as small outbreaks have been reported by individual transplant units. Direct invasion into the skin and soft tissues may also be seen.

Investigation

Gram and Ziehl-Nielsen or Kinyoun stains of specimens are required. *Nocardia* are aerobic Gram-positive organisms, but are weakly acid-fast. Specimens should be inoculated under blood and chocolate agar plates. The organism grows slowly as a fragile

Table 15.19 *Nocardia* species

Nocardia asteroides > 80%
Nocardia otiti discaviaium (*caviae*) 3%
Nocardia farcinica
Nocardia brasiliensis 5% (tropical/subtropical)
Nocardia nova
Nocardia transvalensis

Table 15.20 Clinical features of nocardiosis

Systemic	Acute febrile illness
Abscess (10%)	Skin, muscle, breasts
Joints or bone (5%)	Inflammatory monoarthropathy
Lung (80%)	Cough and dyspnoea, infiltration, nodules, pnemonia, cavities, pleural effusion, empyema
Central nervous system (10–20%)	Multiple abscesses, meninigitis
Nodes (< 5%)	
Liver (< 5%)	
Miscellaneous	Isolated reports of infection in almost any organ

Table 15.21 Investigation of nocardiosis

Chest radiograph → bronchoalveolar lavage, open lung biopsy
Biopsy/curettage of skin and soft tissue lesions
CT of chest and brain
Cerebrospinal fluid examination
Culture: prolonged incubation necessary. Appropriate specialist media required

filamentous branching colony which initially led to misclassification as a fungus. Other more specific culture media will also support the growth of *Nocardia* (Sabouraud's, Lowenstein–Jenson's). An aggressive approach to diagnosis is again important utilizing lavage, biopsy, examination of the cerebrospinal fluid, and aspiration or surgical drainage of any pus (Table 15.21). Serology and skin testing have not yet been developed.

Treatment of nocardiosis

Cotrimoxazole alone or in combination with cefuroxime is usually sufficient. There is no need to reduce or curtail immunosuppression. There appears to be a poor correlation between *in vitro* sensitivity and *in vivo* response. Cefuroxime penetrates to the cerbrospinal fluid well and is of value in central nervous system infections. High-dose cotrimoxazole is needed (8×480 mg/day) and should be continued for at 4–6 months or for 6 weeks after resolution of the disease. In the long term therapy may need to be continued indefinitely at low dose, e.g. 2×480 mg/day. Imipenem is also effective. Where appropriate, surgical excision and drainage should be undertaken. For patients allergic to sulphonamides, amikacin, imipenem, or minocycline can be given.

Prognosis

Before the advent of sulphonamides, mortality was in excess of 80%. With appropriate treatment the mortality for cutaneous disease is virtually zero but central nervous system involvement still carries a significant mortality (40%). Mortality from pulmonary lesions is less at 25–30%.

Prevention

Low-dose cotrimoxazole prophylaxis for *Pneumocystis carinii* does not always appear to be sufficient to prevent *Nocardia* infection (Nampoory *et al.* 1996), although most units report a decrease in the incidence of *Nocardia* after the introduction of cotrimoxazole prophylaxis. Respiratory isolation of patients with pulmonary *Nocardia* on transplant units is recommended.

Immunosuppression during bacterial infections

Most bacterial infections are controlled by phagocytes and macrophages. Apart from steroids, the currently used immunosuppressive agents do not specifically target these processes. Humoral immunity is also less inhibited by the currently available drugs. For most bacterial infections, it does not seem necessary to reduce significantly immunosuppressive agents. Indeed, during the period of stress (septicaemia for example) an increase in the background steroid dose is indicated. The range of antimicrobial agents available is large and the potential for interaction with steroids and other immunosuppressive drugs is great (Table 15.22).

Table 15.22 Antimicrobial drug interactions

Rifampicin	Potent enzyme inducer. Rapid metabolism. Calcineurin-blocking drugs, steroids
Macrolides	Inhibition of cytochrome P-450. Toxic levels. Calcineurin-blocking drugs
Sulphonamides	Synergistic nephrotoxicity, e.g. calcineurin-blocking drugs, aminoglycosides
Fluoroquinolones	Inhibition of cytochrome P-450
Imidazoles	Inhibition of cytochrome P-450 (miconazole > ketoconazole > itraconazole > fluconazole)

Improvements in post-transplant immunological monitoring may help guide the clinician dealing with an infected transplant recipient. A vigorous antiviral response is indicated by an increase in NK cell population, an increase in activated T cells and a reduction in CD69-expressing T cells. A low HLA-DR expression on monocytes may predict sepsis (Haveman *et al.* 1999). Experience with granulocyte colony-stimulating factor, particularly in patients with CMV, indicates that leucopenia may be safely treated without an increase in the risk of acute rejection. For transplant patients with severe infections, it is reasonable to check immunoglobulin levels and sub classes. In a minority of patients, intravenous immunoglobulin may be helpful.

References

Ades L, Akposso K, De Beauregard M-AC, Haymann J-P, Mougenot B, Rondeau E, Srarer J-D. Bacterial endocarditis associated with crescentic glomerulonephritis in the kidney transplant recipient. *Transplantation* 1998 **66**(5): 1.

Aguado JM, Herrero JA, Gavaldá J, Torre-Cisneros K, Blanes M, Rufi G, Moreno A, Gurgui M, Hayek M, Lumbreras C and the Spanish Transplantation Infection Group, Gesitra. Clinical presentation and outcome of tuberculosis in kidney, liver and heart transplant recipients in Spain. *Transplantation* 1997 **63**(9): 1278–1286.

Beaman BL, Beaman L. *Nocardia* species: host–parasitic relationships. *Clinical Microbiology Review* 1994 **I**: 213–264.

Bishara J, Robenshtok E, Weinberger M, Yeshurun M, Sagie A and Pitlik S. Infective endocarditis in renal transplant recipients. *Transplant Infectious Disease* 1999 **1**(2): 138–143.

Dhar JM, Al-Khader AA, Al-Sulaiman M, Al-Hajani MK. Non-typhoid salmonella in renal transplant recipients: a report of twenty cases and review of the literature. *Quarterly Journal of Medicine* 1991 **78**(287): 235–250.

Drobniewski FA and Ferguson J. Tuberculosis in renal transplant units. *Nephrology, Dialysis and Transplantation* 1996 **11**: 768–770.

Drobniewski FA, Ferguson J, Barritt K. Follow up of an immunocompromised contact group of a case of primary tuberculosis on a renal unit. *Thorax* 1995 **50**: 863–868.

Edeltein CL, Jacobs JC, Mooasa MR. Pulmonary complications in 110 consecutive renal transplant recipients. *South African Medical Journal* 1995 **85**: 160–163.

Haveman JW, Van den Berg JW, Van den Berg AP, Mesander G, Sloof MJM, de Leij LHFM and The TH. Low HLA-DR expression on peripheral blood monocytes predicts bacterial sepsis after liver transplantation: relation with prednisolone intake. *Transplant Infections Disease* 1999 **1**(3): 146–152.

Higgins RM, Cahn AP, Porter D, Richardson AJ, Mitchell RG, Hopkin JM, Morris PJ. Mycobacterial infections after renal transplantation. *Quarterly Journal of Medicine* 1978 (286): 145–153.

Jereb JA, Burwen DR, Dooley SW. Nosocomial outbreak of tuberculosis in a renal transplant unit: application of a new technique for restriction fragment length polymorphism analysis of *Mycobacterium tuberculosis* isolate.

John GT, Thomas PP, Thomas M, Jeyaseelan L, Jacob CK, Shastry JCM. A double-blind randomised controlled trial of primary isoniazid prophylaxis in dialysis and transplant patients.

Jurewicz WA, Gunson BK, Ismail T, Ahgrisani L, McMaster P. Cyclosporin A and anti-tuberculous therapy. *Lancet* 1985 **1**: 1343.

Nampoory MRN, Khan ZU, Johny KV, Nessim J, Gupta RK, Al-Muzairai I, Shamhan M, Chugh TD. Nocardiosis in renal transplant recipients in Kuwait. *Nephrology Dialysis and Transplantation* 1996 11: 1134–1138.

Naqvi SA, Hussain M, Askari H, Hashmi A, Hussain Z, Hussain I, Hafiz S, Yazdani I, Rizvi SAH. Is there a place for prophylaxis against tuberculosis following renal transplantation? *Transplantation Proceedings* 1992 24(5): 1912.

Niehues R, Shluter S, Kramer A. Systemic nocardia asteroides infection with endocardial involvement in a patient undergoing immunosuppressive therapy. *Deutsche Medizinische Wochenschrifte* 1996 121: 1390.

Prada JL, Quillanueva JL, Torre-Cisneros J, Rodriguez F, Espinosa M, Anguita M. Endocarditis due to *Coryneibacterium* in a kidney transplant patient. *Nephrology Dialysis and Transplantation* 1994 9: 1185.

Qunibi WY, Al-Sibai MB, Taher S, Hader EJ, De Vol E, Al-Furayh O, Ginn HE. Mycobacterial infection after renal transplantation—report of 14 cases and review of the literature. *Quarterly Journal of Medicine* 1990 77(282): 1039–1060.

Spence RK, Dafoe DC, Rabin G *et al.* Mycobacterial infections in renal allograft recipients. *Archives of Surgery* 1983 118: 356–359.

Thomas PA, Manko MA. Chemoprophylaxis for the prevention of tuberculosis in the immunosuppressed renal allograft recipient.

Tolkoff-Rubin NE, Rubin RH. Urinary tract infection in the immunocompromised host Lessons from kidney transplantation and the AIDS epidemic. *Inflammatory Disease Clinic North America* 1997 11: 707–717.

Tolkoff-Rubin NE, Rubin RH. Urinary tract infections in the compromised. In: Brumfitt W, Hamilton-Miller JMT, Bailey RR (eds) *Urinary tract infection,* 1998 pp. 211–216. Chapman and Hall Medical, London.

Wilson JP, Turner HR, Kirchner KA, Chapman SW. Nocardial infections in renal transplant recipients. *Medicine* 1989 68(1): 38–57.

Yamamoto M, Ogura Y, Sudo K, Hibino S. Diagnostic criteria for disease caused by atypical mycobacteria. *American Review of Respiratory Diseases* 1967 96: 773–778.

16

Fungal and parasitic infections in the renal transplant patient

Jay A. Fishman and Ban-Hock Tan

Introduction

The success of clinical transplantation has been mirrored in the prolonged survival of recipients of organ transplants. Further, the return of allograft recipients to normal activities in the community has enlarged the spectrum of organisms to which these individuals are exposed. Such exposures have contributed to changing patterns of opportunistic infection with a growing variety of uncommon pathogens including fungi, parasites, and viruses that manifest increasing resistance to common antimicrobial therapies. Overall, fungal infection affects 5 to 20% of recipients of solid organ transplants. Fungal and parasitic infections pose particular difficulty in diagnosis for the transplant clinician. Because recipients of solid organ transplants tolerate established infection poorly, early recognition and treatment of infection is critical to disease-free survival.

These infections share a variety of features:

1. A distinction may be made between infections commonly observed in the period immediately following transplantation (i.e. within the first 1 to 2 months) and those observed later in the post-transplant course.
2. Geographical and environmental exposure is critical to most of these infections.
3. Activation is often associated with excessive immune suppression, particularly with corticosteroids which are less important for some other common infections in transplantation (e.g. due to viruses) than for fungal infection.
4. Latency is a common feature of many of the fungi and parasites important to transplantation.
5. The organism must be able to complete its lifecycle within the human host.

The pretransplantation evaluation

Given the importance of the prevention of infection in the transplant recipient, a strategy must be developed for the pretransplant evaluation of transplant candidates to identify unusual risks for the post-transplant period. Some general guidelines include:

1. All known infections must be identified, under control, and preferably eradicated, prior to transplantation. The recipient's serological status, indicative of prior exposure and possible latent infection, should be known for *Toxoplasma gondii* and

Strongyloides stercoralis. As for active infections, evidence for exposure to *Strongyloides* merits pretransplant therapy.

2. In endemic areas, transplants (or transfusions) may provide entry of *T. gondii*, *Trypanosoma cruzi* (Chagas' disease), *Leishmania* spp., *Acanthamoeba*, *Naeglaria*, *Strongyloides stercoralis*, *Taenia* or *Echinococcus* spp. with exacerbation of infection by immune suppression.

3. The patient with recurrent bronchitis, sinusitis, or other recurrent infections treated with multiple courses of antimicrobial agents may be colonized with *Candida* or *Aspergillus* in addition to antimicrobial-resistant bacteria. These patients require radiographic evaluation (CT of chest and sinuses) and often surgical drainage of the sinuses, and eradication of infection to the degree possible before transplantation.

4. Potential donors and recipients require screening for human immunodeficiency virus (HIV) 1 and 2, human T-cell leukaemia virus-1 (HTLV-1), hepatitis A, B, and C, cytomegalovirus (CMV), Epstein–Barr virus (EBV), herpes simplex virus (HSV), varicella zoster virus (VZV), syphilis, and *Toxoplasma gondii*. Screening for HSV, VZV, CMV, and EBV are used as guides for the development of prophylactic strategies after renal transplantation rather than pretransplant therapies (at present). Donor seropositivity for HSV, VZV, EBV, or CMV is not a contraindication to donation, but these infections when active are important cofactors to the activation of other latent infections.

5. Donor infection with certain organisms which have a high propensity to infect anastamotic sites, particularly *Candida* and *Aspergillus*, should be treated, and the resolution of infection documented, prior to procurement.

The risk of fungal and parasitic infections in the transplant recipient

The risk of infection in the organ transplant patient is determined by a semiquantitative relationship between two factors: the epidemiological exposures of the individual and the sum of all of the factors which contribute to the individual's susceptibility (or resistance) to infection, termed the 'net state of immunosuppression'. The net state of immunosuppression is a reflection of all of the factors that contribute to susceptibility to infection. The dose, duration, and temporal sequence in which immunosuppressive drugs are deployed are central to the immune status of the host.

For fungal infections, the presence of colonization and/or of devitalized tissues or fluid collections in the postoperative allograft recipient is critical. Infection related to foreign bodies, devitalized tissues, or fluid collections cannot be cleared while these remain in place (Levin *et al.* 1998; Paya *et al.* 1989). Similarly the prolonged use of steroid therapy or neutropenia will predispose to fungal infection; the allograft recipient who is treated with steroids prior to transplantation is more likely to suffer from *Aspergillus* or *Pneumocystis* infection (including *Pneumocystis carinii* in the 'fungal' category) early after transplantation. The immunological effects of metabolic problems (e.g. protein–calorie malnutrition, uraemia, and, perhaps, hyperglycaemia) and of infection by viruses common to transplant recipients (CMV, EBV, hepatitis B (HBV) and C (HCV), HSV) are described in detail elsewhere (Chapters 10 and 11). The enhanced susceptibility of the diabetic patient to infection with the Mucoraciae merits attention in this regard (Chapter 6). Generally, more

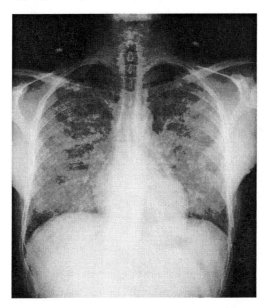

Fig. 16.1 *Pneumocystis carinii* pneumonia in a renal transplant recipient. The patient was admitted for dyspnoea and fever 18 months after living-related renal transplantation. Despite therapy with trimethoprim-sulfamethoxazole, clinical symptoms and the chest radiograph progressed. Lung biopsy revealed simultaneous CMV infection. Ganciclovir therapy allowed resolution of both infections.

than one factor is present in each host; the identification and correction of the relevant factors is central to the prevention and treatment of infection in these hosts.

For fungal and parasitic infections, the specific infections observed in an individual are determined by the nature of the epidemiological exposure (Table 16.1). Such exposures may be quite remote in time and must be identified prior to transplantation. Temporally more distant exposures may include geographically restricted systemic mycoses (*Histoplasma*, *Coccidioides*, *Blastomyces*), *Pneumocystis carinii*, *Toxoplasma gondii*, *Leishmania donovani*, *Strongyloides stercoralis*, or *Trypanosoma cruzi*. Infections of transplant recipients due to these pathogens commonly reflect reactivation of latent infection, but may also represent new, primary infections due to exposures in endemic regions. By contrast, exposures within the hospital in the period immediately surrounding transplantation account for infections due to nosocomial pathogens such as *Aspergillus* spp. and azole-resistant yeasts, as well as bacterial pathogens which often demonstrate antimicrobial resistance. When the air (e.g. in operating rooms, radiology suites, and construction sites), food, equipment, or potable water supply is contaminated with pathogens such as *Aspergillus* spp. or azole-resistant yeasts, clusters of infection in time and space (e.g. by ward or reflecting the common source of the exposures) will be observed.

Timetable of infection after transplantation

Given the relatively standardized management of immunosuppressive regimens after transplantation, those organisms causing infection at various times following transplantation

Table 16.1 Fungal and parasitic infections due to exposures in the community

---

Infections caused by the ingestion of contaminated food or water
  Salmonella spp.
  Cryptosporidium, Microsporidium, Isospora
  Listeria monocytogenes
  Pseudomonas spp., *Legionella* spp., *Serratia* spp.

Systemic mycotic infections: restricted geographical areas
  Histoplasma capsulatum
  Coccidiodiomycosis
  Blastomycosis

Community acquired: ubiquitous saprophytes
  Cryptococcus neoformans
  Nocardia asteroides
  Aspergillus spp.
  Pneumocystis carinii

Endemic parasites
  Strongyloides stercoralis, Trypanosoma cruzi, Leishmania spp.

---

are relatively predictable. For both fungal and parasitic infections, it is useful to divide the post-transplant course into three time periods: the first month post-transplant, the period 1–6 months post-transplant, and the period more than 6 months post-transplant.

In the first month post-transplant, there are two major causes of infection in all forms of organ transplantation. The first is persistence or exacerbation of infections which were present in the donor or the recipient prior to transplantation but which were unrecognized or incompletely treated. Examples of this phenomenon are the reports of transmission of malaria and *Candida* infections via renal allografts (Babinet *et al.* 1991; Johnston 1981; Lefavour *et al.* 1980). The second type of infections are nosocomial infections which reflect postoperative complications (aspiration pneumonitis, wound infections, 'line sepsis') or are related to technical aspects of transplant surgery (devitalized tissues, anastomotic suture lines, haematomas, lymphocoeles, pleural effusions, urinomas). These sites are subject to superinfection and may become the nidus for subsequent infections. Particular risk of nosocomial infection is experienced by patients requiring prolonged ventilatory support and those with diminished lung function, persistent ascites, stents of the urinary tract or biliary ducts, cholesterol emboli, or poorly revascularized graft tissue. In these patients, defects in phagocytic function are predominant and predict infections with *Candida, Aspergillus*, and the Mucoraceae.

In the period 1 to 6 months post-transplant, the nature of infection changes, reflecting a shift towards infection due to pathogens controlled in the normal host by cellular immune mechanisms. While residual problems from the perioperative period may persist, it is during this time period that the traditional 'opportunistic infections' emerge. These include latent infections, particularly the geographical fungal infections (histoplasmosis, coccidioidomycosis, and blastomycosis) and *Pneumocystis carinii* and the protozoa (*T. gondii, Leishmania*, Chagas' disease). Both fungal and parasitic infections present more often in association with viral infection, particularly due to the herpes

(a)

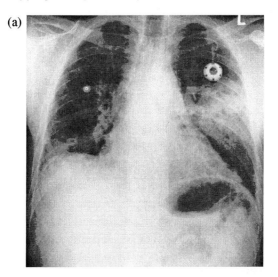

(b)

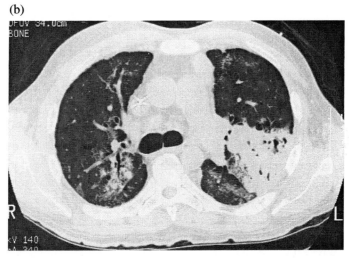

Fig. 16.2 (a) *Aspergillus fumigatus* pneumonia in a renal transplant recipient. The patient was admitted to an outside hospital with fever and chills approximately 9 months after cadaveric renal transplantation. The patient had been treated 1 month earlier for steroid-resistant graft rejection using rabbit thymoglobulin. The patient failed to respond to conventional antimicrobial therapy and underwent chest CT scanning. (b) CT shows dense left-sided infiltrate accompanied by milder right-sided pneumonitis. Bronchoscopy revealed *Aspergillus fumigatus*.

group viruses. The viruses, particularly CMV, serve as important cofactors to many fungal and parasitic infections (George *et al.* 1997). The potential effects of viral infection are diverse and apply not only to CMV but also to HBV, HCV, EBV, and probably to other common viruses as well (respiratory syncytial virus (RSV), human herpesvirus 6 (HHV6), and adenovirus).

There is significant geographical and institutional variation in the occurrence of opportunistic infections during the first 6 months post-transplant. In endemic regions, primary histoplasmosis and coccidioidomycosis, and gastrointestinal infection due to *Isospora, Cryptosporidium* (often in association with unfiltered well or reservoir water), and *Cyclospora* spp., may be seen. At centres with a fixed, high incidence of infections including *Pneumocystis* (rates of 5–10% or higher), low-dose trimethoprim-sulfamethoxazole prophylaxis is a highly effective means of disease prevention for a variety of pathogens including *Pneumocystis, Isospora belli, Toxoplasma*, and *Nocardia*. Similarly, in programmes with a fixed, high incidence of *Aspergillus, Histoplasma*, or azole-resistant yeasts (e.g. in liver transplant recipients) both epidemiological protection (e.g. HEPA-filtered air supply within the hospital), and fungal prophylaxis (as appropriate to the common isolates) may be utilized.

More than 6 months post-transplant, most patients are receiving stable and relatively modest levels of immunosuppression. These patients are subject to common infections acquired in the community (again, with geographical variation) and to unique exposures associated with epidemiological hazards associated with work (e.g. cryptococcosis in urban street sweepers) or hobbies (sporotrichosis, mucormycosis, and aspergillosis in gardeners).

Patients who have less satisfactory graft function generally receive more intensive immunosuppressive therapies. This subgroup of patients is at the greatest risk for infection with such opportunists as *Cryptococcus neoformans*, mucormycosis, dematiaceous (pigmented) fungi or *Nocardia*, and also for more severe community-acquired infections due to influenza or *Listeria*. For this subgroup of patients, prolonged antimicrobial prophylaxis is indicated.

Special factors predisposing to fungal infection

Fungal infection following transplantation has been best studied in relation to lung and liver transplantation, areas in which fungal pathogens often play a major role (Wajszczuk *et al.* 1985; Kusne *et al.* 1988; Paya *et al.* 1989; Nieto-Rodriguez *et al.* 1996; Garcia *et al.* 1998; Singh *et al.* 1997*a*; Hadley and Karchmer 1995). The impact of fungal infection in renal transplantation (up to 5% of recipients) is generally significant in patients receiving higher levels of immunosuppression (chronically) and whom manifest poor graft function, in those with viral coinfection (i.e. CMV), during immunosuppressive treatment of acute graft rejection, and in combined kidney–pancreas transplant recipients (Bach *et al.* 1973; Murphy 1976; Scroggs 1987; Peterson 1981). Excluding *Pneumocystis carinii*, invasive or metastatic fungal infection after all forms of transplantation carries a 30–50% mortality and increases the cost of patient care significantly. Thus, the prevention of these infections is of great importance. The limited number of antifungal antimicrobial agents increases the importance of prevention. Particular problems are posed by the toxicity of amphotericin B, limited experience with and the high cost of lipid-associated formulations of amphotericin, and interactions of the azole-antifungal agents with cyclosporine and tacrolimus.

Major factors associated with increased risks of fungal infection are shown in Table 16.2.

A number of special situations are recognized which affect the incidence of fungal infection. Corticosteroid therapy and CMV infections are associated with the risk of

Table 16.2   Major factors associated with increased risks of fungal infection

Extensive use of broad spectrum antimicrobial agents

Prolonged patient survivals

Excessive immune suppression to prevent graft rejection (notably steroids)

Prolonged pretransplant hospitalizations

Number and duration of vascular, urinary, and surgical drains and catheters (Levin *et al.* 1998)

Decreased serum albumin (nutrition)

Advanced age of the recipient

Renal or hepatic dysfunction after transplantation

Viral coinfection (CMV, HHV6, HCV) (George *et al.* 1997; Dockrell *et al.* 1999)

Bacterial infections

Fungal colonization

Wound infections

Measures of the severity of the illness of the patient—volume of transfusion requirements, duration of stay in intensive care, duration of respiratory support, aspiration pneumonitis

Need for surgical re-exploration or reintervention (retransplantation)

Pneumocystis pneumonia as well as the overall risk of invasive fungal disease. Anastomotic leaks (urinary, vascular, and others) are associated with *Candida* infections, particularly candidaemia without a clear source. Gastrointestinal invasion including ulceration is often due to *Candida* and other yeasts, but often in association with viral infection (CMV or herpes simplex) or coinfection with *Helicobacter pylori*. Older patients receiving mycophenolate mofetil instead of azathioprine may have an increased incidence of fungal infection (Meier-Kriesche *et al.* 1999).

Of particular interest is the importance of fungal infections following pancreatic and kidney–pancreas transplantation. The diabetic population is known to be susceptible to colonization and infection with a variety of fungi including *Candida* spp. and the Mucoraciae. The effects of enteric versus bladder drainage of the pancreas is controversial. The largest published series of 500 kidney–pancreas transplants (Sollinger *et al.* 1998) demonstrated an enzymatic leak in 8–15.5% of patients, intra-abdominal abscess in 2.8%, peritonitis in 11.6%, and wound infection in 8.2%. Of the 388 patients undergoing bladder drainage, 14.2% had intra-abdominal infection in the first year and 16.7% had fungal infections. Patients with enteric drainage had a similar incidence of intra-abdominal infections (12.9%), but fewer fungal infections (7.3%). A smaller series of patients from the same centre (which includes some of the same patients) received immunosuppression with antithymocyte globulin induction, prednisone, cyclosporine, and mycophenolate mofetil (Pirsch *et al.* 1998). In this group, patients receiving enteric drainage of the pancreas had a significantly lower incidence of fungal infection (4%) than a comparable group receiving bladder drainage (17%). This may relate to a significantly higher incidence of CMV infection in the bladder drainage group (21 versus 8%), in addition to exposures to bladder-borne pathogens and/or to the ease of diagnosis of pancreatic infections with bladder drainage. By contrast, Benedetti *et al.* (1996) experienced a 9.2% incidence of intra-abdominal fungal infection after kidney–pancreas transplants, with the rate higher (21%) in enteric-drained versus baldder-drained (10%) transplants. The rate was also higher for combined kidney–pancreas transplants compared with pancreas alone. Fungal infection was associated with graft loss and a high mortality.

Changing patterns of fungal infections

With prolonged survival and improved quality of life of many transplant recipients, the pattern of fungal and parasitic infections has changed. In the first few months after transplantation, during the time of greatest exogenous immune suppression, primary infections are dominated by nosocomially acquired organisms, largely *Aspergillus* and *Candida* spp. Thus, for example, central nervous system infections in transplant recipients are almost uniformly due to disseminated aspergillosis. By contrast, disseminated infection after the first year is increasingly due to the dematiaceous (pigmented) fungi and less commonly due to *Aspergillus* in the absence of neutropenia or prior colonization. Thus, late infections in the transplant population are increasingly caused by 'atypical' fungi (Table 16.3) (Singh *et al.* 1997*b*). These infections are also often atypical in presentation—nodules in the skin or soft tissues, oral lesions, pericardial infiltration—and may be easily confused with tumours or improperly treated in the absence of biopsy and culture data. Some such atypical fungal infections following solid organ transplantation recently treated at the Massachusetts General Hospital are summarized in Table 16.3. Dermatophytosis was detected in 42% of 100 renal transplant recipients in one series from India; these were largely *Tinea cruris* and *Tinea corporis* (Sentamil *et al.* 1999).

Special factors predisposing to parasitic infection

The epidemiology of parasitic infection is unique among the opportunistic pathogens. Those parasitic infections of special importance to the immunosuppressed host share three features: organisms associated with the geographical exposures of the patient, those

Table 16.3 Atypical presentations of fungal infection

Asymptomatic fungal infection (many patients with acute liver failure)*

Cellulitis and nodular skin lesions (Paecilomyces)

Muscle and skin abscesses, pustules (*Fusarium* spp.)

Sinusitis, arthritis, endocarditis, meningitis (*Pseudoallescheria boydii* now *Scedosporium*)

Invasive oesophageal and tracheal disease (*Aspergillus, Candida*)

Hard palate/jaw invasion (Mucoraeciae)

Lung coin lesions or granulomata with *Cryptococcus* or *Hyalohyphomycosis* (blue–green or colourless fungi, e.g. *Penicillium, Fusarium* spp.)

Phaeohyphomycosis (dematiaceous fungi with brown pigments): invasive, infection disseminated from lungs, sinuses, or traumatized skin to CNS, deep tissues (*Aureobasidium pullulans, Exophiala* spp., *Wangiella dermatitidis*

---

*Rolando N *et al.* (1996). *Seminars in Liver Disease*, **16**, 389–402.

organisms which are normally controlled by the (cellular) immune system, and those which can complete their life cycles within the host. Systemic infections due to each of the major protozoan parasites have been described as primary infections resulting from the transplantation of organs or transfusion of blood products from seropositive or actively infected donors into immunosuppressed, naive recipients. Thus, *Toxoplasma gondii*, *Trypanosoma cruzi*, and *Leishmania donovani* have been identified in the immediate post-transplant period. Protozoan infections associated with ingestion (*Cryptosporidium*, *Microsporidium*, *Isospora belli*, *Cyclospora*) or reactivation (*T. gondii*) are generally seen later. Exposure to the blood fluke *Strongyloides stercoralis* is often distant (up to 30 years prior to transplantation) with reactivation in the setting of immune suppression. Urinary schistosomiasis is generally caused by another blood fluke, *Schistosoma hematobium* (although also by other species of schistosomes). While this infection does not reactivate in transplantation, chronic schistosomiasis is a major contributor to renal failure in endemic regions via the development of ureteric obstruction and bacterial reflux. *S. mansoni* and *S. japonicum* may cause hepatic fibrosis and granulomatous disease and contribute to hepatic failure. Similarly, the trematodes or liver flukes which are associated with ingestion of contaminated vegetable matter (*Clonorchia (Opisthorchis) sinensis*, *Dicrocoelium*, *Fasciola*) cannot complete their life cycles within the human host and are not exacerbated by immune suppression. These flukes may cause chronic cholecystitis and cholangitis with liver abscesses ('oriental cholangiohepatitis') necessitating hepatic transplantation in some individuals. *Giardia lamblia* may be exacerbated by hypogammaglobulinaemia, but is not significantly worsened in transplantation. Similarly, a number of reports illustrate the transmission of malaria with renal allografts—but that the disease does not appear to be significantly exacerbated by cellular immune suppression (Babinet *et al.* 1991; Johnston 1981; Lefavour *et al.* 1980; Turkmen *et al.* 1996). Quinine therapy alters cyclosporine levels *in vivo* (Tan and Ch'ng 1991).

General principles in management

Given the inability of immunosuppressed individuals to clear infection efficiently, a number of concepts merit consideration:

1. Inflammatory responses associated with microbial invasion are impaired by immunosuppressive therapy, which results in diminished symptoms and muted clinical and radiological findings. As a result, infections are often advanced (i.e. disseminated) at the time of clinical presentation. Diminished manifestations of infection are manifest in radiological studies as well as in physical signs and symptoms. Thus, clear chest radiographs may reveal diffuse disease in *Pneumocystis* pneumonia or nodular disease with aspergillosis.
2. Altered anatomy following surgery may alter the physical signs of infection and contribute to the susceptibility to infection.
3. Central nervous system (CNS) infection due to fungi is often associated with extraneural infection with the same organism allowing for biopsy and evaluation of established infection without brain biopsy. Occasionally, however, colonization of extraneural sites may confuse diagnosis. By contrast, CNS infection due to parasites is often chronic and extraneural infection may be resolved or difficult to detect.

The use of the CT scan (or MRI of the neuroaxis) is essential for assessing the presence and nature of infectious and malignant processes.

4. Serological tests (antibody assays) are useful primarily for exposures prior to transplantation but rarely of use for the diagnosis of acute infection after transplantation. Patients generally will not seroconvert in a time frame useful for clinical diagnosis. Thus tests which detect proteins (e.g. ELISA, direct immunofluorescence for influenza and respiratory syncytial virus) or nucleic acids (polymerase chain reaction) should be utilized. Tests for fungal and parasite antigens are under development but lack the sensitivity needed for routine use. The value of these tests for most fungi and parasites is uncertain.

5. The 'gold standard' for diagnosis is tissue histology and microbiology. No radiological finding is sufficiently diagnostic to obviate the need for tissue. Further, multiple simultaneous infections are common. Thus, as a routine component of the initial evaluation of transplant recipients with infectious syndromes and for patients failing to respond to appropriate therapy, invasive procedures that provide tissue for culture and for histology are necessary.

6. Antimicrobial agents alone are often inadequate for cure; surgical intervention is often necessary. Synergistic antimicrobial agent therapy must be used when available; however, compromises must often be made based on the inherent toxicities of many antimicrobial agents. The use of second-line agents that allow the progression of infection is unacceptable. Thus, early and precise diagnosis with microbial susceptibility data and optimal antimicrobial therapy are essential to the care of transplant patients.

Infections of special importance in transplantation

Pneumocystis carinii pneumonia

The risk of infection with *Pneumocystis* is greatest in the first 6 months after transplantation and during periods of increased immunosuppression (Fishman 1995, 1998*a*,*b*; Lufft *et al.* 1996). The natural reservoir of infection remains unknown. Aerosol transmission of infection has been demonstrated by a number of investigators in animal models and clusters of infections have developed in clinical settings including between HIV-infected persons and renal transplant recipients (Chave *et al.* 1991; Bazinsky and Phillips 1969). Activation of latent infection remains a significant factor in the incidence of disease in immunocompromised hosts. In the solid organ transplant recipient, chronic immune suppression that includes corticosteroids is most often associated with pneumocystosis. Bolus corticosteroids, cyclosporine, or coinfection with CMV may also contribute to the risk for *Pneumocystis* pneumonia (Arend *et al.* 1996).

In patients not receiving trimethoprim-sulfamethoxazole (or alternative drugs) as prophylaxis, most transplant centres report an incidence of *Pneumocystis carinii* pneumonia of ~10% in the first 6 months post-transplant. There is a continued risk of infection in three overlapping groups of transplant recipients:

(1) those who require higher than normal levels of immune suppression for prolonged periods of time due to poor allograft function or chronic rejection;

(2) those with chronic CMV infection; and

(3) those undergoing treatments which increase the level of immunodeficiency such as cancer chemotherapy or neutropenia due to drug toxicity (Hardy *et al.* 1984).

The occurrence of *Pneumocystis* infection is highly associated with CMV infection, possibly because of an inhibitory effect of CMV on alveolar macrophage function, systemic immune suppression, and possibly via improved growth of *P. carinii* on CMV-infected alveolar epithelium (Fishman 1998, Bozzette *et al.* 1992). The expected mortality due to *Pneumocystis* pneumonia is increased in patients on cyclosporine when compared to other immunocompromised hosts.

The hallmark of infection due to *P. carinii* is the presence of marked hypoxaemia, dyspnoea, and cough with a paucity of physical or radiological findings. In the transplant recipient, *Pneumocystis* pneumonia is generally acute to subacute in development. In patients receiving lung transplants, the rate of asymptomatic isolation of *P. carinii* approaches two-thirds of the total in some series. Of these, up to half are expected to develop symptomatic disease without treatment. For other transplants, 5–12% of unprophylaxed patients will develop pneumocystosis.

The chest radiograph may be entirely normal or develop the classical pattern of perihilar and interstitial 'ground glass' infiltrates (Fishman 1994). Microabscesses, nodules, small effusions, lymphadenopathy, asymmetry, and linear bands are common. Chest CT will be more sensitive to the diffuse interstitial and nodular pattern than routine radiographs. The nodularity seen in transplanted lungs due to *Pneumocystis* may be mimicked by rejection (and is also seen in intravenous drug abusers). The clinical and radiological manifestations of *P. carinii* pneumonia are virtually identical to those of CMV. Indeed, the clinical challenge is to determine whether both pathogens are present. Significant extrapulmonary disease is uncommon in the transplant recipient. Atypical *Pneumocystis* infection (radiographically or clinically) may be seen in patients who have coexisting pulmonary infections or who develop disease while receiving prophylaxis with pentamidine or atovaquone.

The therapy of *P. carinii* pneumonia has been reviewed elsewhere (Fishman 1998*a,b*; Bozzette *et al.* 1995; Branten *et al.* 1995; Hughes *et al.* 1994). Early therapy, preferably with trimethoprim-sulfamethoxazole (TMP-SMZ) is preferred (Hughes *et al.* 1974; Hughes 1987). However, few renal transplant patients will tolerate full-dose TMP-SMZ for prolonged periods of time. This reflects both the false elevation of creatinine due to trimethoprim, and the toxicity of sulfa agents for the renal allograft. Hydration and the gradual initiation of therapy may help. Alternative therapies are less desirable, but have been used with success including: intravenous pentamidine, atovaquone, clindamycin with primaquine or pyrimethamine, and trimetrexate (Falloon *et al.* 1991; Hughes *et al.* 1993, 1994; Toma *et al.* 1989). The use of short courses of adjunctive steroids is useful in transplant recipients as in AIDS patients—with the caveat that the taper must be guaged against the risk of rejection as well as relapsed pulmonary inflammation.

The importance of preventing *Pneumocystis* infection cannot be overemphasized. While low-dose TMP-SMZ or other prophylactic agents are well tolerated in this patient population, as was noted, treatment doses of TMP-SMZ or pentamidine are associated with a high rate of toxicity, particularly renal and hepatic. Alternative prophylactic strategies, including dapsone, atovaquone, inhaled or intravenous pentamidine, are less effective than TMP-SMZ, but useful in the patient with significant allergy to sulfa drugs (Fishman 1998*a*,*b*; Saukkonen *et al.* 1996). Primary infection and relapses with aerosolized pentamidine have been observed (Bradburne *et al.* 1989). Clindamycin/ primaquine has also been used as an alternative combination (Barber *et al.* 1996; Black *et al.* 1994). Newer agents, including the echinocandin lipopeptides and pneumocandins, are in clinical trials (Balkovac *et al.* 1992; Morris *et al.* 1994).

Aspergillus

Invasive aspergillosis generally involves the lungs, often with metastatic infection to the brain and/or liver. *Aspergillus* infection often presents as primary, nosocomially acquired infection or as an invader of tissues already damaged by surgery or by prior illness. The picture of primary, disseminated infection presents as focal, macronodular pulmonary infiltrates (with haematogenous spread to liver, spleen, kidney, and/or brain). More often, *Aspergillus* secondarily infects an area of parenchymal pneumonitis with progressively focal and macronodular infiltrates with early cavitation. CT scans will often discern nodules with a 'halo' in areas of persistent pulmonary infection. Disseminated disease may be subtle—mild abnormalities of liver chemistry, new seizures, or tachypnoea are often ascribed to alternative aetiologies.

The risk of invasive pulmonary aspergillosis appears to be about 50% once the respiratory tract, including the sinuses or trachea, is colonized. 'Pre-emptive' antifungal therapy, usually with amphotericin B, may be indicated when such colonization is noted in patients prior to or during the acute phase of high-dose immunosuppression. A similar strategy is used at centres in which the incidence of nosocomial fungal infection exceeds 5–10%. The clinical presentation is usually one of fever and systemic toxicity, with a variable occurrence of such respiratory symptoms as cough, dyspnoea, tachypnoea, and pleurisy. Most patients have metastatic disease at the time of diagnosis, with the brain and skin (intravenous catheter sites) being relatively common sites for metastatic infection. Isolated nodules in the central nervous system are generally due to *Aspergillus* in the early period after transplantation and to other fungi beyond 1 year post-transplant. The clinical course is determined by the pathological features of this infection—a necrotizing bronchopneumonia with vascular invasion, leading to the three cardinal features of invasive pulmonary aspergillosis—issue infarction, haemorrhage, and metastases. Amphotericin B remains the cornerstone of therapy, with the roles of lipid-associated amphotericin preparations, itraconazole, voriconazole, and other newer agents, as yet ill defined. In general, lipid-associated amphotericin is reserved for patients with progressive renal dysfunction, true intolerance of amphotericin B (rare), or in patients failing to resolve infection due to susceptible fungi on other therapies. Some caution must be used with these agents in the therapy of peritoneal infections, brain infection, and in the lungs where clinical responses are more variable than in hepatic or wound-associated infections.

Cryptococcus neoformans

Cryptococcal infection begins with the lung as the portal of entry for disseminated infection, particularly to the central nervous system. Pulmonary cryptococcosis in transplant

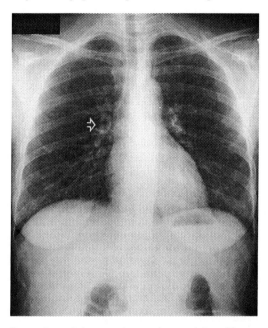

Fig. 16.3 Cavitary disease (arrow) in a renal transplant recipient 15 years after cadaveric renal transplantation. Bronchoalveolar lavage was negative for pathogens. Transbronchial biopsy revealed *Mycobacterium avium intracellulare*-complex while lymph node biopsy revealed *Cryptococcus neoformans*. Cryptococcal antigenaemia assay and PPD skin tests were negative. Both infections responded to therapy.

patients is usually asymptomatic or minimally symptomatic. The most common presentations are asymptomatic pulmonary nodules or lymph node enlargement on routine chest radiograph. Occasionally, a subacute consolidation with influenza like symptoms may be noted. This may occur in association with therapy for graft rejection or following steroid therapy or CMV infection (Bernstein *et al.* 1987). Asymptomatic nodules are aggressively pursued, with pre-emptive fluconazole or amphotericin therapy administered in order to prevent subsequent systemic or neurological disease. Cryptococcal meningitis may present with virtually any cerebrospinal fluid (CSF) formula. All transplant patients with meningitis should have serum and CSF cryptococcal antigen studies performed. The clinical response to therapy must be documented by resampling of the CSF after an appropriate (2-week minimum) period with therapy prolonged (4–6 months of oral fluconazole) beyond the time of documented cure.

Candida and the yeasts

While significant infections due to yeasts are uncommon, increasingly *Candida albicans* is found as a coinfecting agent of abscesses related to infections associated with pancreatitis or urinary leaks or lymphocoeles in the early postoperative patient. Many patients are colonized with *Candida* spp., which contaminate sputum cultures and vascular access catheter sites of the neck and chest. It is, therefore useful to give prophylaxis with oral, non-absorbable antifungal agents (clotrimazole or nystatin) while patients are receiving high-dose immunosuppression or broad-spectrum antimicrobial therapy. Vaginal overgrowth is similarly reduced by the judicious use of topical antifungal agents during periods of increased risk. Although candidal isolation from sputum cultures is common, cases of pulmonary invasion are vanishingly rare, and such cultural results should not, by themselves, lead to other therapy or an aggressive diagnostic programme.

The routine use of azole antifungal agents has shifted the spectrum of yeasts which colonize the transplant recipient towards *C. kreusei*, *C. glabrata*, and occasionally to *Penicillium* or more unusual organisms. As a result, wound infections, sputum, skin infections, vascular line-related infections, and/or cultures obtained from drainage (Jackson–Pratt or other) or percutaneous aspirates increasingly contain 'non-*Candida albicans* yeasts' which are of uncertain significance and generally have reduced susceptibility to fluconazole or itraconazole. This is a particular problem during infection of pancreas allografts with pancreatitis. These infections will require surgical debridement with amphotericin or newer azole (voriconazole) therapy for cure.

Toxoplasma gondii

Serological evidence suggests that up to 70% of all individuals have been exposed to *Toxoplasma gondii*. In Europe, seroprevalence approaches 75%, while estimates in the United States vary from 5 to 40%. *Toxoplasma* causes significant infection only infrequently outside the immunocompromised host. The important role of infection of the CNS by this organism complicates both diagnosis and treatment. This problem is further compounded by the lack of reliable and reproducible serological tests for use in immunocompromised individuals.

Toxoplasmosis occurs with four distinct clinical presentations: congenital, acquired in immunocompetent individuals, disseminated in immunocompromised individuals, and as reactivation of latent infection within the eye (ocular toxoplasmosis). In the transplant recipient, toxoplasmosis is usually due to the reactivation of latent infection in the absence of a limiting immune response. Acute infection in this population generally results from organ transplantation with disease due to dissemination from the transplanted organ or the direct infusion of contaminated blood or blood products (Rose 1983; Herb *et al.* 1978; Hakin *et al.* 1986). The occurrence of toxoplasmosis in a seronegative individual in the absence of organ or blood transfusion is uncommon. The serological status of organ donors should be assessed prior to transplantation, although significant degrees of infection occur only in heart transplant recipients or in recipients of other organs from individuals with undiagnosed, acute infection (Nicod 1996).

Because of the large number of protean manifestations of toxoplasmosis, this infection must be considered in the differential diagnosis of many systemic illnesses in the immunocompromised host. The non-AIDS immunosuppressed patient is likely to have some of the systemic manifestations of toxoplasmosis seen in the immunocompetent host. A 'mono'-like prodrome with fever and lymphadenopathy may precede other manifestations. In this setting, disseminated infection will involve the brain, liver, lungs, bone marrow, heart, spleen, and other organs. Multiple brain lesions are common. The presentation of toxoplasmosis as encephalitis, with diffuse CNS impairment or multiple focal neurological deficits, is described but is uncommon in transplant recipients. However, acute pulmonary or lymph node infections have been seen in our centre. Recipients who develop infections are generally seronegative recipients of seropositive organs.

The diagnosis of infection due to *Toxoplasma* is difficult, most notably in the immuno-compromised individual, in whom early diagnosis is most important and serological tests are least helpful. Demonstration of the tissue cyst form of the organism or of a positive serum IgG level suggests the possibility of infection due to *T. gondii*, but does not prove toxoplasmosis. Tissue cysts persist in the brain, lung, liver, lymph nodes, heart, and spleen for years after acute infection. The presence of trophozoites in lymph node, blood, brain, CSF, or other tissues during acute infection, or the demonstration of an acute (IgM) immune response to the organism, is needed for confirmation (Araujo and Remington 1980). The lumbar puncture is non-diagnostic in most cases. The CSF will have slightly elevated protein levels and few white blood cells. These patients will have a normal to slightly decreased glucose concentration in the CSF; hypoglycorrachia is usually associated with the rupture of organisms directly into the CSF. In the immuno-deficient host, rapid progression of disease or atypical presentations may necessitate tissue diagnosis. Most such patients will fail to demonstrate a timely rise in IgM serum titre. Demonstration of relatively enhanced antibody production in the CSF has been associated with *Toxoplasma* encephalitis. Conversely, cardiac and heart–lung transplant recipients may demonstrate significant titres even without acute infection. In addition to meningoencephalitis, encephalomyelitis, or mass effect due to brain abscess, the patient may present with pneumonitis, myocarditis, or signs of hepatitis. In cardiac transplant recipients, infection may be confused with allograft rejection or viral myocarditis. Biopsy is essential for diagnosis and has the added advantage of identifying other potentially treatable processes. *Toxoplasma gondii* trophozoites are occasionally found in lung lavage or lung biopsy sample from patients with pneumonitis.

Initial therapy for *T. gondii* infection should include a reduction in the immunosup-pressive therapy, when possible. A synergistic combination of antibiotics including pyrimethamine and sulfonamide or clindamycin is favoured for *Toxoplasma* infection. Data from AIDS patients suggest that oral clindamycin may be used in place of high-dose intravenous drug (Fishman 1998*a,b*; Haverkos 1987; Kovacs 1984). The most common sulfonamide used is sulfadiazine, but it is interchangeable with trisulfapyrimi-dine for this purpose (Haverkos 1987). Other sulfonamides are not equally effective. It must be noted that renal and other transplant recipients tolerate full-dose sulfa-drug therapy poorly. Lower doses and serum drug levels must be used to decrease the inci-dence of nephrotoxicity in all patients on calcineurin inhibitors. The main limitation of therapy is drug toxicity with discontinuation of therapy associated with relapse. Newer therapies that have promise include atovaquone, trimetrexate, and the new macrolides roxithromycin, azithromycin, and clarithromycin in combination with sulfonamide or pyrimethamine (Allegra *et al.* 1987). These latter agents have the advantage of excellent tissue penetration in excess of serum levels. Atovaquone appears to have activity against tissue cysts. In AIDS patients with toxoplasmosis, some early relapses have been seen with the macrolide regimens.

Cryptosporidium species

Cryptosporidium is a protozoan parasite that can cause severe and persistent diarrhoea in transplant patients, often in association with CMV infection (Fishman 1995; Soave and Armstrong 1986; Soave and Johnson 1988; Wolfson *et al.* 1985; Roncoroni *et al.* 1989) *Cryptosporidium* has been recognized as a common cause of enteritis worldwide in immunocompetent hosts. *Cryptosporidium* has been detected in up to 5% of immunologically normal individuals experiencing gastroenteritis or chronic malabsorption (Shepherd *et al.* 1988). In the individual with diarrhoea containing *Cryptosporidium*, other organisms are often detected including amoebae, CMV, *Giardia lamblia*, *Isospora belli*, and adenovirus. Immunocompromised individuals, including bone marrow and solid organ transplant recipients, may develop severe and unremitting gastrointestinal and gallbladder infection (Current *et al.* 1983; DuPont 1985; Connolly *et al.* 1981). Despite its growing importance, the pathogenesis of cryptosporidiosis has not been clarified. Symptomatic disease is generally associated with infection of the proximal small bowel. The hepatobiliary tree may serve as a reservoir for reinfection in the immunocompromised host.

Organisms are generally transmitted by faecal–oral contamination. Waterborne transmission has also been demonstrated often in association with contamination of well-water or reservoirs (Hayes *et al.* 1989). Spread occurs between animals and between humans and animals. Human-to-human spread causes the epidemics seen occasionally in day-care centres and in families. Studies in immunocompetent patients demonstrate that a range of 1.5–10% of diarrhoeal diseases are caused by cryptosporidiosis. The Massachusetts General Hospital experience has noted that about 3% of individuals with significant diarrhoeal illness will have *Cryptosporidium* identified in their stools in the absence of other known pathogens (Wolfson *et al.* 1985). Clustering of cases appears to occur during later summer and the autumn.

The patient presents with watery diarrhoea, abdominal pain, anorexia, nausea and vomiting, fever, and myalgias. Stool examination reveals watery stool without blood or white cells, with intermittent shedding of large number of cryptosporidial oocysts. Infection of the gallbladder is common. Organisms may continue to be shed after the resolution of symptoms and disease may recur in the absence of therapy. The right upper quadrant localization of abdominal symptoms may suggest acute cholecystitis. The gallbladder may be dilated, with thickened walls and dilated bile ducts. Cytomegalovirus is an important differential consideration in addition to, or as the primary agent, instead of *Cryptosporidium*.

Diagnosis may be made non-invasively by stool testing. Because oocysts are similar in size to yeasts, identification of *Cryptosporidium* requires special staining (Weber *et al.* 1992). Organisms and typical histopathology are better seen in the small bowel where infection may be patchy. Our experience suggests a synergistic injury between cytomegalovirus and *Cryptosporidium*.

There is no useful therapy for cryptosporidiosis other than treatment of coinfections and reduction in overall immunosuppression. Nutritional and fluid support may be necessary. Antimotility agents have not been demonstrated to be effective. Paromomycin with or without azithromycin often produces symptomatic improvement with some reduction in organism burden. Preliminary encouraging results with the macrolide spiramycin have not been consistently reproducible (Moskovitz *et al.* 1988; Portnoy *et al.* 1984). Alpha-difluoromethyl-ornithine (DFMO) also has demonstrated some palliative effect on infection, but toxicities (largely bone marrow depression) have limited its use. Animal studies using hyperimmune sera against *Cryptosporidium* or bovine colostrum are encouraging (Louie *et al.* 1987).

Isospora belli

Isospora belli is a coccidian protozoan that infects the gastrointestinal tract of immuno-compromised individuals. Isosporiasis is a common cause of diarrhoeal disease in tropical regions, but is found worldwide. The common forms of disease are due to *I. belli* and occasionally *I. hominis*. Both are normally of low pathogenicity. In industrialized regions, these organisms can cause or contribute to disease in immunocompromised individuals. The patient presents with watery, non-bloody diarrhoea with nausea, abdominal pain, and weight loss. Systematic signs (headache, malaise, myalgias, fever) are often present. Prolonged infection may cause malabsorption. The infection is self-limited in the normal host, clearing in 4–6 weeks. Isosporiasis responds to therapy with oral trimethoprim-sulfamethoxazole (TMP-SMZ) and is generally prevented by routine prophylaxis with this agent. Other 'successful' therapies may be useful in part because of the treatment of other concomitant infections. Patients may continue to excrete organisms long after the successful completion of therapy. This observation probably supports the use of prophylactic therapy in symptomatic immunocompromised hosts.

Strongyloides stercoralis

Strongyloides stercoralis is a nematode that infects almost 100 million people worldwide (Genta 1989). This parasitic helminth can complete its entire life cycle within the human host allowing for persistent and occasionally lifelong infection. In the immunocompromised host, dissemination of worms beyond the gastrointestinal tract produces the life-threatening 'hyperinfection syndrome' (Ingra-Siegman *et al.* 1981; Purtilo *et al.* 1974). The presence of a persistent carrier state greatly enlarges the at-risk population for severe disease during periods of immunosuppression. Chronic infections have persisted for over 30 years (Mansfield *et al.* 1996). The exact components of the immune system responsible for the prevention of disease or the reduction of the severity of infection are not known.

Acute gastrointestinal infection will generally produce epigastric fullness or pain and, in some individuals, diarrhoea and malabsorption. Passage of larvae through the lungs may produce eosinophilic pneumonia or 'Loeffler's syndrome' or milder manifestations of dyspnoea, cough, bronchospasm, and fever. Most of these individuals will have a peripheral blood eosinophilia. Gram-negative septicaemia and necrotizing pneumonia may occur numerous times without specific treatment of the underlying worm infection (Scoggin and Call 1977; Scowden *et al.* 1978). Gram-negative meningitis is a common complication of strongyloidiasis; larvae are infrequently detected in the meninges or CSF of affected patients. The complications associated with dissemination reflect both a large worm burden and the effects of organisms accompanying the migrating nematodes. Local and systemic infections and allergic responses may be seen to both the worms and the 'passenger' bacteria from the gut. Bacterial superinfection as a complication of strongyloidiasis is equally common in normal and in immunocompromised individuals, supporting the presumption that bacterial infection is a function of worm penetration, rather than of the underlying immunodeficiency state. The mechanism of such superinfection is unknown, but superinfection occurs in one-third to one-half of individuals with disseminated infection.

The predilection of this organism for the lungs and for the CNS is manifested most impressively with disseminated infection in immunocompromised individuals—the hyperinfection syndrome. Dissemination has been observed in association with cancer, CMV infection, corticosteroid therapy, and acute increases in the level of immunosuppression in transplant recipients, including tacrolimus and cyclosporine (Berger *et al.* 1980; Cruz *et al.* 1966; Fagundes *et al.* 1971; Fowler *et al.* 1982; Hoy *et al.* 1981; Myers 1976; Palau and Pankey 1997; Nucci 1982; Nolan 1981). Pulmonary bacterial superinfection occurs in the setting of small-airway obstruction secondary to entrapped worms. Pneumonitis is generally accompanied by abdominal crisis: severe abdominal pain with ileus, small bowel obstruction, and occasionally septic shock. Hepatic failure has been reported; CNS involvement may include eosinophilic meningitis, altered mental status, coma, or focal neurological deficits. Polymicrobial bloodstream infection may be seen and includes the entire range of gut flora, including *Candida*. Cavitary pulmonary lesions may develop, and transient rashes or skin swelling of the buttocks or lower abdomen may be noted. Peripheral blood eosinophilia is variably observed. Mortality with disseminated infection generally exceeds 75% and is usually due to Gram-negative sepsis. Because the consequences of disseminated *Strongyloides* are so grave, pre-emptive treatment should be considered prior to elective immune suppression in patients with exposures to endemic regions. In seropositive transplant recipients, therapy with ivermectin or thiabendazole should be given in the pretransplant period (Naquira *et al.* 1989). All transplant patients infected with *Strongyloides* should be treated. Uncomplicated gastrointestinal infections may be treated successfully with thiabendazole. A number of other drugs are of less certain efficacy, including mebendazole, cambendazole, and albendazole.

Chagas' disease

Trypanosoma cruzi is a protozoan that infects humans during a blood meal by the reduvid bug. Up to 20 million people are infected worldwide, including up to 40–50% of the population of endemic areas of Central and South America. Cases related to blood transfusion have been reported in the United States and Canada, as well as in endemic areas. The organisms develop intracellularly, releasing aflagellates that enter new cells and repeat the cycle. *Trypanosoma cruzi* has a particular predilection for muscle (including cardiac) and neuroglial cells, and produces local inflammation with lymphocytes, macrophages, and plasma cells. In addition to reduvid infection, infection has occurred as a result of organ transplantation and via blood transfusion.

The major complications of Chagas' disease are cardiac arrhythmias or conduction defects with congestive heart failure. Gastrointestinal involvement may appear as megacolon or megaoesophagus. Latent infection may be reactivated by immune suppression, including individuals who are the recipients of infected organ grafts.

Leishmaniasis

Leishmaniasis is caused by organisms of the protozoan *Leishmania* and takes three clinical forms—visceral, cutaneous, and mucosal. A single *Leishmania* species can produce different clinical syndromes, and each of the syndromes can be caused by more than one species. Case reports of leishmaniasis in patients infected with HIV and in recipients of solid-organ transplants have highlighted the problem of leishmaniasis as an opportunistic infection (Clauvel *et al.* 1986; Montalban *et al.* 1989; Berenguer *et al.* 1998; De Letona *et al.* 1986; Lamas et *al.* 1987). Visceral leishmaniasis is typically caused by *L. donovani* in India and Africa, by *L. infantum* in the Mediterranean, and by *L. chagasi* in Latin America. Occasionally, a *Leishmania* species that is associated mainly with cutaneous disease (e.g. *L. mexicana*) is found in a patient with visceral leishmaniasis.

Recrudescence of visceral leishmaniasis (caused by *Leishmania donovani*) is associated with immunosuppression. Asymptomatic carriage for many years has been reported in patients who had moved away from areas of *L. donovani* transmission with reactivation of visceral leishmaniasis while on immunosuppressive therapy (Badaro 1986; Broeckaert *et al.* 1979). Van Orshoven *et al.* (1979) described visceral leishmaniasis in a renal transplant recipient without recent exposure to an area endemic for leishmaniasis. One case of cutaneous leishmaniasis has been described in a heart transplant recipient (Golino *et al.* 1992). Abdulrahman *et al.* (1998) described a Sudanese renal transplant recipient with a tongue ulcer that was culture positive for *L. donovani*, the only report in the literature of mucosal leishmaniasis in a transplant recipient. All subsequent descriptions in solid-organ transplant recipients have been of visceral disease (Hoeber *et al.* 1993). The clinical manifestations of visceral leishmaniasis in solid-organ transplant recipients resemble those in non-transplant patients (otherwise immunocompetent hosts) including fever, malaise, anorexia, and weight loss often in association with hepatosplenomegaly, pancytopenia, and hypergammaglobulinaemia.

The interval between the transplant and the illness that leads to the diagnosis of leishmaniasis is variable, with reports ranging from 2 months to 7 years after transplantation. Berenguer *et al.* (1998) found that the median time between transplantation and diagnosis of infection was 8 months. An episode of rejection prior to the diagnosis of leishmaniasis has been commonly reported (Orofino 1992; Portoles *et al.* 1994; Ma *et al.* 1979). The diagnosis of leishmaniasis in transplant recipients generally requires an invasive procedure. Bone marrow aspiration is often performed as a part of the evaluation for pancytopenia. Culture of the marrow aspirate for the parasite in the classical NNN media should be requested. Liver biopsies have been used in small numbers of solid organ transplant recipients (Hoeber *et al.* 1993; Hoseini 1995).

The therapies available for the treatment of leishmaniasis are suboptimal. Immunosuppression should be decreased. Most transplant recipients with leishmaniasis have been treated with pentavalent antimony salts for visceral disease (Berenguer *et al.* 1998). Side-effects are common, including pancreatitis (van Orshoven *et al.* 1979; Donovan *et al.* 1990; *Halim et al.* 1993; Moroni 1995; Berenguer *et al.* 1998; Gomez-Campdera

1998). Alternative therapies include allopurinol and ketoconazole, pentamidine, and amphotericin B (including the newer lipid-associated amphotericin formulations). Clearance of infection is often delayed and relapse after treatment has been reported, requiring multiple courses of therapy.

References

Abdulrahman AA, Saleem M, Ibrahim EA and Gramiccia M (1998). Leishmaniasis of the tongue in a renal transplant recipient. *Clinical Infectious Disease* 27, 1332–1333.

Aguardo JM, Plaza J, Escudero A (1986). Visceral leishmaniasis in renal-transplant recipient. *Journal of Infection* 13, 301–302.

Allegra CJ, Chabner BA, Tuazon CU, Ogata-Arakaki D, Baird B, Drake JC, Simmons T, Lack EE, Shelhamer JH, Balis F, Walker R, Kovacs JA, Lane HC and Masur H (1987). Trimetrexate for the treatment of *Pneumocystis carinii* pneumonia in patients with the acquired immunodeficiency syndrome. *New England Journal of Medicine* 317, 978–985.

Araujo FG, Remington JS (1980). Antigenemia in recently acquired acute toxoplasmosis. *Journal of Infectious Diseases* 141, 144–150.

Arend SM, Westendorp RG, Kroon FP, van't Wout JW, Vandenbroucke JP and van (1996). Rejection treatment and cytomegalovirus infection as risk factors for *Pneumocystis carinii* pneumonia in renal transplant recipients. *Clinical Infectious Disease* 22, 920–925.

Babinet J, Gay F, Bustos D, Dubarry M, Jaulmes D, Nguyen L and Gentilini M (1991). Transmission of *Plasmodium falciparum* by heart transplant. *British Medical Journal* 303, 1515–1516.

Bach MC, Adler JL, Breman J, *et al.* (1973). Influence of rejection therapy on fungal and nocardia infections in renal-transplant recipients. *Lancet*, 1, 180–184.

Balkovac JM, Black RM, Hammond ML, Heck JV, Zambias RA, Abruzzo G, Bartizal K, Kropp H, Trainor C, Schwartz RE, McFadden DC, Nollstadt KH, Pittarelli LA, Powles MA and Schmatz DM (1992). Synthesis, stability, and biological evaluation of water-soluble prodrugs of a new echinocandin lipopeptide. *Journal of Medical Chemistry* 35, 194–198.

Barber BA, Pegram PS and High KP (1996). Clindamycin/primaquine as prophylaxis for *Pneumocystis carinii* pneumonia. *Clinical Infectious Disease* 23, 718–722.

Barkholt L, Ericzon BG, Tollemar J, Malmborg AS, Ehrnst A and Wilczek H (1993). Infections in human liver recipients, different patterns early and late after transplantation,. *Transplant International* 6, 77–84.

Bazinsky JH, Phillips JE (1969). *Pneumocystis* pneumonia transmission between patients with lymphoma. *Journal of the American Medical Association* 209, 1527.

Benedetti E, Gruessner AC, Troppmann C, Papalois BE, Sutherland DE, Dunn DL and Gruessner RW (1996). Intra-abdominal fungal infections after pancreatic transplantation, incidence, treatment, and outcome. *Journal of the American College of Surgeons* 183, 307–316.

Berenguer J, Gomez-Campdera F, Padilla B, Rodriguez-Ferrero M, Fernando A, Santiago M and Fernando V (1998). Visceral leishmaniasis (kala-azar) in transplant recipients., case report and review. *Transplantation* 65, 1401–1404.

Berenguer J, Moreno S, Cercenado E, de Quiros JCLB, de la Fuente AG, Bouza E (1989). Visceral leishmaniasis in patients infected with human immunodeficiency virus (HIV). *Annals of Internal Medicine* 111, 129–132.

Berger R, Kraman S, Paciotti M (1980). Pulmonary strongyloidiasis complicating therapy with corticosteroids. *American Journal of Tropical Medicine and Hygiene* 29, 31–34.

Berman JD (1997). Human leishmaniasis, clinical, diagnostic, and chemotherapeutic developments in the last 10 years. *Clinical Infectious Disease* 24, 684–703.

Bernstein B, Flomenberg P, Letzer D (1987). Disseminated cryptococcal disease complicating steroid therapy for *Pneumocystis carinii* pneumonia in a patient with AIDS. *Southern Medical Journal* 87, 537–538.

Black JR, Feinberg J, Murphy RL, Fass RJ, Finkelstein D, Akil B (1994). Clindamycin and primaquine therapy for mild-to-moderate episodes of *Pneumocystis carinii* pneumonia in patients with AIDS (ACTG 044). *Clinical Infectious Disease* 18, 905–913.

Bozzette SA, Arcia J, Bartok AE, *et al.* (1992). Impact of *Pneumocystis carinii* and cytomegalovirus on the course and outcome of atypical pneumonia in advanced human immunodeficiency virus disease. *Journal of Infectious Diseases* 165, 93–98.

Bozzette SA, Finkelstein DM, Spector SA, Frame P, Powderly WG, He W, Phillips L, Craven D, Van der Horst C, Feinberg J and NIAID AIDS Clinical Trials Group (1995). A randomized trial of three antipneumocystis agents in patients with advanced human immunodeficiency virus infection. *New England Journal of Medicine* 332, 693–699.

Bradburne PM, Bettensohn DB, Opal SM, McCool FD (1989). Relapse of *Pneumocystis carinii* pneumonia in the upper lobes during aerosol pentamidine prophylaxis. *Thorax* 44, 591–593.

Branten AJ, Beckers PJ, Tiggeler (1995). Pneumocystis carinii pneumonia in renal transplant recipients. *Nephrology, Dialysis, and Transplant*ation 10, 1194–1197.

Broeckaert A, Michielsen P, Vandepitte J (1979). Fatal leishmaniasis in renal-transplant patient. *Lancet* 2, 740–741.

Casadevall A, Perfect JR (1998). *Cryptococcus neoformans.* ASM Press, Washington, DC.

Chave J, David S, Wauters J, Francioli P (1991). Transmission of *Pneumocystis carinii* from AIDS patients to other immunosuppressed patients, a cluster of *Pneumocystis carinii* pneumonia in renal transplant recipients. *AIDS* 5, 927–932.

Clauvel JP, Couderc LJ, Belmin J, Daniel MT, Rabian C, Seligmann M (1986). Visceral leishmaniasis complicating acquired immunodeficiency syndrome (AIDS). *Transactions of the Royal Society of Tropical Medicine and Hygiene* 80, 1011.

Collins LA, Samore MH, Roberts MS, *et al.* (1994). Risk factors for invasive fungal infections complicating orthotopic liver transplantation. *Journal of Infectious Diseases* 170, 644–52.

Connolly GM, Dryden MS, Shanson DC, *et al.* (1988). Cryptosporidial diarrhea in AIDS and its treatment. *Gut* 29, 593–597.

Cruz T, Reboucas G, Rocha H (1966). Fatal strongyloidiasis in patients receiving corticosteroids. *New England Journal of Medicine* 275, 1093–1096.

Current WL, Reese NC, Ernst JV, *et al.* (1983). Human cryptosporidiosis in immunocompetent and immunodeficient persons. Studies of an outbreak and experimental transmission. *New England Journal of Medicine* 308, 1252–1257.

De Letona JM, Vasquez CM, Maestu RP (1986). Visceral leishmaniasis as an opportunistic infection. *Lancet* 1094.

Denning DW, Evans EG, Kibbler CC, Richardson MD, Roberts MM, Rogers TR, Warnock DW, Warren RE (1997). Guidelines for the investigation of invasive fungal infections in haematological malignancy and solid organ transplantation. *European Journal of Clinical Microbiology and Infectious Diseases* 16, 424–436.

Dockrell DH, Mendez JC, Jones M, Harmsen WS, Ilstrup DM, Smith TF, Wiesner RH, Krom RA, Paya CV (1999). Human herpesvirus 6 seronegativity before transplantation predicts the occurrence of fungal infection in liver transplant recipients. *Transplantation* 67, 399–403.

Donovan KL, White AD, Cooke DA, Fisher DJ (1990). Pancreatitis and palindromic arthropathy with effusions associated with sodium stibogluconate treatment in a renal transplant recipient. *Journal of Infection* 21, 107–110.

DuPont HL (1985). Cryptosporidiosis and the healthy host. *New England Journal of Medicine* 312, 1319–1320.

Fagundes LA, Busato O, Brentano L (1971). Strongyloidiasis, fatal complication of renal transplantation. *Lancet* ii, 439–440.

Falloon J, Kovacs J, Hughes W, *et al.* (1991). A preliminary evaluation of 566C80 for the treatment of *Pneumocystis* pneumonia in patients with the acquired immunodeficiency syndrome. *New England Journal of Medicine* 325, 1534–1538.

Fernandez-Guerrero ML, Aguado JM, Buzon L, *et al.* (1987). Visceral leishmaniasis in immunocompromised hosts. *American Journal of Medicine* 83, 1098–1102.

Fishman JA (1994). Radiologic approach to the diagnosis and management of *Pneumocystis carinii.* In: Walzer P (ed) *Pneumocystis carinii pneumonia.* Marcel Dekker, New York, pp. 415–438.

Fishman J (1995). *Pneumocystis carinii* and parasitic infections in transplantation. *Infectious Disease Clinics of North America* 9(4), 1005–1044.

Fishman JA (1998a). Prevention of infection due to *Pneumocystis carinii. Antimicrobial Agents and Chemotherapy* 42, 995–1004.

Fishman JA (1998b). Treatment of infection due to *Pneumocystis carinii. Antimicrobial Agents and Chemotherapy* 42, 1300–1314.

Fishman JA and Rubin RH (1998). Infection in organ transplant recipients. *New England Journal of Medicine* 338, 1741–1751.

Fowler CG, Lindsay I, Lewin J, Sweny P, Fernando ON, Moorhead JF (1982). Recurrent infestation with *Strongyloides stercoralis* in a renal allograft recipient. *British Medical Journal* 285, 1394.

Garcia S, Roque J, Ruza F, Gonzalez M, Madero R, Alvarado F, Herruzo R (1998). Infection and associated risk factors in the immediate postoperative period of pediatric liver transplantation, a study of 176 transplants. *Clinical Transplantation* 12, 190–197.

Gasser RA Jr, Magill AJ, Oster CN, Franke ED, Grogl M, Berman JD (1994). Pancreatitis induced by pentavalent antimonials during treatment of leishmaniasis. *Clinical Infectious Disease* 18, 83–90.

Genta RM (1989). Global prevalence of strongyloidiasis. Critical review with epidemiologic insight into the prevention of disseminated disease. *Review of Infectious Diseases* 11, 755–767.

George MJ, Snydman DR, Werner BG, Griffith J, Falagas ME, Dougherty NN, Rubin RH (1997). The independent role of cytomegalovirus as a risk factor for invasive fungal disease in orthotopic liver transplant recipients. *American Journal of Medicine* 103, 106–113.

Golino A, Duncan JM, Zeluff B, DePriest J, McAllister HA, Radovancevic B, Frazier OH (1992). Leishmaniasis in a heart transplant recipient. *Journal of Heart and Lung Transplantation* 11(4 Pt 1), 820–3.

Hadley S, Karchmer AW (1995). Fungal infections in solid organ transplant recipients. *Infectious Disease Clinics of North America* 9(4), 1045–1074.

Hadley S, Samore MH, Lewis WD, Jenkins RL, Karchmer AW, Hammer SM (1995). Major infectious complications after orthotopic liver transplantation, and comparison of outcomes in patients receiving cyclosporine or FK506 as primary immunosuppression. *Transplantation* 59, 851–859.

Hakin M, Esmore D, Wallwork J, *et al.* (1986). Toxoplasmosis in cardiac transplantation. *British Medical Journal* 292, 1108–1109.

Halim MA, Alfurayh O, Kalin ME, Dammas S, Al-Eisa A, Damanhouri G (1993). Successful treatment of visceral leishmaniasis with allopurinol plus ketoconazole in a renal transplant recipient after the occurrence of pancreatitis due to stibogluconate. *Clinical Infectious Disease* 16, 397–9.

Hardy AM, Wajszczuk CP, Suffredini AF, *et al.* (1984). *Pneumocystis carinii* pneumonia in renal transplant patients treated with cyclosporin and steroids. *Journal of Infectious Diseases* 149, 143–147.

Haverkos HW (1987). Assessment of therapy for toxoplasma encephalitis. *American Journal of Medicine* 82, 907.

Hayes EB, Matte TD, O'Brien TR, *et al.* (1989). Large community outbreak of cryptosporidiosis due to contamination of a filtered public water supply. *New England Journal of Medicine* **320**, 1372–1376.

Herb HM, Jontofsoh R, Loffler HD, *et al.* (1978). Toxoplasmosis after renal transplantation. *Clinical Nephrology* **8**, 529–532.

Herne N (1980). Mediterranean kala-azar in two adults treated with immunosuppressive agents. *Revue de Medecine Interne* **1**, 237–240.

Hoeber FF, Lerut JP, Reichen J, Zommermann A, Jaeger P, Malinverni R (1993). Visceral leishmaniasis after orthotopic liver transplantation, impact of persistent splenomegaly. *Transplant International* **6**, 55–57.

Holzer BR, Gluck Z, Zambelli D, Fey M (1985). Transmission of malaria by renal transplantation. *Transplantation* **39**, 315–317.

Hoy WE, Roberts NJ, Bryson MF, Bowles C, Lee JCK, Rivero AJ, Ritterson AL (1981). Transmission of strongyloidiasis by kidney transplant. *Journal of the American Medical Association* **246**, 1937–1939.

Hughes WT (1987). *Pneumocystis carinii pneumonitis.* CRC Press, New York.

Hughes WT, McNabb PC, Makres TD, *et al.* (1974). Efficacy of trimethoprim and sulfamethoxazole in the prevention and treatment of *Pneumocystis carinii* pneumonitis. *Antimicrobial Agents and Chemotherapy* **5**, 289–293.

Hughes WT, Feldman S, Chaudhary SC, Ossi MJ, Cox F, Sanyal SK (1978). Comparison of pentamidine isethionate and trimethoprim-sulfamethoxazole in the treatment of *Pneumocystis carinii* pneumonia. *Journal of Pediatrics* **92**, 285–291.

Hughes W, Leoung G, Kramer F, Bozzette SA, Safrin S, Frame P, Clumeck N, Masur H, Lancaster D, Chan C, Lavelle J, Rosenstock J, Falloon J, Feinberg J, LaFon S, Rogers M, Sattler F (1993). Comparison of atovaquone (566c80) with trimethoprim-sulfamethoxazole to treat *Pneumocystis carinii* pneumonia in patients with AIDS. *New England Journal of Medicine* **328**, 1521–1527.

Hughes W, Killmar J, Oz H (1994). Relative potency of 10 drugs with anti-*Pneumocystis carinii* activity in an animal model. *Journal of Infectious Diseases* **170**, 906–911.

Igra-Siegman Y, Kapila R, Sen P, *et al.* (1981). Syndrome of hyperinfection with *Strongyloides stercoralis. Review of Infectious Diseases* **3**, 397–407.

Jacobs F, Depierreux M, Goldman M, *et al.* (1990). Role of bronchoalveolar lavage in diagnosis of disseminated toxoplasmosis. *Review of Infectious Diseases* **13**, 637–641.

Johnston DA (1981). Possible transmission of malaria by renal transplantation. *British Medical Journal* **282**, 780.

Kusne S, Dumer JS, Singh N, *et al.* (1988). Infections after liver transplantation. An analysis of 101 consecutive cases. *Medicine (Baltimore)* **67**, 132–143.

Lamas S, Orte L, Parras F, Garcia Larana J, Matesanz R, Ortuno J (1987). Non-fatal leishmaniasis in a renal transplant recipient. *Nephron* **45**, 71.

Lefavour GS, Pierce JC, Frame JD (1980). Renal transplant-associated malaria. *Journal of the American Medical Association* **244**, 1820–1821.

Levin AS, Costa SF, Mussi NS, Basso M, Sinto SI, Machado C, Geiger DC, Villares MC, Schreiber AZ, Barone AA, Branchini ML (1998). *Candida parapsilosis* fungemia associated with implantable and semi-implantable central venous catheters and the hands of healthcare workers. *Diagnostic Microbiology and Infectious Disease* **30**, 243–249.

Louie E, Borkowsky W, Klesius PK, *et al.* (1987). Treatment of cryptosporidiosis with oral bovine transfer factor. *Clinical Immunology and Immunopathology* **44**, 329–334.

Lufft V, Kliem V, Behrend M, Pichlmayr R, Koch KM, Brunkhorst R (1996). Incidence of Pneumocystis carinii pneumonia after renal transplantation. *Transplantation* **63**, 421–423.

Ma DDF, Concannon AJ, Hayes J (1979). Fatal leishmaniasis in renal-transplant patient. *Lancet* ii, 311–312.

Mansfield LS, Niamatali S, Bhopale V, Volk S, Smith G, Lok JB, *et al.* (1996). *Strongyloides stercoralis*, maintenance of exceedingly chronic infections. *American Journal of Tropical Medicine and Hygiene* 55, 617–624.

Meier-Kriesche HU, Firedman G, Jacobs M, Mulgaonkar S, Vaghela M, Kaplan B (1999). Infectious complications in geriatric renal transplant patients, comparison of two immunosuppressive protocols. *Transplantation* 68, 1496–1502.

Meyers AM, Shapiro DJ, Milne FJ, *et al.* (1976). *Strongyloides stercoralis* hyperinfection in a renal allograft recipient. *South African Medical Journal* 50, 1301–1302.

Montalban C, Martinez-Fernandez R, Calleja JL, *et al.* (1989). Visceral leishmaniasis (kala-azar) as an opportunistic infection in patients with the human immunodeficiency virus in Spain. *Review of Infectious Diseases* 11, 655–660.

Morgan JS, Schaffner W, Stone WJ (1986). Opportunistic strongyloides infection in renal transplant recipients. *Transplantation* 42, 518–524.

Morris SA, Schwartz RE, Sesin DF, Masurekar P, Hallada TC, Schmatz DM, Bartial K, Hensens OD, Zink DL (1994). Pneumocandin DO, a new antifungal agent and potent inhibitor of *Pneumocystis carinii*. *Journal of Antibiotics* 47, 755–764.

Moskovitz BL, Stanton TL, Kusmierek JJ (1988). Spiramycin therapy for cryptosporidial diarrhoea in immunocompromised patients. *Journal of Antimicrobial Chemotherapy* 22, 189–191.

Moulin B, Ollier J, Bouchouareb D, Purgus R, Olmer M (1992). Leishmaniasis, a rare cause of unexplained fever in a renal graft recipient. *Nephron* 60, 360–362.

Naquira C, Jiminez G, Guerra JG, *et al.* (1989). Ivermectin for human strongyloidiasis and ohter intestinal helminths. *American Journal of Tropical Medicine and Hygiene* 40, 304–309.

Nicod LP (1996). Infectious complications of lung and heart-lung transplantation. *Revue des Maladies Respiratoires* 13 (suppl. 5), S41–S47.

Nieto-Rodriguez JA, Kusne S, Manez R, Irish W, Linden P, Magnone M, Wing EJ, Fung JJ, Starzl TE (1996). Factors associated with the development of candidemia and candidemia-related death among liver transplant recipients. *Annals of Surgery* 223, 70–76.

Nolan TJ, Schad GA (1996). Tacrolimus allows autoinfective development of the parasitic nematode *Strongyloides stercoralis*. *Transplantation* 62, 1038.

Nucci M, Portugal R, Pulcher W, Spector N, Ferreira SB, de Castro MB, Noe R, de Oliveira HP (1995). Strongyloidiasis in patients with haematologic malignancies. *Clinical Infectious Diseases* 21, 675–7.

Palau L, Pankey GA (1997). Strongyloides hyperinfection in a renal transplant patient receiving cyclosporine, possible *Strongyloides stercoralis* transmission by kidney transplant. *American Journal of Tropical Medicine and Hygiene* 57, 413–415.

Paya CV, Hermans PE, Washington JA II, *et al.* (1989). Incidence, distribution, and outcome of episodes of infection in 100 orthotopic liver transplantations. *Mayo Clinic Proceedings* 64, 555–564.

Pirsch JD, Odorico JS, D'Alessandro AM, Knechtle SJ, Becker BN, Sollinger HW (1998). Posttransplant infection in enteric versus bladder-drained simultaneous pancreas-kidney transplant recipients. *Transplantation* 66, 1746–1750.

Portnoy D, Whiteside ME, Buckley E III, *et al.* (1984). Treatment of intestinal cryptosporidiosis with spiramycin. *Annals of Internal Medicine* 101, 202–204.

Portoles J, Prats D, Torralbo A, Herrero JA, Torrente J, Barrientos A (1994). Visceral leishmaniasis: a rare cause of opportunistic infection in renal transplant patients in endemic areas. *Transplantation* 57, 1677–1679.

Purtilo DT, Meyers WM, Connor DH (1974). Fatal strongyloidiasis in immunosuppressed patients. *American Journal of Medicine* 56, 488–493.

Roncoroni AJ, Gomez MA, Mera J, *et al.* (1989). *Cryptosporidium* infection in renal transplant. *Journal of Infectious Diseases* **160**, 559.

Saukkonen K, Garland R, Koziel H (1996). Aerosolized pentamidine as alternative primary prophylaxis against Pneumocystis carinii pneumonia in adult hepatic and renal transplant recipients. *Chest* **109**, 1250–1255.

Scoggin CH, Call NB (1977). Acute respiratory failure due to disseminated strongyloidiasis in a renal transplant recipient. *Annals of Internal Medicine* **87**, 456–458.

Scowden EB, Schaffner W, Stone WJ (1978). Overwhelming strongyloidiasis. *Medicine* **57**, 527–544.

Sentamil Selvi G, Kamalam A, Ajithados K, Janaki C, Thambiah AS (1999). Clincial and mycological features of dermatophytosis in renal transplant recipients. *Mycoses* **42**, 75–78.

Shepherd RC, Reed CL, Sinha GP (1988). Shedding of oocysts of *Cryptosporidium* in immuno-competent patients. *Journal of Clinical Pathology* **41**, 1104–1106.

Singh N, Gayowski T, Wagener M, Marino IR, Yu VL (1996). Pulmonary infections in liver transplant recipients receiving tacrolimus. *Transplantation* **61**, 396–401.

Singh N, Arnow PM, Bonham A, Dominguez E, Paterson DL, Pankey GA, Wagener MM, Yu VL. (1997*a*). Invasive aspergillosis in liver transplant recipients in the 1990s. *Transplantation* **64**, 716–20.

Singh N, Chang FY, Gayowski T, Marino IR (1997*b*). Infections due to dematiaceous fungi in organ transplant recipients, case report and review. *Clinical Infectious Disease* **24**, 369–374.

Soave R, Armstrong D (1986). *Cryptosporidium* and cryptosporidiosis. *Review of Infectious Diseases* **8**, 1012–1023.

Soave R, Johnson WD Jr (1988). *Cryptosporidium* and *Isospora belli* infections. *Journal of Infectious Diseases* **157**, 225–229.

Sollinger HW, Odorico JS, Knechtle SJ, D'Alessandro AM, Kalayoglu M, Pirsch JD (1998). Experience with 500 simultaneous pancreas-kidney transplants. *Annals of Surgery* **228**, 284–96.

Tan HW, Ch'ng SL (1991). Drug interaction between cyclosporine A and quinine in a renal transplant patient with malaria. *Singapore Medical Journal* **32**, 189–190.

Toma E, Fournier S, Poisson M, *et al.* (1989). Clindamycin with primaquine for *Pneumocystis carinii* pneumonia. *Lancet* **1**, 1046–1048.

Turkmen A, Sever MS, Ecder T, Yildiz A, Aydin AE, Erkoc R, Eraksoy H, Elgedez U, Ark E (1996). Post-transplant malaria. *Transplantation* **62**, 1521–1523.

Van Orshoven AB, Michielsen P, Vandepitte J (1979). Fatal leishmaniasis in renal-transplant patient. *Lancet* **ii**, 740–741.

Wajszczuk CP, Dummer JS, Ho M, *et al.* (1985). Fungal infections in liver transplant recipients. *Transplantation* **40**, 347–353.

Weber R, Bryan RT, Owen RL, *et al.* (Enteric Opportunistic Infections Working Group) (1992). Improved light-microscopical detection of microsporidia spores in stool and duodenal aspirates. *New England Journal of Medicine* **326**, 161–166.

Wolfson JS, Richter JM, Waldron MA, *et al.* (1985). Cryptosporidiosis in immunocompetent patients. *New England Journal of Medicine* **213**, 1278–1282.

PART III

PREVENTION AND MANAGEMENT

17

Control of infection in the renal unit

Jon Stratton, Alan Macdonald, and Ken Farrington

Introduction

In this chapter we review the current guidelines for infection control and relate this to the renal population. Patients in a renal unit are a unique population because of the combination of their susceptibility to infection, the range of organisms to which they may be exposed (Table 17.1), and the duration of exposure to hospital environments and other renal patients. Infections may be endogenous (arising from the patient's own flora) or exogenous (acquired from the hospital environment or from other patients by cross-infection, often from the hands of healthcare workers). Infection control in the renal unit properly addresses the risks of both endogenous and exogenous infections. To prevent new infections in renal patients and healthcare workers requires that infection control

Table 17.1 The range of micro-organisms within a renal unit

Source of infection	Organisms
Endogenous	*Staphylococcus aureus* *Staphylococcus epidermidis*, e.g. IV line infections, CAPD peritonitis *Escherichia coli* *Klebsiella* spp. *Proteus* spp.
Exogenous: from health care workers and other patients	Methicillin-resistant *Staphylococcus aureus* (MRSA) Vancomycin-resistant enterococci (VRE) Multiply-resistant Gram-negatives species: *Klebsiella*, *Enterobacter, Citrobacter, Serratia, Pseudomonas, Acinetobacter, Stenotrophomonas* (formerly *Xanthomonas*) *maltophilia*, e.g. bacteraemia *Clostridium difficile* Rarely—*Listeria, Nocardia* (renal transplant patients)
Airborne transmission	*Mycobacterium tuberculosis* Varicella zoster virus—chickenpox
From blood products or equipment	Blood-borne viruses: HBV, HCV, hepatitis D (delta) virus, HIV

Abbreviations: IV, intravenous; CAPD, continuous ambulatory peritoneal dialysis; HBV, hepatitis B virus; HCV, hepatitis C virus; HIV, human immunodeficiency virus.

policies and procedures, together with antibiotic policies, are not only understood and adhered to by healthcare workers (and patients, where appropriate), but are also reviewed and refined regularly by multidisciplinary audit.

The susceptibility of renal patients to infection is increased because uraemia reduces immunity. Immunosuppressive therapy for glomerulonephritis and renal transplant can further decrease immunity. Insertion of and repeated handling of intravenous lines, Tenchkoff catheters, in-dwelling urinary catheters, and repeated fistula needling increases the potential for contact with micro-organisms. Antibiotic treatment disrupts the normal flora and may lead to selection in favour of and/or acquisition of more resistant micro-organisms making treatment of subsequent infection more problematic.

Renal patients when first seen are likely to have come from another ward within the hospital or from another hospital, sometimes having spent time in an intensive care unit. Those attending a renal dialysis unit are regularly exposed to this busy and sometimes cramped hospital environment and may be further exposed to fellow dialysis patients in buses or ambulances that transport them to and from the unit. Patients on continuous ambulatory peritoneal dialysis (CAPD) have similar but less intense exposure to the risks of exogenous infections, but run the extra risk of endogenous (or exogenous) exit site infection and/or CAPD peritonitis.

Principles of infection control

Lives can be saved directly by preventing infection. Multiresistant organisms have already become established within the hospital community and cases of methicillin-resistant *Staphylococcus aureus* (MRSA) and vancomycin-resistant enterococci (VRE) are increasing. Outbreaks caused by multiresistant Gram-negative organisms such as *Enterobacter*, *Serratia*, *Klebsiella*, *Stenotrophomonas* (old name *Xanthomonas*), and *Actinobacter* species are also being increasingly reported. There is evidence that employing the appropriate aseptic and hygienic techniques and avoiding excessive and inappropriate use of antibiotics can prevent these multiresistant infections. The SENIC study highlighted the importance of infection control in the prevention of infection.[1]

The principle of infection control is to limit the spread of organisms from the source (such as an infected wound, the nose, or faeces of an asymptomatic colonized patient, contaminated food, equipment, or fluid) to other previously unaffected patients, thereby preventing infection or colonization. This can be achieved by:

1. Eliminating the source of infection. This is accomplished by topical or systemic treatment of the colonized or infected individual, sterilization of equipment, and the cleaning and/or disinfection of contaminated material or surfaces.
2. Inhibiting the transfer of infection from potential or actual sources to unaffected patients. The isolation of infected patients and barrier nursing provide mechanical barriers. Aseptic procedures and no-touch dressing techniques are also important. Hand washing between patients is a professional duty.
3. Enhancing a patient's resistance to infection. Antibiotic prophylaxis may be useful in some circumstances. Examples are the use of prophylactic cotrimaxazole to reduce the incidence of *Pneumocystis carinii* infection in immunosuppressed individuals and the nasal clearance of *Staphylococcus aureus* by topical mupirocin which may reduce the

incidence of CAPD exit site infection. Control of the disease process can also be beneficial, for instance, diabetic patients with poor control have increased risk of infection.

General measures

Organization of infection control

The control of infection team, which includes the infection control doctor and specialist nurses, has a major role in communicating with staff, advising them on infection control issues, and ensuring that the policies and procedures developed by the hospital control of infection committee are implemented. It has the vital responsibility of responding to outbreaks of infection. Surveillance, audit of infection control procedures, risk assessment, and education and training of staff are other essential roles. Each department within the hospital needs to develop effective links with the team. This is particularly relevant for the renal unit.

Quality assurance and improvement

Surveillance 'the continued scrutiny of all aspects of recurrence and spread of a disease that are pertinent to effective control' has a potentially huge role in the control of infection.[2] Computer-based systems that allow synthesis of laboratory and clinical data can facilitate realization of that potential. Data thus generated, together with the results of audits of infection control procedures and other information from clinical audit and incident investigation, provide the material for quality assurance and the potential for quality enhancement (Fig. 17.1).

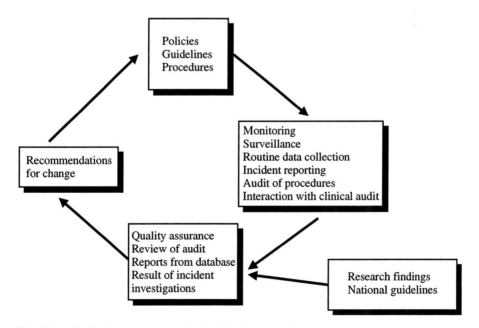

Fig. 17.1 Quality improvement cycles in infection controls.

General hospital policies

There are a number of hospital-wide policies which are applicable to all clinical areas. These may need extending to meet the needs of particular departments.

Disposal of waste

The hospital must comply with the requirements of the local waste regulatory authority.[3] Adequate staff training is essential. Segregation of waste is the key to safe waste disposal (Table 17.2). Sharps containers should not be overfilled, they should be sealed with adhesive when three-quarters full. Advice should be sought from the radiation protection officer about the disposal of radioactive waste.

Disinfection and sterilization procedures

Sterilization means the destruction and removal of all micro-organisms and spores. It is required for instruments and dressings that come into direct contact with open wounds or sterile body sites. Methods used are autoclaving (using steam under pressure at 132 °C), dry heat (generated in ovens at 160 °C), exposure to ethylene oxide gas, and prolonged immersion in gluteraldehyde.

Disinfection means the removal or destruction of sufficient numbers of potentially harmful micro-organisms to make the equipment safe to use. The simplest method is washing with hot water and detergents followed by drying. Disinfectants should only be used when this simple method is inadequate and sterilization is not required. Storage and use of disinfectants such as gluteraldehyde and hypochlorite are governed by the COSHH (Control of Substances Hazardous to Health) regulations. Disinfectants for use on the skin and mucous membranes (e.g. chlorhexidine, povidone iodine, and cetrimide) are known as antiseptics.

Isolation policies

Isolation is used to prevent transfer of micro-organisms from the infected patient to other hosts (source isolation). The degree of isolation required depends on knowledge of the likely routes of transmission of the particular infecting micro-organism. Standard isolation is required for protection against infective agents whose routes of transmission

Table 17.2 Segregation of waste

Types of waste	Examples	Disposal
Clinical waste	Soiled dressings, disposable waste, human and animal tissue	Yellow plastic bags for incineration
Sharps	Needles, ampoules, razors, broken glass	Sealed sharps containers placed in yellow plastic bag for incineration
Glass and aerosol cans		Plastic bins—not for incineration
General, domestic-type waste	Used paper towels, flowers, general kitchen	Black plastic bag—landfill disposal
Food waste		Swill bins—disposal in waste disposal unit in catering department

are by direct contact, air and dust (e.g. meningococcal meningitis, *Streptococcus pyogenes*, chicken pox and herpes zoster). Excretion, secretion, and blood isolation is used for protection against organisms whose transmission is by body fluids (e.g. diarrhoeal illnesses, hepatitis A, B, and C). Strict isolation is required to combat the spread of highly transmissible infections (e.g. viral haemorrhagic fevers). Protective isolation is required for patients who are at greatly increased risk of infection because of their underlying disease or its therapy (e.g. agranulocytosis, immune deficiency, severe burns). The details of these different procedures are beyond the scope of this review.[4]

Universal precautions

A policy of universal precautions should be followed when dealing with all blood and body fluids. These precautions are principally designed for the protection of healthcare staff. The precautions concentrate on identifying high-risk procedures rather than high-risk individuals:

1. Disposable latex gloves must be worn when touching blood and body fluids and handling items which these fluids may have soiled.
2. Gloves must be changed between patients and the hands washed immediately after removal of gloves.
3. Gloves should be powder free. This reduces the likelihood of sensitization. Starch powder may also increase bacterial environmental contamination.[5]
4. Hands and other skin surfaces must be washed immediately after any contamination with blood or body fluids.
5. All potentially contaminated sharps must be disposed of immediately into a sharps disposal bin.

Handwashing

Washing hands with hot water and soap removes transient micro-organisms but has little effect on the resident skin flora. In most situations handwashing with soap is all that is ne essary to prevent cross infection to protect patients and staff from acquiring infection. Alcohol-based handrubs provide a rapid microbicidal action. They do not penetrate organic material, and are therefore of use on visibly clean hands. Alcohol handrubs prevent the regrowth of resident microflora for several hours. Surgical scrubs contain antiseptic and remove both transient and resident skin micro-organisms and reduce the regrowth of resident flora.

Hand washing is the single most important measure for the prevention of spread of infection in ward areas. Hand washing is a professional duty. Hands should be washed thoroughly at the beginning of a shift, nails cleaned, and fresh cuts covered. Hands should be washed again before moving from one patient to the next. Staff caring for immunocomprised patients should use chlorhexidine skin cleanser or a similar agent at the start of the shift and alcohol chlorhexidine solution between patients.

Antibiotic policy

There are several advantages in having an agreed antibiotic policy within the hospital:

1. To ensure patients receive effective antibiotic therapy.
2. To reduce the rate of appearance of resistant organisms.

3. To reserve the use of certain groups of antibiotics for particular infections or types of patient and thereby prolong the useful life of those agents.
4. To restrict the use of some potentially toxic agents and thereby limit the incidence of adverse reactions.
5. To control cost.

The antibiotic resistance pattern within hospitals is constantly changing, requiring that such policies be reviewed regularly. The use of antibiotics is commonplace within the renal unit and the decision to target specific organisms rather than provide broad-spectrum cover is a common therapeutic dilemma made more difficult by emerging resistance to antibiotics. The House of Lords Select Committee on Science and Technology has stated its conviction that resistance to antibiotics and other anti-infective agents constitutes 'a major threat to public health'.[6]

Blood products

Use of blood products is frequently necessary in the renal population. The screening of blood by the transfusion service ensures high standards. Limiting blood transfusion is also important to reduce the antigenic exposure of potential transplant recipients. Maintaining adequate haematinic levels and an adequate erythropoietin prescription in the setting of an adequate dialysis regime can reduce transfusion requirements. Inappropriate anaemia needs to be formally and rigorously investigated in order to avoid the need for unnecessary transfusions.

Problems with particular organisms

In this section we will discuss the principles of infection control, which are common to all areas of the renal unit, focusing on the control of blood-borne viruses, MRSA, VRE, and reduction of unnecessary prescribing of antibiotics.

Blood-borne viruses

Introduction

Hepatitis B virus (HBV) and hepatitis C virus (HCV) are endemic within renal units in many parts of the world. The incidence of HIV infection varies from centre to centre, being non-existent in some and affecting up to 40% of some American dialysis populations.[7] These viruses have a major impact on the dialysis patient not least since actively replicating viruses virtually eliminate the possibility of future transplantation. The potential for viral transfer of blood-borne viruses puts healthcare workers at risk. Worldwide, at least 64 healthcare workers have acquired HIV through exposure at work, many have acquired hepatitis B, and there is also evidence of hepatitis C transmission. It is the responsibility of senior medical staff and managers within a renal unit to ensure that adequate training takes place to ensure safe practices within the unit.

Transmission from one individual to another is most likely when the virus is replicating and the viral load is high. HIV transmission has only been reported from blood, blood products, semen, vaginal secretions, donor organs, and breast milk. HBV is mainly transmitted by blood and sexual contact and perinatally. HCV is mainly transmitted by blood but also by sexual contact and perinatally. Units have reported a varied prevalence of 3.9 to 71%.[8] Hepatitis D infection occurs, but not independently of HBV. It is known that hepatitis G is a blood transmissible virus but its natural history is not yet fully understood. It is unlikely to be as significant as HIV, HBV, or HCV.

Screening

For dialysis patients in renal units in the United Kingdom, the recommendations are for testing every 6 months for HBV and HCV. The frequency of testing for HIV is dependent on the patient's risk factors, the incidence in the elderly being extremely low.

Vaccination

Hepatitis B vaccination is available, but the response rate in dialysis patients is low (around 40% of those completing a course). With a further booster dose this may increase (to 60%), but a significant proportion remain unprotected. Doubled doses used in the vaccination schedule have been reported to improve the response rate further to 92%. The new and recombinant vaccines using intradermal injections are more expensive and report a protection rate of around 70%. Immunization prior to the development end-stage renal failure and initiation of dialysis is the recognized aim. Even in moderate to severe renal failure (serum creatinine levels of about 300 μmol/litre) the success rate is poor.[9] The use of booster doses at 5-yearly intervals has been recommended for responders (hepatitis B surface antibody titres > 100 IU/ml).[10] For the non-immune responders, further booster or boosters may be given and the response rechecked.

Patients

Standards in renal units are not uniform across the world, and new or returning patients who have been dialysed in a non-British unit should be regarded as infected. This should involve isolation for the duration of the incubation period of HBV (5 months). Monthly testing of hepatitis serology during this time is required. Those patients dialysed within the United Kingdom need not be isolated, but screening should be still instituted.

Staff

Sharps and needlestick injuries are the most common vehicles of transmission of blood-borne viruses to healthcare workers. Other routes of transmission include blood splash to mucous membranes and human bites. There is no evidence that blood-borne viruses can be transmitted by blood contact with intact skin or by non-bloody urine or faeces. The hepatitis B antibody status of healthcare workers, including temporary workers, should be checked prior to their commencing work in the haemodialysis unit. For those that are non-immune, a vaccination programme needs to be undertaken and the response rates checked as appropriate. Non-responders should be checked for HBV infection and given booster doses as needed.

Any needlestick injury should be immediately reported, and the individual's immune status rechecked. HBV postexposure prophylaxis should be considered (Table 17.3) but there is no postexposure prophylaxis for HCV.[11] HIV contacts should be managed according to current local postexposure prophylaxis procedures. The healthcare worker

Table 17.3 PHLS Hepatitis Sub-Committee HBV prophylaxis for reported exposure incidents[11]

HBV status of person exposed	Significant exposure			Non-significant exposure	
	HbsAg-positive source	Unknown source	HbsAG-negative source	Continued risk	No further risk
≤one dose HB vaccine pre-exposure	Accelerated course of HB vaccine*, HBIG×1	Accelerated course of HB vaccine*	Initiate course of HB vaccine	Initiate course of HB vaccine	No prophylaxis, reassure
≥two doses HB vaccine pre-exposure	One dose of HB vaccine followed by second dose 1 month later	One dose of HB vaccine	Finish course of HB vaccine	Finish course of HB vaccine	No prophylaxis, reassure
Known responder to HB vaccine	Consider booster dose of HB vaccine	Consider booster dose of HB vaccine	Consider booster dose of HB vaccine	Consider booster dose of HB vaccine	No prophylaxis, reassure
Known non-responder to HB vaccine	HBIG×1. Consider booster dose of HB vaccine	HBIG×1. Consider booster dose of HB vaccine	No HBIG. Consider booster dose of HB vaccine	No HBIG. Consider booster dose of HB vaccine	No prophylaxis, reassure

*Accelerated course: vaccine doses spaced at 0, 1, and 2 months.
HB, hepatitis B; HBIG,

need not avoid continuing to perform exposure-prone procedures pending serological follow-up since the risk to the patient is very small. Healthcare workers found to be infected with a blood-borne virus should be referred for urgent specialist review and must remain off work until serological markers show that they are no longer infectious.

In 1993 the United Kingdom Department of Health stated that healthcare workers who believe they that they may have been infected by HIV must seek medical advice and, if appropriate, diagnostic HIV antibody testing.[12] Healthcare workers infected with HIV may not perform exposure-prone invasive procedures, including haemodialysis.

Equipment and environment

Hepatitis B transmission between patients is well recognized. Infected dialysis patients need to be dialysed in a segregated area with dedicated nurses and limited cross-patient care. Hepatitis C transmission is largely blood-borne within a dialysis unit, although transmission between patients has been reported, particularly when the prevalence within a unit is high.[13] It has recently been suggested that universal precautions without segregation are effective in preventing transmission although this is disputed.[8,14] It is, however, recommended that the same dialysis machine should not be used for infected and non-infected patients. HIV-positive-specific machines are said to be unnecessary. Currently information regarding the safety of reuse is lacking, but there is a risk to staff of unnecessary exposure whilst sterilizing this equipment. Reuse of dialysers in this setting should not be practised. HIV-positive patients should probably use semi-permanent central lines for dialysis access rather than a fistula. On all virally infected patients venous pressure isolators should be changed between patients.

MRSA

Introduction

Recent guidelines have been published.[15] Penicillinase-stable β-lactams, e.g. flucloxacillin, have been the mainstay of antimicrobial therapy for over 35 years and are active against penicillin-resistant *Staphylococcus aureus*. Emergence of strains resistant to flucloxacillin was reported soon after the start of antibiotic use, these are referred to as methicillin-resistant *Staphylococcus aureus* (MRSA). MRSA has a propensity for affecting debilitated patients, and cross-infection can occur with as few as 40 organisms on a healthcare worker's hand. Handwashing between patients is a professional duty. Epidemic strains (i.e. those affecting two or more hospitals) within the United Kingdom have been numbered sequentially EMRSA 1–16. Each strain has its own laboratory characteristics. The most prevalent strains in British hospitals are currently EMRSA 3, 15, and 16. Each EMRSA can acquire mupirocin resistance by acquisition of the *mup4* gene, by cross-colonization of resistant strains, or prolonged or repeated mupirocin treatment courses; this is increasingly prevalent in renal units.[16]

MRSA is as pathogenic as MSSA (methicillin-sensitive *Staphylococcus aureus*). It can cause infections ranging from trivial skin infections to endocarditis and pneumonia. Until 1991, 1.5% of reported systemic *S. aureus* bacteraemias were MRSA. This percentage has since increased: in 1996 21% were MRSA and in 1997, 31.7%.[17]

Patients

Patients in the renal unit are susceptible to MRSA and the prevalence within renal patients has increased. Previous hospitalization, intravascular lines, pressure sores, underlying disease, and recent antibiotics are all risk factors for acquisition. The perineum is a main carriage site of MRSA but is inconvenient for routine screening. The nose, perineum, or groin, any skin lesions, and manipulated sites are the most frequently infected sites. EMRSA 16 is more likely to colonize the throat and cause lower respiratory tract infections. EMRSA- 15 is more likely to cause infections of the urinary tract. The United Kingdom Department of Health emphasizes that patient care should not be compromised by MRSA status and that patients with MRSA should not be denied admission to nursing or residential homes.

Staff

MRSA rarely causes infection in healthy people or their families. Transient carriage is common after treating contaminated patients. Nurses have been shown to carry MRSA in their noses and on their fingers at the end of a shift, and yet be clear of MRSA the following morning.[18] In cases of sustained healthcare worker infection, the individual may be advised by the infection control team to remain off duty while being treated. Those with chronic skin problems like eczema and psoriasis may be difficult to manage if colonized with MRSA and ultimately may have to be counselled for a career change.

Screening

Patients admitted from other hospitals, including hospitals abroad, from nursing or residential homes, or those known to have been colonized or infected previously by MRSA should be screened for MRSA. They should barrier nursed (and possibly isolated) until the results are known.

Treatment

The treatment of MRSA will depend on the site infected and the characteristics of the patient (Boxes 17.1 and 17.2). Control programmes can be successful for both patients and staff. The isolation of affected individuals plays a large part in the control of infection, but it must not be allowed to influence detrimentally the care of the patient. Within the isolation environment, handwashing, gloves, aprons, and designated equipment will all restrict the spread from the isolation facility. When screening highlights an infected person in a ward believed to be clear of MRSA the aim is to limit the infection to this person and attempt eradication of the infection. Ward patients and staff may need to be screened and the infected individuals isolated either in cubicles or in a designated area in the ward. At the entrance to the infected area, an alcohol hand rub should be available. Colonized staff may need to be excluded from the ward. The timing of staff screening is important so as to not to detect the transient carriers. This should be at the start of a shift.

Environment

When MRSA is endemic, the infection control team should be involved to coordinate a strategy. Control measures should be reinforced. The single most important initiative is to

Box 17.1: Treatment of clinical methicillin-resistant *Staphylococcus aureus* (MRSA) infections[15]

Infected skin lesions

- Cover infected or colonized lesions (e.g. wounds, pressure sores) with an antiseptic (e.g. chlorhexidine, povidine) dressing.
- Small lesions: apply mupirocin (2.0%) in polyethylene glycol base up to three times daily for no more than 7–10 days. Avoid prolonged or repeated courses, which encourage selection of mupirocin resistance in *Staphyloccocus aureus*.
- Raw areas or burns: consider mupirocin in a paraffin base (plus systemic therapy as indicated). Avoid mupirocin in polyethylene glycol: systemic absorption of the vehicle risks nephrotoxicity.
- Accompanying measures to eradicate carriage (e.g. in the nose or on the skin or perineum) (see Box 17.2).

Systemic infections

- Obtain appropriate samples for culture and antibiotic sensitivity testing.
- Treatment of severe infections is urgent; first-line antibiotic therapy should be with a glycopeptide administered intravenously:

EITHER vancomycin by intravenous infusion (monitor plasma concentrations: maximum peak (2 h postinfusion) concentration 30 mg/litre, maximum trough (predose) concentration 10 mg/litre).

- Adults: 500 mg over at least 60 min every 6 h or 1 g over at least 100 min every 12 h.
- Neonate: 15 mg/kg initially, then 10 mg/kg every 8–12 h.
- Child (over 1 month): 10 mg/kg every 6 h.

OR teicoplanin by intravenous infusion (maintain trough concentration above 10 mg/litre)

- Adults: 400 mg initially, then 200 mg daily (severe infections 400 mg every 12 h for three doses, then 400 mg daily).
- Neonate: initially single dose 16 mg/kg by intravenous infusion, then 8 mg/kg daily by intravenous infusion.
- Child (over 2 months): initially 10 mg/kg every 12 h for three doses by intravenous injection or infusion, then 6 mg/kg daily.

In patients who are not severely ill, oral therapy may be suitable depending upon the susceptibility of the organism, e.g. rifampicin (0.6–1.2 g daily in two or four divided doses) PLUS sodium fusidate (usual adult dose 500 mg every 8 h). Ciprofloxacin or a macrolide or trimethoprim are other alternatives (see text concerning emergence of resistance).

Box 17.2: Guidelines for the treatment of MRSA carriers*[15]

Nasal carriage

- Apply mupirocin 2% in a paraffin base (Bactroban Nasal) to each nostril three times daily for 5 days.
- MRSA strains with low-level resistance to mupirocin (MIC 8–256 mg/litre) may still respond.
- Culture nasal swab 2 days after treatment; if positive, repeat the treatment once and check also for throat carriage.
- If nasal swab remains positive, or the strain shows mupirocin resistance, consider alternative topical treatment (e.g. 0.5% neomycin + 0.1% chlorhexidine cream (Naseptin), or 1% chlorhexidine cream).
- Avoid repeated courses of mupirocin and the topical use of antibiotics that may be required for systemic use (e.g. fusidic acid, gentamicin).

Skin carriage

- Daily antiseptic bathing for 5 days (repeated if necessary), e.g. with 4% chlorhexidine, 2% triclosan, or 7.5% povidone iodine.
- Wash hair twice weekly with an antiseptic shampoo/detergent.
- Hexachlorophane 0.33% powder for axillary or groin carriage (avoid on broken skin and in neonates).
- Consider use of emollients, and seek dermatological advice, for patients with skin disorders or fragile skin.

Throat carriage

- Significance in relation to spread is unclear. May be difficult to eradicate.
- If there is clear evidence of transmission, consider a single 5-day course of oral treatment with either rifampicin plus fusidic acid or, for susceptible organisms, ciprofloxacin (with the fully informed consent of the carrier).

*The decision to treat patients or staff carriers will depend on the clinical setting and severity of the outbreak, and should be guided by the medical microbiologist and infection control physician.

improve handwashing between patients either with liquid soap and water or with alcohol hand rub. Nursing and medical staff should wear aprons. Extensive handling of the patient requires aprons and includes coverage of back and shoulders. Visitors do not need to wear aprons but should wash their hands on leaving. Staff should wear gloves and wash their hands when leaving. Masks are needed only for exfoliative conditions and during chest physiotherapy. The door should be kept closed when not in use. Antiseptics (triclosan, chlorhexidine) and alcohol hand rub should be available for staff hand disinfection.

Dedicated stethoscopes and sphygmomanometers should be available. Linen should be marked. On discharge the room including the door should be washed with detergent with particular attention to equipment and chairs and horizontal surfaces. A general improvement of hygiene on the ward effectively concentrates the mind in establishing the discipline required to control this infection. Additional steps in reducing contact with uninfected patients, where possible, as well as reviewing antibiotic guidelines should be addressed. MRSA-positive staff should be treated with the same regime as patients.

Vancomycin-resistant enterococci

Overview

Vancomycin-resistant enterococci (VRE) are becoming increasingly prevalent. HICPAC (the Hospital Infection Control Practices Advisory Committee) is a working party formed to draw up initial guidelines on VRE with the aim of education and drafting treatment options.[19] They cite an increased risk with previous vancomycin treatment and/or multimicrobial therapy, severe underlying disease or immunosuppression, intra-abdominal surgery, in-dwelling urethral or central venous catheters, and having been treated on an intensive care or transplant ward. Enterococci are found in the normal gastrointestinal tract. Most infections are considered to be endogenous but transmission from patient-to-patient directly or indirectly via the hands of personnel or contaminated equipment is also possible. The *vanA* gene is plasmid borne and confers high-level resistance to vancomycin and teicoplanin. It can be transferred *in vitro* from enterococci to a variety of Gram-positive organisms including *S. aureus*. HICPAC suggested that preventing and controlling the spread of VRE can only be achieved if the following elements are addressed:

1. Prudent use of vancomycin by clinicians.
2. Education of hospital staff about vancomycin resistance.
3. Early detection and reporting of vancomycin resistance by the hospital microbiology laboratory.
4. Immediate implementation of appropriate infection control measures to prevent person-to-person transmission of VRE.

Vancomycin resistant strains of *S. haemolyticus* have already been reported as have strains of VISA (vancomycin-intermediate *S. aureus*) from Japan, the United States, and Europe.

Patients

Screening for VRE should be reserved for those considered high risk (see above) and should take the form of rectal swabs or faecal screening for those in hospital longer than 7 days. Three separate negative swabs, each a week apart, are necessary before a patient can be deemed to be clear of infection. Some advocate no screening or screening only those patients with diarrhoea, to prevent environmental contamination, as there is no accepted means of eradicating colonization. VRE colonization in the community has been documented, possibly acquired from poultry given avoparcin, a glycopeptide.[20]

Staff

For general care, gloves are worn when in contact with the patient and aprons must also be worn. Handwashing after every contact is essential. Alcohol hand rub is the most effective agent. Door knobs, medical and nursing equipment, plates, and cups can be colonized and dedicated non-critical equipment should be available for the sole use of VRE-infected patients.[21] Screening of all the patient contacts may be required, and the notes of infected patients should be highlighted. Advice on treatment should be sought from the hospital microbiologist. Intermittent temporary dialysis lines and removal of the number of in-dwelling catheters may need to be instituted in order to aid clearance of the pathogen. Prevention of VRE generation is centred around the controlled use of vancomycin. HICPAC has advised on this issue (Table 17.4). Acquisition of VRE necessitates a different approach, the aim being containment of the infection. Education is helpful in preventing nosocomial transmission. Prompt notification of the infection to staff looking after the patient is critical. Congregation of VRE patients together or individually in single rooms will isolate the infection and aid awareness of the problem. With the exception of 3% hydrogen peroxide, most disinfectants appear to be active against VRE.[22]

Clostridium difficile

Clostridium difficile is an anaerobic spore-forming Gram-positive rod. It causes antibiotic-associated diarrhoea or colitis and occasionally, a fulminant pseudomembranous colitis.

Table 17.4 HICPAC guidelines for the prescription of vancomycin[19]

Vancomycin should be restricted to	
Gram-positive organisms	β-lactam resistant organisms. Patients allergic to β-lactam antimicrobials
Antibiotic associated colitis	Failure to respond to metronidazole therapy. Severe and potentially life threatening
Prophylaxis	Infective endocarditis in those at serious risk. Surgery with prosthesis insertion in institutions with a high incidence of MRSA or methicillin-resistant *S. epidemidis*
HICPAC has discouraged the use in the following circumstances	
Prophylactic use	Routine surgical prophylaxis against infection of in-dwelling vascular catheters. Routine prophylaxis for patients on CAPD or HD
Febrile patients	Empirical use in neutropenic febrile patients. Treatment in response to a positive blood culture that may be a contaminant, e.g. a single positive bottle when others are negative. Continued empirical use in patients who are culture negative. Treatment for β-lactam sensitive organisms in patients with renal failure
Other uses	Selective decontamination of the digestive tract. Eradication of MRSA colonization. Primary treatment of antibiotic-associated colitis. In topical applications or irrigations

Immunocompromised, elderly, and renal patients are at particular risk. Spread between susceptible patients is the most common route of acquisition. *Clostridium difficile* toxin can often be detected in the faeces of infected individuals. Avoidance of excessive use of broad-spectrum antibiotics, and adequate hand hygiene reduce the risk of an outbreak of infection. Treatment is by oral metronidazole or oral vancomycin.

Other organisms

Coliforms including *Klebsiella*, *Enterobacter*, *Serratia*, and *Proteus* spp. form part of the normal colonic flora. Extensive use of antibiotics encourages skin colonization and the emergence of gentamicin-resistant strains. Contamination of the hands of healthcare workers and contamination of equipment are the usual routes of transmission.

Pseudomonas spp and the related *Xanthomonas maltophilia* are not normal skin commensals, but are common pathogens in moist environments. Susceptible colonized patients may develop severe systemic infections. Avoidance of excessive use of broad-spectrum antibiotics, adequate hand hygiene, and adequate disinfection of equipment are important means of preventing the spread of infection.

Haemodialysis unit

Overview

The fact that all dialysis patients do not regularly and frequently acquire nosocomial infection is a testament to the procedures that are in place in dialysis units and the quality of staff training. No other area within a hospital carries out invasive and potentially hazardous procedures on the scale that a dialysis unit is required to do. Up to four patients will use a single dialysis machine in a single day. A coordinated and efficient approach is the essential to maintain control of both the safety and infection aspects within a unit.

Patients

The haemodialysis patient is susceptible to numerous threats of developing sepsis. The greatest threat is related to access. Whenever possible vascular access should be obtained using an arteriovenous fistula. The alternatives of semipermanent and temporary catheters generally reduce effective dialysis and have a substantially increased rate of infection. Infections are uncommon in fistulae and PTFE grafts. Semipermanent lines should be placed under sterile conditions. With the emergence of VRE, vancomycin should not be used for prophylaxis, despite its convenience. Silver-coated lines have been developed to try and reduce the rate of line infections, though there is little definite evidence of benefit.[23] Antibiotic-impregnated central vein catheters with rifampicin and minocycline are in development and short-term results look promising. The antimicrobial effect is limited to 4 weeks.[24] The predominant pathogens in line sepsis are *Staphylococcus* spp. *Pseudomonas*, *Enterobacter*, and streptococci are less common. Once line colonization has occurred, antibiotics need to penetrate the biofilm formed over inserted foreign material to achieve clearance of the organism. A prospective study has shown the progression from line colonization to a peripheral bacteraemia is almost inevitable and occurs 5–26 days later. Within 16 weeks of placement, virtually all the lines are colonized.[25] Antibiotic locks may be of benefit in association with intravenous treatment.[26] Removal of catheters is required when there is a delayed response to treatment. The development of Tesio catheters has lead to a reduced incidence of septic episodes and a reduced incidence of exit site infections at the same time as producing better flows than other semipermanent catheters.[27]

Staff

Good infection control in a dialysis unit requires an adequate number of trained staff. Shortcuts in protocols lead to breakdown in infection control procedures. The problem can be minimized by avoiding excessive workloads. Adequate training of staff reduces the complication rate of potentially hazardous procedures. The dialysis unit should not be used as a corridor. Patients waiting to be dialysed, or those who have just finished should be accommodated in a separate area from those dialysing. A member of staff should be appointed as a safety officer with responsibility for recording incidents and protocol violations within the unit. Ultimate responsibility lies with the senior medical staff.[28]

Equipment and environment

To avoid contact with blood, barriers such as gloves and waterproof dressings are effective and should be used when dealing with patients, cleaning machines, sterilizing equipment, and dealing with spillages. Gloves need to be changed between patients. In theatre more than 50% of injuries occur to the non–dominant index finger, 20% occurring to the operator's assistant. Double gloving does not prevent sharps injuries, but does lead to a six-fold decrease of inner glove puncture; it may also reduce the inoculated blood volume. Particular care needs to be taken when new operators are trained. Glove use should be mandatory and gloves should be of the European Standard 455. Face shields are more appropriate than glasses in the haemodialysis setting.

Maintaining a clean and ordered department can reduce the potential for infection transmission. Sharps bins should not be allowed to become more than three-quarters full and safe procedures should be followed for the disposal of waste. Spillages should be promptly cleaned (Table 17.5).[28]

Sharps are used much more frequently in the dialysis unit than any other department in the hospital. The potential for viral inoculation is high (e.g. 0.001 ml of blood can transmit hepatitis B infection) and simple measures can reduce the risks significantly. Needles should not be resheathed and needle and syringe should be disposed of as a single unit.

Table 17.5 Dealing with spillages

Small spills	Chlorine releasing granules then paper towels
Large spills	Paper towels first then 1% hypochlorite
Skin	Wash off under running tap

Water

Exposure and risk

The haemodialysis patient is exposed to huge volumes of water. In a single week the average dialysis patient is exposed to about 300 litres compared with an average person's exposure of about 15 litres. Furthermore in normal circumstances the portal of entry is the gastrointestinal tract, which can afford a selective barrier to unwanted materials, whilst in the haemodialysis patient exposure is via a non-selective membrane. Modern haemodialysis techniques employing highly permeable membranes entail large volumes of dialysis fluid entering the patient during the procedure by back-filtration or by direct infusion during haemofiltration procedures. Unless steps are taken to ensure that high-quality water is produced for use in haemodialysis and unless water quality is monitored rigorously and regularly, patients face potentially serious risks. The major risks are from inorganic material such as aluminium, copper, zinc, calcium, fluoride, sulphate, and nitrate, organic materials such as chloramines, and microbiological contaminants.

Standards of water quality

The Association for the Advancement of Medical Instrumentation (AAMI) have set standards for water quality.[29] AAMI standards for inorganic and organic contaminants have been adopted widely. There have been moves though to recommend higher standards for bacterial counts and endotoxin levels, particularly for use in high-flux haemodialysis and haemodiafiltration. Recently the British Renal Association has adopted the more rigorous standard of the European Pharmacopoeia.[10] Using modern water treatment techniques ultrapurity can be achieved and standards will probably become tighter (Table 17.6).

Water treatment

A variety of techniques are used in combination to produce water of sufficient quality for haemodialysis. Filters play a key role, removing large particulates, bacteria, viruses, and endotoxins. Activated carbon is used to remove contaminants such as chlorine, chloramines, hypochlorites, and chloroform by absorption. Bacterial proliferation can occur in carbon beds and downstream equipment must be positioned which is capable of removing bacteria and endotoxins. Reverse osmosis utilizes forced solvent flow across

Table 17.6 Standards for water dialysis

	Endotoxin (LAL) (Eu/ml)	Microbial count (TVC) (cfu/ml)
AAMI	<10	<200
European Pharmacopoeia	<0.25	<100
Achievable purity	<0.125	<5

AAMI=Association for the Advancement of Medical Instrumentation; LAL=limulus amoebocyte lysate test; TVC=total viable count; cfu=colony-forming units; Eu=European units a semipermeable membrane under hydrostatic pressure. The process removes a wide spectrum of contaminants such as large organic material, bacteria, and ionic species. Ion-exchange resins exchange particular ion species on the resin for others in the feed water. Water softeners are an example, exchanging sodium ions for calcium and magnesium ions in the hard water feed. Bacterial colonization is possible, and downstream ultrafilters or ultraviolet irradiators are required. These devices can be deployed in series to produce ultrapure water, which is stored in a holding tank. Stagnation in the holding tank is avoided by recirculating held water round the distribution ring, which should contain an ultraviolet irradiator to maintain bacteriological quality. Figure 17.2 illustrates such a system for producing ultrapure water.

Monitoring water quality

Routine sampling from multiple points in the system is necessary at regular intervals to ensure chemical and microbiological quality is maintained. Typically this should include weekly estimates of total viable count (TVC) and estimates of endotoxins levels by limulus amoebocyte lysate (LAL) assay in samples taken from the distribution ring return. Routine disinfections need to be supplemented when TVC or LAL action limits are exceeded during the monitoring process. Using these tightly monitored systems, clinical incidents of pyrogenic reaction or water-borne septicaemia should be diminishingly rare and any episode requires vigorous investigation.

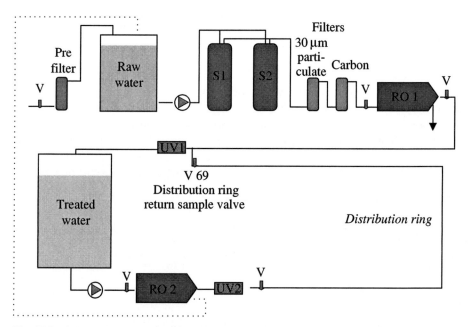

Fig. 17.2   Schematic systems for the production of ultrapure water for haemodialysis: S, softener; RO, reverse osmosis unit; V, sample valve; UV, ultraviolet lamps.

Predialysis protocol

A wide area surrounding the fistula should be cleaned with 0.5% chlorhexidine in 70% ethyl alcohol. Local anaesthetic can be applied before cannulation. Areas of infection around the fistula must be given a wide berth. Semipermanent catheters should be treated with extreme care to avoid introducing infection. Caps should not be reused. The limbs of the access should be cleaned with 0.5% chlorhexidine in 70% ethyl alcohol.

Postdialysis protocol

Following dialysis, the circuit should be removed and double yellow bagged. Blood-stained linen should be placed in red alginate stitched bags and then a red plastic bag, heavily blood-soaked linen should be placed in a yellow bag for incineration. Disposable dialysers should be transported in yellow bags and incinerated. The techniques for reuse are discussed below. During dismantling and washing, staff should wear plastic aprons and gloves. A 0.1% chlorine-releasing solution should be used for routine cleaning, both in the general unit and areas where hepatitis patients are dialysed. The machines should be washed with 0.1% hypochlorite solution and clamps and dialysis holders should be soaked for 30 min in hypochlorite solution (60 min is corrosive). Blind connections to the dialysis circuit with pressure monitors need to be sterile to avoid contamination. Direct contamination of venous pressure monitors may occur. Dirty gauges must be cleaned and sterilized with ethylene oxide or replaced.

Reuse of dialysers

Since its first description in 1964 the techniques of the dialyser reuse have improved. The advantages include improved biocompatibility, reduced first use reactions, and reduced exposure to reactive material in new dialysers, as well as the obvious cost reduction. There are inherent risks in attempting to reuse a dialyser designed for a single procedure but with appropriate environmental and processing controls the risks may be reduced or eliminated. Failure of these protocols may lead to septicaemia, endotoxaemia, and under-dialysis. Dialyser reuse does not seem to have a consistent effect on overall mortality figures. Other factors such as prudent use of dialysis prescription and correction of anaemia are probably more important.[30] Reuse of dialysers is not recommended for patients with active systemic infection, including hepatitis, because of an increased risk of cross-infection. Epidemiological studies have not shown that reuse is associated with a higher prevalence of HBV.[31] HCV infection is not a contraindication, though additional precautions are recommended. The incidence of HCV infection is lower in units that have a separate room for reprocessing the dialysers of positive patients. The incidence may be lower in techniques involving the use of peracetic acid.[32] For detailed descriptions of the reprocessing we refer the reader to other sources but here consideration will be given to the use of universal precautions, disinfection, and water requirements.[33]

Universal precautions

The area in which reprocessing is undertaken should be separate from the main unit with good ventilation. It should be possible to complete the entire procedure within that area.

A clean and clear label should be placed on each reprocessed dialyser stating the patient's name, number of uses, date of last reprocessing, and original and residual total fibre volume. Before reuse of a dialyser the label must be rechecked by two members of staff and preferably also the patient. Routine testing of sample dialysers is recommended for disinfectant and bacterial counts on each shift. The dialyser should be adequately rinsed prior to the reconnection of the patient. Data relating to the reuse technique should be collected and audited on a regular basis.

Disinfection

The chemicals used in reprocessing generally achieve disinfection rather than sterilization. The most commonly used agents are peracetic acid, formaldehyde, and glutaraldehyde (Table 17.7). Peracetic acid is gradually replacing formaldehyde as the most popular agent. The disinfectant is infused into the blood and dialysate compartments, and when at least four compartment volumes are infused, more than 90% of the prescribed concentration should be achieved. The disinfectant is drained and the dialyser rinsed just prior to the next dialysis session. Heat sterilization of polysulfone dialysers at temperatures of 105 °C for 20 h is an alternative method. A residue of disinfection fluid within the dialyser may lead to pain at the access site, dyspnoea, hypotension, and haemolysis on reuse. Septicaemia on dialysis is equally common in reprocessing units and single-use units.[33] The main causes of septicaemia in reprocessing centres are contaminated water and inadequate disinfectant concentrations. Published reports of these occurrences have usually incriminated a breakdown in the unit's protocols pertaining either to the processing strategies or quality control. Quality control must be meticulous to protect staff and patients from infection and disinfectant exposure. The use of automated systems does not reduce the need for vigilance.

Table 17.7 Disinfectants used in reprocessing dialysers

Disinfectant	Storage*	Advantages	Disadvantages
Formaldehyde	24h/4%/20°C	Cheap and efficacious. Stable formula	Offensive smell. Asthma and contact dermatitis. Anti-N abs and haemolysis. Noxious fumes with bleach. Potential patient sensitization
Peracetic acid	11h/1%/20°C	Less hazardous Less noxious	Dialyser reduction. Reacts with bleach. Weekly solute production required
Glutaraldehyde	1h/0.75%/20°C	Historical use	Lower reuse rates achieved
Heat	20h/–/105°C	No chemical residues Dialyser K_{uf} increased	Polysulfone dialysers only. Limited availability

*Minimum time/concentration/temperature.
K_{uf} = ultrafiltration coefficient.

Intravenous iron

Intravenous iron therapy is used regularly in dialysis units to maintain patients iron stores. Iron is an essential requirement for bacterial multiplication. An excess of iron in the body may increase the risk for infection. At times of infection the prescription of intravenous iron should be suspended, as there is evidence that in end-stage renal failure the iron adversely affects the function of macrophages and T and B lymphocytes thereby increasing infection.[34]

Continuous ambulatory peritoneal dialysis

Overview

The unique feature of infection control in a continuous ambulatory peritoneal dialysis (CAPD) unit is its dependence on patient training and compliance. The onus is therefore on the physicians and nurses to ensure adequate training. Inadequate patient selection or training, or poor compliance with the procedure, will usually manifest as a high incidence of peritonitis or exit site infection and reduced technique and patient survival. Dialysis technique and host defence against infection are of paramount importance.

Patients

MRSA screening is recommended prior to CAPD catheter insertion, especially if the patient has been in contact with ward patients. If a patient is found to be MRSA-positive on screening the standard regime can be used (Box 17.2) with added cover of 4% aqueous chlorhexidine total body wash on operation day. Attention to the positioning of the exit site is important. The conventional exit site lies within the confines of the lower abdomen. In obese patients drooping folds of skin may cause a catheter to overhang the groin on standing. This can lead to increased risk of infection. A swan-neck catheter has been developed which opens onto the chest wall. In obese patients use of such a catheter may reduce the incidence of exit site infections.[35]

CAPD patients on immunosuppressive drug therapy have a greater incidence of peritonitis, more frequent hospital admissions, more days off CAPD, and more frequent need for catheter removal. Thus CAPD is not considered a desirable method of dialysis in this group of patients (Table 17.8).[36] HIV-positive patients have a survival rate of 58% at 1 year and 54% at 2 years. Patients with advanced disease fare less well, having higher hospitalization rates. Peritonitis rates are higher in HIV-positive CAPD patients. Infection control

Table 17.8   Immunosuppression and CAPD outcome

Events per year per person	Peritonitis	Hospital admissions	Days off CAPD	PD catheter removal
Immunosuppressed (146)	1.77	0.64	8.5	28%
Non-immunosuppressed (39)	0.67	0.23	1.7	10%

in this population will consist of the universal procedures described elsewhere with special attention to the disposal of the effluent dialysate.[37] HIV- and HBV-positive patients on CAPD produce potentially infective effluent. Appropriate disposal is essential.[38]

Nasal carriage of *S. aureus* will increase the incidence of both exit site infection and Gram-positive peritonitis. Eradication is possible with topical mupirocin and the incidence of exit site infections is significantly reduced. The peritonitis rate is lowered, though not significantly. Overall this process is expensive and may not be considered cost-effective.[39]

Staff

CAPD staff have a lower probability of coming into contact with a patient's body fluids than haemodialysis staff. Safety precautions remain important, and vigilance should not be reduced.

Equipment and environment

Scrupulous exit site care can reduce the rate of exit site infections. A silver ring placed at the base of a peritoneal dialysis catheter does not convey protection against infection, neither does the use of povidine iodine powder spray at the exit site.[40,41] Covering the exit site with a dressing film after iodine application may, however, be beneficial. Daily exposure and dressing does not reduce the infection rate.[42] Cyclical rifampicin (5 days out of 3 months) or daily mupirocin application to the exit site may reduce the incidence of catheter infection and peritonitis with *S. aureus*.[43] There is probably no significant difference between single and dual cuffs in CAPD catheters in terms of catheter survival, episodes of peritonitis, or exit site infections in adults.[44] Once exit site infections have occurred cuff shaving can be effective in eliminating up to 50% of *S. aureus* infections and 100% of *S. epidermidis* infections. It is ineffective in eliminating Gram-negative exit site infections. Replacement of CAPD catheters for tunnel infection or exit site infection in a single-stage procedure has an 85 % success rate. The disconnect dialysis system has been established as the preferred peritoneal dialysis system over the single bag method. The higher purchase price of the disconnect system is more than offset by the reduction in incidence of peritonitis.

Procedures

Catheter insertion

The insertion of a Tenchkoff catheter is an obvious potential portal of entry for infection. Covering of the procedure with antibiotics is recommended. Vancomycin is unnecessary for this and the suggested prophylaxis is with cefuroxime, a single intravenous dose prior to catheter insertion.[45]

CAPD techniques

Hands should be washed with chlorhexidene skin cleanser (Hibiscrub) or alcohol chlorhexidine (Hibisol). Gloves should be worn for any procedure involving exit site or tubing.

The connector site must be sprayed, or wiped with 70% alcohol and allowed to dry before and after any disconnection/reconnection procedure. The exit site should be cleaned daily with povidone iodine or chlorhexidene, and covered with a dry dressing. Leaving more than 10 cm of catheter length from the exit site will prevent unnecessary movement of the catheter within its tunnel. The exit site should not be immersed during bathing.

Transplantation

The renal transplant recipient is particularly vulnerable to infection, predominantly because of the need for immunosuppression to prevent graft rejection. Infections often arise due to organisms already carried by the patient. There is now thought to be no need for strict protective isolation in the immediate postoperative period. Cross-infection can be prevented by adherence to the principles and practices outlined earlier in this chapter. Infection can also be transplanted with the graft and there should be extensive screening of the donor and donor organs. Prophylactic use of antimicrobial agents may also be helpful at the time of transplantation, and afterwards cotrimaxazole is commonly used to prevent opportunist infection with *Pneumocystis carinii* and *Nocardia*. These and other issues will be fully covered in the chapters on transplantation.

The renal ward

Figure 17.3 depicts the renal ward at the centre of a complex microbiological web which encompasses all of the potential problems outlined in earlier sections. Vigilant application of the principles of infection control discussed above is required to ensure that patients receive the safe and effective care in this environment to which they are entitled.

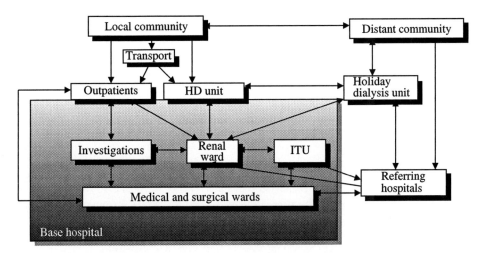

Fig. 17.3 Microbiological environment of the renal unit.

References

1. Haley RW, Morgan WM, Culver DH, White JW (1985). Update from the SENIC project. Hospital infection control: recent progress and opportunities under prospective payment. *Am J Infect Control* **13**(3): 97–108.
2. Beneson AS (1985). *Control of communicable diseases in man*, 14th edn. American Public Health Association, Washington, DC.
3. Health Services Advisory Committee (1982). *The safe disposal of clinical waste*, HN (82) 22. HMSO, London.
4. Philpott-Howard J and Casewell M (1994). *Hospital infection control. Policies and practical procedures*. WB Saunders, London.
5. Dave J, Wilcox MH, Kellett M (1999).Glove powder: implications for infection control. *J Hosp Infect* **42**(4): 283–5.
6. House of Lords Select Committee on Science and Technology (1998). *Resistance to antibiotics and other antimicrobials*. Stationary Office, London.
7. Tokars JI, Alter MJ, Miller E, Moyer LA, Favero MS (1997). National Surveillance of dialysis associated diseases in the United States—1994. *ASAIO J* **43**(1): 108–19.
8. Weghitt TG (1999). Blood borne virus infections in dialysis units—a review. *Rev Med Virol* **9**(2): 101–9.
9. Koher H, Arnold W, Renschin G *et al.* (1984). Active hepatitis B vaccination of dialysis patients and staff. *Kidney Int* **25**: 124–8.
10. The Renal Association (1997). *Treatment of adult patients with renal failure*, 2nd edn. Royal College of Physicians, London.
11. PHLS Hepatitis Subcommittee (1992). *CDR Review 1992* **2**: R97–R101.
12. Department of Health (1993). *AIDS/HIV infected health care workers: guidance on the management of infected health care workers*, EL(93)24.
13. Irish DN, Blake C, Christophers J, Craske JE, Burnapp L, Abbs IC, MacMahon EM, Muir P, Banatvala JE, Simmonds P (1999). Identification of hepatitis C virus seroconversion resulting from nosocomial transmission on a haemodialysis unit: implications for infection control and laboratory screening. *J Med Virol* **59**(2): 135–40.
14. Pereira JG, Levey AS (1997). Hepatitis C virus infection in dialysis and renal transplantation. *Kidney Int* **51**: 981–99.
15. The combined working party of the British Society for Antimicrobial Chemotherapy, the Hospital Infection Society and the Infection Control Nurses Association (1998). Revised guidelines for the control of methicillin-resistant *Staphylococcus aureus* infection in hospitals. *J Hosp Infect* **39**: 253–290.
16. BSAC/HIS/ICNA working party (1999). *Revised guidelines on the control of MRSA in hospitals*. Cafferkey MT, Hone R, Keane CT (1988). Sources and outcome for methicillin-resistant *Staphyloccus aureus* bacteraemia. *J Hosp Infect* **11**: 136–143.
17. Speller DC, Johnson AP, James D, Marples RR, Chalet A, George RC (1997). Resistance to methicillin and other antibiotics in isolates of *Staphylococcus aureus* from blood and cerebrospinal fluid, England and Wales 1989–1995. *Lancet* **350**(9074): 323–5.
18. Cookson N, Peters B, Webster M, Phillips I, Rahman M, Noble W (1989). Staff carriage of epidemic methicillin-resistant Staphylococcus aureus. *J Clin Microbiol* **27**: 1471–1476.
19. Hospital Infection Control Practices Advisory Committee (1995). Recommendations for preventing the spread of vancomycin resistance. *Infect Control Hosp Epidemiol* **16**(2): 105–13.
20. Bates J (1997). Epidemiology of vancomycin resistant enterococci in the community and the relevance of farm animals to human infection. *J Hosp Infect* **37**(2): 89–101.
21. Warnick F (1997). Vancomycin resistant enterococcus. *Clin J Oncol Nurs* **1**(3): 73–7.

22. Saurina G, Landman D, Quale JM (1997). Activity of disinfectants against vancomycin-resistant *Enterococcus faecium*. *Infect Control Hosp Epidemiol* 18(5): 345–7.

23. Trerotola SO, Johnson MS, Shah H, Kraus MA, MuKuslsy MA, Ambrosius WT, Harris VJ, Snidow JJ (1998). Tunneled haemodialysis catheters; use of silver coated catheter for prevention of infection—a randomised study. *Radiology* 207(2): 491–6.

24. Raad I, Hanna H (1999). Intravascular catheters impregnated with antimicrobial agents: a mile-stone in the prevention of blood stream infections. *Support Care Cancer* 17(6): 386–90.

25. Dittmer ID, Sharp D, MuNulty CA, Williams AJ, Banks RA (1999). A prospective study of central venous haemodialysis catheter colonizarion and peripheral bacteraemia. *Clin Nephrol* 51(1): 34–9.

26. Chang JM, Tsai JC, Hwang SJ, Chuen HC, Guh JY, Lai YH (1997). Treatment of permcath-related sepsis in uraemic patients. *Kao Hsiung I Hsueh Ko Hsueh Tsa Chih* 13(3): 155–61.

27. Prabhu PN, Kerns SR, Sabatelli FW, Haawkins IF, Ross EA (1997). Long-term performance and complications of the Tesio twin catheter system for haemodialysis access. *Am J Kidney Dis* 30(2): 213–18.

28. Ayliffe GAJ, Lowbury EJL, Geddes AM, Williams JD (1993). *Control of hospital infection. A practical handbook*, 3rd edn. Chapman and Hall Medical, London.

29. Association for the Advancement of Medical Instrumentation (1982). *American standard for haemodialysis systems* RD-5. Arlington, Virginia.

30. Collins AJ, Ma JZ, Constantini EG, Everson SE (1998). Dialysis unit and patient characteristics Associated with reuse practices and mortality: 1989–1993. *J Am Soc Nephrol* 19(11): 2108–17.

31. Tokars JI, Alter MJ, Favero MS, Moyer LA, Bland LA (1993). National surveillance of dialysis associated diseases in the United States, 1991. *ASAIO J* 39(4): 966–75.

32. dos Santos JP, Loureiro A, Centoroglo-Neto M, Pereira BJ (1996). Impact of dialysis room and reuse strategies on the incidence of hepatitis C virus infection in haemodialysis units. *Nephrol Dial Transplant* 11(10): 2017–22.

33. Miles AM, Friedman EA (1996). Dialyzer reuse—techniques and controversy. *Replacement of renal function by dialysis*, revised 4th edn. Kluwer Academic, Dordrecht, pp. 454–71.

34. Patruta SI, Horl WH (1999). Iron and infection. *Kidney Int Suppl* 69: S125–S130.

35. Twardowski ZJ, Prowanr BF, Nichols WK, Nolph KD, Khanna R (1998). Six year experience with swan-neck presternal peritoneal dialysis catheter. *Perit Dial Int* 18(6): 598–602.

36. Andrews PA, Warr KJ, Hicks JA, Cameron JS (1996). Impaired outcome of continuous ambulatory peritoneal dialysis in immunosuppressed patients. *Nephrol Dial Transplant* 11(6): 1104–8.

37. Tebben-JA, Rigsby MO, Selwyn PA, Brennan N, Kliger A, Finkelstein FO (1993). Outcome of HIV infected patients on continuous ambulatory peritoneal dialysis. *Kidney Int* 44(1): 191–8.

38. Scheel P Jr, Malan M (1996). Disposal of dialysate in HIV positive patients: an update. *Adv Renal Replacement Ther* 3(4): 298–301.

39. Davey P, Craig AM, Hau C, Malek M (1999). Cost-effectiveness of prophylactic nasal mupirocin in patients undergoing peritoneal dialysis based on a randomised, placebo controlled trial. *J Antimicrob Chemother* 43(1): 105–12.

40. SIPROCE study group (1997). Efficiency of a silver ring in preventing exit site infections in adult PD patient: results of the SIPROCE study. Silver ring prophylaxis of the catheter exit site. *Adv Perit Dial* 13:227- 32.

41. Wilson AP, Lewis C, O'Sullivan H, Shetty N, Neild GH, Mansell M (1997). The use of povidine iodine in exit site care for patients undergoing continuous peritoneal dialysis (CAPD). *J Hosp Infect* 35(4): 287–93.

42. Tanaka S (1996). Sealing the catheter exit site with dressing film and its effectiveness in preventing exit-site infection: bacterial culture. *Adv Perit Dial* 12: 214–17.

43. Bernardini J, Piraino B, Holley J, Johnston JR, Lutes R (1996). A randomised trial of *Staphylococcus aureus* prophylaxis in peritoneal dialysis patients: Mupirocin calcium ointment 2% applied to the exit site versus cyclic oral rifampicin. *Am J Kidney Dis* 27(5): 695–700.
44. Eklund B, Honaken E, Kyllonen L, Salmela K, Kala AR (1997). Peritoneal dialysis access: Prospective randomised comparison of single-cuff and double-cuff straight Tenckhoff catheters. *Nephrol Dial Transplant* 12(12): 2664–6.
45. Wikdahl AM, Engman U, Stegmayr BG, Sorenssen JG (1997). One-dose cefuroxime iv. and i.p. reduces microbiological growth in PD patients are catheter insertion. *Nephrol Dial Transplant* 12(1): 157–60.

18

Prevention and treatment of infections in vascular access

Mrinal K. Dasgupta

Introduction

The haemodialysis patient is continually susceptible to infection, vascular access providing a convenient avenue for bacterial entry. Environmental and autochthonous Gram-positive bacteria are the primary pathogens, although fungal and Gram-negative infections are not rare. Of the three types of long-term vascular access—the native arteriovenous fistula, the prosthetic arteriovenous graft, and the plastic central venous double-lumen catheter—the fistula is least likely to become infected.[1-6] However, as there are more and more patients who have no available sites for vascular access or who have started dialysis suddenly without the time for a planned fistula or graft implantation, the central venous catheters are becoming more widely used, and it is for this reason that the rate of infection in haemodialysis patients is steadily increasing.[7-12] Untreated infections lead to bacteraemia and distant metastases, fatal conditions in immunocompromised haemodialysed patients.[12,13] The treatment of infections and, more importantly, their prevention are thus topics which have received considerable attention in the literature of late, and many of the proposed and current protocols are still being debated.[4,5,10,11,13-16] The strategy is essentially to minimize the risk of contamination, to establish methods for early diagnosis, and to treat the infection with appropriate antibiotics as soon as possible. This chapter aims to discuss infections and to suggest preventive measures in relation to each type of vascular access.

Prevention

The key to reducing the incidence of access-related infections is an experienced team that participates in education in infection control, in developing local policies, in implementing continuous quality improvement, and in communicating with patients (see Fig. 18.1). Efforts to prevent infection begin when a patient is selected for dialysis. Immuno-compromised patients, anaemics, and those with a history of bacteraemia are at a high risk of developing access-related infection.[8,12,13,17] These patients should be monitored regularly for infections because early diagnosis and treatment prevent systemic spread of a localized endovascular infection. In the case of anaemia, one might also consider treating this disorder (and maintaining haemoglobin at or around 11 g/dl) as a measure of preventing infection.[17]

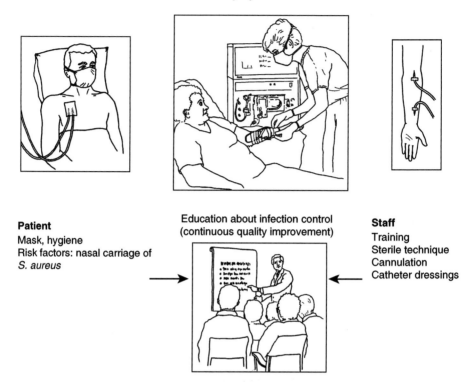

Patient
Mask, hygiene
Risk factors: nasal carriage of
S. aureus

Education about infection control
(continuous quality improvement)

Staff
Training
Sterile technique
Cannulation
Catheter dressings

Fig. 18.1   Several steps in vascular access infection control with special emphasis on continuous
quality improvement.

Whatever form of access is used, each must be surgically placed, and several patients
contract infections during this process. Prophylactic antibiotics are usually administered.[3] Once dialysis has begun, every type of access can become infected. In haemodialysis, the incidence of metastatic complications like osteomyelitis, endocarditis, arthritis,
etc. ranges from 8.7 to 50%, the highest risk of infection being with *Staphylococcus
aureus*.[12,13] The first choice for access is the arteriovenous fistula, because its complete
internalization and protection by the skin renders it the least susceptible to sepsis, the
rate of infection varying between 1 and 4%.[1,2] Theoretically, half of the patients selected
for dialysis ought to have fistulae, but in reality only one-tenth or one-fifth of haemodialysis patients have this form of access in the United States (European and Canadian
patients are more likely to have fistulae than are American ones).[17,18] Naturally, fistula
sites can become 'exhausted', in the sense that all of the suitable sites for fistula creation
have been used, and so dialysis patients who have been dialysed on fistula for several
years graduate to a graft or a catheter. But the reason for the rarity of fistula access in new
patients is that a large proportion of them are either elderly (and thus rarely have vascular access sites appropriate for fistula creation) or are diabetic (and might have peripheral
vascular disease and/or neuropathy). Additionally, several centres have inadequate
predialysis planning, the result of which is that over half of their new dialysis patients

have come through as emergencies. Since a fistula requires between 2 and 3 months to mature and to handle the volume of blood flow for dialysis, it cannot be used in patients who need immediate treatment for advanced azotaemia. Increasingly, therefore, the arteriovenous graft and the double-lumen dialysis catheters are being used in long-term dialysis access.[8–14]

The arteriovenous graft is ready for cannulation in between 2 and 4 weeks, and is still less susceptible to infection than is the catheter because, like the fistula, it resides underneath the surface of the skin. But the graft's PTFE (polytetrafluoroethylene) plastics promote adhesion by biofilms, and the consequence is that, of the 11 to 20% of arteriovenous grafts that become infected, many of them are colonized with pathogens resistant to antibiotics.[3,4] The silastic catheter is most prone to bacterial colonization as it lacks a protective endothelial lining, and its rate of infection does change with the duration of use and with the type of catheter.[19–22] Some catheters have cuffs whose Dacron promotes natural fibrosis, a protective shield against bacterial entry from the exit site. Consequently, the incidence of bacteraemia is higher in non-cuffed temporary catheters (from 1.6 to 7.7 per thousand catheter days) than it is in those with cuffs.[23,24] There are claims that the frequency of infection is lower with the tunnelled cuffed catheter (approximately 0.2 to 0.5 bacteraemias per thousand catheter days) but these have been refuted with another study that reports 3.9 bacteraemias per thousand catheter days (a rate of infection equivalent to that of non-tunnelled catheters).[10,11,13] These statistics suggest that the source of infection is not exclusively surface catheter colonization (and subsequent migration of bacteria towards the cuff), but rather intraluminal and even extraluminal colonization. Various factors contribute to infection, and one of the least regarded is time. The longer a catheter is kept within the patient, the greater the colonization of the catheter surface.[10–14,17] In short, the use of a catheter is discouraged, although the choice of access does depend on the situation of the individual patient. If a catheter must be inserted, then only trained professionals should be permitted to do so, and an in-dwelling catheter should not be used for more than 6 weeks, as its use in long-term access increases the risk of infection in haemodialysis.

The next step is to educate the patient and the dialysis staff in infection control.[25,26] The standard sterile technique for vascular access is to insist that both the patient and the staff wash their hands before the procedure, that the staff and the patient wear masks and gloves during the connecting and disconnecting steps, that the patient wears a mask during dialysis with a catheter, that all catheter exit site dressings are done with a touch of povidone iodine ointment and dry gauze (to prevent exit-site infections), and that only trained professionals are permitted to touch the access site and to cannulate.[27] The education of staff must be a continuous process. Initially, one should teach staff about how to cannulate as recommended by national guidelines, and how to identify the early signs of infection: redness, swelling and pus.[16,26] If any one of these is present, one should take skin swabs and blood samples for culturing, and change the dressing with each dialysis for patients with central venous catheters. It is imperative that the vascular access should not be used for any other purpose, such as giving fluids or intravenous alimentation, and also that an appropriate dose of anticoagulants is administered. Thrombosis of an arteriovenous graft or catheter is a condition of vascular blockage which results from insufficient administration of anticoagulants, its relevance to bacteria being that aggregates of blood are almost always sources of infection.[28] Lastly, incidences of infections, their outcomes, and their management should be recorded in each centre, and such data should be analysed periodically in relation to regional and national data for benchmarking. Discussions with staff regarding the trends in infection will help to identify specific problems and insufficiencies that require more attention, and which should be reviewed with the patients.

Because it is potentially a major cause of access infections, and because there is much controversy about how this problem should be best treated, nasal carriage of *Staphylococcus aureus* deserves special mention. To diagnose the nasal carriage of *S. aureus* involves taking periodic cultures from patients' noses, especially those who have previously had infections caused by nasal *S. aureus*.[29-31] But cultures are expensive, and several centres have tested the efficacy of prophylactic mupirocin treatment in preventing infections.[32,33] The cyclical nasal application of mupirocin is indeed successful, but because this sort of treatment encourages the formation of mupirocin-resistant *S. aureus* strains, and because patients find intranasal application of an ointment uncomfortable and are reluctant to administer this ointment intranasally, the debate continues about how much money should be allocated to nasal *S. aureus* detection.[32-34] A recent multicentre study has concluded that nasal *S. aureus* is not an independent risk factor for infection: although otherwise well designed, this study used a follow-up period of only 6 months, and analysed its data with a Cox model which cannot be accepted as definitive.[17] As further prospective studies of nasal *S. aureus* and its effect on vascular access infections are needed to resolve the controversy of how best to treat it, it is advisable to administer prophylactic mupirocin ointments in those patients who have repeatedly tested positive for nasal *S. aureus*, and who are at a high risk of developing access infections.[17] In the past some physicians have recommended the cyclical use of rifampicin to treat nasal *S. aureus*.[31] Randomized clinical trials show convincingly that the cyclical use of oral rifampicin is as effective as that of intranasal mupirocin, and that patients are much less reluctant about treatment.[31] However, in addition to discolouring contact lenses, rifampicin interacts with commonly used medications (like warfarin, β-adrenergic blockers, enalapril, phenytoin, cyclosporin, oral contraceptives, quinidine, verapamil, and digoxin) to make the antibiotic potentially toxic to dialysed patients. As a result, the use of rifampicin is strongly discouraged.

Total prevention of infection in haemodialysis patients with arteriovenous grafts or double-lumen catheters is not possible, but significant reductions in the rate of infection can be achieved with sterile technique, early diagnosis, and education of patients and staff in infection control. Predialysis planning with the creation of an arteriovenous fistula remains the ideal solution to the problem of vascular access infections.

Management

Diagnosis

The first manifestation of infection on the surface of the skin is usually a local swelling around the access, pain, and sometimes localized signs of phlebitis. As with any other endovascular sepsis, bacteraemia and distant metastases will follow if the local infection remains untreated.

The diagnosis of bacteraemia is first by examination and then by culture. Fever begins with bacteraemia, and if fever persists in a haemodialysed patient for no other obvious clinical reason, it is likely due to bacteraemia caused by an access-related infection. The final diagnosis, however, is by blood culture, the blood being drawn conventionally through the access line. Ideally, the blood sample should be taken not only from the access line but also from the peripheral vein so that the growth of the same bacteria can be confirmed from both the cultures, indicating that the source of infection is the vascular access. Discordant results between the two cultures may indicate a focus of infection different from the access. Also, for research purposes, a quantitative culture showing at least a four-fold difference in the growth of bacteria between the access line and the peripheral sample is required to confirm the diagnosis.[35] Clinically, blood cultures should be repeated after 48 to 96 h, regardless of whether the patient remains febrile after antibiotic therapy or not. One week after the course of antibiotics is completed, the physician should culture blood samples from both sites to determine whether all of the bacteria have indeed been eradicated, and whether metastatic infections have occurred.[13,21] Undiagnosed and untreated bacteraemia will result in the spread of infection to distant sites causing arthritis, osteomyelitis, and endocarditis (distant metastases). In severely immunocompromised patients, these conditions would be fatal. In fact, recurrent or unexplained fever despite a course of antibiotics, particularly in a patient who had been treated for *S. aureus* vascular infection should be thoroughly investigated for metastatic complications.[13,21]

As discussed above, the risk of infection varies with the use of different types of access, the type of organism involved, and the immune status of the host. An infected fistula usually responds to antibiotic therapy, whereas catheters and grafts cannot usually be salvaged solely with antibiotic therapy (because resistant biofilm bacteria adhere to plastics). The following sections give recommendations for infection management specific to the type of vascular access used.

Treatment of infections of the arteriovenous fistula

For local superficial infections not involving the fistula, the treatment should involve local antibiotics. Actual fistula infections and bacteraemia should be treated like endovascular infections with intravenous antibiotics for 6 weeks, starting with both Gram-positive and Gram-negative coverage, and changing to the appropriate antibiotic after the culture results are obtained. Such a lengthy period of antibiotic treatment is recommended to eradicate bacteria from the vascular track and to prevent distant metastases. The response to antibiotic therapy is generally quite good, and surgical removal of the fistula is rarely required.[1,2,7] However, in the event of clinical signs of septic emboli, the fistula should be removed.[16]

Treatment of infections of the arteriovenous graft

The treatment of arteriovenous graft infections always requires graft removal as adherent bacteria cannot be fully eradicated because they easily develop resistance to routine dosages of antibiotics.[4,19,20,36,37] Local graft infections without bacteraemia should be treated with oral or intravenous antibiotics. However, once antibiotic therapy has started, it is best to resect the local infected part of the graft (based on culture results from the local site), and then reconnect the uninfected graft material. Parenteral antibiotic treatment should be given to check systemic spread and to clear the vascular track (original site of graft and source of infection), in keeping with the principles of treating an endovascular infection. Bacteraemia is treated with the use of intravenous antibiotics, and extensive infection of the access requires total removal of the graft.[4,16,36] The intravenous antibiotics used are always determined by the type of organism and are thus based on culture results. The duration of antibiotic therapy is usually a minimum of 3 to 6 weeks after the removal of the infected graft. With *S. aureus* and fungi, for example, 6 weeks of treatment is recommended because their strong affinity for colonizing plastics make them difficult to eradicate and very likely to produce metastatic infections.

Treatment of infections of the central venous double-lumen catheter

General principles

The double-lumen dialysis catheter is made of silastic rubber (or polyurethane) which promotes thrombus formation and bacterial colonization with biofilms (bacteria encased in a sheath of polysaccharides that renders them resistant to routine antibiotic therapy).[19,20,28,37] As a result, treatment with antibiotics will be unsuccessful unless the catheter is removed and replaced. In practice, as these catheters are used in situations where an access site is exhausted, inaccessible, or unavailable, it may be difficult to remove the catheter.[7–12] Dialysis with a catheter must continue, even if it is only to allow the maturation of a graft or fistula. Different and desperate attempts at catheter salvage have been reported in the literature.[10,13,15,18,21–24] There is no real consensus about a general approach to management, and the following guideline, based on current literature, is proposed with the understanding that a delay in catheter removal could result in death (as one is dealing with endovascular sepsis), especially if the patient has other comorbid conditions.

Treatment of local exit site infections

Local exit site infections are predominantly caused by lax adherence to sterile technique (e.g. such as not wearing masks and gloves during dressing changes or during dialysis connections), particularly with patients or nurses who are nasal carriers of *S. aureus*.[12–16,26,30–33] Skin bacteria can also extend into the exit site to create infection.[27] The local exit site infection is indicated by pus underneath the dressings of the catheter exit site and by associated induration of the local tissue. The patient is usually asymptomatic except that some tenderness may be present if there is any tunnel involvement. These infections should be treated with local applications of mupirocin or other antibiotics, and with proper dressing changes.[16,26] Systemic antibiotics are not required unless signs of bacteraemia and/or tunnel infections are noted.

Treatment of systemic infections or bacteraemia

Bacteraemia is treated with intravenous antibiotics for at least 3 weeks. The catheter is usually removed if fever does not subside, if the second culture (after between 48 and

Catheter infections with bacteraemia

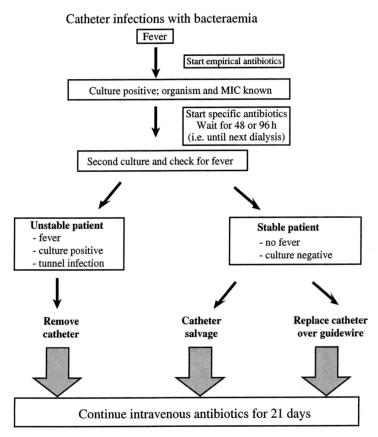

Fig. 18.2   A systematic approach to managing catheter-related systemic infections (bacteraemia) in both haemodynamically stable and unstable patients.

96 h) remains positive, or if there is evidence of tunnel infections (see Fig. 18.2).[13,16,17,21] In any case, so that dialysis can continue, most physicians attempt to salvage catheters with antibiotic management and by replacing the catheter over a guidewire.[13,21,38]

In immunocompromised patients. If infection of the vascular access remains untreated in immunocompromised patients, it will spread metastatically with potentially fatal conse-quences. With immunocompromised patients, antibiotic therapy should start when bacteraemia is diagnosed, and the catheter should be removed if there is persistent fever.[13,21] Even if fever subsides, if the second culture is positive the catheter should be removed and the patient investigated for metastatic infection.[13,21]

In haemodynamically stable patients with no other complications. The same method of therapy is followed for haemodynamically stable patients. If the culture is negative and fever subsides in between 48 and 96 h, one can attempt to replace the catheter over a guidewire or to continue antibiotic therapy to salvage the original catheter.[11,13,21,38,39] Catheter salvage has been reported by some to be very effective, and by others to be of questionable merit (with only 25 to 31% of salvage by antibiotic treatment being successful).[11,21,39] One should remember that results are difficult to interpret because studies report data based on cases from different centres, because there is no uniform protocol of study, and because a randomized, scientific, and safe study is difficult to do under the circumstances. However, a recent multicentre prospective study has demonstrated convincingly that antibiotic salvage of catheters failed in 68% of cases, and that, in a follow-up period of 3 months, only 16% of catheters could be successfully salvaged by antibiotic treatment (i.e. with no recurrence of infection).[13] This study also reported that the patients whose bacteraemia (fever) responded to antibiotic therapy after between 48 and 72 h had no increased evidence of distant metastases of infection (like arthritis, osteomyelitis, endocarditis) in relation to those whose fever did not subside in this short period.[13] This implies that if one uses the same protocol for infection management as the group which conducted this study, then one can attempt to salvage the catheter in patients whose fever subsides in between 48 and 96 h because they are least likely to have metastatic infections. In all other patients, one should remove the catheter, and insert a new one over a guidewire.[38] Antibiotic administration should be continued intravenously for 3 weeks after replacement of the catheter. The infection-free survival rate of catheters thus replaced is around 90% in 45 days, and it has also been reported that this replacement procedure does not increase the frequency of complications due to distant infections.[38] Since the catheter is the only avenue of access for many patients on haemodialysis, this procedure of catheter replacement enables dialysis to continue, and is thus an important recent advance in haemodialysis infection management for patients who fulfil the criteria mentioned above.

Antibiotic treatment for all access infections

Most of the infections are caused by *S. aureus* (between 40 and 77% for catheter access infections), streptococci, and *Pseudomonas*, and there have been recent reports of enterococci, all of which are either autochthonous or environmental.[4,7,8,13,17] Empirical therapy should begin by covering both Gram-positive (antistaphylococcal) and Gram-negative bacteria. An antibiotic—and its dosage—should be selected definitively based on culture results. It is important to note that with dialysis catheters all bacteraemia should be treated with antibiotics for at least 21 days, regardless of whether the catheter is being replaced or not.

Empirical therapy

Administration of vancomycin and gentamicin is the first choice of antibiotics for suspected infection and bacteraemia in vascular grafts. Vancomycin is given intravenously in a dose of 20 mg/kg on a weekly basis after the haemodialysis session. When using a dialyser with a large surface area or high-flux dialysis, the effective blood level of vancomycin should be monitored to maintain a trough level of 15 mg/litre or alternately to use 500 mg of vancomycin intravenously after each dialysis. The dose of gentamicin is between 1 and 2 mg/kg intravenously after each dialysis session. Gentamicin levels should be monitored for a peak greater than 7 μg/ml and for a trough less than 1 μg/ml. It should be noted that gentamicin has systemic side-effects, particularly ototoxicity. Due to concerns about vancomycin-resistant enterococci (VRE) infections, instead of vancomycin, cephalosporins like cefazolin (between 1 and 2 g intravenously) can be given in a single dose after dialysis. This is practiced in many centres and is probably safe; however, there are still no pharmacokinetics data for a single dose of cefazolin in dialysis patients reported in the literature. The final selection of antibiotics is, of course, guided by the microbiological culture and antibiotic sensitivity results. The duration of antibiotic treatment will depend on the type of bacteria and the type of access, as discussed below.

Specific antibiotic therapy

S. aureus infection are treated with vancomycin (20 mg/kg) once a week postdialysis intravenously for 6 weeks, or with cefazolin (between 1 and 2 g) after each dialysis intravenously. The vancomycin dose should be 500 mg every run if a high-flux dialyser is being used. For MRSA, vancomycin is the drug of choice.

Pseudomonas infections are treated with gentamicin as above. Once a culture reports that *Pseudomonas* is the pathogen, one should remove the catheter and use two antibiotics sensitive against that particular strain of *Pseudomonas*. Antibiotic therapy should be continued for 3 weeks.

Enterococcal infections are treated with a combination of vancomycin and gentamicin (as given above). To avoid vancomycin-resistant enterococci, vancomycin should be replaced with ampicillin (in a 1 g loading dose, followed by 500 mg every 6 h for the next 3 weeks).

Patients with fungaemia should have all catheters removed immediately, and be treated with amphotericin B with an intravenous dosage of 0.5 mg/kg/day. The catheter should be removed. A total of 500 mg of amphotericin B is needed, and a higher total dose is required for patients with diabetes mellitus or patients receiving steroids and hyperalimentation. In non-neutropenic patients, fluconazole should be given at a dose of between 200 and 400 mg orally daily to combat fungaemia due to *Candida albicans*. Fluconazole is not effective against *Candida* species other than *C. albicans*. For fungi other than *C. albicans*, flucytosine can be administered orally at a dose of 1000 mg/day. The antifungal treatment should be continued for 6 weeks after removal of the catheter.

The duration of antibiotic treatment for bacteraemia

The duration of antibiotic treatment for bacteraemia is still a controversial topic, and one about which there is no published consensus. From the above discussion, it is obvious that the length of antibiotic treatment really depends on the kind of access, the degree of colonization, and the consequent response of the access to antibiotic therapy. Bacteraemia can be a fatal condition if untreated, and the safest approach remains that which focuses on eradicating all of the bacteria and which thus prevents distant and/or recurrent infections.[13,17,21] A summary of the recommended duration of antibiotic therapy and of the expected response to treatment is given for each kind of access in Table 18.1.

The future of infection prevention in haemodialysis

As more and more patients are dialysed with central venous catheters, it is becoming obvious that the silastic rubber is prone to infection, and, due to colonization by

Table 18.1   Treatment of bacteraemia in vascular access

	AV fistula	AV graft	Catheter
Duration of IV antibiotic treatment	6 weeks	Between 3 and 6 weeks*	3 weeks
Response to antibiotic treatment	Good[†]	Poor[†]	Poor[†]
Removal or replacement of access	Removal often unnecessary	Resection always. Replacement in some cases	Removal in unstable patients. Replacemnt in stable patients. Antibiotic salvage attempted in stable patients meeting specific criteria

IV = intravenous; AV = arteriovenous.

*Most patients can be treated with antibiotics for 3 weeks, but in cases of *Staphylococcus aureus* and fungal infections, 6 weeks of treatment is necessary to prevent distant metastases.

[†]A 'good' response is one in which antibiotic treatment is sufficient to control the infection of the access, and removal or replacement are unnecessary. With AV grafts and catheters, the prognosis is 'poor' because biofilm colonization and subsequent antibiotic resistance necessitate removal and replacement of the catheter or graft.

resistant biofilm, always will be. Modifications have been made to the standard dialysis technique and catheters, with varying degrees of success. The antibiotic lock—in which vancomycin or ciprofloxacin (100 mg/ml in 5% sodium heparin) were injected into each catheter lumen between two haemodialysis sessions—was reportedly effective but unpopular.[21] Biomaterials that resist colonization and adhesion by biofilm bacteria are currently being sought. Recent efforts have been made to use an antibiotic-bonded catheter to prevent bacteraemia.[40,41] One such study describes the effects of using central venous catheters coated with rifampin and minocycline to be very success-ful in eliminating catheter colonization, while another study reported that the similar use of an antiseptic-impregnated catheter (chlorohexadine silver sulphadiazine) reduced the frequency of catheter-related infection.[40,41] Although the results of these randomized clinical trials are encouraging, these catheters were used for short-term temporary central venous access in patients who were not being dialysed. Silver-coated catheters have been created with the novel technology of ion-beam assisted deposits of silver on the surface of the silicone rubber.[42,43] The biocompatibility of these catheters has been investigated in several models of peritoneal dialysis, and it was determined that the catheters are indeed safe and have antibacterial properties.[44] There is, however, some concern about the silver released because it is taken up by macrophages, as demonstrated in an experimental longitudinal study in a rabbit model of peritoneal dialysis.[45] Further long-term studies with silver catheters are needed before they can be used routinely to reduce the incidence of access-related infec-tions. With both the antibiotic lock and with the antibiotic-bonded and silver-coated catheters, one is also presented with the grave problem of antibiotic resistance.[21,40,41,44]

Conclusion

Although the central venous double-lumen catheter is the access most susceptible to infection, current trends in the haemodialysis patient population are obliging dialysis physicians to use the catheter increasingly in permanent access. Infections are best prevented by sterile technique and infection control, education, benchmarking, and the use of an arteriovenous fistula or an arteriovenous graft. The management of infections varies with the type of access that has developed sepsis. Local infections are easily treated with local antibiotics, but bacteraemia and distant metastasis can result if infections are untreated. With the fistula, bacteraemia is not common, and most such infections are treated with antibiotics; the arteriovenous graft can become infected as well with adherent biofilm strains that are resistant to routine antibiotic therapy, and these generally require a partial or complete removal of the graft; the catheter is most likely to become infected, and, in most cases, it seems best to remove the colonized catheter and to replace it with another. Catheter salvage is possible under certain circumstances, and a recent study has described the group of patients most likely to respond favourably to catheter salvage and antibiotic therapy. As more patients are using the central venous catheter for dialysis access, it is becoming obvious that the silastic rubber must be replaced or altered to make its surface less prone to biofilm colonization. These issues have been reviewed recently.[46] Some of the suggested new alternatives to the silastic catheter are promising in that they are biocompatible and have antibacterial properties, but most have potential disadvantages (like increased bacterial resistance, possible systemic toxicity) that can only become apparent with long-term studies. At this point, the best solution to the problem of access infections is to develop a strong predialysis programme, and to ensure that most patients use an arteriovenous fistula for haemodialysis access.

References

1. Kherlakian G.M., Roedersheimer L.R., Arbaugh J.J., Newmark K.J., King L.R. (1986). Nine years' experience with internal arteriovenous fistulas for haemodialysis: Study of some factors influencing results. *Am J Surg*, **152**, 238–246.
2. Dunlop M.G., Mackinlay J.Y., Jenkins A.M. (1986). Vascular access: experience with brachiocephalic fistula. *Ann R Coll Surg Engl*, **68**, 203–206.
3. Odurny A., Slapak M. (1984). The use of Goretex (P.T.F.E.) for angio-access for chronic haemodialysis: the place of perioperative antibiotics. *Br J Clin Prac*, 134–137.
4. Bhat D.J., Tellis V.A., Kohlberg W.I., Driscoll B., Veith F.J. (1980). Management of sepsis involving expanded polytetrafluoroethylene grafts for haemodialysis access. *Surgery*, **87**, 445–450.
5. Suchoki P., Conlon P., Knelson M., Harland R.C., Schwab S.J. (1996). Silastic cuffed catheters for haemodialysis vascular access: thromolytic and mechanical correction of HD catheters malfunction. *Am J Kidney Dis*, **28**, 379–386.
6. Boyle M.J., Gawley W.F., Hickey D.P., Drumm J., Murphy D.M., Hanson J.S., Glacken P. (1997). Experience using the Quinton Permcath for haemodialysis in the Irish Republic. *Nephrol Dial Transplant*, **12**, 1934–1939.
7. U.S. Renal Data System. X. (1995). The cost effectiveness of alternative types of vascular access and the economic cost of ESRD. *Am J Kidney Dis*, **26**, S140–S156.

8. U.S. Renal Data System. VI. (1995). Causes of death. *Am J Kidney Dis*, **26**, S93–S102.

9. Kaufman J.L. (1995). The decline of the autogenous haemodialysis access site. *Semin Dial*, **8**, 59–61.

10. Dryden M., Samson A., Ludlam H., *et al.* (1991). Infective complications associated with the use of Quinton permcath for long-term vascular access for haemodialysis patients. *J Hosp Infec*, **19**, 257–262.

11. Moss A., Vasilakis C., Holley J., *et al.* (1990). Use of silicone dual-lumen catheter with a Dacron cuff as a long-term vascular access for haemodialysis patients. *Am J Kidney Dis*, **16**, 211–215.

12. Kessler M., Hoen B., Mayeux D., *et al.* (1993). Bacteraemia in patients on chronic haemo-dialysis. *Nephron*, **64**, 95.

13. Marr K.A., Sexton D.J., Conlon P.J., Corey G.R., Schwab S.J., Kirkland K.B. (1997). Catheter-related bacteraemia and outcome of attempted catheter salvage in patients under-going haemodialysis. *Ann Intern Med*, **127**, 275–280.

14. Hoen B, Kessler M, Hestin D, Mayeux D. (1995). Risk factors for bacteria infections in chronic haemodialysis adult patients: a multicentre prospective survey. *Nephrol Dial Transplant*, **10**, 377–381.

15. Raad I.I., Hohn D.C., Gilbreath B.J., Suleiman N., Hill L.A., Bruso P.A., *et al.* (1994). Prevention of central venous catheter-related infections by using maximal sterile barrier precautions during insertion. *Infec Control Hosp Epidemiol*, **15**, 231–238.

16. NKF-DOQI (1997). Clinical practice guidelines for vascular access. *Am J Kidney Dis*, **30** (suppl. 3), S179–S200.

17. Hoen B., Paul-Dolphin A., Hestin D., Kessler M. (1998). EPIBACDIAL: a multi centre prospective study of risk factors for bacteraemia in chronic haemodialysis patients. *J Am Soc Nephrol*, **9**, 869–876.

18. Widus D.W. (1993). Permanent vascular access: A nephrologist's view. *Am J Kidney Dis*, **21**, 457–458.

19. Dasgupta M.K., Ward K., Noble P., Larabie M., Costerton J.W. (1994). Development of bacterial biofilms on silastic catheter materials in peritoneal dialysis fluid. *Am J Kid Dis*, **23**, 709–716.

20. Raad I., Costerton J.W., Sabharwal U., Sacilowski M., Anaissie E., Bodey G.P. (1993). Ultrastructural analysis of indwelling vascular catheters: a quantitative relationship between luminal colonization and duration of placement. *J Infect Dis*, **168**, 400–407.

21. Capdevilla J.A., Segarra A., Planes A.M., Ramirez-Arellano M., Pahissa A., Piera L., Martinez-Vazquez J.M. (1993). Successful treatment of haemodialysis catheter-related sepsis without catheter removal. *Nephrol Dial Transplant*, **8**, 231–234.

22. Read I., Darouiche R., Hachem R., Sacilowski M., Bodney G.P. (1995). Antibiotics and prevention of microbial colonization of catheters. *Antimicrob Chemother*, **39**, 2397–2400.

23. Uldall P.R., Merchant N., Woods F., Yarworski U., Vas S. (1981). Changing subclavian haemodialysis canulas to reduce infection (Letter). *Lancet*, **1**, 1373.

24. Chessbrough J.S., Finch R.G., Burden R.P., *et al.* (1986). A prospective study of the mechanisms of infections associated with haemodialysis catheters. *J Infect Dis*, **154**, 579–589.

25. Kaplowitz L.G., Comstock J.A., Landwehr D.M., Dalton H.P., Mayhall C.G. (1988). A prospective study of infections in haemodialysis patients: patient hygiene and other risk factors for infection. *Infect Control Hosp Epidemiol*, **9**, 534–541.

26. Department of Health and Human Services, Centers for Disease Control (1995). Draft guideline for prevention of intravascular device related infections. Part I. Intravascular device-related infections: An overview, and Part 2. Recommendations for prevention of intra-vascular device-related infections. Notice of comment period. *Fed Regist*, **60**, 49 978–50 006.

27. Levin A., Mason A.J., Jindal K.K., Fong I.W., Goldstein M.B. (1991). Prevention of haemodialysis subclavian vein catheter infections by topical povidone iodine. *Kidney Int*, 40, 934–938.
28. Barzaghi A., Dell'Orto M., Rovelli A., *et al.* (1995). Central venous catheter clots: incidence, clinical significance and catheter care in patients with haematologic malignanacies. *Pediatric Haematol Oncol*, 12, 243–246.
29. Ena J., Boelaert J.R., Boyken L.D., Van Landuyt H.W., Godard C.A., Herwaldt L.A. (1994). Epidemiology of *Staphylococcus aureus* infections in patients on haemodialysis. *Infect Control Hosp Epidemiol*, 15, 78–81.
30. Goldblum S.E., Reed W.P., Which J.A., Goldman R.S. (1978). *Staphylococcus* carriage and infections in haemodialysis patients. *Dial Transplant*, 7, 1140–1148.
31. Yu V.L., Goetz A., Wagener M., Smith P.B., Rihs J.D., Hanchett J., Zuravleff J.J. (1986). *Staphylococcus aureus* nasal carriage and infections in patients on haemodialysis. *New Engl J Med*, 315, 91–96.
32. Glowacki L.S., Hodsman A.B., Hammerberg O., Meraw J., McNeill V., Card M.L., Potters H., McGhie K., Stitt L.W. (1994). Surveillance and prophylactic intervention of *Staphylococcus aureus* nasal colonization in a haemodialysis unit. *Am J Nephrol*, 14, 9–13.
33. Boelaert J.R., Van Landuyt H.W., Godard C.A., Daneels R.F., Schurgers M.L., Matthys E.G., De Baere Y.A., Gheyle D.W., Gordts B.Z., Herwaldt L.A. (1993). Nasal muporicin ointment decreases the incidence of *Staphylococcus aureus* bacteraemias in heamodialysis patients. *Nephrol Dial Transplant*, 8, 235–239.
34. Layton M.C., Patterson J.E. (1994). Mupirocin resistance among consecutive isolates of oxacillin-resistant and borderline oxacillin resistant *Staphylococcus aureus* at a university hospital. *Antimicrob Agents Chemother*, 38, 1664–1667.
35. Capdevila J.A., Planes A.M., Palomer M., Gasser I., Almirante B., Pahissa A., Crespo E., Martinez-Vazquez J.M. (1992). Value of differential quantitative blood cultures in the diagnosis of catheter related sepsis. *Eur J Clin Microbiol Infect Dis*, 11, 403–407.
36. Cheng B.C., Cheng K.K., Lai S.T., Yu T.J., Kuo S.M., Weng Z.C., *et al.* (1992). Long-term results of PTFE graft for haemodialysis vascular access. *J Surg Assoc ROC*, 25, 1070–1076.
37. Dasgupta M.K., Costerton J.W. (1989). Significance of biofilm adherent bacterial microcolonies on Tenckhoff catheter of CAPD patients. *Blood Purif*, 7, 144–145.
38. ZShaffer D. (1995). Catheter-related sepsis complicating long-term tunneled central venous dialysis catheters: management by guidewire exchange. *Am J Kidney Dis*, 25, 593.
39. Swartz R.D., Messana J.M., Boyer C.J., Lunde N.M., Weitzel W.F., Hartman T.L. (1994). Successful use of cuffed central venous haemodialysis catheters inserted percutaneously. *J Am Soc Nephrol*, 4, 1719–1725.
40. Raad I., Darouiche R., Dupuis J., Abi-Said D., Gabrielli A., Hachem R., *et al.* (1997). Central venous catheters coated with minocycline and rifampin for prevention of catheter-related colonization and bloodstream infections. *Ann Intern Med*, 127, 267–274.
41. Maki D.G., Stolz S.M., Wheeler S., Mermel L.A. (1997). Prevention of central venous catheter-related bloodstream infection by use of an antiseptic-impregnated catheter. *Ann Intern Med*, 127, 257–266.
42. Sioshansi P. (1994). New process for surface treatment of catheters. *J Artif Organ*, 18, 266–271.
43. Baumber R., Mestres P., Sioshansi P. (1994). New surface treated catheters for blood access (abstract). *J Am Soc Nephrol*, 5, 406.
44. Dasgupta M.K. (1997). Silver-coated catheters in peritoneal dialysis. *Perit Dial Int*, 7, 142–145.

45. Dasgupta M.K., Larabie M., Nation P. (1997). Migration of silver-laden macrophages after implantation: a cause of concern for long-term use of silver-coated catheters (abstract)? *Perit Dial Int*, **17**, S43.
46. Nassar G.M., Ayus J.C. (2001). Infectious complication of hemodialysis access. *Kidney Int*, **60**, 1–13.
47. Webb A., Abdalla M., Russell G. (2001). A protocol of urokinase infusion and warfarin for the management of the thrombosed haemodialysis catheter. *Nephrol Dial Transplant*, **16**, 2075–2078.
48. Wardowski T. (1998). High-dose intradialytic urokinase to restore the patency of permanent central vein hemodialysis catheters. *Am J Kidney Dis*, **31**, 841–847.
49. Tranter S.A., Donoghue J. (2000). Brushing has made a sweeping change: use of the endo-luminal Fas brush in haemodialysis central venous catheter management. *Aust Crit Care*, **13**, 10–13.
50. O'Riordan E., Conlon P.J. (1998). Hemodialysis catheter bacteraemia: evolving strategies. *Curr Opin Nephrol Hypertens*, **7**, 639–642.

19

Infections complicating diseases of the feet in renal patients

M.E. Edmonds and A.V.M. Foster

Introduction

Many of the amputations in patients with renal impairment are the result of infections complicating diseases of the feet. Diabetic foot infections are the commonest presentation of sepsis in the lower limbs of patients with renal insufficiency and are usually preceded by foot ulceration which may reach an incidence of 26% in patients with diabetic nephropathy.[1] Microalbuminuria is an independent risk factor for diabetic foot ulcers in type 2 diabetes as is a low creatinine clearance.[2] Patients presenting with pedal infections often have mild to moderate abnormalities of renal function and proteinuria is an established risk factor for amputation.[3-5] As well as increased morbidity, the combination of diabetes and uraemia has also been associated with mortality from sepsis; 17% of deaths in diabetic patients admitted to 28 German dialysis centres were due to septicaemia, mostly originating from diabetic foot problems.[6] However, even in uraemic diabetic renal patients, ulceration, amputation, and death are not inevitable.

The aim of this chapter is to enable practitioners in renal medicine to take control of foot problems and foot infections and to give enough simple practical information to enable outcomes to be improved. Because infection and amputation are often late events in the natural history of the renal foot and are nearly always complications of pre-existing disease, prevention of foot lesions is a crucial part of management. Early recognition of the at-risk foot, the prompt institution of preventive measures, and the provision of rapid and intensive treatment to control infection and achieve rapid healing can reduce the number of amputations in diabetic patients with renal disease.[7]

As diabetic patients are the most prone to develop foot sepsis, much of the emphasis in this chapter will be on the management of the diabetic foot which is the area of expertise of the authors.[8] We describe a simple staging system for the natural history of the diabetic foot. This has been developed to provide practitioners with a framework for diagnosis and management. It involves classifying the lower limb into the neuropathic or neuroischaemic foot, dividing the natural history of the foot into six distinct stages, and finally providing a simple plan of management for each stage, within a multidisciplinary framework.

Classification

There are five important risk factors for foot ulceration: neuropathy, ischaemia, deformity, callus, and oedema.[8]

For practical purposes, the diabetic renal foot can be divided into two distinct entities: the neuropathic foot and the ischaemic foot. However, neuropathy is nearly always found in association with ischaemia, and the ischaemic foot is best called the neuroischaemic foot. The purely ischaemic foot, with no concomitant neuropathy, is rarely seen in diabetic renal patients and its management is the same as for the neuroischaemic foot. It is always essential to differentiate between the neuropathic and the neuroischaemic foot as their management will differ.

Infection often complicates ulceration in both the neuropathic and neuroischaemic foot. It is responsible for considerable tissue necrosis in the renal foot and this is the main reason for major amputation.

The neuropathic renal foot

The neuropathic renal foot is warm, numb, and well perfused, with bounding pulses due to arteriovenous shunting, and distended dorsal veins. Sweating is diminished due to autonomic neuropathy, the skin is dry and prone to fissuring, and any callus will be hard and dry. The toes are clawed and the arch of the foot raised, leading to high pressure points on the sole of the foot, which is the common site of neuropathic ulceration, often associated with neglected callus.

Although renal osteodystrophy is less common in diabetic renal failure than other forms of renal failure, the renal diabetic neuropathic foot is prone to other bone and joint problems, especially the Charcot foot, which can cause severe deformity and subsequent ulceration leading to severe sepsis.[9] Thompson *et al.* found a 20% incidence of neurotrophic skeletal disease in diabetic transplant recipients but no Charcot joints and no evidence of neuropathy in non-diabetic transplant recipients.[10]

The neuroischaemic renal foot

The neuroischaemic renal foot is a cool pulseless foot with poor perfusion. It almost invariably has neuropathy. It can be a deceptively healthy pink or red colour. Oedema is common and may be secondary to cardiac or renal impairment. Intermittent claudication and rest pain are often absent because of neuropathy and the distal distribution of arterial disease. Plantar ulceration is rare, but ulcers are found around the margins of the foot. In the presence of infection or if tissue perfusion is critically diminished the neuroischaemic renal foot can develop gangrene with alarming rapidity.

The natural history of the diabetic renal foot

The natural history of the diabetic renal foot can be divided into six stages.[8]

- Stage 1: The patient does not have the risk factors of neuropathy, ischaemia, deformity, callus, and oedema which render him or her vulnerable to foot ulcers. Some patients with diabetes and non-diabetic renal disease will fall into this category but the majority of patients with diabetic nephropathy will have some of the risk factors as described below in stage 2. Diabetic nephropathy is the major cause of renal failure in diabetes, but approximately 10% of diabetic patients develop renal failure from other causes. These patients are less prone to foot problems than those with diabetic nephropathy.

- Stage 2: The foot is still intact but the patient has developed one or more of the risk factors for ulceration.
- Stage 3: The foot has a skin breakdown. This is usually an ulcer, but may include some minor injuries such as blisters, splits, or grazes which are portals of entry for infection. Any break in the skin of the foot of a renal patient should be regarded as a pivotal event on the road to amputation. Foot problems should receive treatment before renal replacement therapy is undertaken as sepsis and gangrene are contra-indications for renal transplantation.
- Stage 4: The ulcer has developed infection with the presence of cellulitis which can complicate both the neuropathic and the neuroischaemic renal foot.
- Stage 5: Necrosis has supervened. In the neuropathic foot, infection is usually the cause; in the neuroischaemic foot, infection is still the most common reason for tissue destruction although ischaemia contributes. However, the renal foot has a particular propensity for developing necrosis following trauma even in the absence of infection and ischaemia. The reasons for this are not entirely clear.
- Stage 6: The foot cannot be saved and will need a major amputation, after which the remaining foot will be at great risk of amputation.

Every renal patient can be placed into one of these stages and the appropriate management strategies then carried out. In stages 1 and 2, the emphasis is on prevention of ulceration. In stage 3, the presentation and management of foot ulceration is discussed. Finally, stages 4 and 5 address complications of foot ulceration, notably, cellulitis, and necrosis.

Multidisciplinary management

It is always necessary to take control of the renal foot to prevent progression to a higher stage, and management will be considered under the following headings: wound control, microbiological control, vascular control, metabolic control, mechanical control, and educational control.

Successful management of the renal foot needs the expertise of a multidisciplinary team. No one person can take control. Members of the team will include the physician, podiatrist/chiropodist, nurse, orthotist, radiologist, and surgeon.[11] It is helpful if the team works closely together, within the focus of the renal unit, and also meets regularly for ward rounds and radiography conferences. Each team member should be available quickly in an emergency. Some roles may overlap, depending on local expertise and interest.

Stage 1: normal foot

Presentation

By definition, the stage 1 foot does not have the risk factors for foot ulcers; so the diagnosis of stage 1 is made by screening patients and excluding risk factors. All diabetic renal feet should therefore be screened for these risk factors including neuropathy and ischaemia, and checked at every clinic visit. The screening procedure is described below. Regular screening of diabetic renal feet prevents amputation.[7]

Examination may also reveal common foot problems such as thickened nails, dry skin, fissures, blisters, fungal infections, and minor traumas which should be treated by a podiatrist. Verrucae are rare in diabetic renal transplant patients: at King's College hospital only two of 50 such patients had foot warts. We have seen secondarily infected periungual granulomas masquerading as ingrowing toenails in a non-diabetic renal transplant recipient which resolved when cyclosporin A was discontinued: all the toes were involved.

Neuropathy

Almost all patients with diabetic nephropathy have evidence of both small and large fibre loss in the feet, although the degree of damage is extremely variable. Small fibre loss predominates leading to loss of pain and thermal sensation before the large fibre modalities (light touch or vibration) are blunted. In a series of 56 patients with diabetic nephropathy attending King's College Hospital, the mean thermal threshold was 19.4±9.8 °C, range 5–30 °C, normal range 3.6–9.8 °C, and the mean vibration threshold was 22.5±15 V, normal range 3.1–10.2 V in the feet. Patients with neuropathy will feel no pain to warn them of the presence of infection and may continue to walk freely on an infected foot which results in rapid spread of sepsis. Renal patients should be screened regularly for neuropathy since sensation may only become impaired later in the course of their nephropathy. A simple inexpensive tool for detecting neuropathy is the monofilament.*[8]

Degeneration of sudomotor fibres leads to reduction in sweating which results in dry skin with plaques of hard callus that readily crack and cause ulceration. Autonomic dysfunction has been documented in patients with chronic renal failure of various aetiologies and virtually all patients with diabetic nephropathy have grossly abnormal autonomic function, although symptoms are variable.[12] In 41 patients attending with diabetic nephropathy, variation of heart rate with deep breathing was abnormal in fewer than 10 (mean value 2.7±2.3 beats/min).[14]

Ischaemia

The most important manoeuvre for detecting ischaemia is the palpation of the foot pulses. A small hand-held Doppler can be used to confirm the presence of pulses and to quantitate the vascular supply.† Absence of pulses and an ankle-brachial pressure index of less than 1 confirms ischaemia.

Medial calcification gives an artificially elevated systolic pressure, even in the presence of ischaemia. It is thus difficult to assess the diabetic foot when the pulses are not palpable, but the pressure index is greater than 1. It is then necessary to use other methods to assess flow in the arteries of the foot, such as examining the pattern of the Doppler arterial waveform or measuring transcutaneous oxygen tension or toe systolic pressures.[8]

---

*These can be obtained from Promedics Orthopaedic and Electrical Products, Clarendon Road, Blackburn, Lancashire BB1 9TA, UK.
†MultiDopplex, Huntleigh Diagnostics Huntleigh Healthcare, Unit 35, Portmanmoor Road, Cardiff CF24 5HN, UK.

Most diabetic renal patients have medial arterial calcification. The most striking feature is the presence of extensive digital arterial calcification which occurs on both feet and hands and is often associated with the occurrence of digital gangrene. Of 80 patients with diabetic nephropathy who had received a transplant, 11 developed digital gangrene and all had severe digital calcification.[13]

Deformity

Deformity often leads to bony prominences associated with high mechanical pressures on the overlying skin and ulceration. Deformity should be recognized early and accommodated in properly fitting shoes before ulceration occurs. Deformed Charcot feet are particularly prone to ulceration and infection.

Callus

This is a thickened area of epidermis which develops at sites of high pressure and friction and will ulcerate if neglected.

Oedema

Oedema is a major factor predisposing to ulceration, and often exacerbates a tight fit inside poorly fitting shoes. It also impedes healing of established ulcers and delayed healing puts the patient at increased risk of infection.

Management

Although the foot is not at risk, the following components of multidisciplinary management are still important to prevent the development of ulceration.

Mechanical control

Mechanical control is based upon wearing the correct footwear. Therefore, advice about footwear purchase is necessary and patients should be told the principles of good footwear.[8]

Metabolic control

Hyperglycaemia, hypertension, hyperlipidaemia, and smoking are risk factors for neuropathy, ischaemia, and, indirectly, via cardiac and kidney impairment, to oedema of the feet. Thus, tight control of blood glucose, blood pressure, and blood lipids is extremely important for preserving neurological and cardiovascular function. Patients should be advised to stop smoking.

Educational control

Many renal patients with diabetes behave in a reckless way as exemplified by walking barefoot, wearing unsuitable shoes, and picking their feet. In a group of 50 renal transplant diabetic patients treated at King's College Hospital, 31 patients suffered 86 episodes of trauma to their feet despite having been educated in foot care.[7] Advice on basic foot care, including nail-cutting techniques, the first aid treatment and early reporting of minor injuries and other foot problems, and the purchase of suitable shoes, should be given to all renal patients, and outcomes will be improved if the feet are checked regularly by the patients themselves.

Stage 2: the high risk foot

Presentation

The foot has developed one or more of the risk factors for ulceration: neuropathy, ischaemia, deformity, callus, and oedema. It is important to detect patients who have developed these factors by a regular screening examination (as described above).

Management

Mechanical control

Callus, dry skin, and fissures secondary to neuropathy should be treated by the podiatrist. Diabetic renal patients should never use proprietary corn and callus removers.

Deformities

Deformities in the neuropathic foot tend to render the sole vulnerable to ulcers, requiring special insoles, whereas in the neuroischaemic foot the margins need protection, and appropriately wide shoes should therefore be advised. Renal patients with risk factors should be assessed by an orthotist.[8]

Vascular control

Patients with absent foot pulses should have the ankle-brachial pressure index measured to confirm ischaemia and to provide a baseline, so that subsequent deterioration can be detected. If a patient has rest pain, disabling claudication, or the pressure index is below 0.5, then they already have severe ischaemia and should be referred for a vascular opinion. All diabetic patients with evidence of peripheral vascular disease may benefit from antiplatelet agents.

Metabolic control

Even though neuropathy or ischaemia may now be present, progression may be checked by treating hyperglycaemia, hypertension, hyperlipidaemia, and smoking. Oedema may complicate both the neuropathic and the neuroischaemic foot. Its main cause will be impaired cardiac and renal function which needs to be optimized.

Educational control

Because lost protective pain sensation is so prevalent in renal patients they need advice on how to protect their feet from mechanical, thermal, and chemical trauma. Renal patients must be warned that they lack sensitivity and should establish a habit of regular inspection of the feet so that problems can be detected quickly and help sought early.

Most diabetic renal patients will have retinopathy and if vision is impaired then patients will need help with early detection of foot problems.

Stage 3: the ulcerated foot

Presentation

It is essential to differentiate between ulceration in the neuropathic foot compared with that in the neuroischaemic foot.

Neuropathic ulcer

Trauma is the most common cause of ulceration in renal transplant patients but neglected callosity also frequently causes ulceration.[7] Tissue autolysis occurs below the plaque of callus and results in a small cavity filled with serous fluid that eventually breaks to the surface with ulcer formation. Twenty-five per cent of patients with diabetic nephropathy will develop neuropathic ulceration.[13] Dimensions of neuropathic ulcers are deceptive, and it is always important to probe an ulcer as this may reveal hidden depths, and also reveal a sinus down to bone suggesting osteomyelitis.

Infection may supervene at any time and will take the patient into stage 4. It is especially serious in immunosuppressed transplant patients. Galen's signs may be diminished and the patient will not complain of pain.

Neuroischaemic ulcer

Ischaemic ulceration usually occurs on the margins of the foot as a result of minor trauma from tight ill-fitting shoes. Ischaemic ulcers present as an area of yellow slough with a rim of erythema. Infection often complicates ischaemic ulcers and sepsis may spread rapidly through the foot, especially in the immunosuppressed transplant patient. Infection can lead to a digital vasculitis with thrombosis.

Management

The aim should always be to close the ulcer as quickly as possible, thereby lessening the risk of infection complicating the foot.

Mechanical control

In the neuropathic foot rapid healing can be achieved by the immediate application of some form of cast to reduce the plantar pressures. Various casts are available and include the Aircast, total contact cast, and Scotchcast boot.[8,15,16] If these are not available the foot should be offloaded with crutches and wheelchair. When the ulcer has healed the aim should be to prevent recurrence. The patient should be fitted with cradled insoles which are designed to redistribute weight bearing away from the vulnerable pressure areas and at the same time provide a suitable cushioning. These insoles usually need to be accommodated in bespoke shoes.[17] An orthotist can also supply suitable extra-depth shoes to protect the vulnerable margins of neuroischaemic feet.

Wound control

Debridement. Debridement is the most important part of wound control and is best carried out with a scalpel. It removes callus and enables the true dimensions of the ulcer to be perceived. Drainage of exudate and removal of dead tissue renders infection less likely. Debridement enables a deep swab to be taken for culture.

Dressings. Sterile, non-adherent dressings should cover all ulcers to protect them from trauma, absorb exudate, reduce infection, and promote healing. There is no evidence from large studies that any dressing is better or worse than any other; however, dressings should be lifted every day to ensure that problems or complications are detected quickly, especially in patients who lack protective pain sensation.

Microbiological control

The ulcerated renal patient is at great risk of infection as there is a portal of entry for invading bacteria. In the presence of neuropathy and ischaemia and uraemia the inflammatory response is impaired. Renal transplant patients' immunosuppression renders them at increased risk of infection and may reduce the signs and symptoms of infection. Many renal patients lack protective pain sensation which would otherwise automatically force them to rest. Uniform agreed practice on the place of antibiotics in the clinically non-infected ulcer has not been established, but it is important to maintain close surveillance of the ulcer to detect infection which would be an indication for antibiotic therapy.

Vascular control

If ulcers in the renal neuroischaemic foot fail to heal despite optimum treatment, the reason may be ischaemia. A careful vascular assessment is necessary. Angioplasty is a valuable treatment to improve arterial flow and is indicated for the treatment of arterial stenoses as well as arterial occlusions of less than 10 cm in length. If lesions are too widespread for angioplasty, then arterial bypass may be considered.[8] Once perfusion of the foot is increased, the patient's capacity to mount an inflammatory response and combat foot infection will improve.

Metabolic control

It is important to make sure that systemic, metabolic, or nutritional disturbances which retard healing of ulcers and render the patient susceptible to infection are minimized.

Stage 4: foot ulcer and cellulitis

Presentation

Infection is caused by organisms which invade the ulcer from the surrounding skin. Staphylococci and streptococci are the most common pathogens.[18] However, infections due to Gram-negative and anaerobic organisms occur in approximately 50% of patients.[19] Often infection is polymicrobial and the average number of isolates from patients hospitalized with pedal infections is three to five.[19] When staphylococci and streptococci are present together they can combine to produce a rampant cellulitis that extends rapidly through the foot producing marked necrosis within only a few hours. Enzymes from these bacteria are also angiotoxic and cause *in situ* thrombosis of vessels. If both vessels are thrombosed in the toe, then it becomes necrotic and gangrenous and this is probably the basis of so-called 'diabetic' gangrene in which tissue necrosis is seen only a few centimetres away from a bounding dorsalis pedis pulse. However, Gram-negative and anaerobic organisms may also cause *in situ* thrombosis. Both aerobic and anaerobic organisms can rapidly infect the bloodstream and result in life-threatening bacteraemia.

Infected ulcer

Local signs that an ulcer has become infected include colour change of the base of the lesion from healthy pink granulations to yellowish or grey tissue, purulent discharge, unpleasant smell, development of sinuses, undermined edges, or exposed bone. There may also be localized erythema, warmth, and swelling, usually associated with ulceration. In the neuroischaemic foot it may be difficult to differentiate between the erythema of cellulitis and the redness of ischaemia. However, the redness of ischaemia is usually cold, although not always so, and is most marked on dependency whereas the erythema of inflammation is warm.

Cellulitis

When infection spreads there is widespread intense erythema and swelling, and lymphangitis. Regional lymphadenitis, malaise, 'flu-like' symptoms, fever, and rigors may develop. In the presence of neuropathy, pain and throbbing are often absent, but, if present, usually indicate pus within the tissues, and palpation may reveal fluctuance suggesting abscess formation, although discrete abscesses are relatively uncommon in the infected diabetic foot. Often there is a generalized sloughing of the ulcer and surrounding subcutaneous tissues, which liquefy and disintegrate.

Severe infection can also present as a blue–purple discoloration when there is an inadequate supply of oxygen to the soft tissues. This is caused by increased metabolic demands of infection and an inability of the foot to respond to these by increasing blood flow to the area of infection. Blue discoloration can occur in both the neuropathic and also the neuroischaemic foot, particularly in the toes, and in the neuroischaemic foot must not be automatically attributed to worsening atherosclerosis of the leg arteries.

Subcutaneous gas may be detected by direct palpation of the foot and the diagnosis is confirmed by the appearance of gas in the soft tissue on the radiograph. Although clostridial organisms have previously been held responsible for this presentation, non-clostridial organisms are more frequently the offending pathogens: these include *Bacteroides*, *Escherichia*, and anaerobic streptococci.

Only 50% of episodes of severe cellulitis will provoke a fever or leucocytosis.[20] A substantial number of patients with a deep foot infection do not have severe symptoms and signs indicating the presence of deep infection. In most studies of limb-threatening infection in diabetic subjects, only 45–50% had a temperature about 38.5°C. However, when increased body temperature or leucocytosis is present, it usually indicates substantial tissue damage.[21]

Osteomyelitis

Infection of the soft tissues may be complicated by underlying osteomyelitis. If a sterile probe inserted into the ulcer reaches bone this confirms the diagnosis of osteomyelitis. Chronic osteomyelitis of a toe has a swollen, red, sausage-like appearance. In the initial stages, a plain radiograph may be normal, and localized loss of bone density and cortical outline may not be apparent until at least 14 days later. The radionuclide bone scan using technetium-99m diphosphonate is very sensitive but not specific for osteomyelitis. Gallium or indium scans may improve specificity but magnetic resonance imaging may be most helpful in demonstrating loss of bony cortex.[22] The definitive method for diagnosing osteomyelitis is by bone biopsy. However, bone biopsy may cause infection, and false negative biopsies have been described. Therefore there is no gold standard for the diagnosis of osteomyelitis and judgement is still based on clinical symptoms and signs.[21]

All renal patients presenting with cellulitis should have a radiograph of the foot to detect gas in the deep tissues, foreign body, and bony destruction secondary to infection.

Management

Infection in the diabetic renal foot needs full multidisciplinary treatment. It is vital to achieve microbiological, wound, vascular, mechanical, and metabolic control, for if infection is not controlled it can spread with alarming rapidity, causing extensive tissue necrosis and taking the foot into stage 5.

Microbiological control

General principles. Optimum treatment requires antibiotics and removal of sloughy infected tissue by debridement. At initial presentation, it is important to prescribe a wide spectrum of antibiotics because it is impossible to predict the organisms from the clinical appearance. It is therefore vital to send swabs for culture without delay in all stage 4 patients. Deep swabs or tissue should be taken from the ulcer after initial debridement and if the patient undergoes operative debridement then deep tissue should also be sent. Ulcer swabs should be taken at every follow-up visit. It is possible that bacterial species which are usually not pathogenic can cause a true infection in a diabetic foot when part of a mixed flora. As there is a poor immune response of the diabetic patient to sepsis, even bacteria regarded as skin commensals may cause severe tissue damage. This includes Gram-negative organisms such as *Citrobacter*, *Serratia*, *Pseudomonas*, and *Acinetobacter*. When Gram-negative bacteria are isolated from an ulcer swab, they should not be automatically regarded as insignificant.

Blood cultures should also be sent if there is fever and systemic toxicity. Close contact with the microbiologist is advised and it is helpful to do laboratory bench rounds to discuss management.

Antibiotic treatment. Infection in the neuroischaemic renal foot is often more serious than in the neuropathic foot which has a good arterial blood supply; therefore we regard a positive ulcer swab in a neuroischaemic foot as having serious implications, and this influences antibiotic policy.

Antibiotic treatment is discussed both as initial treatment and follow-up: dosage should be determined by the level of renal function and the associated mode of renal replacement therapy. There are few adequately performed randomized studies regarding antimicrobial treatment of foot infections. As a result, antimicrobial treatment is empirical.

The following regime has been developed in our unit based on many years of treating the diabetic foot and significantly reducing amputations.

1. Local signs of infection in the ulcer or mild cellulitis.
    - Initial treatment:
        - These are suitable for outpatient care, but if the patient is ischaemic, elderly, frail, or lives alone, arrange a daily visit from the nurse. Give flucloxacillin, metronidazole, and trimethoprim. If the patient is allergic to penicillin, substitute erythromycin for flucloxacillin. Cellulitis, on the borderline of mild to severe, can be treated with intramuscular ceftriaxone.
    - Follow-up plan (with reference to previous visit's swab):
        - If no signs of infection and no organisms isolated, stop antibiotics but if the patient is severely ischaemic with a pressure index below 0.5 consider continuing antibiotics until healing.
        - If no signs of infection are present but organisms are isolated, focus antibiotics, and review in 1 week.
        - If signs of infection are present but no organisms are isolated, continue the triple antibiotics as above.
        - If signs of infection are still present, and organisms are isolated, focus antibiotic regime according to sensitivities.
        - If methicillin-resistant *Staphylococcus aureus* (MRSA) is grown, but there are no local or systemic signs of infection, use topical mupirocin 2% ointment (if sensitive).
        - If MRSA is grown, with local signs of infection, consider oral therapy with two of the following: sodium fusidate, rifampicin, trimethoprim, or doxycycline, according to sensitivities, together with topical mupirocin 2% ointment.
2. Neuropathic and neuroischaemic renal foot with severe cellulitis
    - Initial treatment
        - Admission for intravenous antibiotics is the treatment of choice for this serious condition.
        - If admission is not possible, then give intramuscular ceftriaxone and oral metronidazole. Trace the distribution of the cellulitis with a marker pen so that extension can be detected and review in 2 days.
        - Patients should be on bedrest at home with daily visits from a district nurse to re-dress the foot and alert the renal unit if the foot is deteriorating.
        - On review as an outpatient, if cellulitis is controlled, continue intramuscular ceftriaxone and oral metronidazole, and review 1 week later.
        - If cellulitis is increasing, then admit for intravenous antibiotics. Quadruple therapy is indicated: amoxicillin, flucloxacillin, metronidazole, and ceftazidime. If patient is allergic to penicillin, replace amoxicillin and flucloxacillin, with erythromycin or vancomycin (with doses adjusted according to serum levels). On admission the foot should be urgently assessed as to the need for surgical debridement (see wound control).
    - Follow up plan
        - The infected foot should be inspected daily to gauge the initial response to antibiotic therapy.
        - Appropriate antibiotics should be selected when sensitivities are available.

- If no organisms are isolated, and yet the foot remains severely cellulitic, then a repeat deep swab should be taken, but the quadruple antibiotic therapy, as above, should be continued.
- If MRSA is isolated, give vancomycin (dosage to be adjusted according to serum levels) or teicoplainin. These antibiotics may need to be accompanied by either sodium fusidate or rifampicin orally.
- Intravenous antibiotic therapy can be changed to the appropriate oral therapy when the signs of cellulitis have resolved.
- Patients should be followed up weekly in the renal unit and antibiotic therapy adjusted as described above.
- Treatment of infected diabetic patients with home intravenous antibiotics may be complicated by systemic *Candida* infections.

Osteomyelitis
- Initial treatment. At first, antibiotics will be given for the contiguous infected ulcer and cellulitis as above.
- Follow up plan. On review, antibiotic selection is guided by the results of deep swabs, but it is useful to choose antibiotics with good bone penetration, such as sodium fusidate, rifampicin, clindamycin, and ciprofloxacin. Antibiotics should be given for at least 12 weeks. Such conservative therapy is often successful, and is associated with resolution of cellulitis and healing of the ulcer. However, if after 3 months' treatment, the ulcer persists, with continued probing to bone which is fragmented on the radiograph, then in the neuropathic renal foot we favour resection of the underlying bone, which often entails toe amputation or removal of metatarsal heads.

Wound control
Diabetic foot infections are almost always more extensive than would appear from initial examination and surface appearance.

It is wise to perform an initial debridement in the diabetic foot clinic so that the true dimensions of the lesion can be revealed and samples obtained for culture. Often callus may be overlying the ulcer and this must be removed to reveal the extent of the underlying ulcer and allow drainage of pus and removal of infected sloughy tissue.

Cellulitis should respond to intravenous antibiotics, but the patient needs daily review to detect evidence of spreading infection. In severe episodes of cellulitis, the ulcer may be complicated by extensive infected subcutaneous soft tissue. At this point, the tissue is not frankly necrotic but has started to break down and liquefy. It is best for this tissue to be removed operatively. The definite indications for urgent surgical intervention are: a large area of infected sloughy tissue, localized fluctuance and expression of pus, crepitus with gas in the soft tissues on radiograph and purplish discoloration of the skin, indicating subcutaneous necrosis.

In the neuroischaemic foot, any surgical debridement needs to be accompanied by an assessment of the arterial perfusion to the foot to evaluate the healing potential of surgical wounds. All of these patients will need urgent vascular investigation.

Vascular control

It is important to explore the possibility of revascularization in the infected neuro-ischaemic foot. Improvement of perfusion will not only help to control infection but will also promote healing of wounds if operative debridement is necessary. Doppler ultrasound studies may initially be carried out, followed by angiography. Alternatively, transfemoral angiography can be performed as the initial procedure.

Mechanical control

Patients should be on bedrest with heel protection with foam wedges.

Educational control

The importance of bedrest, giving complete off-loading of the foot, is paramount. Patients must understand that if they walk on an infected foot they risk losing their leg.

Stage 5: foot ulcer and necrosis

Presentation

This stage is characterized by the presence of necrosis (gangrene), which has grave implications, threatening the loss of the limb.

It is classified as either wet necrosis due to infection or dry necrosis due to ischaemia. Wet necrosis is secondary to a septic vasculitis (see below), associated with severe soft tissue infection and ulceration, and is the commonest cause of necrosis in the diabetic foot. Necrosis can involve skin, subcutaneous, and fascial layers. In the skin it is easily evident but in the subcutaneous and fascial layers it is not so apparent. Often the bluish-black discoloration of skin is the 'tip of an iceberg' of massive necrosis which occurs in subcutaneous and fascial planes, so-called necrotizing fasciitis.

Dry necrosis results from severe ischaemia secondary to poor tissue perfusion from atherosclerotic narrowing of the arteries of the leg, often complicated by thrombus and emboli. This may be acute but is usually chronic.

Digital necrosis is a relatively common problem in patients with advanced diabetic nephropathy. It may result from a septic neutrophilic vasculitis of the digital arteries. If this is diagnosed at an early stage when the toe is discoloured but not frankly black rapid treatment with intravenous antibiotics may save the toe. However, with the background of nephropathy, digital necrosis can occur in the absence of infection. It may be precipitated by trauma and is probably associated with undetected microvascular disease.

Wet necrosis

In wet necrosis, the tissues are grey or black, moist, and often malodorous. Adjoining tissues are infected and pus may discharge from the ulcerated demarcation line between necrosis and viable tissue.

Dry necrosis

Dry necrosis is hard, blackened, mummified tissue and there is usually a clean demarcation line between necrosis and viable tissue. Necrosis presents in both the neuropathic and the neuroischaemic foot and the management is different in both.

Neuropathic foot

In the neuropathic foot, necrosis is invariably wet, and is caused by infection complicating a digital, metatarsal, or heel ulcer, and leading to a septic vasculitis of the digital and small arteries of the foot. The walls of these arteries are infiltrated by polymorphs leading to occlusion of the lumen by septic thrombus.

Neuroischaemic foot

Both wet and dry necrosis can occur in the neuroischaemic foot.

Wet necrosis is also caused by a septic vasculitis, secondary to soft tissue infection and ulceration. However, in the neuroischaemic foot, reduced arterial perfusion to the foot resulting from atherosclerotic occlusive disease of the leg arteries is an important predisposing factor.

Dry necrosis is usually secondary to a severe reduction in arterial perfusion and occurs in three circumstances: severe chronic ischaemia, acute ischaemia, and emboli to the toes.

Severe chronic ischaemia. Peripheral arterial disease usually progresses slowly in the diabetic patient, but eventually a severe reduction in arterial perfusion results in vascular compromise of the skin, often precipitated by minor trauma, leading to blue toes which usually become necrotic unless the foot is revascularized and may become infected.

Acute ischaemia. Blue discoloration leading to necrosis of the toes is also seen in acute ischaemia, which is usually caused either by thrombosis of an atherosclerotic stenosis in the superficial femoral or popliteal artery or emboli from proximal atherosclerotic plaques in the iliac, femoral, or popliteal arteries. It presents as a sudden onset of pain in the leg associated with pallor of the foot, quickly followed by mottling and slate grey discoloration. The diabetic patient may not get paraesthesiae because of an existing sensory neuropathy, which also reduces the severity of ischaemic pain and may delay presentation.

Emboli to the toes. Another cause of necrosis, particularly to the toe, are emboli to the digital circulation originating from atherosclerotic plaques in the aorta and leg arteries. The initial sign may be bluish or purple discoloration which is quite well demarcated but which quickly proceeds to necrosis. If it escapes infection it will dry out and mummify. Microemboli present with painful petechial lesions in the foot that do not blanch on pressure.

Management

Patients should be admitted immediately for urgent investigations and multidisciplinary management.

Wound control

Neuropathic foot. In the renal patient with an infected necrotic neuropathic foot, operative debridement is almost always indicated for wet gangrene. The main principle of treatment is surgical removal of the necrotic tissue, which may include toe or ray amputation (removal of toe together with part of the metatarsal) or, rarely, trans-metatarsal amputation. Although necrosis in the diabetic foot may not be associated with a definite collection of pus, the necrotic tissue still needs to be removed. In the neuropathic foot, there is good arterial circulation and the wound, after debridement, always heals as long as infection is controlled.

Very occasionally, patients may not be suitable for or refuse operation, and the aim would then be to convert wet gangrene into dry by conservative treatment and intravenous antibiotics.

Neuroischaemic foot. In the neuroischaemic renal foot, wet necrosis should also be removed when it is associated with severe spreading sepsis. This should be done whether pus is present or not. In cases when the limb is not immediately threatened, and the necrosis is limited to one or two toes, it may be possible to control infection with intravenous antibiotics and proceed to urgent revascularization and at the same operation perform digital or ray amputation, which should subsequently heal.

If angioplasty or bypass is not possible, then a decision must be made to either amputate the toes in the presence of ischaemia or allow the toes, if infection is controlled, to convert to dry necrosis and autoamputate. Surgical amputation should be undertaken if the toe is painful or if the circulation is not severely impaired, that is, a pressure index greater than 0.5 or a transcutaneous oxygen tension greater than 30 mmHg.[8]

- Operative debridement. Consent should be obtained for the most extensive debridement anticipated, including digital or ray amputation. It is important to remove all necrotic tissue, down to bleeding tissue, as well as opening up all sinuses. Deep necrotic tissue should be sent for culture immediately. Wounds should not be sutured. A foot with a large gaping wound following extensive tissue removal may be lightly held together by winding long strips of paraffin gauze around the foot; however, the strips should be cut through to accommodate swelling and must not prevent drainage of exudate. In the neuropathic foot, irrigation with 2% Milton may be useful for 5 days. Skin grafting may be the best way to achieve healing of large tissue deficits. Ischaemic wounds are extremely slow to heal even after revascularization, and wound care needs to continue as an outpatient in the diabetic foot clinic, but with patience, outcomes may be surprisingly good.
- Autoamputation. Careful sharp debridement is performed along the demarcation line between necrosis and viable tissue to debulk dead tissue, drain pockets of pus, and prevent accumulation of debris. Dry sterile dressings are used to separate necrotic toes from their fellows, for if necrosis is in direct contact with viable tissue, it can spread. Patients should not bathe to ensure that necrotic tissues are kept dry, since moistening necrosis may encourage infection. Such neuroischaemic feet with dry necrosis may remain at stage 5 for many months and are followed up until the necrotic toe drops off to reveal a healed stump.

Microbiological control

Wet necrosis. The microbiological principles of managing wet necrosis are similar to those of the management of infection in stage 4. When the patient initially presents, send off deep wound swabs and tissue specimens for microbiology. Deep tissue taken at operative debridement must also go for culture. Intravenous antibiotic therapy (amoxi-cillin, flucloxacillin, metronidazole, and ceftazidime) should be given.

However, if the patient is allergic to penicillin, then erythromycin or vancomycin (dosage adjusted according to serum levels) may be used instead of amoxicillin and flucloxacillin.

Intravenous antibiotics can be replaced with oral therapy after operative debridement and when infection is controlled. On discharge from hospital oral antibiotics are contin-ued and reviewed regularly in the foot clinic. When the wound is granulating well and swabs are negative then the antibiotics are stopped.

Care should be taken to protect the feet of diabetic renal patients in hospital: of 50 renal transplant patients followed at King's College Hospital five developed heel sores, and three ulcers were caused by antithrombolytic tights after hospital admissions for problems unrelated to the feet.

Dry necrosis. When dry necrosis develops, antibiotics should be prescribed if discharge develops or the wound swab is positive, and continued until there is no evidence of clinical or microbiological infection.

When toes have gone from wet to dry necrosis and are allowed to autoamputate, antibi-otics should only be stopped if the necrosis is dry and mummified, the foot is entirely pain-free, and there is no discharge exuding from the demarcation line. Daily inspection is essential, regular swabs should be sent for culture, and antibiotics should be restarted if the demarcation line becomes moist or swabs grow organisms.

Vascular control

All renal neuroischaemic feet that present with necrosis must have Doppler studies to confirm ischaemia followed by arteriography to show stenoses or occlusions of the arteries of the leg, particularly in the tibial arteries. In wet necrosis, revascularization is necessary to heal the tissue deficit after operative debridement. In dry necrosis, which occurs on the background of severe macrovascular disease, revascularization is necessary to maintain the viability of the limb.

When dry necrosis is secondary to emboli, a possible source should be investigated.

In some patients, increased perfusion following angioplasty may be useful. However, unless there is a very significant localized stenosis in the iliac or femoral arteries, angio-plasty rarely restores to the foot the pulsatile blood flow which is necessary to keep the limb viable in severe ischaemia or to restore considerable tissue deficits secondary to necrosis. This is best achieved by arterial bypass.

Peripheral arterial disease is common in the tibial arteries, and distal bypass with an autologous vein has become an established method of revascularization, in which a conduit is fashioned from either the femoral or popliteal artery down to a tibial artery in the lower leg, or the dorsalis pedis artery on the dorsum of the foot. Patency rates and limb salvage rates after revascularization do not differ between diabetic patients and non-diabetic patients, and a more aggressive approach to such revascularization procedures should be promoted.[23]

Postoperatively, the leg has wounds both where the graft has been inserted and from where the vein has been harvested. Wounds overlying the arterial graft must be kept free from infection otherwise the graft will block. Such wounds need regular cleaning and covering with dry sterile dressings, and any associated necrotic tissue which becomes bulky or moist should be gently debrided.

Postoperative oedema is common and treatment with elevation and diuretics are important. The patient should enter a graft surveillance programme.

Mechanical control

During the peri- and postoperative period, bedrest is essential with elevation of the limb to relieve oedema and heel protection. After operative debridement in the neuroischaemic foot, especially when revascularization has not been possible, non-weight-bearing is advised until the wound is healed. In the neuropathic foot, non-weight-bearing is advisable initially and then off-loading of the healing postoperative wound may be achieved by casting techniques. If necrosis is to be treated conservatively, by autoamputation, which can take several months, then the patient needs a wide-fitting shoe such as a Drushoe to accommodate foot and dressings. Patients should walk as little as possible.

Metabolic control

When patients present with necrosis, against the background of severe infection or ischaemia, they may be very ill and will need close metabolic and haemodynamic monitoring.

Considerable metabolic decompensation may occur, and full resuscitation is required with intravenous fluids and an intravenous insulin sliding scale, which is often necessary to achieve good blood glucose control whilst the patient is infected.

Conclusion

Patients with impaired renal function are at increased risk of developing foot lesions. Once the skin is broken they are at a high risk of developing limb-threatening infection. They thus need very close screening, monitoring, and optimal foot care, especially if they have peripheral neuropathy or peripheral vascular disease.[24,25] Early diagnosis and aggressive treatment of foot infections in the renal patient will lead to a reduction in major amputations.

References

1. Moloney A, Tunbridge WMG, Ireland JT and Watkins PJ. Mortality from diabetic nephropathy in the United Kingdom. *Diabetologia* 1983; **25**: 26–30.
2. Griffiths GD, Wieman TJ. The influence of renal function on diabetic foot ulceration. *Arch Surg* 1990; **125**: 1567–1569.
3. Leichter SB, Allweiss P, Harley J, Clay J, Kuperstein-Chase J, Sweeney G , Kolkin J. Clinical characteristics of diabetic patients with serious pedal infections. *Metabolism* 1988; **37** (suppl. 1): 22–24.
4. Lehto S, Ronnemaa T, Pyorala K, Laakso M. Risk factors predicting lower extremity amputations in patients with NIDDM. *Diabetes Care* 1996; **19**: 607–612.
5. Moss SE, Klein R, Klein BEK. The 14-year incidence of lower extremity amputations in a diabetic population. *Diabetes Care* 1999; **22**: 6951–6959.

6. Koch M, Thomas B, Tschope W, Ritz E. Survival and predictors of death in dialysed diabetic patients. *Diabetologia* 1998; **36**: 1113–1117.
7. Foster AVM, Snowden S, Grenfell A, Watkins PJ, Edmonds ME. Reduction of gangrene and amputations in diabetic renal transplant patients: the role of a special foot clinic. *Diabetic Medicine* 1995; **12**: 632–635.
8. Edmonds ME, Foster AVM. *Managing the diabetic foot*, 2000. Blackwell Science, Oxford.
9. Clohisy DR, Thompson RC. Fractures associated with neuropathic arthropathy in adults who have juvenile onset diabetes. *J Bone Joint Surg* 1988; **70A**: 1192.
10. Thompson RC, Havel P, Goetz F. Presumed neurotrophic skeletal disease in diabetic kidney transplant recipients. *J Am Med Assoc* 1983; **249**: 1317–1319.
11. Edmonds ME, Blundell M, Morris HE, Cotton L, Thomas EM, Watkins PJ. Improved survival of the diabetic foot: the role of a specialised foot clinic. *Quarterly Journal of Medicine* 1986; **232**: 763–771.
12. Ewing DJ, Winney R. Autonomic function in patients with chronic renal failure on intermittent haemodialysis. *Nephron* 1975; **15**: 424–429.
13. Grenfell A, Bewick M, Snowden S, Watkins PJ, Parsons V. Renal replacement for diabetic patients: experience at King's College Hospital 1980–89. *Quarterly Journal of Medicine* 1992; **85**: 861–874.
14. Gilbey SG, Walters H Edmonds ME, Archer AG, Watkins PJ, Parsons V *et al*. Calcification, autonomic neuropathy and peripheral blood flow in patients with diabetic nephropathy. *Diabetic Med* 1989; **6**: 37–42.
15. Coleman WC, Brand PW, Birke JA. The total contact cast: a therapy for plantar ulceration on insensitive feet. *J Am Pod Assoc* 1984; **74**: 548.
16. Burden AC, Jones GR Jones R, Blandford RL.Use of the Scotchcast boot in treating diabetic foot ulcers. *British Medical Journal* 1983; **286**: 1555–1557.
17. Uccioli L, Aldeghi A, Faglia E *et al*. Manufactured shoes in the prevention of diabetic foot ulcers. *Diabetes Care* 1995; **18**: 1376–1378.
18. Lipsky BA. A current approach to diabetic foot infections. *Current Infectious Disease Reports* 1999; **1**: 253–260.
19. Grayson ML. Diabetic foot infections: antimicrobial therapy. In: Eliopoulos GM (ed.) *Infectious disease clinics of North America*, 1995, pp. 143–162. WB Saunders, Philadelphia, PA.
20. Armstrong DG, Lavery LA, Sariaya M, Ashry H. Leukocytosis is a poor indicator of acute osteomyelitis of the foot in diabetes mellitus. *J Foot Ankle Surg* 1996; **4**: 280–283.
21. The International Working Group on the Diabetic Foot. *International consensus on the diabetic foot*, 1999.
22. Longmaid III HE, Kruskal JB. Imaging infections in diabetic patients. In: Eliopoulos GM (ed.) *Infectious disease clinics of North America*, 1995, pp. 163–182. WB Saunders, Philadelphia, PA.
23. Pomposelli FB, Marcaccio EJ, Gibbons GW *et al*. Dorsalis pedis arterial bypass: durable limb salvage for foot ischaemia in patients with diabetes mellitus. *J Vasc Surg* 1995; **21**: 375–38.
24. Ritz E, Koch M, Fliser D, Schwenger V. How can we improve prognosis in diabetic patients with end-stage renal disease? *Diabetes Care* 1999; **22**: B80–B83.
25. Schömig M, Ritz E, Standl E, Allenberg J. The diabetic foot in the dialyzed patient. *J Am Soc Nephrol* 2000; **11**: 1153–1159.

20

Travel and vaccination in renal patients

Aine Burns

Introduction

Patients suffering from renal failure, whether victims of pharmacologically inflicted and/or pathophysiologically mediated immunosupression (Chapter 2) are at greater risk of succumbing to and dying from infectious diseases. Preventive and treatment strategies used in the general population are not as effective in renal patients. The enormous success of renal replacement therapies and particularly renal transplantation over the past three to four decades has led to an explosion in the numbers of 'at-risk' renal patients. Improved patient well-being has also led to an expectancy by patients and their families of travel abroad despite the inherent added risk of infection that this brings. The more widespread use of ever more powerful immunosuppressant drugs will be likely to further increase the susceptibility to infection in renal patients in the future. Thus, our success as renal and transplant physicians combined with the introduction of the Boeing 747 in the 1970s has brought about a number of new dilemmas in respect of travel and vaccination for renal patients. With regard to vaccination there are many factors such as patient age, illness, degree of renal failure, mode and adequacy of dialysis, nutritional status, amount and type of current or previous immunosupression, organ transplantation, vaccine type and design, manufacturing procedures, dose site, method and regimen of administration, and use of adjuncts and immune modulators which may influence responsiveness and therefore efficacy. This chapter will review the currently available information with regard to travel and vaccination in renal patients.

Vaccination in renal patients

There is little doubt that immunization has been of enormous benefit to humankind since its first use over 200 years ago in the fight against smallpox. We already take for granted that patients of our generation do not have to contend with the risk of smallpox and there is currently a realistic expectation that poliomyelitis will be eradicated globally within a few years. It is hoped that measles eradication will follow. The advent of molecular biological techniques of genetic manipulation together with a better understanding of the processes of infection, immunity, and tolerance has led to more and better vaccines becoming available. But despite these advances there is in general an alarmingly poor uptake by healthy individuals within existing immunization programmes which leaves a pool of non-immunized people who pose a considerable risk of preventable diseases to the immunocompromized population in particular. This failure to implement effective programmes of immunization may result in part from apathy about diseases now rarely encountered by family doctors, but there is also considerable ignorance about vaccination together with widespread misinterpretation of the contraindications and exaggerated concerns about the medicolegal consequences of a vaccine reaction.

Impact of chronic renal failure and end-stage renal failure on responses to immunization

Implementing preventive measures to avoid infection in renal patients is clearly very relevant to nephrologists, yet such efforts are less effective than in the general population. Patients with renal impairment and end-stage renal failure have a reduced response to vaccination which is related to the general suppression of the immune system and in particular to impaired cellular immune responses which are especially relevant where the antigenic vaccines require T-cell help for antibody response (e.g. influenza and hepatitis B).[1] Renal patients not only make reduced antibody responses following vaccination but the response is also short-lived when compared with patients with normal renal function. Over 90% of people with normal renal function respond to hepatitis B vaccine; this falls to only 50–60% in the dialysis population.[2] The response to a vaccine is proportional to the degree of renal failure but the mode of dialysis makes little difference.[3,4] There is emerging evidence to suggest that improved adequacy of dialysis may improve immune responsiveness.[5] Others have claimed better responses with newer vaccines and using different modes, frequencies, and doses of vaccine delivered.[6]

Risks associated with vaccination

The risks associated with vaccination in a healthy population are very small. In the United Kingdom in 1995, out of 14 million doses of vaccines distributed there were only 152 reports of reactions classified as serious by the Department of Health, i.e. approximately one per 100 000 distributed doses of vaccine.[7] Many more patients, however, suffer mild side-effects of vaccination such as self-limiting fevers, rashes, or injection site reactions, though it is often difficult to be sure that the reaction is caused by a particular vaccine. In the context of the renal patient, however, these albeit small risks are greater. It is difficult to quantify this increased risk but it has to be viewed against the risks of developing a particular disease and the likelihood of increased morbidity and mortality from that disease in a compromised host. In general, the non-immunized healthy population pose a far greater risk to the renal patient than the vaccine. However, immuno-supressed renal patients are at risk of disseminated infection from certain live vaccines whether administered deliberately or acquired through contact with an individual who is shedding the live attenuated organism postvaccination. There is no evidence to suggest that immune-competent patients with renal failure are at risk of disseminated infection from live attenuated vaccines used in immunization, and although responses to vaccination are poorer than normal some protection is conferred. It is recommended therefore that the immune-competent renal patient and their close contacts should proceed with vaccinations as for the normal population. The length of time which should elapse between withdrawal of immunosuppressive treatment and the administration of live vaccines is debatable. It is probably safe to use live vaccines 6 months after treatment has stopped, but some authorities prefer to wait 1 year, particularly if the amount of immunosuppression the patient has received is high or if the patient has undergone serotherapy with ATG, OKT3, or other monoclonal antibodies.

The greatest fears are with the oral polio and BCG vaccines. Oral poliomyelitis vaccine should not be given to immunosuppressed patients, their children, or household contacts for fear of paralytic poliomyelitis from the vaccine virus. Inactivated poliomyelitis vaccine which is not dangerous should be given instead but it may be ineffective. BCG vaccine is contraindicated in immunosupressed patients. Patients considered at risk of acquiring tuberculosis for the first time or those likely to suffer reactivation of old tuberculosis because of illness or immunosupression should be considered instead for prophylactic treatment with oral isoniazid or an equivalent drug.

Although measles, mumps, and rubella (MMR) are live though attenuated vaccines and should not be administered to immunosuppressed patients, there is no risk of transmission of virus following MMR immunization of contacts, and the children, siblings, and close contacts of such patients should be immunized against these diseases. Similarly, no adverse effects have been reported following MMR vaccination in HIV-positive individuals who are at increased risk from these diseases.

The immunosuppressed patient

The definition of 'immunosuppression' in renal patients is controversial. There is clearly no ambiguity where patients have received an organ transplant and are on immunosupressive treatment. However, other renal patients with impaired renal function demonstrate poor cell-mediated immune responses and are frequently given oral corticosteroids as part of their treatment regimen and are in practice immunosuppressed. Children who receive prednisolone orally or rectally at a daily dose (or its equivalent) of 2 mg/kg/day for at least 1 week or 1 mg/kg/day for 1 month are advised against having live virus vaccines. For adults an equivalent dose of steroids is harder to define, but immunosuppression should be considered in those who receive 40 mg of prednisolone per day for more than 1 week. Administration of live vaccines should be postponed for at least 3 months after immunosuppressive treatment is stopped. Patients receiving lower doses of steroids given in combination with cytotoxic agents or serotherapy (ATG or equivalent poly/monoclonal antibodies designed to decrease cell-mediated immunity) are equally if not more at risk from immunosupression and should therefore not be given live vaccines except under exceptional circumstances. What effect newer agents such as mycophenylate mofetil will have on antibody responses to vaccines is uncertain but animal work suggests that this drug reduces B-cell responses to antigenic stimuli.[8]

Killed inactivated vaccines such as diphtheria, tetanus, pertussis, and inactivated polio vaccine and recombinant antigen vaccines, e.g. hepatitis B, are safe though the immune response is less. Fortunately, most adult renal patients have already been immunized against measles but in the paediatric field measles tragically kills immunosuppressed children each year. The best protection against measles in the immunosuppressed is a high prevalence of immunity in the community minimizing exposure for the patient and their family. It is important that sibling and close contacts of immunosuppressed patients be appropriately immunized. Recipients of measles vaccine are not normally infectious to others, although some people prefer to restrict contact with the immunosuppressed patient for 2 weeks after vaccination. Similarly, close contacts of an immunosuppressed patient who requires polio vaccination should receive inactivated polio vaccine instead of the oral vaccine as discussed above.

At the time of commencement of immunosupression in renal patients serological evidence of immunity or lack of it to measles, mumps, rubella, and chickenpox should be documented. If subsequent exposure to these infections occurs in an antibody-negative individual prophylactic immunoglobulin should be administered as soon as possible, although their value is controversial. Human normal immunoglobulin and specific immunoglobulins for varicella zoster and measles are available. Recently, a live attenuated vaccine against chickenpox has become available and we have used it successfully to immunize two zoster-antibody-negative renal transplant patients whose occupation made exposure to chickenpox likely. It is anticipated that pretransplant vaccination of at-risk zoster-antibody-negative individuals will become the norm in future. In view of the very high morbidity and mortality of chickenpox in the immunosupressed this will undoubtedly be a welcome development.

Response to immunization in organ transplant recipients

Whether a patient will respond to a particular vaccine after organ transplantation clearly varies depending on the vaccine, the degree of immunosupression, and perhaps the immune responsiveness of that individual. Post-transplantation impaired immune responses have been shown for influenza, hepatitis B, and pneumococcal vaccines.[9,10] However, tetanus and inactivated polio vaccinations are well tolerated and induce protective antibody levels (although lower titres than in the normal population). Girndt *et al.* have shown that the level of antibody response to vaccination with tetanus toxoid is poorer in transplant patients than in patients with chronic renal failure or on haemodialysis, although the non-responder rate was much higher in their chronic renal failure (11/20=55%) and haemodialysis (16/23=69%) patient groups compared with either control individuals (15/15=100%) with normal renal function or those with renal transplants (6/7=85%).[11] Interestingly, in this study prior successful vaccination with hepatitis B vaccine was associated with a good response to the tetanus toxoid vaccine in all groups which may imply that an individual's immune responsiveness is more important than the degree of renal impairment, the mode of dialysis, or the presence of immunosupression.[11] For diphtheria, vaccination has been found to be less effective in transplant patients and antitoxin levels decrease rapidly within 1 year of vaccination.[12] A further confounding variable may be the choice of immunosupressive regimen as renal transplant patients receiving azathioprine have been shown to respond better to influenza vaccine than those receiving cyclosporine.[13]

Recommended routine vaccination for adult renal patients

The following section deals with vaccines recommended for First World renal patients not planning to travel abroad.

Influenza

The immune-competent renal patient with significantly impaired or dialysis-dependent renal failure is at increased risk of bacterial superinfections following viral upper respiratory tract infections and community-acquired pneumonias. Influenza viruses are common pathogens and by far the greatest morbidity and mortality from influenza is amongst those with underlying diseases including renal failure and pharmacological immunosuppression. It is recommended that 'at-risk' patients receive influenza vaccination annually. There is now good evidence that immunization of those at high risk reduces hospital admissions and deaths.[14,15] The two types of influenza virus which are responsible for most cases (A and B) are highly infectious and are responsible for upwards of 3000 deaths in the United Kingdom each year, especially in the elderly population. Vaccine development against both viruses has been hampered by 'antigenic drift' (changes in principal antigens) which occurs in both viruses but more so with influenza A than B. Major changes in the virus 'antigenic shift' occur infrequently, but when they occur the new viral subtypes can cause epidemics and pandemics. The World Health Organization monitors influenza viruses throughout the world and makes recommendations about the strains to be included in vaccines for subsequent years. The vaccines are prepared each year. They are derived from chemically inactivated whole viruses which undergo further treatment and purification and are usually a combination of three types (two influenza A and one influenza B). The purification procedures produce two types of vaccine either 'split virus' or 'surface antigen'. Both are equally effective and safe, but the latter contains highly purified antigen prepared from disrupted virus particles. The antibody response to these vaccines is similar to that of the general population, unlike other vaccines in haemodialysis and chronic renal failure patients. Annual influenza vaccination is therefore recommended to all chronic dialysis and chronic renal failure patients.[16] Similarly, most units recommend annual influenza vaccination for all renal transplant recipients.

Pneumococcus

Vaccination against pneumococcal infection is recommended by the United Kingdom Department of Health for all patients, including renal patients, who are at risk of developing pneumococcal infection, although the evidence that pneumococcal vaccination prevents pneumonia, bacteraemia, or meningitis, particularly in immunocompromized patients, is uncertain and the lack of a reliable, readily available test for pneumococcal pneumonia makes interpretation of trial results difficult despite the use of this vaccine in the United Kingdom since 1979. Pneumococcal pneumonia is the most common cause of community-acquired pneumonia, accounting for 5–28% of such infections in the United Kingdom, and the death rate from bacteraemic pneumococcal infection can reach 55%.[17] The immunosupressed renal patient is particularly at risk, but there is also increased risk to diabetic renal patients, those with nephrotic syndrome, hypocomplementaemia, and those with chronic renal failure. A disturbing increase in penicillin and erythromycin resistance of *Stretococcus pneumoniae* in the United Kingdom (1.5% in 1990 to 3.9% in 1995 for penicillin and 2.8% to 8.6% for erythromycin) further emphasizes the need for prevention. The currently available pneumococcal vaccines (Pneumovax II (Pasteur Merieux) and Pnu-Imune (Wyeth)) contain polyssccharide elements from 23 different types of *S. pneumoniae* which should cover more than 90% of likely organisms in the United Kingdom. An estimation of antibody response to pneumococcal vaccine is used as a marker for protective immunity following vaccination. However, there is no agreement on what antibody level protects against pneumococcal disease and antibody responses to only a few of the serotypes are usually measured. A good antibody response (four- to eight-fold increase of antibody titre) in an immunocompetent individual is usually seen by about 4 weeks after vaccination. However, antibody responses are likely to be poor and/or poorly sustained in renal patients. Such patients should therefore be vaccinated as early as possible in the course of a progressive disorder. Previous reports evaluating the 14-valent vaccine in patients with renal diseases have reported weak and delayed immune response in adult patients with renal failure and on dialysis. However, Fuchshuber's group in Cologne, using the newer 23-valent pneumococcal vaccine, observed a four-fold or greater increase in antibody response postvaccination in 83% of their 40 children with chronic renal disease (including patients with nephrotic syndrome, chronic renal failure, those undergoing both haemodialysis and peritoneal dialysis, and renal transplant patients) but only 68% had sustained this response at 6 months and by 1 year fewer than half (48%) had an adequate antibody titre.[6] It is unclear how long pneumococcal vaccination protects against infection, and estimates range from 3–8 years in the normal population. The Department of Health advise revaccination every 5–10 years for individuals with chronic renal failure or nephrotic syndrome but some groups believe that earlier revaccination should be advocated, especially as the concerns regarding risks of revaccination in those with high circulating antibody levels seem to be unjustified.[18] Pneumococcal and influenza vaccination can safely be given at the same time, at a different site.

Hepatitis B

Hepatitis B status needs to be established as early as possible in patients with renal impairment. If hepatitis B surface antigens and core antibodies are negative, hepatitis B vaccination should be embarked upon as soon as it is recognized that the patient is likely to require renal replacement therapy, as responses are likely to diminish with declining renal function.[19] Currently, there are two types of hepatitis B vaccine available: plasma-derived and recombinant. The former was developed from chemically inactivated hepatitis B surface antigen (HBsAg) particles obtained from chronic HBsAg carriers and was licenced in the United States in the early 1980s.[20] Over 90% of normal individuals under 40 years of age would be expected to mount a protective response following vaccination with this plasma-derived hepatitis B vaccine. The antibody response decreases with age to 80% in the elderly.[21] This figure falls further to between 50 and 60% in the dialysis population and is felt, in general, to be proportional to the degree of residual renal function and the age of the patient. More recently, DNA recombinant technology has produced a new vaccine which is produced in yeast and has equivalent immunogenicity to the older vaccine.[22] Virtually all normal individuals who generate an adequate antibody response to this vaccine have long-lasting protective immunity. An antibody titer of >10 IU/litre has been shown to be protective, but titers of >100 IU/litre are known to be more effective and dialysis patients attaining these levels are more likely to retain adequate immunity. In one study of 56 haemodialysis patients given three 40 µg doses of hepatitis B vaccine into the deltoid muscle, 92% of vaccinated patients achieving a maximum antibody response of between 10 and 100 IU/litre had lost their protection compared with only 3% of those who achieved an initial response of >100 IU/litre.[23] Although routine immunization of dialysis patients is recommended, common sense suggests that vaccination should be performed at the earliest opportunity; using this argument together with an augmented vaccination regimen immunization efficacy as high as 82% has been achieved in patients with chronic renal failure (creatinine clearance above 20 ml/min).[24] Other groups using various methods such as reinforced protocols (double doses at more frequent intervals), differing modes of injection (intradermal versus intramuscular), addition of low-dose interleukin 2 by intramuscular injection following the hepatitis B vaccination, and adjuvant immune stimulation to enhance vaccine efficacy in the dialysis population have been less successful. Gluteal injections have also been associated with decreased response rates.[25–32] Recombinant vaccines which contain additional hepatitis B surface antigens (responsible for viral attachment to target cells) compared with conventional hepatitis vaccines may prove to be effective in patients who are vaccine resistant, but whether these confer advantages in the renal population is unknown.[33] The cost and relatively poor success rate of hepatitis B vaccination programmes together with the low incidence of hepatitis B infection in United Kingdom dialysis units has meant that many units no longer follow an aggressive policy of hepatitis B vaccination. Therefore, renal units must be especially vigilant in their daily routines. Hepatitis B surface antigen-positive patients should continue to be dialysed separately from negative patients and special care needs to be paid to patients returning or originating from areas of high hepatitis B prevalence and for 6 months following their return until hepatitis B status can be established with certainty. There is, however, no benefit in repeated booster vaccinations in those patients who do not make a response to four separate administrations of double-dose (40 mg) hepatitis B vaccine administered at 0, 1, 2, and 6 months. Following outbreaks of hepatitis B in dialysis units virus genotyping can help to identify the source and likely route of transmission. In these circumstances specific antihepatitis B human immunoglobulin can be administered but may be of little value in preventing further infection.

In summary, the current consensus (ignoring cost implications) is that all new renal patients who are surface antigen and core antibody negative should receive hepatitis B vaccination as early as possible in the course of their illness. The most effective commonly used regimen in trials to date involves a 40 mg (double) dose administered on four occasions, deep into the deltoid muscles at 0, 1, 2, and 6 or 12 months. If no antibody response develops, then further identical courses of the same vaccine are futile. However, a trial of a low-dose intradermal protocol in non-responders may be worthwhile.[32] Antibody titres can usefully be remeasured at 12–18 months and booster doses of 40 mg can restore protective antibody levels in those who have previously responded. Thereafter, anitbody titres can be remeasured every 1–3 years and further booster doses administered to the responders. Further evidence is needed before other strategies designed to improve immunological response can be recommended.

Tetanus

Infection with *Clostridium tetani* still carries a high mortality. There have been on average 14 notified cases in England and Wales each year since 1985, and vaccination for unprotected persons is recommended. Primary immunization of children is given as part of a triple vaccine with diphtheria toxoid and *Bordetella pertussis* (diphtheria, tetanus, pertussis (DTP)). Two further booster doses are usually recommended before leaving school. Fully immunized patients are usually only given further booster doses following tetanus-prone injuries. Protection is equally important in chronic renal failure and renal transplant patients. However, response to the standard triple tetanus toxoid vaccine (75 IU) in chronic renal failure and dialysis patients is reduced such that only 70% of patients can achieve a protective antibody response. Transplant patients have been reported to achieve antibody responses similar to the normal population. Thus, uraemia appears to be more inhibitory than pharmocological immunosupression in determining the response to tetanus toxoid. It is recommended therefore that the need for and effect of tetanus vaccination should be monitored by antitetanus antibody quantification and in the case of wounds immunization against tetanus should be administered liberally together with antitetanus immunoglobulin if the risk of infection is felt to be high.

Diphtheria

Morbidity and mortality from *Corynebacteria diphtheriae* has virtually disappeared over the past 50 years in developed countries due to successful vaccination. However, epidemics are still occurring particularly in Russia and countries of the former Soviet Union and the few cases reported in the United Kingdom in recent years have nearly all originated in the Indian subcontinent or Africa. Rather alarmingly, however, reports that 38% of blood donors in the United Kingdom are not immune to diphtheria and that decreased immunity occurs with increasing age underline the importance of continuing high levels of uptake of diphtheria vaccine in healthy children and boosting in adulthood if resurgence of this disease either contracted or imported from abroad is to be avoided. Since 1992 a new non-toxigenic variety of diphtheria has been reported in *C. diptheriae vargravis*, which in the healthy population presents merely as a sore throat without signs of toxicity. The relevance of this strain to renal patients is not known but vaccination with the diphtheria toxoid is not likely to prevent or ameliorate infection.

Anthrax

An alum precipitate of antigen is available for immunization but is recommended only for those at risk of exposure to disease, i.e. those involved in the handling of herbivorous animals or their products.

Haemophilus influenzae B (HIB)

Invasive *Haemophilus influenzea* B is almost exclusively a disease of children under 4 and was an important cause of meningitis, epiglottitis, and septicaemia prior to the introduction of HIB immunization. Since then its incidence has fallen sharply such that only one death occurred from this disease in the United Kingdom in 1995. The safety and efficacy of the currently available conjugated bacterial capsule vaccines are exemplary. The conjugate HIB vaccines are not live but contain non-replicating bacterial capsular antigens conjugated to diphtheria or tetanus toxoid or meningococcal membrane proteins. They are therefore safe to use in all renal patients, are recommended for all infants from 2 months of age, and a single dose for splenectomized adults.

Varicella/herpes zoster

A live attenuated virus vaccine is available. Little is known about the response to varicella vaccine in dialysis and chronic renal failure patients. Because of the seriousness of primary infection in transplant recipients most paediatric units actively immunize children on transplant waiting lists. We have successfully vaccinated two zoster-antibody-negative renal transplant recipients who were at high risk of infection by virtue of their professions. No adverse effects were noted and the antibody response was deemed protective in both. Very few adult units seek out and attempt to vaccinate seronegative patients prior to renal transplantation. In view of the severity of primary herpes zoster infections in the immunocompromised host perhaps it is time to review practice now that an effective vaccine is available.

Epstein–Barr virus (EBV)

A new vaccine is currently being evaluated in EBV IgG antibody-negative children awaiting solid organ transplantation. It is hoped that this vaccine will be effective in preventing primary EBV infections and EBV-driven post-transplant lymphoproliferative disorders.

Travel in renal patients

Clearly, the risks associated with travelling abroad depend to a large extent on where the individual patient is travelling to. 'Travellers' diarrhoea' poses a particular risk in Third World countries and malaria in tropical climates. Up to 50% of European travellers spending 3 weeks or more in developing countries develop diarrhoea even if they stay in good quality hotels. The commonest organisms associated with travellers' diarrhoea are enterotoxogenic *Escherichia coli* (which may be part of the normal bowel flora of the local population). *Salmonella, Shigella, Campylobacter*, rotavirus, and the parasite *Giardia lamblia* are all possible culprits. All are transmitted via the faecal-oral route and risk can be minimized by following the rules for eating and drinking safely. Even in infected areas the risk to travellers of, for example, cholera is small if basic common-sense precautions are taken. All renal patients travelling abroad should therefore be advised to maintain scrupulous personal, food, and water hygiene. Patients should only drink, clean teeth, wash salad, and make ice from reputable bottled, boiled, or sterilized water, they should avoid shellfish, unpasturized dairy produce, and dishes containing uncooked eggs and eat only vegetables and fruit which need to be pealed by the consumer. In general, only freshly prepared, well cooked, piping hot food should be consumed.

Other common-sense measures should be taken to avoid obvious problems. Patients should carry a list of their current medications and ensure that they either carry sufficient supplies of drug with them or have secured a reliable source of obtaining these before departing. Ideally, patients should also have a clear 'To whom it may concern letter' outlining their diagnoses, current management, and most recent relevant blood results, together with information which would allow another physician to obtain further information about the patient if necessary. Practical consideration should be given to acquiring adequate insurance cover (which should include adequate funds for repatriation) prior to departure. If appropriate, patients should wear a 'medi-alert' bracelet or similar. Regular haemodialysis patients need to make alternative dialysis arrangements. Some units advise patients undergoing peritoneal dialysis to travel with a 2–4 day supply of antibiotics which can be administered intraperitoneally if the patient develops peritonitis while abroad, thus allowing time to return home for further therapy. Fair-skinned immunosupressed patients should take particular care to reduce the risk of sunstroke and squamous cell carcinomas which are the most common malignancies occurring in renal transplant patients. If sun exposure cannot be avoided then patients should be advised to apply appropriate sun-blocking creams.

Prior to travelling abroad renal patients, particularly those with renal transplants, need to be educated so that if they do suffer bouts of gastrointestinal upset while abroad they follow simple guidelines to avoid dehydration and to ensure adequate intake of vital immunosupressant drugs while ill. Travellers should go prepared with sachets of replacement sugar and salt which can be reconstituted with freshly boiled or bottled water if needed. Patients should be advised to continue to eat if possible as food shortens the illness and lessens the fluid loss. If the diarrhoea does not settle in 48 h or so medical help should be sought.

Nephrotic patients and those with procoagulant tendencies must be aware of the risks of developing venous thrombosis during long journeys by air or bus, particularly where there is little opportunity to move about. In some patients it may be considered worthwhile administering low-molecular-weight heparin or taking asprin to reduce these risks for the duration of the journey. Avoiding alcohol and maintaining a high fluid intake are important simple prophylactic measures.

Malaria

Malaria presents a serious risk for travellers to tropical countries. During 1996 2500 cases were reported to the Malaria Reference Laboratory of the Public Health Laboratory Service for the United Kingdom. Eleven of these patients died. The majority of the cases were due to *Falciparum* malaria. Just over half the total cases were acquired in Africa and one-third in the Indian subcontinent. One-third of cases occurred in settled migrants following visits to their country of origin, which emphasizes the fact that previously acquired immunity is not lifelong. No information is available on how many, if any, of these patients were suffering from renal impairment or were immunosupressed. Nevertheless, renal patients should always follow the so called ABC of malaria prevention: Awareness of the risk, mosquito Bite prevention, appropriate Chemoprophylaxis. In general, drugs used for the prevention of malaria are safe in the usual dosage in advanced renal failure, dialysis, and transplant patients. However, if therapeutic doses are required a reduced dose is recommended if creatinine clearance falls below 20–25 ml/min.

Vaccination for adult renal patients travelling abroad

Hepatitis A

Hepatitis A is transmitted by the faecal-oral route. The incubation period is 15–40 days and the disease is generally mild, but severity increases with age and occasional fulminant cases occur. There is no chronic carrier state and progression to chronic liver damage does not occur. The prevalence of hepatitis A is greater in countries outside northern and western Europe (including Spain, Portugal, and Italy), North America, Australia, and New Zealand. Approximately 15% of cases reported in the United Kingdom are contracted abroad. The Indian subcontinent and the Far East are the areas of highest risk but eastern Europe is also emerging as a high-risk area. The currently available vaccine is a whole virus inactivated with formaldehyde. Protective antibodies persist for 1 year following a single dose. Protection can be extended for up to 10 years following a single booster dose. Vaccination against hepatitis A is recommended when travelling into areas of high prevalence, especially if sanitation is likely to be poor. Testing for hepatitis A antibodies may make vaccination unnecessary but if this is not easily available then vaccination regardless of status is advisable. Postimmunization testing for antibody titres is recommended for the immunosuppressed who may need more than one dose to achieve protection. Patients with chronic liver disease should also be vaccinated because of the potentially lethal deterioration in liver function which could occur with even a mild infection with hepatitis A. If an immunosuppressed renal patient has close contact with a case of hepatitis A then human normal immunoglobulin (HNIG) can give protection for up to 4 months. Similarly, an immunosupressed patient who has not been adequately vaccinated against hepatitis A travelling to an area of high prevalence should be considered for HNIG. HNIG can inhibit antibody response to measles, mumps, and rubella vaccines but not yellow fever, typhoid, or BCG and should be delayed for 3 weeks post-MMR vaccine. If HNIG has already been given 3 months should elapse before giving MMR.

Cholera

Vibrio cholerae is widespread in the Far East, Africa, central South America and a new type 0139 is present in India, Bangladesh, and Thailand. The last indigenous case of cholera occurred in England and Wales over 100 years ago, although occasional imported cases occur. Cholera vaccine gives only limited personal protection and does not prevent spread of the disease. It has therefore been abandoned in most countries and is no longer recommended by the World Health Organization and is therefore not required by any traveller.

Japanese encephalitis

Japanese encephalitis is a mosquito-borne viral encephalitis prevalent throughout southeast Asia and the Far East. Infection may go unrecognized, but severe encephalitis with a mortality of approximately 30% can occur with even greater chance of permanent neurological damage. It is particularly common just after the wet season and in areas where pig farming and rice growing are practiced. A formalin-inactivated whole cell vaccine is available on a named patient basis only. It is recommended for travellers to endemic areas whose stay will be longer than 1 month or those who are likely to be at increased risk because of extensive outdoor activities. However, this vaccine is not advised in renal disease because of the lack of information regarding efficacy and safety. Precautions against mosquitoes are therefore mandatory.

Tick borne encephalitis

This meningoencephalitis is caused by a flavivirus transmitted to humans by the bite of an infected tick or occasionally by ingestion of unpasteurized milk from infected goats. It is endemic in forested parts of Europe and Scandinavia. Fatalities are fortunately relatively rare, occurring in approximately 1% of patients. However, one in 10 patients develops a slowly resolving paresis. Preventative measures include avoiding tick bites, especially in late spring and summer when the ticks are active. An unlicensed inactivated whole cell virus vaccine is available on a named patient basis. It is recommended for travellers who are planning to camp or walk in endemic areas, especially where there is heavy undergrowth during the late spring and summer. No information is available specifically for renal patients but common-sense precautions such as covering arms, legs, and ankles and using insect repellent are advised.

Rabies

Encephalomyelitis caused by acute infection with rabies virus has not been reported to occur indigenously in the United Kingdom since 1902. The United Kingdom has been free from indigenous animal rabies since 1922. Yet occasional cases occur in patients infected abroad. Rabies in animals is endemic throughout Asia, Africa, and Latin America. In Europe foxes are the predominant host but many other animals including horses, dogs, cats, cattle, and deer can become infected and transmit disease to humans. In America concern is growing over the numbers of raccoons, skunks, and bats infected. Transmission is usually by the bite of a rabid animal. Postexposure prophylaxis depends on the prevalence of rabies in the country where exposure occurred and the ownership and condition of the biting animal. Prophylaxis may involve administration of human rabies-specific immunoglobulin and inactivated vaccine. Individual risk assessment is recommended and advice should be sought from national virus reference laboratories Pre-exposure immunization is reserved for those working with animals or bats which may be infected.

Meningococcus

No effective vaccine is available against the commonest B strain of the Gram-negative diplococcus *Neisseria meningitis* prevalent in the United Kingdom. The group C strain has been responsible for approximately one-third of reported isolates, though the recent figures suggest that this has risen to 40%. Group A strains are rare in the United Kingdom but have been responsible for epidemics of disease in other countries. Overall mortality is around 10%. An effective vaccine against group A and C organisms is available and is recommended for asplenic adults and children travelling to areas of increased risk. The vaccine is made from the polysaccharide outer capsule of the diplococcus and is therefore safe in immunocompromised patients. There is little information on the response of renal patients to this vaccine, but it is wise to recommend it to patients who plan to travel (especially if backpacking or living rough or with local communities) in endemic areas where group A infection is endemic. Such areas include sub-Saharan Africa, Delhi, Nepal, and Pakistan.

In November 1999 a new meningococcal C conjugate vaccine immunization programme was launched in the United Kingdom in response to growing concerns about the increased incidence especially amongst 15-, 16-, and 17-year-olds and the recent increase in the percentage of patients with group C meningococcus. The new vaccine overcomes some of the problems encountered with the older vaccine in that it is effective in children under 2 and vaccine-induced immunity lasts 3–5 years. In the first instance the new vaccine was being administered to 15–17-year-olds and to children under 1 year of age. More recently this programme has been extended to all schoolgoing children. It is not known whether this vaccination programme will decrease the carriage rate which for all meningococci varies from 5–11% in adults to 25% in teenagers. It is likely that decreased carriage amongst the healthy population would indirectly protect the immunosuppressed.

Yellow fever

Yellow fever is an acute viral infection spread by the bite of infected mosquitoes or occasionally infected monkeys. Fifty per cent of non-immunized adults die from the acute illness. The disease occurs in South America and tropical Africa. Preventive measures include eradication of mosquitoes, protection from mosquito bites, and vaccination. The latter is compulsory for entry into some countries. The yellow fever vaccine is a live attenuated preparation and therefore is contraindicated in immunosuppressed patients and those with hypogammaglobulinaemia. In healthy individuals a single dose confers immunity in almost 100% of recipients and persists for at least 10 years. Thus, renal patients who have previously been immunized may have some protection. Nevertheless, avoidance of mosquito bites is recommended.

References

1. Rodby, RA., Trenholme, GM. Vaccination in the dialysis patient. *Semin Dial* 1991; 4: 102–106.
2. Buti, M., Viladomiu, L., Jardi, R. Long-term immunogenicity and efficacy of hepatitis B vaccine in haemodialysis patients. *Am J Nephrol* 1992; 12: 144–147.
3. Seaworth, B., Drucker, J., Starling, J., Drucker, R. Stevens, C., Hamilton, J. Hepatitis B vaccines in patients with chronic renal failure before dialysis. *J Infect Dis* 1988; 157: 332–337.
4. Dukes, CS., Street, AC., Starling, JF., Hamilton, JD. Hepatitis B vaccination and booster in pre-dialysis patients: a 4-year analysis. *Vaccine* 1993; 11: 1229–1232.
5. Dacko, C., Holley, JL. The influence of nutritional status, dialysis adequacy, and residual function on the response to hepatitis B vaccination in peritoneal dialysis patients. *Adv Perit Dial* 1996; 12: 315–318.
6. Fuchshuber, A., Kuhnemund, O., Keuth, B., Lutticken, D., Michalk, D., Querfeld, U. Pneumococcal vaccine in children and young adults with chronic renal disease. *Nephrol Dial Transplant* 1996; 11: 468–473.
7. Salisbury, DM, Begg, NT. (ed.). *Immunisation against infectious disease*, pp. 29–33. HMSO, London.
8. Smith, KG., Isbel, NM., Catton, MG., Leydon, JA., Becker, GJ., Walker, RG. Supression of the humoral immune response by mycophenolate mofetil. *Nephrol Dial Transplant* 1998; 13: 160–164.
9. Beyer, WEP., Diepersloot, RJA., Masurel, N., Simoons, M.L., Weimar, W. Double failure of influenza vaccination in a heart transplant patient. *Transplantation* 1987; 43: 319–324.
10. Wagner, D., Wagenbreth, I., Stachacan-Kunstyr, R., Flik, J. Failure of vaccination against hepatitis B with Gen-H-B-Vax-D in immunosuppressed heart transplant recipients. *Clin Investig* 1992; 70: 585–589.
11. Grindt, M., Pietsch, M., Kohler, H., Tetanus immunization and its association to hepatitis B vaccination in patients with chronic renal failure. *Am J Kidney Dis* 1995; 26: 454–460.
12. Huzly, D., Neifer, S., Reinke, P., Schroder, K., Schonfeld, C., Hofmann, T., Bienzle, U. Routine immunization in adult renal transplant recipients. *Transplantation* 1997; 63: 839–845.

13. Veraluis, DJ., Beyer, WEP., Masurel, N., Wenting, GJ., Weimar, W. Impairment of immune response to influenza vaccination in renal transplant recipients by cyclosporine, but not azathioprine. *Transplantation* 1986; **42**: 376–379.
14. Ahmed, AH., Nicholson, KG, Nguyen van Tam, JS., Pearson, JCG. Effectiveness of influenza vaccine in reducing hospital admissions during the 1989–1990 epidemic. *Epidemiol Infect* 1997; **118**: 27–33.
15. Ahmed, AH., Nicholson, KG., Nguyen van Tam, JS. Reduction in mortality associated with influenza vaccine during 1989–90 epidemic. *Lancet* 1995; **346**: 591–595.
16. Grekas, D. *et al.* Influenza vaccination in renal transplant patients is safe and serologically effective. *Int J Clin Pharm Therapy Toxicol* 1993; **31**: 553–566.
17. Marrie, TJ. Community acquired pneumonia. *Clin Infect Disease* 1994; **18**: 501–513.
18. Nichol, KL., MacDonald, R., Hague, M. Side effects associated with pneumococcal vaccination. *Am J Infect Control* 1997; **25**: 223–238.
19. Zanolli, R., Morgese, G. Hepatitis B vaccine: current issues. *Ann Pharmacother* 1997; **31**: 1059–1067.
20. Douglas, RG. The heritage of hepatitis B vaccine. *J Am Med Assoc* 1996; **276**: 1796–1798.
21. Ukena, T., Esber, H., Bessette, R., Parks, T., Crocker, B., Shaw, FE. Site of injection and response to hepatitis B vaccine. *New Engl J Med* 1985; **313**: 579–580.
22. Lindsay, KL., Herbert, DA., Gitnick, GL. Hepatitis B vaccine: low post-vaccination immunity in hospital personnel given gluteal injections. *Hepatology* 1985; **5**: 1088–1090.
23. Peces, R., de la Torre, M., Alcazar, R., Urra, JM. Prospective analysis of factors influencing the antibody response to hepatitis B vaccine in haemodialysis patients. *Am J Kidney Dis* 1997; **29**: 239–245.
24. Miller, E., Alter, MJ., Tokars, JI. Protective effect of hepatitis B vaccine in chronic haemodialysis patients. *Am J Kidney Dis* 1999; **33**: 356–360.
25. West, DJ., Calandra, GB. Vaccine induced immunologic memory for hepatitis B surface antigen; implications for policy on booster vaccination. *Vaccine* 1996; **14**: 1019–1027.
26. Faranna, P., Cozzi, G., Bellone, M., Pedrini, L. Immunization and vaccination protocol in haemodialysis patients with naturally acquired hepatitis B antibody. *Nephron* 1992; **61**: 311–312.
27. Lombardi, M., Pizzarelli, F., Righi, M., *et al.* Hepatitis B vaccination in dialysis patients and nutritional status. *Nephron* 1992; **61**: 266–268.
28. Mitwalli, A. Responsiveness to hepatitis B vaccine in immunocompromised patients by doubling the dose scheduling. *Nephron* 1996; **73**: 417–420.
29. Hollinger, FB. Factors influencing the immune response to hepatitis B vaccine booster dose guidelines, and vaccine protocol recommendation. *Am J Med* 1989; **87**: 36S–40S.
30. Frazer, IH., Jones, B., Dimitrakakis, M., Mcckay, IR. Intramuscular versus low-dose intradermal hepatitis B vaccine. Assesment by humoral and cellular immune response to hepatitis B surface antigen. *Med J Austral* 1987; **146**: 242–245.
31. Ono, K., Kashiwagi, S. Complete seroconversion by low-dose intradermal injection of recombinant hepatitis B vaccine in haemodialysis patients. *Nephron* 1991; **1**: 47–51.
32. Zuckerman, AJ. Appraisal of intradermal immunisation against hepatitis B. *Lancet* 1987; **i**: 435–436.
33. Junkers, P., Devillier, P., Salomon, H., Cerisier, JE., Courouce, AM. Randomised placebo-controlled trial of recombinant interleukin-2 in chronic uraemic patients who are non-responders to hepatitis B vaccine. *Lancet* 1994; **344**: 856–857.

21

Antimicrobial dosing regimens in renal patients

D. Craig Brater

Renal impairment leads not only to the accumulation of endogenous compounds, but can also result in the retention of exogenously administered antibiotics and their polar metabolites, some of which may be active. For many antibiotics, doses must be reduced to attain concentrations similar to those obtained in patients with normal renal function. Several general characteristics of a drug allow prediction as to whether renal dysfunction is likely to mandate changes in dosing. If an antibiotic has a wide therapeutic index, accumulation in patients with renal insufficiency to concentrations severalfold higher than in patients with normal renal function has little, if any, consequence, and dose adjustment can be ignored. Cephalosporins are good examples. In contrast, aminoglycoside antibiotics have such narrow therapeutic ranges that dose adjustment is required.

Patients with renal insufficiency accumulate endogenous organic acids that are normally excreted by the kidney, and these compounds are able to displace acidic drugs, such as penicillin or sulfonamide antibiotics, from albumin binding sites (Depner *et al.* 1980; Gulyassy *et al.* 1986; Reidenberg and Drayer 1984). The likelihood that such an effect will be clinically important is determined by the degree of binding of the antibiotic. Generally, for drugs bound <90%, the magnitude of the effect is so small as to be irrelevant. In contrast, drugs bound >90% may be importantly affected by changes in binding. For example, penicillin is more than 99% bound to albumin. Thus, less than 1% is free in plasma and constitutes the active moiety. In uraemia, what may appear to be a trivial decrease in binding from 99% to 98% actually results in a doubling of the free, unbound concentration from 1% to 2%, a magnitude of change that may be clinically important.

The degree of protein binding also predicts the potential for removal of a drug by dialysis or by haemofiltration. Dialysis can only remove unbound drug; thus, a high degree of binding means that only small, often insignificant, amounts of drug can be removed. As such, drugs that are more than 90% bound to plasma proteins will have negligible removal by dialytic procedures with the exception of haemoperfusion techniques.

The percentage of overall elimination of a drug or active metabolite that occurs via the kidney allows prediction of the potential for clinically important accumulation of antibiotics or metabolites in patients with renal insufficiency. If about 40% or more of an antibiotic dose is excreted in urine, dose adjustment will be needed in patients with renal insufficiency, assuming that the drug in question has a sufficiently narrow therapeutic index to be of concern.

Antibiotics restricted to the extracellular, and particularly the intravascular, compartment are accessible to removal by haemodialysis unless precluded by high degrees of protein binding. Such drugs have small volumes of distribution of the order of total body water or less (i.e. about 0.7 litre/kg). In contrast, a drug with a large volume of distribution implies wide disbursement of drug throughout the tissues. Following this logic, a drug with a small volume of distribution and low protein binding (e.g. aminoglycoside antibiotics) is substantially removed by dialytic procedures and requires supplemental dosing after dialysis. In contrast, an antibiotic with a large volume of distribution, though still able to pass across a dialysis membrane, has so little of the drug in the plasma relative to overall body stores that the amount removed is negligible.

Role of the kidney in antibiotic disposition

Absorption

By several theoretical mechanisms, renal disease could affect antibiotic absorption. For example, slowed intestinal motility could decrease the rate of gastric emptying of medications to small intestinal absorption sites causing a delay in absorption. Changed regional distribution of blood flow could affect absorption from intramuscular or subcutaneous sites. Such effects on drug absorption remain purely speculative; based on current data clinicians may assume that absorption is essentially normal in patients with renal insufficiency. Though not strictly an absorptive process, first-pass metabolism by the intestinal mucosa and liver can influence systemic availability of an antibiotic. By unknown mechanisms, renal insufficiency can reduce non-renal elimination of drugs. For drugs with substantial first-pass elimination, such inhibition could cause greater bioavailability. This phenomenon has been documented with some drugs, none of which are antibiotics.

Distribution

Protein binding of highly bound antibiotics is a major determinant of drug distribution; changed binding of acidic drugs, such as many of the penicillins and sulfonamides, frequently occurs in patients with renal insufficiency. Many acidic drugs are bound to albumin; accumulated endogenous organic acids in patients with renal impairment can displace exogenously administered drugs and thereby increase the proportion of unbound drug in plasma (Depner *et al.* 1980; Gulyassy *et al.* 1986; Reidenberg and Drayer 1984). A popular misconception is that this displacement results in increased concentrations of unbound pharmacologically active drug causing an enhanced effect, including toxicity. In the majority of instances, however, there is no increase in concentration of unbound drug and, therefore, no change in response (Greenblatt *et al.* 1982; Klotz 1976; MacKichan 1989; Tozer 1981). The reason for unbound drug concentrations being unchanged is that for many drugs with low total clearance (obeying so-called 'restrictive' elimination, in which unbound clearance equals intrinsic clearance), clearance of total drug from plasma is directly related to the fraction of unbound drug (Wilkinson 1987):

$$Cl_{total} = fu \times Cl_u$$

where Cl_{total} is clearance, fu is the fraction unbound, and Cl_u is unbound clearance.

Thus, if displacement from albumin causes the unbound fraction to increase, total clearance increases proportionally but unbound or intrinsic clearance is unchanged, resulting in a maintenance of the unbound concentration at its previous level. This similar unbound concentration occurs at a lower total drug concentration; thus, the fraction or percentage unbound is increased, but the concentration unbound is unchanged (Greenblatt *et al.* 1982; Klotz 1976; MacKichan 1989; Tozer 1981). This scenario is true for a number of acidic drugs, many of which are highly protein bound, have low total clearances, and are displaced from albumin binding sites in uraemia. Among antibiotics, timocillin is a good example. In patients with end-stage renal disease displacement occurs but the unbound concentrations is the same. The binding changes described above can influence the calculation of distribution volume. If calculated based on total drug concentration, the volume of distribution may become larger when binding decreases, particularly for drugs that distribute extensively into intracellular sites and therefore have large volumes of distribution (Greenblatt *et al.* 1982; Klotz 1976; MacKichan 1989; Tozer 1981). This observation alone can lead to the false conclusion that loading doses need to be increased. In contrast, the distribution volume of the unbound, pharmacologically active drug is essentially unchanged, meaning that no adjustment of loading dose should be made. Ticarcillin illustrates this phenomenon wherein its volume of distribution relative to total drug concentration increases in patients with end-stage renal disease; since unbound concentration is the same, the volume of distribution relative to unbound ticarcillin is unchanged. Unfortunately, the medical literature concerning changes in drug disposition in patients with renal insufficiency is replete with data ignoring unbound drug concentrations. For highly bound drugs, if disposition parameters for total drug (clearance and volume of distribution) are the only values reported, and if these values are increased in patients with renal insufficiency, one must question whether the effect is solely due to displacement from binding, meaning that disposition parameters for unbound drug may be unchanged and that no alteration in dosing would be indicated.

Metabolism

The proximal nephron is able to metabolize drugs; among other metabolic pathways, the proximal tubule contains mixed function cytochrome P-450 oxidases (CYP), but in lower amounts than the liver. Interestingly, isoforms of CYP appear to be differentially regulated in the kidney relative to the liver (Haehner *et al.* 1996). The proximal nephron also has peptidases that allow it to metabolize proteins, peptides, and some xenobiotics. For example, proximal tubule dipeptidases metabolize imipenem (Barza 1985). As such, if imipenem alone is administered to patients, all antibacterial effect in the urine is lost due to proximal tubular metabolism. To attain efficacy for urinary tract infections, imipenem is administered with cilastatin, which inhibits the dipeptidases allowing sufficient amounts of unchanged imipenem in the urine to kill bacteria (Barza 1985).

In addition to the metabolic roles of the kidney described above, the kidney excretes many drug metabolites formed in the liver. Renal insufficiency does not necessarily mean that drug metabolites will accumulate since other excretory pathways exist, such as biliary excretion. In addition, many drug metabolites presumably have no effects. On the other hand, there are numerous examples of accumulation of metabolites, including those

Table 21.1 Active metabolites of antimicrobial drugs that are eliminated by the kidney

Drug	Active metabolite
Antibacterial agents	
Cephalosporins	
Cefotaxime	Desacetylcefotaxime
Cefoxitin	Decarbamoylcefoxitin
Cephalothin	Desacetylcephalothin
Cephapirin	Desacetylcephapirin
Macrolides	
Clarithromycin	14-hydroxy (R)-clarithromycin
Quinolones	
Ciprofloxacin	Four different metabolites
Fleroxacin	N-demethylfleroxacin
Norfloxacin	Six different metabolites
Pefloxacin	N-desmethylpefloxacin and norfloxacin
Sulfonamides	
Sulfamethoxazole	Acetyl metabolite
Sulfisoxazole	Acetyl metabolite
Antifungal agents	
Itraconazole	Hydroxyitraconazole
Antiviral agents	
Vidarabine	Hypoxanthine arabinoside

of antibiotics, that are pharmacologically active (Table 21.1) (Dutt *et al.* 1994; Verbeeck *et al.* 1981). Some of the metabolites listed exert pharmacological effects similar to those of the parent compound (e.g. desacetylcefotaxime) and in others examples the metabolite has a different pharmacologic profile from the parent drug (e.g. the acetyl metabolite of sulfonamides). It should be apparent that in order to use antibiotics with active metabolites safely in patients with renal insufficiency, one must not only know the pharmacological profile of the parent drug, but also its metabolite(s). In general, one should also try to avoid such drugs in patients with renal disease by selecting alternative agents with similar spectrums of activity but non-renal routes of elimination.

Excretion

Mechanisms by which the kidney excretes drugs are analogous to its normal physiological processes of glomerular filtration, active secretion, and reabsorption, both active and passive. Effects on any of these processes can mandate changes in drug dosing. The most common clinical setting, of course, is renal insufficiency in which both glomerular filtration and active secretion are reduced.

Glomerular filtration

The glomerulus offers no barrier to filtration of the unbound fraction of most drugs, including all antibiotics (Besseghir and Rock-Ramel 1987; Prescott 1972). Glomerular pores allow passage of molecules up to molecular weights of about 65 000 Da, and the vast majority of xenobiotics are approximately two orders of magnitude smaller than that.

For antibiotics that are freely filtered at the glomerulus, such as aminoglycoside antibiotics, renal elimination is quite rapid. For many other antibiotics, binding to serum proteins restricts filtration so that only the unbound fraction can be filtered. For example, in contrast to aminoglycoside antibiotics that have negligible protein binding, many cephalosporins and penicillins are more than 99% bound to albumin. Thus, less than 1% of the drug in plasma is available for filtration and this route of renal excretion is negligible.

The limits to glomerular filtration of a drug, then, are usually not the glomerular barrier itself, but instead are factors that prevent filtration, predominantly binding to macromolecules that are too large to be filtered.

Secretion

The kidney secretes many drugs from blood into urine (Besseghir and Rock-Ramel 1987; Moller and Sheikh 1982; Peters 1960; Prescott 1972; Rennick 1972, 1981; Ullrich 1976; Weiner and Mudge 1964). Separate pathways have been characterized for organic acids and organic bases in the proximal tubule; more recently it has been appreciated that P-glycoprotein is responsible for renal secretion of an increasing list of compounds (Dutt *et al.* 1994).

Antibiotics gain access to secretory sites via the peritubular capillary. If 20% of renal plasma flow is filtered, then the remaining 80% of flow reaches sites of secretion. This process is active since an uphill concentration gradient is generated. Moreover, depriving the proximal tubule of energy also inhibits movement of drugs from the peritubular to the tubular side of the cell (Besseghir and Rock-Ramel 1987; Pritchard and Miller 1996). It appears that the energy necessary for active secretion via all of the identified pathways is ultimately generated by peritubular Na^+, K^+-ATPase since active secretion can be inhibited by ouabain and similar experimental manoeuvres (Besseghir and Rock-Ramel 1987; Burckhardt and Ullrich 1989; Shimada *et al.* 1987).

The efficiency of secretion is quite impressive since substantial secretion occurs for many drugs that are highly protein bound, such as penicillin, meaning that the affinity for transport exceeds that for binding (Hall and Rowland 1985).

In vivo, the active secretion of organic acids accounts for the renal elimination of a large number of compounds, including substantial numbers of antibiotics. Table 21.2 offers examples of antibiotics and potential inhibitors of secretion for which the major component of renal elimination is secretion (Brater 1980). Probenecid is the prototypic inhibitor of organic acid secretion and was specifically developed for this purpose. When penicillin was in short supply, concomitant use of probenecid was developed allowing administration of smaller doses, thereby conserving the antibiotic (Beyer *et al.* 1951). All of the organic acids listed in Table 21.2 can potentially compete with each other for secretion. As such, clinicians must realize the potential for interaction among these drugs and decide whether such an interaction may be clinically important. Ethambutol and amantadine are the only organic base antibiotics that have been shown to be actively secreted. Though not studied, other substrates for this transport pathway listed in Table 21.2 might compete for secretion. Several antimicrobials are substrates for

Table 21.2   Antibiotics and potential inhibitors that are actively secreted by the kidney

Antibiotic	Potential inhibitor
Organic acids	
Cephalosporins (most)	Loop diuretics
Penicillins (most)	Propenecid
Sulphonamides (most)	Thiazide diuretics
Organic bases	
Amantadine	Histamine H_2-antagonists
Ethambutol	Metformin
	Procainamide
	Trimethoprim

P-glycoprotein. In particular, P-glycoprotein keeps protease inhibitors out of the brain and probably contributes to their poor intestinal absorption (Lee and Gottesman 1998; Kim *et al.* 1998). However, there is negligible renal secretion of these drugs so potential ramifications of this pathway insofar as renal elimination is concerned are not important clinically.

Reabsorption

The kidney can both actively and passively reabsorb drugs. Aminoglycoside antibiotics are filtered by the glomerulus and then reabsorbed by the brush border of the proximal tubule via at least two different mechanisms, a carrier-mediated transport system and pinocytotic uptake leading to lysosomal accumulation (Just and Habermann 1977; Just *et al.* 1977; Lipsky *et al.* 1980; Silverblatt and Kuehn 1979; Sokol *et al.* 1989). The net result of these processes is the build-up of intracellular stores of aminoglycosides. This sequestration is such that slow release from intracellular stores allows detection of aminoglycosides in the urine for several weeks after a single dose (Schentag and Jusko 1977). The degree of accumulation might be expected to correlate with the development of nephrotoxicity from aminoglycosides. However, studies have shown that polyaspartic acid blocks experimental gentamicin nephrotoxicity without producing decreases in the intracellular concentrations of gentamicin (Gilbert *et al.* 1989; Ramsammy *et al.* 1989).

Dialysis

Dialytic procedures, including haemofiltration, can remove antibiotics in sufficient amounts to require supplemental dosing. Removal of drugs by continuous arteriovenous haemofiltration or continuous venovenous haemofiltration differs from conventional haemodialysis. Firstly, the pore size of the membrane is larger, allowing drugs of about 5000 Å to be freely filtered. Thus, vancomycin, the size of which limits conventional dialytic removal so that no dose supplementation is needed, is readily removed by these filtration techniques, requiring dose adjustment (Pollard *et al.* 1994; Dupuis *et al.* 1989; Bickley 1988; Matzke *et al.* 1986; DeSoi *et al.* 1992). Secondly; essentially all of the unbound drug in plasma can be removed by these methods. Thus, drug clearance by ultrafiltration is equal to the unbound fraction times the ultrafiltration rate. This simple calculation can be used to estimate whether supplementary antibiotic should be given and the amount.

The amount of many antibiotics removed by dialysis has been quantified in clinical studies. Table 21.3 presents current data that can be used for dosing guidelines (Brater 1994). For antibiotics with negligible removal, no dosing adjustment is needed over and above that which occurs due to the patient's level of renal function. In contrast, for antibiotics where potentially important amounts are removed, a supplemental dose equal to the amount removed can be given at the conclusion of haemodialysis. In patients treated with peritoneal dialysis, the dose can be increased to compensate for the amount of drug removed by the dialytic procedure. Interestingly, most drugs are negligibly removed by peritoneal dialysis (Table 21.3). This observation is in contrast to the substantial absorption of many drugs that occurs when administered with the peritoneal dialysate (Somani *et al.* 1982). For example, 20–25% of a dose of an aminoglycoside antibiotic is removed by peritoneal dialysis; in contrast, instillation of aminoglycosides into the peritoneum results in 50% or more being absorbed systemically. The mechanism of this unidirectional peritoneal transport of drugs has not been explored.

Dosing of antibiotics in patients with renal insufficiency

Loading dose

In some clinical conditions, rapid attainment of therapeutic antibiotic concentrations is desired. Since reaching a steady-state serum concentrations requires four to five times the drug half-life, and since renal impairment may prolong half-life sufficient to render

Table 21.3 Removal of antimicrobial agents by dialysis: per cent of a dose removed during a session of haemodialysis or 24 h of CAPD

Drug	Haemodialysis	CAPD
Antibacterial agents		
Aminoglycosides	50%	20–25%
Spectinomycin	50%	
Carbapenems		
Imipenem	80–90%	Negligible
Cephalosporins		
Cefaclor	33%	
Cefadroxil	50%	
Cefamandole	50%	Negligible (5%)
Cefazolin	50%	20%
Cefipime	40–70%	26%
Cefixime	Negligible(1.6%)	Negligible
Cefmenoxime	16–51%	Negligible (< 10%)
Cefmetazole	60%	
Cefodizime	50%	Negligible (15%)

(continued)

Table 21.3 (continued)

Drug	Haemodialysis	CAPD
Cefonicid	Negligible	Negligible (6.5%)
Cefoperazone	Negligible	Negligible
Ceforanide	20–50%	
Cefotaxime	60%	Negligible (5%)
Cefotetan	Negligible (5–9%)	
Cefotiam	30–40%	
Cefoxitin	50%	Negligible
Cefpirome	32–48%	Negligible (12%)
Cefpodoxime	50%	
Cefprozil	55%	
Cefroxadine	50%	
Cefsulodin	60%	
Ceftazidime	50%	Negligible
Ceftibuten	39%	
Ceftizoxime	50%	Negligible (16%)
Ceftriaxone	40%	Negligible (4.5%)
Cefuroxime	20%	
Cephacetrile	50%	
Cephalexin	50–75%	30%
Cephalothin	50%	
Cephapirin	20%	
Macrolide antibiotics		
Clindamycin	Negligible	Negligible
Dirithromycin	Negligible	
Lincomycin	Negligible	Negligible
Monobactams		
Aztreonam	40%	Negligible
Carumonam	51%	
Moxalactam	30–50%	Negligible (15–20%)
Nitromidazoles		
Metronidazole	45%	Negligible (10%)
Ornidazole	42%	Negligible (6%)
Tinidazole	40%	
Penicillins		
Amdinocillin	32–70%	Negligible (<4%)
Amoxicillin	30%	
Ampicillin	40%	
Azlocillin	30–45%	
Carbenicillin	50%	
Cloxacillin	Negligible	
Dicloxacillin	Negligible	
Methicillin	Negligible	
Mezlocillin	20–25%	24%
Nafcillin	Negligible	
Oxacillin	Negligible	
Penicillin	50%	
Piperacillin	30–50%	Negligible (6%)

Table 21.3   (continued)

Drug	Haemodialysis	CAPD
Temocillin	50%	Negligible
Ticarcillin	50%	Negligible
Polymyxins		
Colistin	Negligible	Negligible
Quinolones		
Ciprofloxacin	Negligible (2%)	Negligible (0.4–1.6%)
Enoxacin	Negligible	
Fleroxacin	Negligible (3–7%)	Negligible (<10%)
Levofloxacin	Negligible	Negligible
Lomefloxacin	Negligible	
Norfloxacin	Negligible	
Ofloxacin	Negligible (15–25%)	Negligible (4–6%)
Pefloxacin	Negligible	
Temafloxacin	Negligible (9.4%)	
Sulfonamides		
Sulfamethoxazole	50%	Negligible (8%)
Trimethorprim	50%	Negligible (7%)
Tetracyclines		
Doxycycline	Negligible	Negligible
Minocycline	Negligible	Negligible
Vancomycin	Negligible	Negligible (15–20%)
Teicoplanin	Negligible	Negligible (5%)
Antifungal agents		
Amphotericin B	Negligible	
Fluconazole	40%	Negligible (18%)
Flucytosine	50%	
Itraconazole	Negligible	Negligible
Ketoconazole	Negligible	Negligible
Miconazole	Negligible	Negligible
Antimalarial agents		
Chloroquine	Negligible	
Mefloquine	Negligible	
Quinine	Negligible	
Antituberculous agents		
Ethambutol	Negligible (12%)	
Isoniazid	75%	
Para-aminosalicylic acid	50%	
Antiviral agents		
Acyclovir	60%	Negligible (<10%)
Amantadine	Negligible	
Didanosine	20–67%	Negligible
Foscarnet	27–58%	
Ganciclovir	Negligible	
Lamivudine	Negligible	
Ribavirin	Negligible (8%)	
Vidarabine	50%	
Zidovudine	Negligible	Negligible

the time of attainment of steady state too delayed for clinical purposes, a loading dose strategy needs to be employed. An example might be a patient with suspected sepsis in whom an aminoglycoside antibiotic is to be given. In patients with normal renal function, the half-life of an aminoglycoside is 2 to 3 h. Thus, dosing every 8 h means steady state is reached with the second dose and no loading dose is needed. In contrast, if the patient's creatinine clearance is 30 ml/min, then the aminoglycoside half-life is 12 h or more and attainment of steady state would take at least 2 days. In this setting, a loading dose is critically important. The loading dose of a drug that is needed is a function of its volume of distribution:

loading dose = desired concentration × volume of distribution.

Values for volume of distribution can be found in standard reference texts, but these sources often ignore changes in this parameter that may occur in patients with renal disease.

Table 21.4 lists antibiotics for which changes in volume of distribution have been documented in patients with renal disease (Brater 1994). For those drugs that are highly protein bound, notation is made as to whether the distribution volume of the pharmacologically active unbound drug concentration is altered. In most instances where unbound drug has been measured, there is no change, and therefore no change in loading dose is required. As discussed previously, adjusting therapy based on findings from total concentration of highly bound drugs can be misleading.

Table 21.4   Volume of distribution of antimicrobial drugs that are altered in patients with renal disease

Drug	V_d^* (litre/kg)	
	Normal renal function	ESRD
Antibacterial agents		
Cephalosporins		
Cefazolin	0.11–0.14	0.17
Cefoxitin	0.27	Increase
Macrolide antibiotics		
Erythromycin	0.6–0.8	1.2
Penicillins		
Azlocillin	0.18	0.3
Timocillin	0.15–0.24	Increase (no change[†])
Quinolones		
Norfloxacin	3.2	1.7
Antifungal agents		
Miconazole	2–3	Decrease

$*V_d$ = volume of distribution.
[†]Data for unbound drug.
ESRD = end-stage renal disease.

Maintenance dose

If the maintenance dose of an antibiotic needs to be decreased in patients with renal insufficiency, one can either decrease individual doses, give 'normal' doses at prolonged intervals, or use a combination. In general, one should adjust the interval to a maximum of 24 h after which the individual dose is also adjusted.

The disposition of many drugs has been studied in patients with renal insufficiency. From such data, dosing guidelines can be derived based on a patient's level of renal function (Brater 1994) (Table 21.5). Once the table is used to decide the amount of dose adjustment required, the clinician needs to decide how to adjust dose, dosing interval, or both. These data can then be coupled with those from Table 21.3 in patients receiving dialysis. Alternatively, one can seek an alternative agent that needs no dose adjustment in patients with renal insufficiency (Table 21.6).

Table 21.5 Maintenance doses of antimicrobial agents in patients with renal insufficiency (relative to normal dose)

Drug	Creatinine clearance (ml/min)		
	> 50	20–50	< 20
Antibacterial agents			
Aminoglycosides	1/3	1/2	1/4
Carbapenems			
Imipenem		1/2	1/4
Meropenem		1/2	1/3
Cephalosporins			
Cefaclor		1/2	1/4
Cefadroxil	1/2	1/4	1/8
Cefamandole	1/2	1/3	1/4
Cefazolin	1/2	1/4	1/6
Cefepime	2/3	1/5	1/8
Cefetamet	1/2	1/4	1/8
Cefixime		1/2	1/3
Cefmenoxime	1/2	1/4	1/6
Cefmetazole	2/3	1/2	1/3
Cefodizime			1/2
Cefonicid	1/2	1/5	1/10
Ceforanide	1/2	1/3	1/5
Cefotaxime		1/2	1/4
Cefotetan	1/2	1/4	1/10
Cefotiam		3/4	1/2
Cefoxitin	1/2	1/4	1/6
Cefpirome		1/2	1/4
Cefpodoxime		1/4	1/8
Cefprodoxime	1/2	1/3	1/5
Cefprozil			1/2

(continued)

Table 21.5 (continued)

Drug	Creatinine clearance (ml/min)		
	>50	20–50	<20
Cefroxadine		1/2	1/4
Cefsulodin	1/2	1/4	1/10
Ceftazidime	1/2	1/5	1/10
Ceftibuten	1/2	1/6	
Ceftizoxime	1/2	1/4	1/10
Cefuroxime		1/2	1/4
Cephacetrile	1/2	1/4	1/10
Cephalexin		1/3	1/10
Cephalothin	2/3	1/2	1/6
Cephapirin		1/2	1/3
Cephradine		1/3	1/10
Loracarbef	1/2	1/4	1/10
Chloramphenicol and thiamphenicol			
Thiamphenicol	1/2	1/3	1/10
Macrolide antibiotics			
Clarithromycin			1/3
Lincomycin		1/2	1/3
Roxithromycin			1/2
Monobactams			
Aztreonam	1/2	1/3	1/4
Carumonam	2/3	1/3	1/6
Moxalactam	1/2	1/3	1/10
Penicillins			
Amdinocillin		1/2	1/4
Amoxicillin		1/2	1/6
Ampicillin	1/2	1/4	1/10
Azlocillin		1/2	1/4
Carbenicillin	1/3	1/5	1/10
Methicilin		1/2	1/4
Mezlocillin	1/2	1/4	1/8
Penicillin		1/5	1/8
Piperacillin		1/2	1/3
Ticarcillin	1/2	1/3	1/4
Timocillin		1/2	1/4
Polymyxins			
Colistin	1/2	1/3	1/6
Polymyxin B	Avoid	Avoid	Avoid
Quinolones			
Ciprofloxacin			1/2
Enoxacin	1/2	1/3	1/4
Fleroxacin	3/4	1/2	1/3
Levofloxacin			1/6
Lomefloxacin			1/6
Norfloxacin			1/2

Table 21.5 (continued)

Drug	Creatinine clearance (ml/min)		
	>50	20–50	<20
Ofloxacin			1/2
Sparfloxacin			1/2
Temafloxacin	3/4	1/2	1/4
Sulfonamides			
Sulfamethoxazole			1/2
Sulfisoxazole	3/4	1/2	1/4
Trimethoprim			1/2
Tetracyclines			
Tetracycline		1/3	1/10
Urinary bacteriostatics			
Cinoxacin			1/10
Fosfomycin			1/4
Vancomycin-like agents			
Teicoplanin		1/2	1/3
Vancomycin	2/3	1/2	1/10
Antifungal agents			
Fluconazole		1/2	1/3
Flucytosine	1/2	1/3	1/4
Miconazole			1/3
Terbinafine			1/2
Antimalarial agents			
Chloroquine	1/2	1/5	1/10
Quinine		1/2	1/3
Antiparasitic agents			
Pentamidine		Undefined	
Antituberculous agents			
Cycloserine		Undefined	
Ethambutol		1/2	1/3
Isoniazid			1/2
Para-aminosalicylate		Undefined	
Antiviral agents			
Acyclovir		1/2	1/5
Amantadine	1/2	1/5	1/10
Cidofovir		Undefined	
Didanosine			1/3
Foscarnet		Undefined	
Ganciclovir	1/2	1/5	1/10
Lamivudine		1/3	1/6
Penciclovir		1/2	1/4
Rimantadine			1/2
Stavudine		1/5	1/10
Vidarabine		Undefined	
Zalcitabine		1/2	1/4
Zanamivir		Undefined	
Zidovudine			1/2

Table 21.6 Antimicrobial agents, the elimination of which is not affected by renal insufficiency

Antibacterial agents	Cephalosporinis
	Cefoperazone
	Cefpiramide
	Ceftriaxone
	Macrolides
	Azithromycin
	Clindamycin
	Dirithromycin
	Erythromycin
	Josamycin
	Miocamycin
	Rosaramicin
	Nitroimadazoles
	Benznidazole
	Metronidazole
	Misonidazole
	Nimidazole
	Ornidazole
	Tinidazole
	Penicillins
	Cloxacillin
	Dalfopristin/quinupristin
	Dicloxacillin
	Flucloxacillin
	Nafcillin
	Oxacillin
	Quinolones
	Difloxacin
	Grepafloxacin
	Moxifloxacin
	Pefloxacin
	Trovafloxacin
	Tetracyclines
	Doxycline
	Minocycline
Antifungal agents	Amphotericin
	Griseofulvin
	Itraconazole

Table 21.6   (continued)

	Ketoconazole
	Terbinafine
Antihelminthic agents	Albendazole
	Ivermectin
	Levamisole
	Mebendazole
	Oxamniquine
Antimalarial agents	Amodiaquine
	Artemether/artesunate
	Halofantrine
	Hydroxychloroquine
	Mefloquine
	Primaquine
	Pyrimethamine
Antiparasitic agents	Allopurinol riboside
	Atovaquone
	Nifurtimox
	Nitazoxanide
	Secnidazole
Antituberculous agents/drugs used for leprosy	Capreomycin
	Clofazimine
	Dapsone
	Ethionamide
	Pyrazinamide
	Rifabutin
	Rifampin
	Rifapentine
	Thiiacetazone
	Viomycin
Antiviral agents	Abacavir
	Cladribine
	Indinavir
	Nelfinavir
	Ribavirin
	Ritonavir
	Saquinivir
	Spiramycin

References

Barza, M. (1985). Imipenem: First of a new class of beta-lactam antibiotics. *Annals of Internal Medicine*, **103**: 552–560.

Besseghir, K., Rock-Ramel, F. (1987). Renal excretion of drugs and other xenobiotics. *Renal Physiology*, **10**: 221–241.

Beyer, K.H., Russo, H.F., Tillson, E.K., Miller, A.K., Verwey, W.F., Gass, S.R. (1951). 'Benemid', p-(di-n-Propylsulfamyl)-benzoic acid: Its renal affinity and its elimination. *American Journal of Physiology*, **166**: 625–639.

Bickley, S.K. (1988). Drug dosing during continuous arteriovenous hemofiltration. *Clinical Pharmacy*, **7**: 198–206.

Brater, D.C. (1980). The pharmacological role of the kidney. *Drugs*, **19**: 31–48.

Brater, D.C. (1994). *Pocket manual of drug use in clinical medicine*, 7th edn. Improved Therapeutics, Indianapolis.

Burckhardt, G., Ullrich, K.H. (1989). Organic anion transport across the contraluminal membrane–Dependence on sodium. *Kidney International*, **36**: 370–377.

Data, J.L., Nies, A.S. (1974). Dextran 40. *Annals of Internal Medicine*, **81**: 500–504.

Depner, T.A., Gulyassay, P.F., Stanfel, L.A., Jarrard, E.A. (1980). Plasma protein binding in uremia: Extraction and characterization of an inhibitor. *Kidney International*, **18**: 86–94.

DeSoi, C.A., Sahm, D.F., and Umans, J.G. (1992). *American Journal of Kidney Diseases*, **4**: 354–360.

Drayer, D.E. (1976). Pharmacologically active drug metabolites: Therapeutic and toxic activities, plasma and urine data in man, accumulation in renal failure. *Clinical Pharmacokinetics*, **1**: 426–443.

Dupuis, R.E., Matzke, G.R., Maddux, F.W., O'Neil, M.G. (1989). Vancomycin disposition during continuous arteriovenous hemofiltration. *Clinical Pharmacy*, **8**: 371–374.

Dutt, A., Heath, L.A., Nelson, J.A. (1994). P-glycoprotein and organic cation secretion by the mammalian kidney. *Journal of Pharmacology and Experimental Therapeutics*, **269**: 1254–1260.

Gilbert, D.N., Wood, C.A., Kohlhepp, S.J., Kohnen, P.W., Houghton, D.C., Finkbeiner, H.C., Lindsley, J., Bennett, W.M. (1989). Polyaspartic acid prevents experimental aminoglycoside nephrotoxicity. *Journal of Infectious Diseases*, **159**: 945–953.

Greenblatt, D.J., Sellers, E.M., Koch-Wester, J. (1982). Importance of protein binding for the interpretation of serum or plasma drug concentrations. *Journal of Clinical Pharmacology*, **22**: 259–263.

Gulyassy, P.F., Bottini, A.T., Stanfel, L.A., Jarrard, E.A., Depner, T.A. (1986). Isolation and chemical identification of inhibitors of plasma ligand binding. *Kidney International*, **30**: 391–398.

Haehner, B.D., Wrighton, S.A., Gorski, J.C., Vandenbranden, M., Watkins, P.B., Janardan, V., Hall, S.D. (1996). The bimodal distribution of midazolam activity and protein content in human kidney. *Molecular Pharmacology*, **50**: 52–59.

Hall, S., Rowland, M. (1985): Influence of fraction unbound upon the renal clearance of furosemide in the isolated perfused rat kidney. *Journal of Pharmacology and Experimental Therapeutics*, **232**: 263–268.

Just, M., Habermann, E. (1977). The renal handling of polybasic drugs. 2. *In vitro* studies with brush border and lysosomal preparations. *Naunyn Schmeidebergs Archives of Pharmacology*, **300**: 67–76.

Just, M., Erdmann, G., Habermann, E. (1977): The renal handling of polybasic drugs. 1. Gentamicin and aprotinin in intact animals. *Naunyn Schmeidebergs Archives of Pharmacology*, **300**: 57–66.

Kim, R.B., Fromm, M.F., Wandel, C., Leake, B., Wood, A.J.J., Roden, D.M., *et al.* (1998). The drug transporter P-glycoprotein limits oral absorption and brain entry of HIV-1 protease inhibitors. *Journal of Clinical Investigation*, 101: 289–294.

Klotz, U. (1976). Pathophysiological and disease-induced changes in drug distribution volume: Pharmacokinetic implications. *Clinical Pharmacokinetics*, 1: 204–218.

Lee, C.G.L., Gottesman, M.M. (1998). HIV-1 protease inhibitors and the MDR1 multidrug transporter. *Journal of Clinical Investigation*, 101: 287–288.

Lipsky, J.J., Cheng, L., Sacktor, B., Lietman, P.S. (1980). Gentamicin uptake by renal tubule brush border membrane vesicles. *Journal of Pharmacology and Experimental Therapeutics*, 215: 390–393.

MacKichan, J.J. (1989). Protein binding drug displacement interactions. Fact or fiction? *Clinical Pharmacokinetics*, 16: 65–73.

Matzke, G.R., O'Connell, M.B., Collins, A.J., Keshaviah, P.R. (1986). Disposition of vancomycin during hemofiltration. *Clinical Pharmacology and Therapeutics*, 40: 425–30.

Moller, J.V., Sheikh, M.I. (1982). Renal organic anion transport system: Pharmacological, physiological, and biochemical aspects. *Pharmacology Reviews*, 34: 315–358.

Peters, L. (1960). Renal tubular excretion of organic bases. *Pharmacology Reviews*, 12: 1–35.

Pollard, T.A., Lampasona, V., Akkerman, S., Tom, K., Hooks, M.A., Mullins, R.E., *et al.* (1994). Vancomycin redistribution: Dosing recommendations following *high-flux* hemodialysis. *Kidney International*, 45: 232–237.

Prescott, L.F. (1972). Mechanisms of renal excretion of drugs (with special reference to drugs used by anaesthetists). *British Journal of Anaesthesia*, 44: 246–251.

Pritchard, J.B., Miller, D.S. (1996). Renal secretion of organic anions and cations. *Kidney International*, 49: 1649–1654.

Ramsammy, L.S., Josepovitz, C., Lane, B.P., Kaloyanides, G.J. (1989). Polyaspartic acid protects against gentamicin nephrotoxicity in the rat. *Journal of Pharmacology and Experimental Therapeutics*, 250: 149–153.

Reidenberg, M.M., Drayer, D.E. (1984). Alteration of drug-protein binding in renal disease. *Clinical Pharmacokinetics*, 9 (suppl. 1): 18–26.

Rennick, B.R. (1972). Renal excretion of drugs: Tubular transport and metabolism. *Annual Review of Pharmacology and Toxicology*, 12: 141–156.

Rennick, B.R. (1981). Renal tubule transport of organic cations. *American Journal of Physiology*, 240: F83–F89.

Schentag, J.J., Jusko, W.J. (1977). Renal clearance and tissue accumulation of gentamicin in man. *Clinical Pharmacology and Therapeutics*, 22: 364–370.

Shimada, H., Moewes, B., Burckhardt, G. (1987). Indirect coupling to Na$^+$ of p-aminohippuric acid uptake into rat renal basolateral membrane vesicles. *American Journal of Physiology*, 253: F795–F801.

Silverblatt, F.J., Kuehn, C. (1979). Autoradiography of gentamicin uptake by the rat proximal tubule cell. *Kidney International*, 15: 335–345.

Sokol, P.P., Huiatt, K.R., Holohan, P.D., Ross, C.R. (1989). Gentamicin and verapamil compete for a common transport mechanism in renal brush border membrane vesicles. *Journal of Pharmacology and Experimental Therapeutics*, 251: 937–942.

Somani, P., Shapiro, R.S., Stockard, H., Higgins, J.T. (1982). Unidirectional absorption of gentamicin from the peritoneum during continuous ambulatory peritoneal dialysis. *Clinical Pharmacology and Therapeutics*, 32: 113–121.

Tozer, T.N. (1981). Concepts basic to pharmacokinetics. *Pharmacology and Therapeutics*, 12: 109–131.

Ullrich, K.J. (1976). Renal tubular mechanism of organic solute transport. *Kidney International*, **9**: 134–148.

Verbeeck, R.K., Branch, R.A., Wilkinson, G.R. (1981). Drug metabolites in renal failure: Pharmacokinetic and clinical implications. *Clinical Pharmacokinetics*, **6**: 329–345.

Weiner, I.M., Mudge, G.H. (1964). Renal tubular mechanisms for excretion of organic acids and bases. *American Journal of Medicine*, **36**: 743–762.

Wilkinson, G.R. (1987). Clearance approaches in pharmacology. *Pharmacological Reviews*, **39**: 1–47.

INDEX

References to figures are in bold, those to tables are in italics.